D1686664

MEDICAL RADIOLOGY
Diagnostic Imaging

Editors:
A. L. Baert, Leuven
M. F. Reiser, München
H. Hricak, New York
M. Knauth, Göttingen

J. Stoker (Ed.)

MRI of the Gastrointestinal Tract

With Contributions by

R.G.H. Beets-Tan · A. S. Borthne · J. M. Froelich · V. Goh · S. I. Gonçalves · S. Gourtsoyianni
S. Halligan · S. Kinner · S. Kirchhoff · A. Laghi · D. M. J. Lambregts · T. C. Lauenstein
K. S. Lee · A. Lieneman · D. J. Lomas · R. N. Low · M. Maas · C. Matos · A. J. Nederveen
V. Panebianco · N. Papanikolaou · M. A. Patak · G. Pelle · I. Pedrosa · M. Pezzullo
C. Pierre-Jerome · C. S. Reiner · A. M. Riddell · J. Stoker · N. J. Taylor · S. A. Taylor
D. J. M. Tolan · R. Tutuja · D. Weishaupt · K.-U. Wentz · C. von Weymarn · M. Wissmeyer
M. L. W. Ziech · F. M. Zijta

Foreword by

A. L. Baert

With 265 Figures in 505 Separate Illustrations, 43 in Color and 19 Tables

Springer

Jaap Stoker, MD, PhD
Professor of Radiology
Department of Radiology
Academic Medical Center
University of Amsterdam
Meibergdreef 9
1105 AZ Amsterdam
The Netherlands

Medical Radiology · Diagnostic Imaging and Radiation Oncology
Series Editors:
A. L. Baert · L. W. Brady · H.-P. Heilmann · M. Knauth · M. Molls · C. Nieder

Continuation of Handbuch der medizinischen Radiologie
Encyclopedia of Medical Radiology

ISBN: 978-3-540-85531-6   e-ISBN: 978-3-540-85532-3

DOI: 10.1007/978-3-540-85532-3

Springer Heidelberg Dordrecht London New York

Medical Radiology · Diagnostic Imaging and Radiation Oncology ISSN 0942-5373

Library of Congress Control Number: 2009931699

© Springer-Verlag Berlin Heidelberg 2010

This work is subject to copyright. All rights are reserved, whether the whole or part of the material is concerned, specifically the rights of translation, reprinting, reuse of illustrations, recitation, broadcasting, reproduction on microfilms or in any other way, and storage in data banks. Duplication of this publication or parts thereof is permitted only under the provisions of the German Copyright Law of September 9, 1965, in its current version, and permission for use must always be obtained from Springer-Verlag. Violations are liable for prosecution under the German Copyright Law.

The use of general descriptive names, registered names, trademarks, etc. in this publication does not imply, even in the absence of a specific statement, that such names are exempt from the relevant protective laws and regulations and therefore free for general use.

Product liability: The publishers cannot guarantee the accuracy of any information about dosage and application contained in this book. In every individual case the user must check such information by consulting the relevant literature.

Cover design: Publishing Services Teichmann, 69256 Mauer, Germany

Printed on acid-free paper

9 8 7 6 5 4 3 2 1

Springer is part of Springer Science+Business Media (www.springer.com)

Foreword

It is my great pleasure and privilege to introduce another volume, published in our book series *Medical Radiology – Diagnostic Imaging*, and which is devoted to MR imaging of the Gastrointestinal Tract.

The editor Dr. J. Stoker, an internationally leading gastrointestinal radiologist, has been involved since many years in basic and translational clinical research of the challenging field of MR imaging of the GI tract, an organ system that offers considerable technical difficulties for obtaining acceptable image quality, even with modern MRI technology.

Recent technical progress in equipment design, as well as in computer hardware and software laid the base for the full development of MRI of the GI tract as a clinical tool for routine radiological imaging.

This book is one of the first publications to offer a state of the art and comprehensive overview of the meticulous examination techniques and the specific sequences, which are essential for optimal image quality in MR imaging of the GI tract. It further covers in depth the actual diagnostic role of MRI in the management of Crohn's disease, rectal cancer, and diseases of the anus, which are already well-established clinical applications of this modality. Finally, it also explores new clinical frontiers for the study of the GI tract such as dynamic MRI, perfusion and diffusion MRI, and high-field imaging.

The short preparation period for this volume ensures the reader that the very last advances in our knowledge of this rapidly evolving field could be included in this new volume.

The clear and informative text, the numerous, well-chosen illustrations of superb technical quality as well as the traditional Springer excellent standards of design and lay out make this outstanding work a reference handbook for all certified general and gastrointestinal radiologists. Also, radiologists in training will find it very useful for improving their knowledge and their skills. Referring physicians such as gastroenterologists and abdominal surgeons will benefit from it to improve the clinical management of their patients.

I am greatly indebted to the editor J. Stoker for his efficient and brilliant editorial work as well as for the judicious choice of the contributing authors, all well-known and internationally recognized experts in the field, who wrote the 19 individual chapters.

It is my sincere wish and my firm conviction that this unique book will meet great success with the readership of our book series *Medical Radiology – Diagnostic Imaging*.

ALBERT L. BAERT
Series Editor

Preface

Magnetic resonance imaging (MRI) of the gastrointestinal tract was not an upfront obvious development as the gastrointestinal tract is a challenging organ system for MRI. Obtaining good image quality of a tube with a few millimeter thin wall is demanding, while peristalsis and respiration further increase difficulties. These hurdles have been largely overcome by hardware and software improvements.

At present, MRI is an important diagnostic technique of especially small bowel (e.g. Crohn's disease), colon (e.g. rectal cancer), and anus. The combination of high intrinsic contrast resolution, lack of ionizing radiation, and no invasiveness is crucial for this role.

Now MRI techniques widely used in other fields, such as diffusion and perfusion MRI, make their way to clinical application in MRI of the gastrointestinal tract. Also dynamic MRI and MRI of motility have been introduced. MRI of the gastrointestinal tract at high field is studied.

The book is intended as an up to date overview of MRI of the gastrointestinal tract. Initial technical chapters are followed by clinical orientated chapters of all parts of the gastrointestinal tract and closely related structures. By presenting both basic and advanced knowledge, this book is intended to be instructive for the novice while simultaneously offering experienced practitioners further insights into the value of MRI of the gastrointestinal tract. I hope that readers will find this book useful when starting or improving their use of MRI in patients with gastrointestinal diseases.

I thank all the distinguished experts in the field who contributed to this book. I am very pleased that they were willing to share their insights and expertise. I thank Professor Baert for his invitation to contribute a book dedicated to *MRI of the gastrointestinal tract* for the renowned *Medical Radiology* series. Ursula Davis, her successor Daniela Brandt, and colleagues at Springer are thanked for the always timely and friendly communication and very effective production process.

I thank my secretary Annemarie van der Woestijne for her help during the preparation of this book.

Amsterdam, The Netherlands   Jaap Stoker

Contents

Technique 1

1. MRI of the Gastrointestinal Tract: Coils, Sequences, Techniques 3
   DAVID J. LOMAS

2. MRI of the Gastrointestinal Tract at High-Field Strength 21
   AART J. NEDERVEEN and SONIA I. GONÇALVES

3. Contrast Media for MRI of the Gastrointestinal Tract 33
   ARNE S. BORTHNE and CLAUDE PIERRE-JEROME

4. Dynamic Contrast-Enhanced and Diffusion-Weighted
   MRI of the Gastrointestinal Tract 51
   VICKY GOH and N. JANE TAYLOR

Clinical Application 65

5. MRI of the Esophagus and Stomach 67
   ANGELA M. RIDDELL

6. MRI of Upper GI Tract Motility 81
   VALERIA PANEBIANCO, GIUSEPPE PELLE AND ANDREA LAGHI

7. MRI of the Duodenum 93
   CELSO MATOS and MARTINA PEZZULLO

8. MRI of the Small Bowel: Enterography 117
   MANON L.W. ZIECH and JAAP STOKER

9. MRI of the Small Bowel: Enteroclysis 135
   NICKOLAS PAPANIKOLAOU and SOFIA GOURTSOYIANNI

10. MRI of the Small Bowel: Clinical Role 149
    DAMIAN J.M. TOLAN, STUART A. TAYLOR, and STEVE HALLIGAN

11. MRI of the Colon (MR Colonography): Technique 173
    SONJA KINNER and THOMAS C. LAUENSTEIN

12. MRI of the Colon (Colonography): Results 185
    FRANK M. ZIJTA and JAAP STOKER

13	**MRI of the Rectum** 205
	Doenja M.J. Lambregts, Monique Maas and Regina G. H. Beets-Tan

14	**MRI of Bowel Motility** 229
	Michael A. Patak, Constantin von Weymarn, Klaus-Ulrich Wentz, Radu Tutuja, Michael Wissmeyer, and Johannes M. Froelich

15	**MRI of the Peritoneum** 249
	Russell N. Low

16	**MRI of Adhesions and Small Bowel Obstruction** 271
	Andreas Lienemann and Sonja Kirchhoff

17	**MRI of Acute Conditions of the Gastrointestinal Tract** 283
	Karen S. Lee and Ivan Pedrosa

18	**MRI of the Pelvic Floor** 315
	Caecilia S. Reiner and Dominik Weishaupt

19	**MRI of the Anus** 329
	Steve Halligan and Stuart Taylor

Subject Index 347

List of Contributors 353

Technique

MRI of the Gastrointestinal Tract: Coils, Sequences, Techniques

DAVID J. LOMAS

CONTENTS

1.1 Introduction 4
1.2 **Coils** 4
1.2.1 Requirements 4
1.2.2 Multicoil Receive Arrays 4
1.2.3 Endoluminal Coils 5

1.3 **Sequences** 5
1.3.1 Requirements 5
1.3.2 Echoplanar (EPI) 6
1.3.3 RARE (TSE, FSE) 6
1.3.4 Single Shot RARE (TSE, FSE)/Single Shot Half-Fourier RARE (HASTE, SSFSE) 8
1.3.5 Balanced SSFP (True-FISP, FIESTA, Balanced FFE) 9
1.3.6 Spoiled Gradient Echo (FLASH, SPGR, T1FFE) 10
1.3.7 Breath-Hold Interpolated 3D T1W (VIBE, LAVA, FAME, THRIVE) 11
1.3.8 Hydrographic Projection Imaging 12
1.3.9 Fat Suppression 13
1.3.10 Dynamic Acquisition 14
1.3.11 Diffusion-Weighted Imaging 15
1.3.12 Perfusion Imaging 16

1.4 **Techniques** 16
1.4.1 Requirements 16
1.4.2 Pharynx and Esophagus 17
1.4.3 Stomach 17
1.4.4 Small Bowel 17
1.4.5 Colon 17
1.4.6 Rectum and Anus 17

References 18

KEY POINTS

Successful MRI of the GI tract requires an understanding of the anatomical and physiological challenges along with the technical basis of MRI. Receiver coils need to be purpose-designed for adequate coverage and efficient to provide good signal. Increasingly, designs take account of parallel acceleration techniques, which can improve volume coverage and temporal resolution. Conventional sequences are still used where motion artifacts are limited but GI tract imaging predominantly relies on fast breath-hold imaging. These methods now provide a range of contrast and high-quality diagnostic images with either breath-hold or subsecond acquisitions that can freeze many sources of motion artifacts. Refinements provide effective fat suppression, hydrographic projection imaging similar to traditional X-ray fluoroscopy, and high-quality sectional images that demonstrate the bowel lumen, wall, and extramural tissues. Interpolated 3D T1w breath-hold sequences used with antiperistaltic pharmacologic agents provide for pre- and postintravenous gadolinium imaging that can encompass whole sections of the GI tract. Dynamic imaging is possible by using balanced gradient echo and/or single-shot half-Fourier spin echo sequences that can illustrate organ filling and emptying in the GI tract and evaluate both normal and abnormal GI tract physiology. Diffusion-weighted and perfusion imaging techniques are becoming widely available and provide quantification parameters to apply to the GI tract.

DAVID J. LOMAS, MD
Department of Radiology, University of Cambridge and Addenbrooke's Hospital, Hills Road, Cambridge, CB2 0QQ, UK

1.1 Introduction

The gastro-intestinal tract presents all imaging methods with well-known technical challenges, including physiological motion (e.g. swallowing, gastric, and small bowel peristalsis) (KELLOW 1986); the complexity, inaccessibility, and variability of the tubular anatomical components; the simultaneous intraluminal juxtaposition of gas, solids, and liquids; and the presence of extrinsic motion related to blood flow and respiration. The disease processes that develop in the human GI tract create further imaging challenges as the disease patterns and morphology vary. The imaging may need to be optimised to demonstrate predominantly intra-luminal (e.g. polyps), mural (e.g. wall inflammation, tumor or stricture) or extramural (e.g. fistula formation, endometriosis, adjacent organ tumors) disease changes depending on the clinical presentation and the region of the tract under investigation. During the last century, X-ray-based imaging successfully addressed these challenges with a range of strategies that have become routinely practised techniques in hospitals worldwide. These include the use of bowel preparation methods, oral and tube delivered contrast media, the use of static and fluoroscopic (dynamic) imaging along with postural changes often aided by tilting examination tables.

Given these challenges, it is no surprise that the gastro-intestinal tract is one of the last body systems to be successfully imaged by MRI. This is partly due to the technical capability and limitations of MRI as well as the competing performance of other X-ray-based imaging modalities, including most recently developed multidetector CT. During the 1990s, improvements in MR hardware led to a substantial improvement in the ability to image the GI tract and this has now been demonstrated successfully on a wide variety of MRI systems. The majority of research developments and clinical applications have used 1.5 T 50–60 cm diameter closed cylindrical bore systems. These provide a good compromise of field strength, related artifacts, volume coverage, and gradient performance. Higher field strength systems have also been used successfully but present a range of additional challenges, addressed in more detail in Chap. 2. This chapter will focus on the technical requirements and strategies that have been developed for supporting high-quality MR imaging of the GI tract. In this application as in most others, MR image quality is a compromise of many factors, not the least of them being the spatial and temporal resolution, both of which must be exploited for imaging the GI tract.

1.2 Coils

1.2.1 Requirements

Receiver coils are an integral part of MRI and for GI tract imaging the major requirements are for adequate volume coverage, RF homogeneity, and signal-to-noise ratio (SNR). In an ideal MRI system, all the imaging would be obtained using the body coil built into the cylindrical bore of the system, but in practice, although this usually provides good homogeneity and volume coverage, it provides inadequate SNR on both 1.5 T and 3 T systems. This results in compromised image quality and it is well known that inadequate SNR will also degrade contrast to noise ratio (CNR) which is often crucial for diagnosis (CONSTABLE and HENKELMAN 1991). Modern MRI systems now rely almost exclusively on multicoil surface receive arrays (ROEMER et al. 1990) for abdominal and pelvic imaging. Although these have spatially varying RF sensitivity, which results in signal reduction with distance from the coil surface, they can double the overall SNR when compared with the intrinsic body coil. This is particularly important in bowel imaging as it permits short enough acquisitions for breath-hold imaging. The early multicoil "torso" and "cardiac" arrays had relatively small fields of view cranio-caudally (e.g. 20–30 cm) that limited their use to either the abdomen or pelvis but not both without time-consuming repositioning. These arrays are appropriate for esophageal or pelvic imaging, but more recently larger arrays have been introduced (Fig. 1.1) that cover the abdomen and pelvis (e.g. 40–44 cm cranio-caudally), essential for imaging the whole of the large and small bowel efficiently.

1.2.2 MultiCoil Receive Arrays

At the time of writing, most commercial body receive arrays comprising between 8 and 16 coil elements with separate or multiplexed receiver channels. Thirty-two channel arrays are becoming available commercially, but it is not yet clear whether the use of 64 and 128

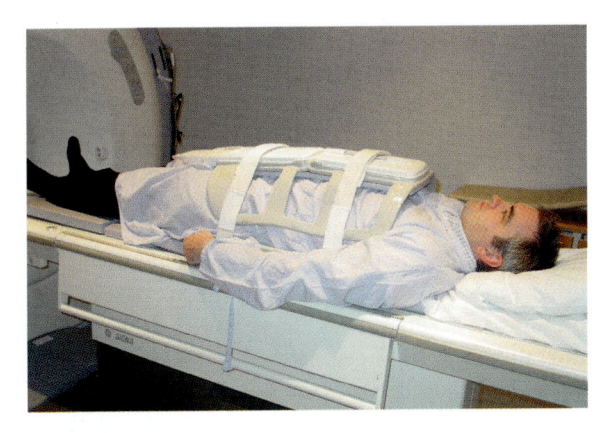

Fig. 1.1. A typical flexible multi-element receiver array with sufficient superior–inferior coverage for the whole abdomen and pelvis

channel arrays will offer gains that justify the complexity, cost, and increased risk of mechanical failure. In general, increasing channel and coil number creates problems in achieving adequate radiofrequency depth penetration but brings the benefit of facilitating parallel imaging reconstruction techniques. These techniques partially replace phase encoding with spatial sensitivity encoding related to the coil geometry. This can improve temporal resolution and reduce some artifacts but parallel receive acceleration reduces the SNR and is therefore probably most usefully exploited for optimizing imaging on higher field systems (3T and above). The use of acceleration in two directions simultaneously facilitates more rapid 3D imaging, but at the present time it has not been possible to achieve 3D imaging with adequate spatial resolution and volume coverage in the subsecond range needed to freeze bowel peristalsis. The two main early methods utilize the spatial sensitivity information to create the replaced phase encode information slightly differently. Sensitivity encoding (SENSE) applies this information in "image" space after the Fourier reconstruction of "K" space (Pruessmann et al. 1999), whereas the simultaneous acquisition of spatial harmonics (SMASH) method (Sodickson and Manning 1997) performs this step within "K" space before Fourier reconstruction.

Another challenge for parallel techniques for bowel imaging is the requirement for calibration images to generate the spatial sensitivity maps. The early implementations acquired these calibration images separately at the beginning of an examination but for GI tract imaging subsequent signal variations owing to contrast medium and bowel motion could invalidate these images creating artifacts in the reconstruction process. More recently, self- or auto-calibrating techniques have been developed that are more appropriate for imaging the GI tract (Griswold et al. 2002; Brau et al. 2008).

1.2.3
Endoluminal Coils

Endoluminal coils have been introduced for upper gastrointestinal – primarily esophageal – imaging and anorectal imaging. The limited experience with these coils mainly concerns anorectal imaging. Saddle geometry or phased array coils are used with dedicated cylindrical coils for anal imaging (Stoker et al. 1999). The higher local spatial resolution of endoluminal coils has to be weighted against the discomfort, costs, and limited availability. Thereby, with present external multicoil receive arrays high-resolution images are obtained as well. The main application of endoluminal anorectal MRI is in the detection of subtle internal openings in fistula-in-ano and evaluating fecal incontinence (see Chap. 19). Endoluminal coils are also studied for their role in staging esophageal and gastric cancer (see Chap. 5).

1.3
Sequences

1.3.1
Requirements

Virtually all the sequences used successfully to image the majority of the GI tract need to acquire their data within a tolerable breath-hold – for most people this is a maximum of 15–20 s (hyperventilation is helpful in increasing this maximum to some extent). This effectively rules out using most of the conventional slow imaging sequences using spin or gradient echoes that take several or more minutes to acquire. Breath-hold or faster imaging is necessary first to avoid blurring or interleaving artifact from respiratory-related abdominal motion. Secondly, gastric and small bowel peristalsis although relatively slow is unpredictable, so gating methods are impractical and to freeze this motion each image has to be acquired in less than a second, unless antiperistaltic agents are used. Currently, only 2D imaging sequences are fast enough to provide this type of subsecond acquisition. At these speeds, acceptable image quality can be obtained even during free breathing but breath-holding or respiratory triggering is often employed to avoid interleaving artifacts and unpredictable volume coverage.

All of the 3D strategies currently used acquire the data for each image over longer time periods (e.g., 10–20 s) and are therefore prone to blurring artifacts from peristaltic motion unless pharmacological agents, e.g., hyoscine bromide or glucagon are administered to transiently paralyse the bowel. Antiperistaltic agents have been widely used with X-ray contrast and endoscopy techniques to both relax and paralyze the bowel. Over the years, there has been some debate about the efficacy and duration of action of these agents for the small bowel. This has been studied using dynamic MRI of the small bowel, which demonstrated that glucagon has a longer duration of action (up to 3 times longer) and is more effective at achieving paralysis of the whole small bowel than hyoscine bromide agents (FROEHLICH et al. 2005, 2009). In comparison, hyoscine bromide based agents have proven more effective at relaxing the large bowel and have been routinely used in most MR colonography studies.

The exceptions to the situation described above are the rectum and perineum where conventional 2D and 3D spin-echo imaging sequences can be used over several minutes to improve spatial resolution. This is because motion-related artifacts are much reduced owing to the relatively static nature of the surrounding pelvic and perineal soft tissues. In practice, even in this part of the GI tract most traditional spin-echo sequences have been replaced by multishot RARE imaging as described below. This is because higher spatial resolutions can now be achieved in the same or less imaging time overall.

An overview of imaging acquisition sequences is given below, which concentrates on rapid imaging sequences that can provide adequate image quality within a 15–20-s breath-hold or less. Where possible, generic sequence names have been used largely conforming to those used in the MR physics community (BERNSTEIN et al. 2004). These are summarized in outline protocols in Table 1.1, which provides a cross-reference for the vendor "trade" names that are often more widely used. In addition, a brief introduction to hydrographic and dynamic imaging is given along with an overview of diffusion weighted and perfusion imaging that are being increasingly used for evaluation of particularly GI tract tumors.

1.3.2
Echoplanar (EPI)

Echoplanar imaging was originally the only imaging sequence that could acquire data fast enough to freeze bowel motion and several pioneering early publications on MR of the GI tract used this approach (EVANS et al. 1993). EPI was introduced early in the development of MRI (MANSFIELD 1977) and consists of an echotrain generated by alternating refocusing readout gradients. Utilizing high receiver bandwidths allows subsecond imaging but the alternating readout gradients effectively multiply any phase errors related to magnet or other inhomogeneity. As a result, EPI is particularly prone to susceptibility artifacts and even with optimizsation may show geometric distortions and signal losses close to air tissue interfaces (Fig. 1.2). This is markedly different to the performance of echotrain spin-echo sequences discussed below.

The development of improved fast spin and gradient echo techniques during the 1990s has largely superseded EPI for structural and dynamic imaging of the bowel. Recently, EPI has found a new niche in relation to diffusion weighted imaging (DWI) for which it has particular benefits. DWI is being applied to several regions of the GI tract both for routine clinical and research use and is discussed below and in more detail in Chap. 4.

1.3.3
RARE (TSE, FSE)

Early MR imaging was limited by the long acquisition times of conventional spin and gradient echo sequences in all body areas and to overcome this Hennig introduced "fast" T2w spin echo imaging in the late-1980s with the "rapid acquisition with relaxation enhancement" or RARE sequence now better known as fast spin-echo (FSE) or turbo spin-echo (TSE) (HENNIG et al. 1986). This relies on the use of multiple refocusing 180° pulses to generate multiple readout echoes after the initial excitation. In practice, vendors routinely use less than 180° refocusing (typically optimized at 130–155°) pulses to reduce power deposition. The refocusing pulse train makes these sequences particularly resistant to off-resonance artifacts and magnetic field inhomogeneities, especially helpful at gas–tissue interfaces, which are a frequent feature of GI tract imaging.

The early forms of this sequence were only practical with short echo trains owing to the limited gradient performance then available. This was because long interecho spacing caused marked variation of the signal amplitudes in K space, which resulted in spatial frequency filtering – visible on the images as blurring in the phase encode direction. This effect is most

Table 1.1. Overview of the main fast imaging sequence types and nomenclature

2D or 3D	2D	2D	2D	2D	3D	3D
Generic name	RARE	Single-shot half-Fourier RARE	Hydrographic projection RARE	Balanced SSFP	Balanced SSFP	Interpolated 3D T1w
Trade names	TSE/FSE	HASTE, SSFSE, EXPRESS, FASE	Any RARE sequence in single shot mode	True-FISP, FIESTA, balanced FFE, balanced SARGE, true-SSFP	True-FISP, FIESTA, balanced FFE, balanced SARGE, true-SSFP	VIBE, FAME, LAVA, THRIVE
Acquisition time per section	0:1 min	0:1	0:1	0:1	0:10–0:25	0:10–0:25
Total acquisition time (min:s)	0:1	0:1–0:25	0:1	0:10–0:25	0:10–0:25	0:10–0:25
Section thickness (mm)	5–10	5–10	10–100	2–10	2–4	3–6
Number of actual sections		16–30	1 (can be more)	1–30	8–32	8–32
TE or TE effective (ms)	60–90	60–90	600	1.5–2.5	1.5–2.5	1.5
TR (ms)	0	800–2,000	4,000–10,000	4.0–5.5	4.0–5.5	3.0–4.0
Fat suppression	N	N (Y)	Y	N	N	Y
Excitation flip angle (refocusing) (degrees)	(130–180)	(130–180)	(130–180)	50–70	50–70	10–15
Echotrain length	Single or multi-shot full Fourier	Single-shot half-Fourier	Single-shot half or full Fourier	N/A	N/A	N/A
Parallel acceleration (×)	1	1–2	1–2	1–2	1–4	1–4
"Cine" version possible	Yes if single shot	Yes	Yes	Yes	No	No
Antiperistaltic needed	No if single shot	No	No	No	Yes	Yes

Matrix and voxel sizes have been omitted for simplicity, but are typically 256 × 256 or larger and for large FOV coronal imaging 512 × 256 is commonly achieved. Smaller matrices may be needed to achieve good temporal resolution with "cine" sequences. Echotrain lengths relate to the number of phase encode steps required to fill K space. This means that for a 256 × 256 acquisition single-shot full-Fourier acquisition, the echotrain would be 256 long, whereas single-shot half-Fourier would have an echotrain approximately 128 long. Multishot sequences have widely varying echotrains but are usually full-Fourier and typical variations for a 256 × 256 matrix would include 32 shots with an 8 echotrain, 16 shots with a 16 echotrain or 8 shots using a 32 echotrain. Actual TEs and TRs are manufacturer-dependent and influenced by other parameters, especially field of view and section thickness. Receiver bandwidths also directly influence many of these parameters but are omitted for simplicity. Fat suppression techniques may include spectral, inversion recovery or combined methods as appropriate. The use of parallel techniques varies with manufacturer and radiologist acceptance in respect of image quality

noticeable in tissues and materials with a short T2 value because their amplitude decays away quickly following the initial excitation. In the RARE sequence, these smaller amplitude "late" echoes are typically placed in the periphery of K space resulting in less "information" in the high spatial frequencies used to

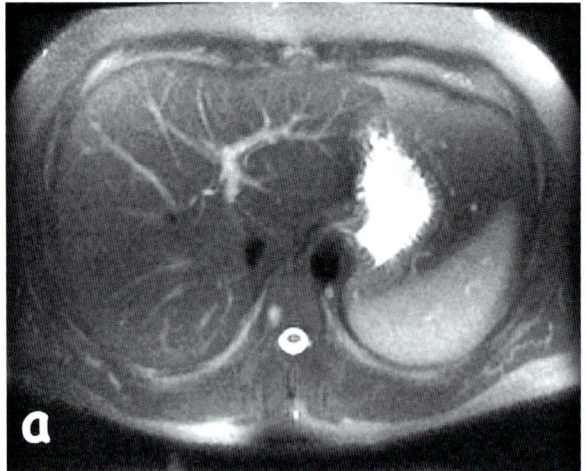

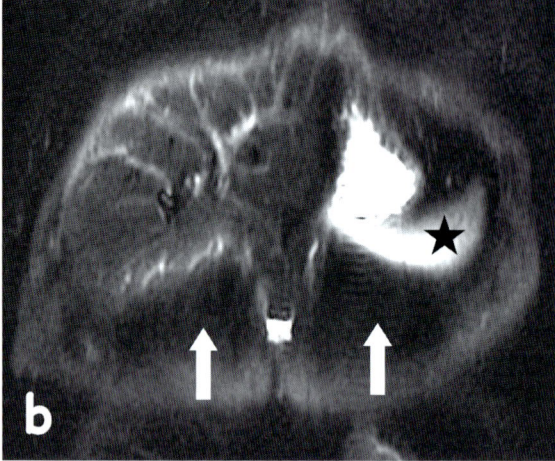

Fig. 1.2. Images obtained at the same level in a volunteer using single shot echotrain techniques and similar parameters, both taking approximately 500 ms to acquire: (**a**) single-shot half-Fourier RARE (**b**) single shot half-Fourier EPI. Note the signal loss posteriorly (*arrows*) in the EPI image resulting from the susceptibility effect of the air in the adjacent posterior sulci of the lungs and the geometric distortion creating a reduction in spleen size (*asterisk*). The RARE image is resistant to these effects owing to the 180° refocusing pulses

generate the sharp edges and boundaries in an MR image (Constable and Gore 1992). Many early implementations of this sequence suffered from these blurring artifacts in the phase encode direction (Fig. 1.3). This problem was initially reduced by using short echo trains, which meant that multiple "shots" or repetitions had to be used to fill K space. This initially made RARE an impractical sequence for breath-hold imaging in the abdomen and pelvis but in this multishot form they are still widely used for high spatial resolution imaging of the rectum and perineum as well as structural imaging of the esophagus.

Compared with conventional spin-echo sequences, RARE-based sequences also have enhanced fat signal owing to the reduction of the J coupling effect, and altered contrast owing to both the use of heterogeneous echo times in K space and magnetisation transfer effects resulting from multiple RF pulses being played out close together both spatially and temporally (Bernstein et al.). The contrast alterations are more difficult to quantify but essentially RARE sequences with long echo trains (e.g. single shot sequences described below) demonstrate a substantial "bias" toward long T2w materials (Hennig et al. 1996) so that these materials appear high signal (bright) in the image. This is one of the reasons why water-based contrast media are so effective with these sequences. It also explains why, when used with a shorter effective TE, they are limited in their discrimination between shorter T2 materials such as when detecting malignant liver lesions.

1.3.4
Single Shot RARE (TSE, FSE)/Single Shot Half-Fourier RARE (HASTE, SSFSE)

During the mid- to late-1990s, "single shot" versions of the RARE sequence became feasible owing to the use of improved gradient performance and higher receiver bandwidths to reduce inter-echo spacing. These sequences had an immediate positive impact on GI tract imaging as they could acquire multiple images within a breath-hold and in most cases each image is obtained within a second, freezing both respiratory and most bowel peristaltic motion. Early versions employed half-Fourier techniques (Semelka et al. 1996) that relied on the symmetry of K space so that only half of K space needed to be collected (in practice just over 50% is required for the reconstruction to operate properly, e.g., typically 132 echoes are collected for a 256 matrix study). Virtually, all modern 1.5 T systems are now also capable of full Fourier (i.e. a full echo-train, 256 echoes in the example above) single-shot acquisitions within approximately 1–2 s. Half-Fourier reconstruction is still widely employed as it retains the advantages of a shorter echo-train – faster per image acquisition (usually subsecond, essential for freezing bowel peristalsis) and less RF power deposition – but at the expense of a reduction in SNR. One side effect of reducing the inter-echo spacing to a minimum is degradation in the accuracy of slice selection, which can lead to cross-talk effects between adjacent sections. On modern

Fig. 1.3. RARE imaging and spatial frequency blurring. Single shot half-Fourier RARE images of a phantom using inter-echo spacing of 6 ms in the upper image and 18 ms in the lower image. Note the marked blurring in the phase encode direction (*left – right*) in the lower image owing to the signal amplitude reductions for the echoes placed in the periphery of K space. The effect is worse for materials with shorter T2 values and is largely overcome by reducing the echospacing as much as possible

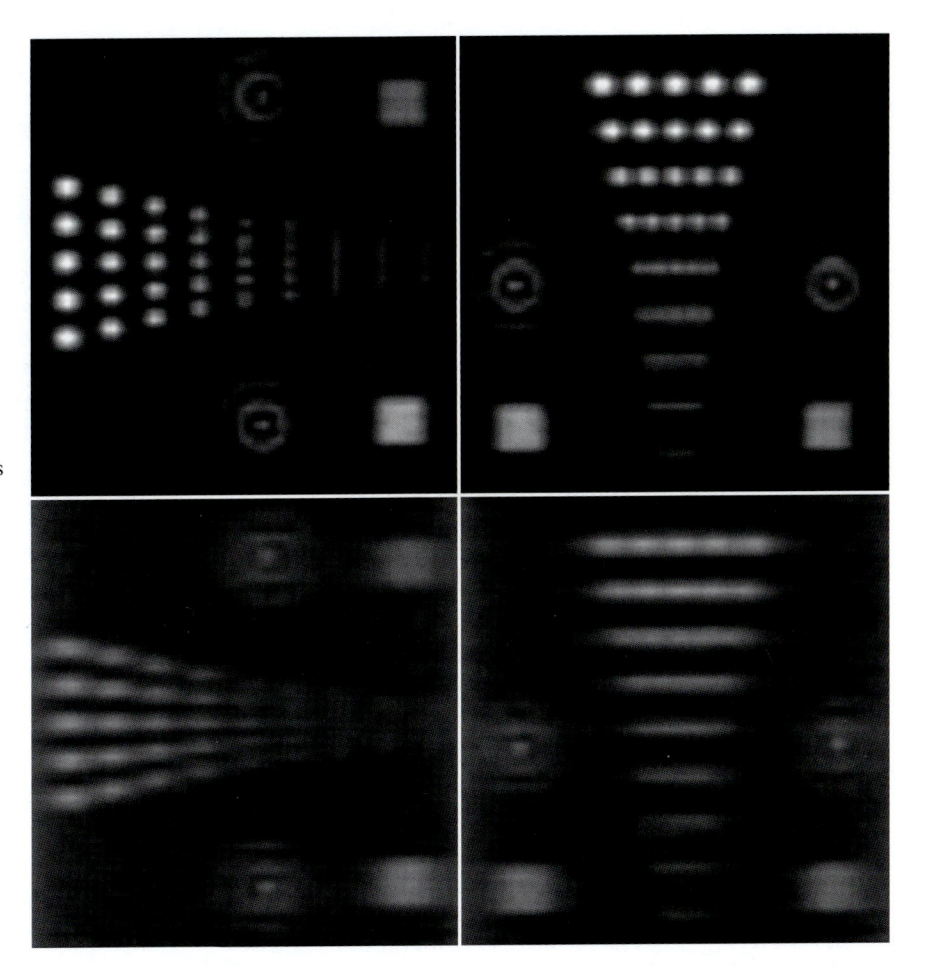

systems using higher receiver bandwidths, it is usually possible to obtain multiple sections covering a tissue volume in a single breath-hold. Where relatively short TRs are employed (1.5 s or less) with sequentially acquired contiguous sections, the cross-talk leads to incomplete signal recovery – most prominent in long T1 materials such as fluid. This is visible as reduced fluid signal intensity affecting intraluminal signal and contrast in the GI tract as well as in bile and urine. This can be overcome by interleaving sections in the acquisition order or extending the TR when repeated views of the same section are required (e.g., using hydrographic techniques as described below). These sequences have become widely used for breath-hold GI tract imaging, particularly where the bowel wall is of interest, e.g., the small and large bowel. To freeze bowel peristalsis, the half-Fourier forms are widely used as they can easily achieve the subsecond acquisitions required. In projection hydrographic form, they are also widely used to monitor filling or emptying of a portion of the GI tract as described below.

1.3.5
Balanced SSFP (True-FISP, FIESTA, Balanced FFE)

Versions of this signal-efficient balanced gradient echo sequence have been available for some years (OPPELT et al. 1986) and used for both neurological and cardiac imaging in particular. It was initially developed as a fast relatively T2* weighted sequence that worked well over small fields of view and which generated good bright blood vascular images. The "balanced" nature of the sequence avoids the signal instability problems of other gradient echo sequences when operated with a short TR. In 2D forms, multiple images can be obtained within a breath-hold and each image can be obtained in less than a second – freezing both bowel peristalsis and respiratory motion. The contrast generated is a complex function of several parameters including the TE, TR, and flip angle as well as the T1 and T2 of the materials being imaged. The "balancing" of all the applied gradients used in the sequence makes it very efficient and therefore ideal for rapid breath-hold imaging, but the early versions suffered from banding artifacts related

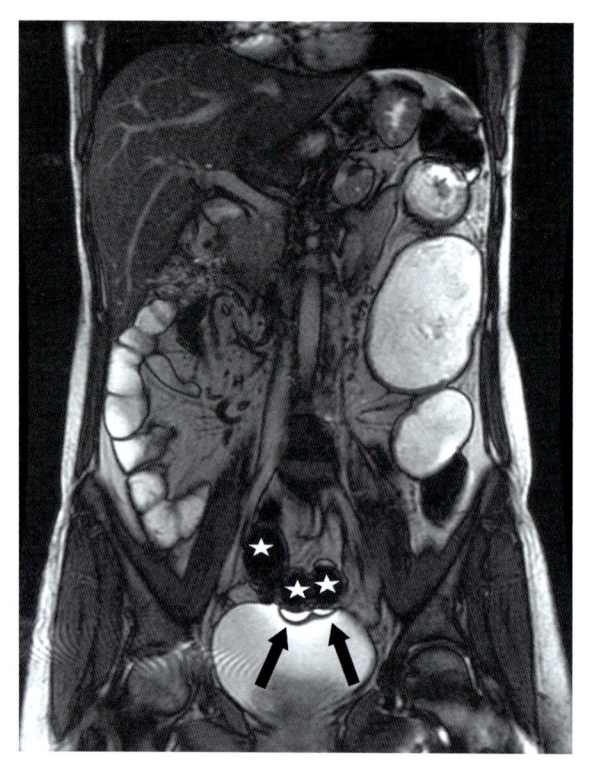

Fig. 1.4. bSSFP susceptibility artifacts. A coronal image covering the whole abdomen and pelvis in a patient with Crohns disease. In the pelvis, the gas-filled sigmoid (*asterisk*) has created a "signet ring" susceptibility related artifact (*arrows*) at the edges of the bowel, which overlaps the bladder. These arise mainly in the frequency direction from the disturbance of the magnetic field homogeneity at the tissue–gas interfaces

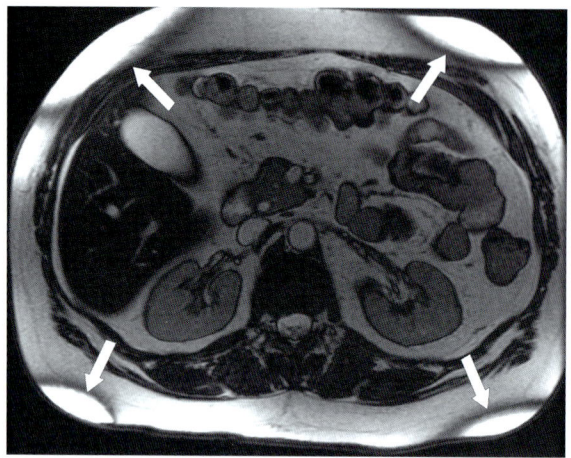

Fig. 1.5. bSSFP banding artifacts. Black band artifacts (*arrows*) are present in the subcutaneous fat at the four quadrants of this axial image arise from abrupt phase transitions owing to phase accumulation related to the magnetic field homogeneity and the repetition time (TR). Apart from reducing the TR, most solutions to this problem require acquisition times longer than a breath-hold

to magnetic field inhomogeneity which, in virtually all magnet designs, is more noticeable over large fields of view – such as those used in GI tract imaging. This sequence is also prone to local magnetic field or susceptibility artifacts which are particularly common at gas–tissue interfaces. Developments over the last decade have reduced the so-called "banding" artifacts to allow good quality imaging of the GI tract although the susceptibility artifacts are more difficult to overcome and may lead to misinterpretation unless recognized (Fig. 1.4). In general terms, the banding artifacts (Fig. 1.5) arise from phase accumulation during the acquisition. This is a result of using alternating sign radiofrequency excitation pulses that maximize the SNR. The phase accumulation evolves during the TR (so is worse with longer TRs) and is also influenced by the heterogeneity and overall strength of the static magnetic field. Reducing the artifacts requires a short TR as well as good static magnetic field homogeneity, along with high quality and stable gradient amplifier design and performance. These requirements become more demanding at higher field strength and the basis of these artifacts and other potential solutions are discussed in further detail in Chap. 2. Typically, for GI tract imaging this sequence is operated with parameters providing predominantly T2* contrast so that most fluids appear high signal when compared with most other soft tissues, which are of intermediate signal. A particular advantage of this sequence is the short TE, which means that bulk motion in fluid (e.g., within the, gut lumen) rarely creates artifacts when compared with single-shot RARE-type sequences. Detailed optimization of the parameters for this sequence has been described for small bowel imaging with water-based contrast media (GOURTSOYIANNIS et al. 2001). This sequence has become very widely used for imaging the small bowel and for dynamic imaging and with antiperistaltic agents can also be employed effectively in 3D versions.

1.3.6
Spoiled Gradient Echo (FLASH, SPGR, T1FFE)

During the late-1980s and early 1990s, as part of the drive to reduce acquisition times to within a breath-hold, the conventional simple gradient echo sequences were used with short TRs (e.g., 200 ms or less). Initially, this did not work well and resulted in unstable steady-state transverse magnetization, which created severe image artifacts. Although this could be addressed by using "rewinder" gradients between repetitions (this is the basis of most "fast" gradient echo sequences with a mixture of T2 and T1 weighting) or more carefully balanced gradient approaches (e.g., bSSFP as described above), they proved unsuitable for obtaining a fast acquisition with predominantly T1 weighting. This problem was eventually solved by the introduction of so-called "spoiling" techniques that destroyed any "residual" transverse magnetisation after each TR, resulting in a relatively T1 weighted image. This was achieved successfully either using spoiling gradients (FLASH, Turbo-FLASH) or radiofrequency spoiling (SPGR, FSPGR). Both these approaches can be used to obtain multiple sections within an acceptable breath-hold and are very widely available on commercial MRI systems. However, they still use a relatively long TR of 100–200 ms to achieve adequate T1 weighting, which means that every image is still acquired over some 15–20 s depending on the acquisition parameters. This means these sequences are only really effective for breath-hold GI tract imaging when antiperistaltic agents are used. Subsequent refinement of these sequences using partial or "fractional" echo methods has allowed for shorter echo times with improved slice coverage and the ability to acquire multiple echoes (Fast SPGR, TurboFLASH). A feature of gradient echo sequences is the cyclic variation of water and fat signals with echo time and that at particular (field-dependent) recurring time intervals the two signals either combine and are in "in phase" or oppose each other and are "out of phase". This feature is widely used to detect the presence of water fat mixtures in for example the bone marrow or liver parenchyma and the ability of the "fast" versions of this sequence to acquire both the in and out of phase echo images in the same breath-hold.

The more recent development of interpolated centric ordered short TR 3D sequences as described below has largely superseded these initial spoiled gradient echo version as they are more efficient and generally more resistant to breath-hold failures. However, where the newer 3D T1w gradient echo sequences are not available, these more conventional 2D T1w versions provide an alternative, particularly for pre- and postintravenous gadolinium contrast agent based imaging.

1.3.7
Breath-Hold Interpolated 3D T1W (VIBE, LAVA, FAME, THRIVE)

Although 3D T1w gradient echo sequences have been available for some time for MR angiography (MRA) and neuroimaging, their application in the abdomen and pelvis was limited until the mid-1990s when optimised sequences were developed (ROFKSY et al. 1999). Initially, MRA sequences were employed for colonic imaging using gadolinium (LUBOLDT et al. 1997), but they were subsequently optimized to provide some background tissue contrast rather than the complete background suppression desirable for MRA. These optimized sequences achieved acceptable spatial resolution and image quality within a breath-hold and utilized features from contrast enhanced MR angiography sequences, such as centric ordering and fat suppression. These help make the imaging less likely to suffer from respiratory-related artifacts if, for example, a patient cannot maintain a breath-hold throughout the whole of an acquisition. In addition they employ both in-plane and through-plane volume interpolations to further improve image quality. Typically, they are used pre- and postintravenous gadolinium administration. Utilised at 50–70 s postinjection there is usually good enhancement visible in the bowel wall (Fig. 1.6). In the last few years, improved multi-echo acquisitions with

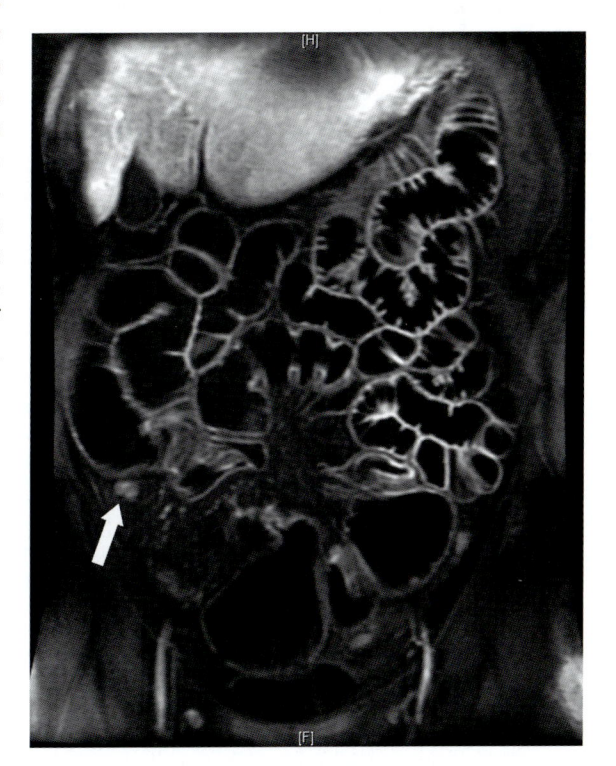

Fig. 1.6. Interpolated 3D T1w coronal imaging following intravenous antiperistaltic (hyoscine bromide) and gadolinium contrast medium administration during a small bowel MR enteroclysis study. The use of fat suppression improves the delineation of the normally enhancing small bowel wall and folds. This patient with Crohns disease also has clearly visible enhancing mesenteric lymph nodes (*arrow*)

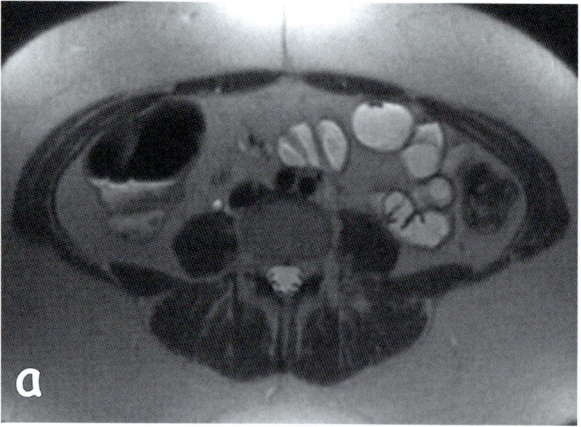

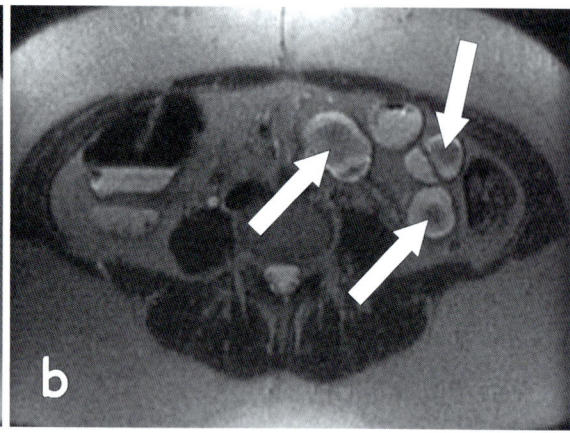

Fig. 1.7. Single shot half-Fourier RARE flow void artifacts. Two axial images using an effective echo time of 60 ms obtained during breath-holding. Note the loss of signal centrally in the lumen (*arrows*) on the thinner section 3-mm image (**a**) compared with the relatively unaffected 10-mm image (**b**). Bulk fluid motion during the echo time results in the excited fluid losing signal either by moving out of the image section or because the fluid motion causes spin dephasing within each voxel. This is less frequently observed in thicker sections and with in-plane motion but is exacerbated with longer effective echo times such as used in hydrographic projections (see Fig. 1.8)

phase correcting reconstruction algorithms have provided the ability to generate both in and out of phase images along with separate water and fat images for each section of a whole imaging volume within a single breath-hold. These approaches can provide near-optimal fat suppression (MA 2004; REEDER et al. 2005) and improved gradient performance has provided other enhancements in image quality.

1.3.8
Hydrographic Projection Imaging

It was appreciated in 1988 that by reversing the phase encode order for RARE imaging, it was possible to obtain images at very long echo times that emphasized those tissues or materials with a long T2 value (HENNIG et al. 1986). This is particularly the case for fluids and many body fluids have a long T2 value similar to water, which allows for their selective imaging using this technique. These materials are ideally suited to this technique as the slow T2 decay of fluids also reduces the recognized problem of spatially frequency blurring described above. Hydrographic imaging with RARE sequences has a particular limitation in bowel imaging related to bulk fluid motion during the long readout echo times. If "excited" fluid moves out of the slice during the long echo time of an acquisition, then a signal void may result that may simulate an intraluminal lesion. This may also occur with relatively short effective echo times and if there is in-plane motion within the fluid leading to spin dephasing within the image voxels (Fig. 1.7). Such signal voids are exacerbated by using thin sections perpendicular to the direction of motion with long effective echo times and conversely can be partially overcome by using thick slab imaging. Alternatively, antiperistaltic agents will reduce motion in the intraluminal fluid and reduce the artifact. Thick slab or "projection" imaging of fluids is effective as the signal from other background tissues with shorter T2 values decays away rapidly leaving just the fluid-filled structures visible in the resulting image volume (LAUBENBERGER et al. 1995). Such projection hydrographic imaging is now used widely in MRCP examinations but has also found use in sialography, and renography. This approach has become widely used for the GI tract and demonstrated in the stomach and colon but has been mainly utilized for the small bowel (UMSCHADEN et al. 2000). Combined with water-based contrast, this approach can be used to observe the whole of a bowel segment (stomach, small bowel or colon) during filling or emptying by repeatedly imaging the same thick slab or section encompassing the relevant segment. The sub-second acquisitions will freeze the bowel motion and if respiratory gated or breath-held allow for a dynamic "cine" like display of the filling or emptying process. A potential disadvantage of repeated acquisitions in the same location is the long T1 recovery time that is required to maintain the SNR. Although "fast recovery" techniques can partly overcome this (MAKKI et al. 2002), it means that the

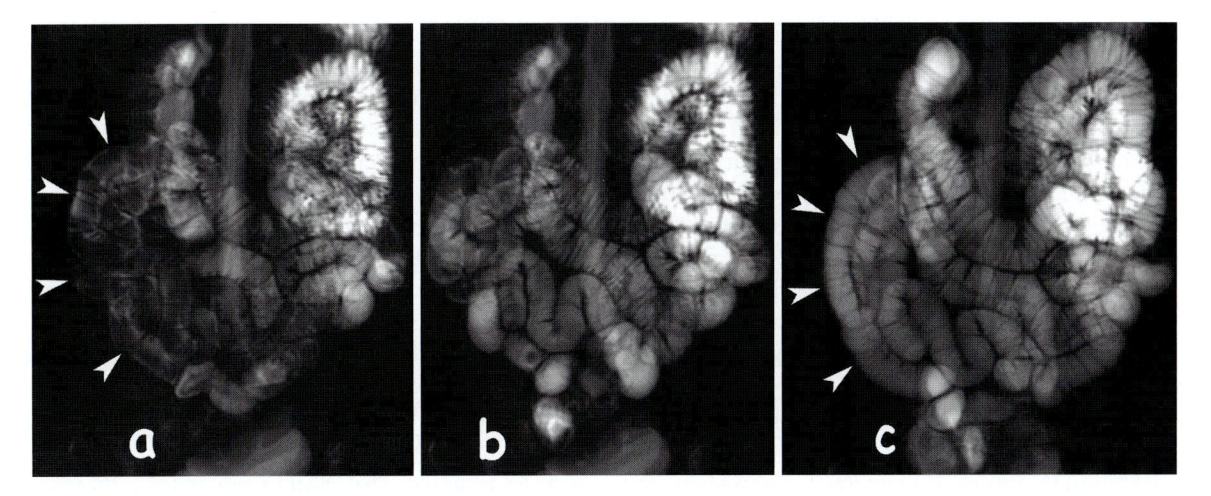

Fig. 1.8. Hydrographic projection images during MR enteroclysis obtained with single-shot half-Fourier RARE using an effective echo time of 600 ms and a section thickness of 10 cm. Three images (**a–c**) at different timepoints in a series of 60 obtained during filling of the small bowel. Note how the demonstration of the distal ileum (*arrowheads*) improves as the small bowel fills and the movement of the fluid in the small bowel slows. No antiperistalstic agents were needed as the images are acquired in less than one second. Respiratory gating reduces respiratory artifact and misregistration allowing the sequence to be viewed as a "cine" to aid detection of abnormal small bowel

sequential images often need to be at least several seconds and more optimally at 6–10 s intervals to allow good signal recovery. Even at this slow frequency diagnostic, quality images of the bowel can be relatively easily obtained (Fig. 1.8) and used not just to monitor filling or emptying but directly for diagnosis.

1.3.9 Fat Suppression

Effective fat suppression is used in several situations for GI tract imaging, in particular pre- and post-gadolinium T1w sequences and also when detecting fluid tracks and fistulae in the perineum with T2w imaging. There are two main strategies for achieving fat suppression, spectral methods, and inversion recovery methods and these are also combined in some sequences. Spectral fat suppression relies upon the difference in resonant frequency between water and fat (typically 220 Hz at 1.5 T) and the use of "spectrally selective" radiofrequency excitation pulses. This approach is very specific but prone to artifacts resulting from static field inhomogeneity (so the effect is often uneven over large fields of view) and at lower field strength requires very good RF pulse design to achieve sufficient "selectivity." It has the advantage of being relatively easy to add to many sequences as a preparation phase so that adding fat suppression is a relatively simple change for clinical protocols as and when needed. Immediately before the main acquisition, a frequency-selective RF pulse excites just the lipid protons creating signal in the transverse plane, which is then immediately destroyed using "killer" gradients. The main acquisition then proceeds as normal but there are only water protons left to excite – resulting in reduced fat signal in the resulting images. Inversion methods rely on the short T1 value of lipid and work by inverting the initial longitudinal magnetisation of the lipid to a negative value and waiting (the inversion time TI) for it to return to zero (the null point). At that specific moment in time, the "readout" part of the sequence is applied so that no signal is returned from the short T1 fat. This method gives very good even fat suppression but can be misleading particularly in the presence of met-hemoglobin, which also has a short T1 value. Therefore, occasionally the products of hemorrhage can be misinterpreted as fat. STIR (short tau inversion reovery) sequences are based on this inversion approach and demonstrate T2-like contrast although they are predominantly T1w sequences. This is because all the water proton signals are also inverted and are read-out when still "negative" so that short T1 materials produce a lower signal than long T1 materials – the reverse of normal T1w images. This constraint of fixing the inversion time to the T1 of fat also reduces the overall SNR in the sequence, although this can partly be offset by integrating the inversion approach with a RARE sequence creating a fast or turbo STIR sequence. Various combinations of spectral and inversion time approaches have been used to try and combine the best features of each approach. Fast3D T1w gradient echo sequences, discussed above, often use a combined approach for fat suppression. This is because of the need for a short TR that does not allow sufficient time for a long inversion time or for increasing the RF power burden. Typically, a spectrally selectively pulse inverts the lipid signals for several repetitions (and lines of K space) with the echoes obtained at the optimal inversion time for fat suppression being placed at the centre of K space for maximum fat suppression effect.

1.3.10 Dynamic Acquisition

X-ray fluoroscopy is widely used for GI examinations to evaluate dynamic physiological events such as swallowing, gastric emptying, small bowel peristalsis, and defecation. In addition, this is frequently combined with the use of contrast medium and posture changes to improve the delineation of a particular region, e.g., small bowel to detect subtle strictures. MRI system vendors have yet to develop a fully integrated approach that allows for equivalent in-room control, display, and data acquisition combined with postural changes for GI tract imaging. Decubitus views are possible but often difficult owing to the presence of surface coil arrays attached to the patient, which in some cases cannot be rotated.

In the meantime, several approaches have been proposed to try and obtain similar information using predominantly the breathing-independent sequences SSFP and single-shot half-Fourier RARE. These strategies an be implemented using most modern systems and although they lack the flexibility of a truly interactive fluoroscopy system they allow observation of function and in the small bowel allow improved evaluation of strictures and their distensibility.

As described in hydrographic imaging above, it is possible to obtain relatively slow (2–10 s intervals) "dynamic" imaging of small bowel filling or gastric emptying by repeatedly acquiring images in the same fixed location. This approach can be speeded up by using short effective TE single shot half-Fourier RARE methods with thinner section to image materials with faster recovery time, e.g., to allow visualization of the bowel wall. Although versions that can image at 3–5 frames per second have been developed, the short TRs lead to loss of contrast from fluids but they may still be useful, for example, in functional imaging of the pelvic floor during straining (Fletcher et al. 2003).

bSSFP sequences have proven more promising for dynamic imaging using water-based contrast agents as they have a short enough TE/TR to freeze the majority of motion within the bowel lumen and can be used to image serially in the same location without significantly degrading the SNR. These sequences have been widely used in "cine" form for cardiac imaging and adapted by several groups for GI tract imaging. Two main approaches have been used with standard clinical MRI systems, first a breathing-independent cine acquisition, which typically acquires sequential images at a single location. Second, multisection multiphase acquisitions can be obtained during sequential breath-holds (Fig. 1.9). These stacks of images obtained at the same location can then be resorted to generate "cine" like multiphase imaging at each location. In both cases, the advantage is the ability to observe the bowel at different phases of peristalsis, which can be helpful for both confirming the diagnosis of a stricture and evaluating its severity. This is a difficult area to evaluate technically in terms of the impact on diagnosis but several recent papers have indicated the value of emulating traditional X-ray "fluoroscopic" approaches (Buhmann-Kirchhoff et al. 2008).

Although most modern MRI systems offer some sort of interactive interface, none of these offer the sort of integration required to provide the ease of use familiar to users of X-ray fluoroscopy tables. Several research groups working on interventional MRI systems have adapted the capabilities of existing MRI systems to allow for varying degrees of interactivity, particularly navigation of an imaging plane through a 3D volume in real-time and simultaneous manipulation of several contrast parameters (Makki et al. 2002; Graves et al. 2009). Improved MR system architectures are required to allow for real-time switching of parameters and for appropriately responsive methods of controlling the MR system during a GI tract examination. These techniques may in the future allow for the real exploitation of some of the advantages of MRI, which can image in any plane and deploy a wide range of soft tissue contrast valuable for detecting GI tract pathology. The potential to make an MRI system operate more

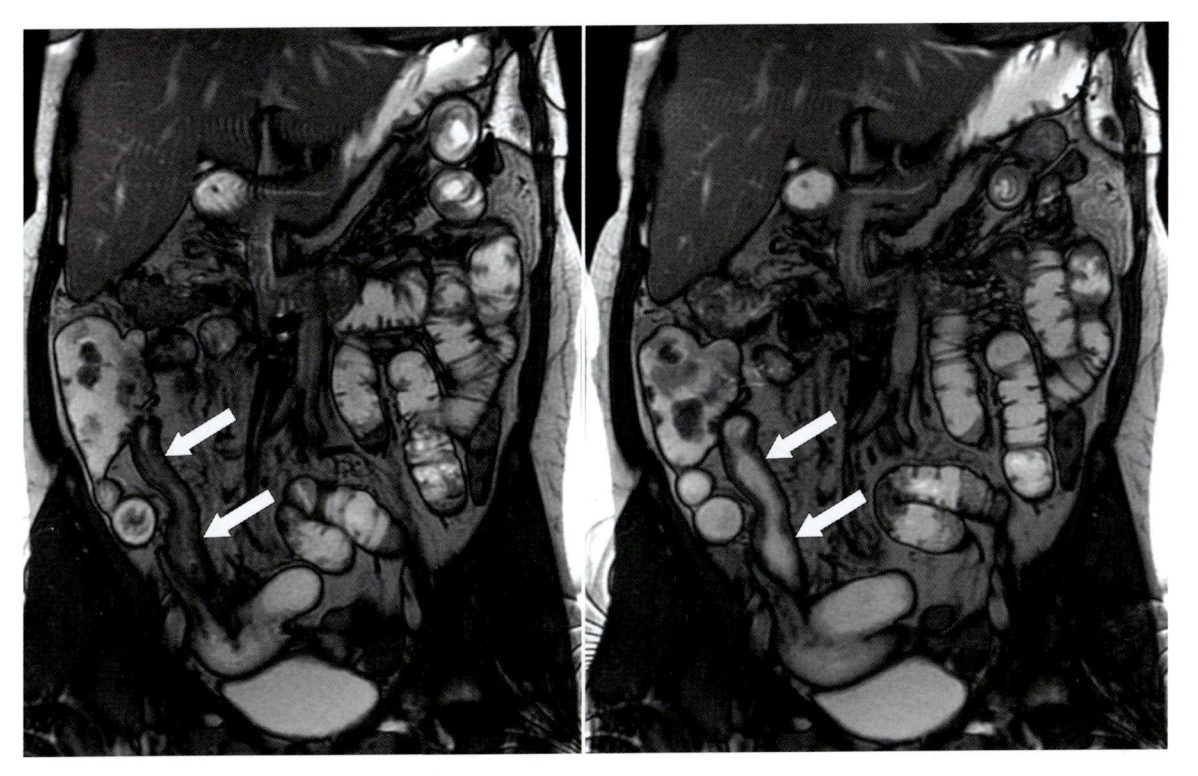

Fig. 1.9. Multiphase, multisection bSSFP dynamic imaging during MR enteroclysis. Ten sequential stacks of 2D bSSFP were acquired coronally covering the small bowel using separate breath-holds immediately after the contrast medium reached the terminal ileum. These can then be reordered to allow scrolling through the ten images acquired at the same location but at different phases of peristalsis. The two images displayed demonstrate the variation in lumen size in an affected terminal ileum (*arrows*) that can be demonstrated using this "pseudo-cine" approach

like a real-time ultrasound system (Holsinger 1999) is becoming more feasible as the computing power and MR system designs evolve.

1.3.11
Diffusion-Weighted Imaging

Diffusion is the random motion of molecules within a medium and, in the presence of a magnetic field gradient, the diffusion of water molecules will accelerate the dephasing of their proton spins. In biological tissues, diffusion may occur equally in all directions (isotropic diffusion) or vary with direction (anisotropic diffusion) for example in neurons. Rapid diffusion leads to rapid spin dephasing and a measurable signal loss. This effect occurs with virtually all MRI sequences but is often negligible or masked by other effects. It is possible to increase the effect by applying bipolar sensitizing gradients in one or more directions of interest. These sensitising gradients can be added to a wide range of sequences but in clinical practice are most widely used with spin-echo prepared single shot echoplanar imaging. This is to ensure a very fast acquisition that is relatively insensitive to other motion, particularly "bulk" tissue motion (related to breathing, etc.), which could mask the diffusion effect. At body temperatures, free water protons will diffuse approximately 30 µm in 50 ms, which in biological tissues is larger than most cell diameters. In body tissues cellular structure, adjacent organelles, and both intracellular and extracellular molecules will all effectively restrict the motion of water molecules in vivo although this process is still not fully understood. The size of the bipolar gradients can be varied to influence the sensitivity to motion and these are expressed as "b" values. The analysis of images based on several of these values generates the apparent diffusion coefficient that is often "mapped" onto structural imaging. Widely used in the brain for detecting early strokes and tracking neuronal fibre tracts, this concept is increasingly being used in body imaging. At low "b" values, the effects of tissue perfusion influence the analysis and it is also clear that materials with a long T2 value may create artifacts owing to a "shine through" effect. There has been particular oncological interest in the use of this technique not only to improve the detection and characterization of lesions but also as a biomarker in solid tumors for early detection of treatment response and this is an area of active research. See chapter 4 for more details.

1.3.12
Perfusion Imaging

Perfusion imaging with MRI has been mainly used for evaluating brain pathologies and, to a lesser extent, tumors in a range of body organs. The majority of methods use a similar approach to CT-based perfusion methods using analysis of the first pass of an injected intravenous bolus of a contrast agent. Gadolinium media are commonly used, but unlike CT, the relationship between MRI signal and concentration of contrast agent is nonlinear. This factor along with several other variables means this technique needs very careful attention to detail if repeatable and reliable results are to be obtained. Several different T1w acquisition methods have been used, initially with standard SPGR and FSPGR sequences outlined above. To increase temporal resolution and acquire images fast enough to accurately sample the variation of contrast medium concentrations, short TR sequences with "saturation" or inversion preparation pulses have been developed. In addition, the baseline T1 values of the tissues or fluids being measured have to be initially determined to derive accurate estimates of the contrast medium concentrations. Most published work has used multicompartment pharmacokinetic models to derive several perfusion-related parameters used to characterize perfusion in soft tissues. Complexities arise from the requirement for an arterial input function and typically the need to estimate both a high concentration arterial input and a lower concentration tissue value. Much of the work relating to the GI tract has used qualitative evaluation of enhancement for evaluating mural perfusion changes, for example in Crohns disease. More recently, in solid GI tract tumors, perfusion techniques have been investigated using more formal quantification for tumor characterization and as a potential prognosis and treatment response marker. Several national and international groups are working on standardizing these techniques so that they can be applied reliably and repeatably across different vendor platforms and institutions (Table 1.1). See chapter 4 for more details.

1.4
Techniques

1.4.1
Requirements

Virtually, all current techniques rely on an intraluminal contrast medium to improve the delineation of the bowel wall, lumen and extraluminal tissues. The passage of a "bolus" of contrast medium is often diagnostically valuable in demonstrating that normal distension of the relevant segment of the GI tract can be achieved. These requirements are of course identical to the demands for conventional X-ray contrast radiography and not surprisingly many of the MR-based techniques parallel earlier X-ray-based approaches. Both negative and positive contrast intraluminal media have been employed for GI imaging (Wesbey 1985; Lomas 1999). Although initially short T1 (positive) contrast media were demonstrated with T1w imaging usually with fat saturation, more recently negative contrast media have been used combined with intravenous gadolinium to generate the contrast between enhancing bowel wall and dark lumen. Both negative (e.g., gas) and positive (e.g., water-based media) have been used with proton density and T2w imaging sequences. These media and their applications are discussed in more detail in Chap. 3. The role of intravenous gadolinium varies with technique but in general has been used to help identify mural lesions, wall thickening and focal collections – in a similar fashion to CT and iodinated contrast medium.

It should be noted that currently MRI is primarily used to detect chronic GI tract pathology – conditions such as malignancy and inflammatory bowel disease. Multidetector CT dominates the diagnosis of acute GI tract conditions such as perforation, intestinal obstruction and intra-abdominal collections. As MRI techniques improve, this balance is expected to shift in future years (see Chap. 17) and this will influence the optimal techniques used for imaging the GI tract. A brief introduction to the key aspects of technique in relation to the different parts of the GI tract follows. Subsequent chapters will address these issues in further detail.

1.4.2
Pharynx and Esophagus

Structural imaging of the oropharynx is often considered part of neuroradiology, whereas the functional imaging of deglutition is part of the GI tract. The diagnostic imaging of swallowing abnormalities is currently an area where MRI is currently unable to provide adequate temporal and spatial resolution to detect the subtle structural (esophageal webs) and functional abnormalities that can arise. X-ray video fluoroscopy using 25–50 frames per second acquisition is still required (Kendall et al. 2000), although palatal function related to phonation and sleep apnoea has been evaluated successfully with MRI.

The esophagus is frequently imaged using conventional sequences for demonstration of mural lesions such as tumors. There has been relatively little literature on dynamic evaluation of oesophageal function. Although the temporal resolution is less critical than for the oro-pharynx, this is still a challenging area as the anatomy of the esophagus makes it difficult to achieve complete coverage without using thick sections. Projection imaging would seem appropriate but the RARE-based approaches using hydrographic techniques are generally too slow to reliably capture a contrast bolus passing through the lumen. Cine bSSFP methods are fast enough (Barkhausen et al. 2002), but demand very accurate positioning and therefore often require multiple acquisitions to achieve good coverage. Functional assessment is also limited by the fact that swallowing has to be performed in a prone or supine position rather than the more desirable erect position.

1.4.3
Stomach

Gastric imaging for tumors has been achieved using rapid breath-hold acquisitions as well as more conventional sequences that are often acquired to evaluate the adjacent organs such as the liver. Gastric function was described and evaluated in the 1980s using echoplanar-based sequences and then again in the 1990s using both RARE (Bilecen et al. 2000) and bSSFP approaches. 2D and 3D strategies for evaluating gastric function and emptying have been described and gastric peristalsis is generally slow enough to permit successful imaging with either technique.

1.4.4
Small Bowel

Small bowel imaging with MRI developed initially with water-based methods and both oral and nasojejunal tube delivery of contrast media. Filling is well demonstrated using a hydrographic approach and many groups use antiperistaltics when the small bowel is filled to allow for 3D breath-hold imaging with both spatially interpolated bSSFP and T1w sequences the latter pre- and postintravenous gadolinium. A more functional assessment can be obtained acquiring multisection multiphase 2D imaging when the small bowel is almost completely filled. These images then provide the option of sequential viewing at each sectional level to evaluate the peristalsis and distension of different loops of bowel. In future, the ability to rapidly switch the imaging capability from hydrographic imaging to bSSFP and navigate to a bowel loop of interest may become feasible but currently the majority of MR systems do not provide this capability in a responsive enough fashion to be clinically useful.

1.4.5
Colon

MRI of the large bowel has been demonstrated successfully with both gas and fluid contrast media and in general RARE-type sequences have been used to observe and confirm filling, followed by an antiperistaltic agent and breath-hold imaging most commonly with pre- and postgadolinium-enhanced 3D T1w sequences. In common with CT colonography, a variety of tagging strategies have been investigated to reduce or avoid the burden of preprocedure bowel cleansing. Although MRI has several potential advantages over CT, particularly the lack of ionizing radiation, the overall performance has not improved on CT and the examinations currently take longer and are less easy to perform than CT. Future developments using specific contrast media may make MR colonography a more practical proposition for widespread clinical use.

1.4.6
Rectum and Anus

Structural rectal imaging has been optimized for demonstrating tumor in relation to the rectal wall and the surgically important surrounding meso-rectal fat and related fascial planes. In this region, respiratory, vascular and peristaltic artifacts are much less likely and the techniques are optimised using longer acquisition times and conventional multishot RARE imaging to achieve high spatial resolution imaging. In general, moderately T2w imaging is used to discriminate tumor from the adjacent smooth muscle with thin sections where possible, perpendicular to the axis of the involved rectum. Although there have been advocates of specific intraluminal contrast media, these have not gained wide acceptance. Perineal imaging for fistula and ischio-anal fossa abnormalities is well established and most sites rely on fat suppressed thin section T2w imaging in multiple planes but particularly axial and coronal planes. T2w imaging without fat suppression allows good evaluation of the normal anatomical structures such as the anal sphincter muscles. There are advocates of both matched unenhanced and/or enhanced T1w imaging for improving the delineation of abscesses and confirming the presence and location of inflamed fistula tracks. Endoanal coils have been used and can be helpful in patients with (cryptoglandular) fistula-in-ano and in fecal incontinence. Functional imaging of the pelvic floor during straining and defecation has been achieved using a range of media such as ultrasound gel as a water-based agent with both sequential T2w single-shot RARE or bSSFP techniques for observation.

References

Barkhausen J, Goyen M, von Winterfeld F, et al (2002) Visualization of swallowing using real-time TrueFISP MR fluoroscopy. Eur Radiol 12(1):129–133

Bernstein MA, King KF, Zhou XJ (2004) Handbook of MRI pulse sequences. Elsevier, Amsterdam

Bilecen D, Scheffler K, Seifritz E, et al (2000) Hydro-MRI for the visualization of gastric wall motility using RARE magnetic resonance imaging sequences. Abdom Imaging 25: 30–43

Brau AC, Beatty PJ, Skare S, et al (2008) Comparison of reconstruction accuracy and efficiency among autocalibrating data-driven parallel imaging methods. Magn Reson Med 59(2):382–395

Buhmann-Kirchhoff S, Lang R, Kirchhoff C, et al (2008) Functional cine MR imaging for the detection and mapping of intraabdominal adhesions: method and surgical correlation. Eur Radiol 18(6):1215–1223

Constable RT, Gore JC (1992) The loss of small objects in variable TE imaging: implications for FSE, RARE, and EPI. Magn Reson Med 28:9–24

Constable RT, Henkelman RM (1991) Contrast, resolution, and detectability in MR imaging. J Comput Assist Tomogr 15: 297–303

Evans DF, Lamont G, Stehling MK, et al (1993) Prolonged monitoring of the upper gastrointestinal tract using echo planar magnetic resonance imaging. Gut 34:848–852

Fletcher JG, Busse RF, Riederer SJ, et al (2003) Magnetic resonance imaging of anatomic and dynamic defects of the pelvic floor in defecatory disorders. Am J Gastroenterol 98(2): 399–411

Froehlich JM, Daenzer M, von Weymarn C, et al (2009) Aperistaltic effect of hyoscine N-butylbromide versus glucagon on the small bowel assessed by magnetic resonance imaging. Eur Radiol 19:1387–1393

Froehlich JM, Patak MA, von Weymarn C, et al (2005) Small bowel motility assessment with magnetic resonance imaging. J Magn Reson Imaging 21(4):370–375

Gourtsoyiannis N, Papanikolaou N, Grammatikakis J, et al (2001) MR enteroclysis protocol optimization: comparison between 3D FLASH with fat saturation after intravenous gadolinium injection and true FISP sequences. Eur Radiol 11:908–913

Griswold MA, Jakob PM, Heidemann RM, et al (2002) Generalized autocalibrating partially parallel acquisitions (GRAPPA). Magn Reson Med 47(6):1202–1210

Hennig J, Nauerth A, Friedburg H (1986) RARE imaging: a fast imaging method for clinical MR. Magn Reson Med 3(6): 823–833

Holsinger AE, Wright RC, Riederer SJ, et al (1990) Real-time interactive magnetic resonance imaging. Magn Reson Med 14:547–553

Kellow JE, Borody TJ, Phillips SF, et al (1986) Human interdigestive motility: variations in patterns from esophagus to colon. Gastroenterology 91:386–395

Kendall KA, McKenzie S, Leonard RJ, et al (2000) Timing of events in normal swallowing: a videofluoroscopic study. Dysphagia 15:74–83

Laubenberger J, Büchert M, Schneider B, et al (1995) Breathhold projection magnetic resonance-cholangio-pancreaticography MRCP): a new method for the examination of the bile and pancreatic ducts. Magn Reson Med 33(1):18–23

Lomas DJ (1999) The potential for MRI of the small bowel. Imaging 11:161–169

Luboldt W, Bauerfeind P, Steiner P, et al (1997) Preliminary assessment of three-dimensional magnetic resonance imaging for various colonic disorders. Lancet 349(9061): 1288–1291

Ma J (2004) Breath-hold water and fat imaging using a dual-echo twopoint Dixon technique with an efficient and robust phase-correction algorithm. Magn Reson Med 52:415–419

Makki M, Graves MJ, Lomas DJ (2002) Interactive body magnetic resonance fluoroscopy using modified single-shot half-Fourier rapid acquisition with relaxation enhancement (RARE) with multiparameter control. J Magn Reson Imaging 16:85–93

Mansfield P (1977) Multiplanar image formation using NMR spin echoes. J Phys C: Solid State Phys 10:L55–L58

Oppelt A, Graumann R, Barfuss H, et al (1986) FISP: a new fast MRI sequence. Electromedica 54:15–18

Pruessmann KP, Weiger M, Scheidegger MB, et al (1999) SENSE: sensitivity encoding for fast MRI. Magn Reson Med 42(5):952–962

Reeder SB, Hargreaves BA, Yu H, et al (2005) Homodyne reconstruction and IDEAL water-fat decomposition. Magn Reson Med 54:586–593

Roemer PB, Edelstein WA, Hayes CE, et al (1990) The NMR phased array. Magn Reson Med 16:192–225

Rofsky NM, Lee VS, Laub G, et al (1999) Abdominal MR imaging with a volumetric interpolated breath-hold examination. Radiology 212:876–884

Semelka RC, Kelekis NL, Thomasson D, et al (1996) HASTE MR imaging: description of technique and preliminary results in the abdomen. J Magn Reson Imaging 6: 698–699

Sodickson DK, Manning WJ (1997) Simultaneous acquisition of spatial harmonics (SMASH): fast imaging with radiofrequency coil arrays. Magn Reson Med 38:591–603

Stoker J, Rociu E, Zwamborn AW, Schouten WR, Laméris JS (1999) Endoluminal MR imaging of the rectum and anus: technique, applications, and pitfalls. Radiographics 19(2): 383-98 (Mar–Apr)

Umschaden HW, Szolar D, Gasser J, et al (2000) Small-bowel disease: comparison of MR enteroclysis images with conventional enteroclysis and surgical findings. Radiology 215: 717–725

Wesbey GE, Brasch RC, Goldberg HI, et al (1985) Dilute oral iron solutions as gastrointestinal contrast agents for magnetic resonance imaging; initial clinical experience. Magn Reson Imaging 3:57–64

MRI of the Gastrointestinal Tract at High-Field Strength

Aart J. Nederveen and Sonia I. Gonçalves

CONTENTS

2.1 Principal Problem of High Field MRI 21
2.1.1 Tissue Relaxation Rates 22
2.1.2 Susceptibility 22
2.1.3 Contrast Agents 23
2.1.4 Chemical Shift Artifacts 23
2.1.5 B1-Inhomogeneity Artifacts 24
2.1.6 SAR Limitations 24
2.1.7 SSFP Banding Artifacts 25

2.2 Changes to Accomodate These Problems 28
2.2.1 Improvement Using Parallel and Fast Imaging Techniques 28
2.2.2 Solving the Banding Artifact at 3 T 30

References 30

KEY POINTS

High-field imaging of the GI tract at 3 T can be very *attractive* in terms of signal to noise ratio (SNR) when compared with 1.5 T imaging. However, several issues need to be addressed and a direct transition of sequences used at 1.5–3 T is not possible. The main constraints in 3 T imaging are related to changes in tissue *T1* and *T2* relaxation parameters, susceptibility artifacts, changes in efficiency of contrast agents, chemical shift artifacts, B1-inhomogeneity artifacts, specific absorption rate (SAR) limitations, and steady-state free precession (SSFP) banding artifacts. In general, a careful adjustment of sequence parameters is needed to avoid these artifacts. The use of parallel imaging techniques is more beneficial at 3 T when compared with 1.5 T because by reducing scan time SAR problems often present at 3 T can be avoided. For reducing B1-inhomogeneity, hardware adjustments are needed. Banding artifacts generated in SSFP-sequences pose a severe limitation to the clinical use of these sequences. Though methods exist to overcome this problem, a satisfactory solution has not been proposed so far.

2.1 Principal Problem of High-Field MRI

The use of high-field whole-body MRI systems, i.e. 3 Tesla (T) MRI scanners, has become increasingly popular since its introduction in the beginning of the 2000s decade. The clinical applications range from brain to musculoskeletal imaging (Barth et al. 2007). However, several different problems are associated with imaging at 3 T and a direct transition from 1.5 to 3 T is not possible. In particular, aspects related to pulse sequence design, such as timings, radiofrequency

Aart J. Nederveen, PhD
Sonia I. Gonçalves, PhD
Department of Radiology, Academic Medical Center, Amsterdam, The Netherlands

pulses, and specific absorption rate (SAR) issues have to be considered when imaging at 3 T. Furthermore, experience gained, for example, in imaging the brain at 3 T does not necessarily apply to improved abdominal imaging (Hussain et al. 2005; Merkle et al. 2006; Merkle and Dale 2006; Patak et al. 2007; Schindera et al. 2006). This is because many of the problems that are associated with imaging at 3 T are region-specific. The main constraints in 3 T imaging are related to changes in tissue $T1$ and $T2$ relaxation parameters, susceptibility artifacts, changes in efficiency of contrast agents, chemical shift artifacts, B1-inhomogeneity artifacts, SAR limitations, and steady-state free precession (SSFP) banding artifacts.

2.1.1
Tissue Relaxation Rates

Several studies (Bazelaire et al. 2004; Stanisz et al. 2005) on the variation of $T1$ and $T2$ relaxation parameters at 3 T showed that the longitudinal relaxation parameter $T1$, increases with magnetic field strength by sometimes as much as 38% for liver tissue (Bazelaire et al. 2004) or 62% in gray matter. However, the range of parameter variation among different studies may be quite wide because of the dependence on the $T1$ and $T2$ measuring methods. The increase in Larmor frequency from 64 MHz at 1.5 T to 128 MHz at 3 T causes an efficiency decrease in the energy transfer between spins and lattice, thus causing the increase in $T1$ values at 3 T (Bazelaire et al. 2004). In addition to the absolute changes in $T1$, the relative differences in $T1$ parameters among different tissues, change from 1.5 to 3 T. This causes an additional confounding effect when comparing $T1$-weighted images obtained at 1.5 and 3 T using the same contrast parameters such as time to repeat (TR). Because of the aforementioned differences, the contrast in both sets of images will not be comparable.

The transverse relaxation parameter $T2$ has been reported by several studies (Bottomley et al. 1984; Stanisz et al. 2005) to be essentially independent of the magnetic field strength. However, the study of Bazelaire et al. (2004), where $T1$ and $T2$ measurements were performed in vivo, reported a decrease in $T2$ values of the order of 8%. This decrease might be partially explained by the diffusion of water molecules in the neighborhood of paramagnetic molecules such as hemoglobin in deoxygenated blood. The spins in water molecules experience small local field inhomogeneties in the vicinity of these molecules and as a consequence, a shortening of $T2$ is observed. These effects, though small, tend to increase with field strength and therefore it is very likely that they become visible at 3 T while at 1.5 T they remain essentially unnoticed.

The change in $T1$ and $T2$ relaxation parameters at 3 T implies the decrease of $T1$ contrast in $T1$-weighted images or the decrease in the signal-to-noise ratio (SNR) of $T2$-weigthed images, if time to echo (TE) and TR parameters are used that are identical to the ones used at 1.5 T.

A greater additional source of concern at 3 T is the change in the $T2^*$ relaxation value. At high field, the sphere of homogeneity (Vlaardingerbroek et al. 1999) of the magnetic field is smaller. This, together with increased difficulties in shimming and increased tissue susceptibility effects cause a significant decrease in $T2^*$, which becomes apparent in gradient-echo sequences, in general, and in SSFP sequences, in particular, where the contrast is weighed by $T1/T2$ ratio (see Sect. 2.1.7) and also by magnetic field inhomogeneities through $T2^*$.

2.1.2
Susceptibility

The magnetic susceptibility of a substance can be defined as its ability to become magnetized in response to an external magnetic field. In the vicinity of interfaces between tissues with different susceptibilities (e.g., air-soft tissue and bone-soft tissue interfaces), there are micro-variations in the magnetic field, which cause among others, in-plane image distortion, localized areas of high and low intensity, as well as localized signal drops due to local shortening of $T2^*$. This series of image artifacts are referred to as tissue susceptibility artifacts and they increase with field strength (Bernstein et al. 2006; Soher et al. 2007). In practice, they are found in gas-filled bowel, since the susceptibility of air is much lower than that of soft-tissue, or near metallic implants since the susceptibility of metal is much higher than that of tissue. The effects of the field variations introduced by interfaces between tissues with different susceptibilities depend, however, on the type of sequence. Thus, echo-planar imaging (EPI), which consists of acquiring several gradient echoes in each TR, each of these echoes corresponding to a different phase encoding step, suffers much more from susceptibility artifacts than fast gradient-echo imaging sequences. In addition, the effects of susceptibility artifacts on magnetization preparation prepulses such as inversion recovery or fat saturation can cause a decrease in the efficiency of these prepulses because the spins affected by the local field inhomogeneities may fail to be tipped by the prepulse.

2.1.3
Contrast Agents

The action of contrast agents also changes with increasing field strength because not only the tissue relaxation times but also the relaxivity R of the contrast agent changes. The effect of the contrast agent in the $T1$ relaxation parameter of a given tissue is given by (BERNSTEIN et al. 2006; SOHER et al. 2007):

$$\frac{1}{T_{1,C}} = \frac{1}{T_1} + R\,C, \quad (2.1)$$

where

$T_{1,C}$ is the longitudinal relaxation in the presence of a concentration C of contrast agent;

T_1 is the longitudinal relaxation in the absence of contrast agent.

For chelated gadolinium contrast agents, there is only a decrease of 5–10% in relaxivity when going from 1.5 to 3 T. When compared with the variations observed in $T1$ parameters, the relaxivity variation is very small. This implies that for the same contrast concentration C, the relative change in $T1$ parameters is larger at 3 T because the term $1/T_1$ is smaller. When comparing images obtained at 1.5 and 3 T using the same contrast concentration, the image obtained at 3 T shows more contrast difference, which means that less contrast has to be administered at 3 T to obtain images equivalent to those obtained at 1.5 T. An additional important point is that the increase in contrast effectiveness at 3 T should be considered when clinically evaluating images and increased contrast in certain areas should not be interpreted as pathological.

Another category of contrast agents are the superparamagnetic iron oxides (SPIOs) and ultra small superparamagnetic iron oxides (USPIOs). These types of contrast agents are composed of ferrites consisting of magnemite and magnetite (Fe_2O_3, Fe_3O_4), which show superparamagnetic behavior (COROT et al. 2006). They have been introduced for hepatic imaging and are nowadays extensively used not only in liver studies but also in molecular imaging (BULTE and KRAITCHMAN 2004). The effect of (U)SPIOs on $T1$ image contrast is similar to that described in (2.1) for chelated gadolinium contrast agents with the difference that the relaxivity of (U)SPIOs is higher and is dependent on the aggregation of the contrast agent. However, the principal effect of (U)SPIO's is $T2^*$ effect, i.e. the strong decrease of $T2^*$ due to the magnetization difference between different voxels within the image, which results from the inhomogeneous distribution of the contrast agent. This magnetization difference becomes important for (U)SPIOs due to the high magnetic susceptibility of iron oxide. At higher field strengths, the $T2^*$ effect increases due to higher intra-voxel dephasing, which implies that the use of (U)SPIOs is more efficient at 3 T than at 1.5 T.

2.1.4
Chemical Shift Artifacts

The chemical shift artifacts occur due to the difference in the resonance frequencies of H^1 spins in water and fat molecules and they are divided into chemical shift artifacts of the first and second kinds. Chemical shift artifacts of the first kind originate directly from the difference in precession frequencies, estimated to be approximately equal to 3.5 ppm (SOHER et al. 2007), and they occur along the frequency encoding and slice selection directions. The difference in resonance frequencies is directly proportional to the field strength and therefore this type of artifact becomes more problematic at 3 T where the frequency difference is equal to 440 Hz. The chemical shift causes a misregistration of fat, which appears as a dark band toward the lower part of the readout gradient field and as a bright band toward the higher part of the readout gradient field. Such artifact can be easily seen around the kidneys but is also present at the boundary of the GI tract and it can occupy from one to several pixels in the image. At 3 T the width of these bands doubles, which means that at a constant field of view (FOV) and spatial resolution, the receiver bandwidth must be doubled in order to reduce the artifacts to a size compared with those obtained at 1.5 T. This bandwidth increase comes at the expense of a decrease in the signal-to-noise ratio (SNR) by approximately 30% (HAACKE et al. 1999). In clinical practice, however, this type of artifact is not very problematic and therefore the noise considerations associated with RF pulse bandwidth broadening rarely have to be considered.

The chemical shift artifact of the second type results from the intravoxel phase cancellation during readout originated by the presence of water and fat molecules in the same voxel. Contrary to the chemical shift of the first kind, it can be seen along all voxels in a fat–water interface and is therefore not restricted to the frequency encoding direction. The size of this type of artifact does not change with field strength but the echo times have to be adjusted when imaging at 3 T in order to account for the higher resonance frequency, which causes the water and fat spins to appear in and out-of-phase at different moments when compared with what happens at 1.5 T. In the 3 T case, the spins appear in-phase at $2.2 + i \times 2.2$ ms and out-of-phase at $1.1 + i \times 2.2$ ms, where i is an integer larger or equal than 1, whereas at 1.5 T the spins appear out-of-phase at $2.2 + i \times 4.4$ ms. Thus, in order to capture in-phase or out-of-phase images at 3 T, the echo times have to be halved.

2.1.5
B1-inhomogeneity Artifacts

Contrary to chemical shift or susceptibility artifacts, which exist both in 1.5 and 3 T and only become more apparent at 3 T because of the increased SNR, there are other artifacts such as B1 inhomogeneity and standing wave artifacts, which are specific of high field strength MRI. The increase in field strength is associated with an increase in resonance frequency, which implies a concomitant increase in the RF pulse frequency. This frequency change caused various technical problems related to coil design (DUENSING and FITZSIMMONS 2006), which had to be optimized to achieve a homogeneous B1 field. B1 field homogeneity is crucial for $T2$-weigthed pulse sequences such as turbo spin echo (TSE) images and artifacts due to B1 inhomogeneities often arise in images obtained with these protocols (SCHICK et al. 2005).

Another problem inherent to the higher frequency of the RF pulse is the shortening of B1 wavelength. The high dielectric constant of tissue (water) causes the B1 wavelength to decrease from 234 cm in free space to approximately 30 cm in the body. The latter is of the order of magnitude of the field of view (FOV) of many body imaging protocols and therefore artifacts resulting from the generation of standing waves within the FOV can occur. These artifacts consist of strong signal variations across the image where areas of high signal intensity occur where there is constructive interference and areas of signal drop coincide with areas of destructive interference. These artifacts become more pronounced in larger areas of the body and, therefore, imaging of the abdomen can particularly be affected by this type of artifact. One solution to this problem lies in improving coil design and RF transmission (ALSOP et al. 1998; TOMANEK et al. 1997; VAUGHAN et al. 2004). Examples of such solutions are the combination of several RF transmit coils whereby the phase and amplitude of the signal emitted by each coil are adjusted to obtain an homogeneous B1 field (THESEN et al. 2003) or by parallel RF transmission (KATSCHER et al. 2006). An additional possibility is to obtain a homogeneous B1 field by means of passive coupling of coils (SCHMITT et al. 2005). In the latter solution, the current induced in a local coil during excitation is used to improve the homogeneity of the B1 field. Another type of solution is to place a cushion of dielectric material over the region to be imaged to avoid the generation of standing wave interference patterns. The cushion is made of a gel with a high dielectric constant mixed with gadolinium in order to suppress the signal from the gel itself.

Conductivity effects also tend to increase B1 field inhomogeneity. These effects happen in the neighborhood of highly conductive tissue such as ascites where current is induced by the rapidly changing RF field. The induced current tends to oppose the RF field, therefore causing local signal drops in the image.

Figure 2.1 illustrates the effect of B1-inhomogeneity in the abdomen. In healthy volunteer (panel A), only a small effect can sometimes be visible (see arrow), whereas in a patient with liver cirrhosis, portal hypertension, and ascites (panel B), the effect can be much larger because of the shielding effect of fluids, making the entire image useless. In the panels C and D, the result of B1-shimming using multitransmit parallel RF transmission is shown.

2.1.6
SAR Limitations

Specific absorption rate (SAR) is a measure of the energy deposition in the human body and at 3 T, limitations in this parameter play an important role. Quantitatively, the SAR is given by:

$$\text{SAR} = \left(\frac{\tau}{TR}\right) N_P N_S \frac{\sigma |E|^2}{2\rho} \quad (2.2)$$

where

τ is the RF pulse duration;
TR is the sequence repetition time;
N_p is the number of pulses;
N_s is the number of slices;
σ and ρ are tissue conductivity and density, respectively;
$|E|$ is the amplitude of the induced electric field within the tissue.

This second equation shows that if the main field is increased from 1.5 to 3 T and all other parameters

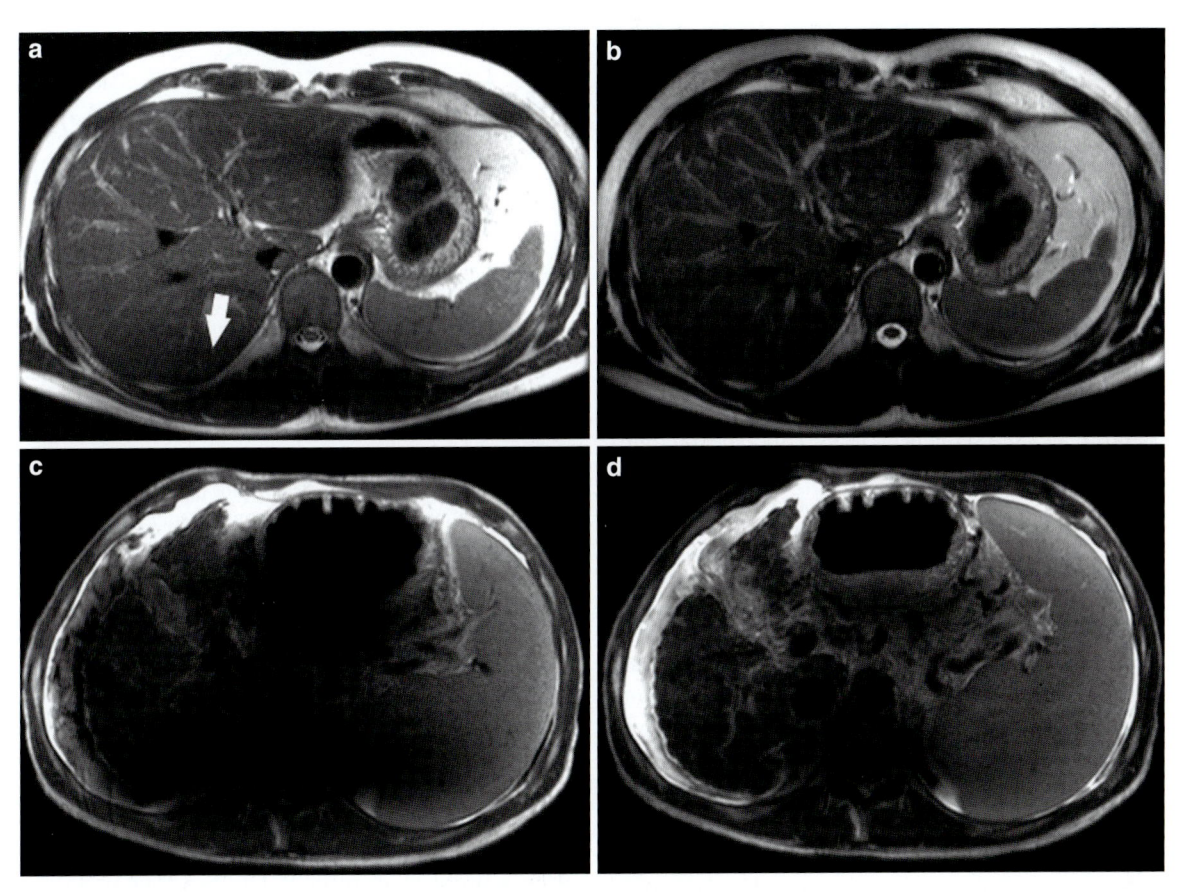

Fig. 2.1. Illustration of the effect of B1-inhomogeneity in the abdomen (courtesy Bonn University, Germany and Philips Medical Systems, Best, The Netherlands). A normal liver is visualized in (**a**) with B1-inhomogeneity indicated by an *arrow*. (**c**) Shows a patient with liver cirrhosis, portal hypertension, and ascites. Here, the effect can be much larger due to the shielding effect of fluids, making the entire image useless. (**b** and **d**) Show the effect of B1-shimming using parallel RF transmission (multitransmit)

remain constant, then the SAR increases by a factor of 4. This can potentially cause an increase in tissue temperature, which has to be taken in consideration in safety issues of pulse sequence design at 3 T to keep the temperature increase below 1°C. Thus, SAR aspects frequently introduce limitations in the use of sequences such as spin echo (SE) or balanced SSFP (Scheffler and Lehnhardt 2003) that often work close to SAR limits.

2.1.7
SSFP Banding Artifacts

Pulse sequences falling under the classification of balanced (b-)SSFP sequences such as b-FFE (balanced fast field echo), True-FISP (fast imaging with steady-state precession), and FIESTA (fast imaging employing steady-state acquisition) have become popular in the last years. They belong to the class of rapid gradient-echo sequences where in each *TR*, the magnetization reaches the same state thus implying that the signal is acquired in steady state, this process having been described for the first time by Carr (1958) as SSFP. In a given *TR*, the RF pulse rotates the magnetization by a given angle θ and in the course of *TR*, the magnetization will undergo longitudinal and transverse relaxation. Furthermore, the transverse magnetization will experience a certain amount of (spatially dependent) dephasing β due to the applied gradients and magnetic field inhomogeneities. After a number of *TR*s typically equal to $5 \times T1/TR$, the magnetization reaches a steady state.

In addition to b-SSFP sequences, the most important steady-state sequences (Chavhan et al. 2008) are *T1*-FFE (FLASH, SPGR) and *T2*-FFE (PSIF, SSFP) and they differ in the type of gradient switching pattern that determines the amount of dephasing in each *TR*, which characterizes the type of steady state that is reached and results in different types of contrast. In quantitative terms, the amount of dephasing in each *TR* is given by:

$$\beta(\vec{r}, TR) = \gamma \delta B_0(\vec{r}) TR + \gamma \vec{r} \cdot \int_0^{TR} \vec{G}(t) dt, \quad (2.3)$$

where

γ is the gyromagnetic ratio;
$\delta B_0(\vec{r})$ is the magnetic field inhomogeneity at position $(\vec{r})$;
$\vec{G}(t)$ is the applied gradient at time instant t.

From all SSFP sequences, b-SSFP has special interest because of the much higher signal that is obtained even at very short *TR*s (smaller than 10 ms) when compared with *T1*-FFE or *T2*-FFE (HAACKE et al. 1999). The difference of b-SSFP with respect to *T1*-FFE and *T2*-FFE is that the gradients are fully balanced in each *TR*. This implies that the amount of dephasing in each *TR* is only dependent on the magnetic field inhomogeneities since the second term of the right-hand side of (2.2) is zero. A direct consequence of this is that b-SSFP is insensitive to (constant velocity) flow (VLAARDINGERBROEK and DEN BOER 1999).

Let us consider for simplification that the first RF pulse in the b-SSFP sequence is applied in a situation of thermal equilibrium. This implies that $\vec{M}_0 = M_0 \vec{z}$ and under these circumstances the steady-state magnetization M_{SS} at the end of each *TR* is:

$$M_{SS} = \frac{M_0(1-E_1)E_2 \sin\theta}{d} \sqrt{(1-2E_2\cos\beta + E_2^2)}, \quad (2.4)$$

where

$$E_1 = e^{-\frac{TR}{T1}}, \quad E_2 = e^{-\frac{TR}{T2}};$$

θ is the flip angle;
β is the dephasing caused by the resonance offset as given in (2.3);
d is defined as

$$d = (1-E_1\cos\theta)(1-E_2\cos\beta) - E_2(E_1-\cos\theta)(E_2-\cos\beta). \quad (2.5)$$

A detailed mathematical derivation of (2.4) and (2.5) can be found in HAACKE et al. (1999) or VLAARDINGERBROEK and Den Boer (1999). From (2.4), it is seen that M_{SS} varies periodically as a func-

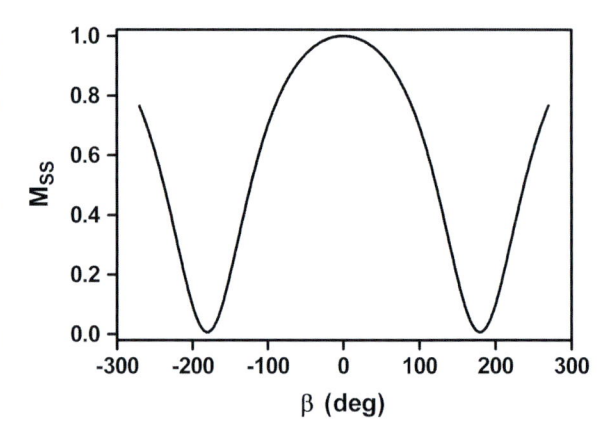

Fig. 2.2. Plot of the transverse magnetization in steady state (M_{SS}) as a function of phase offset (β) for the b-SSFP where the phase alternation of RF pulses was considered. Flip angle = 50° and *TR* = 10 ms, *TE* = 5 ms. Signal loss occurs at specific phase offsets

tion of β as illustrated in Fig. 2.2 where a flip angle of 50° was considered and the RF pulse was applied alternatively along the positive and negative directions of the x-axis, i.e. in each *TR* the accumulated phase of the transverse magnetization is $\beta + 180°$.

Because β is spatially dependent, the appearance of bands of varying signal intensity in the images is often a problem in b-SSFP. The banding artifact is characterized by large signal drops in locations where β is equal to ±180° and at 3 T this problem becomes very serious because the B0 inhomogeneities are larger and shimming is therefore less efficient and often unable to prevent these artifacts. As a consequence, the clinical application of b-SSFP at 3 T remains limited until now.

The banding artifacts of b-SSFP at 3 T become quite prominent. To illustrate this, images obtained in a phantom are presented in Fig. 2.3 for both at 1.5 and 3 T using identical *TR*, *TE*, and flip angle. The phantom contains several tubes with different *T1*-values. The desired contrast is present for both field strengths. However, at 3 T the banding artifact is much more prominent. At 1.5 T, the areas without bands is roughly two times larger than at 1.5 T. In practice, the banding artifact at 3 T severely constrains the clinical use of this sequence in the abdominal region due to the enhanced susceptibility effects, which aggravate magnetic field inhomogeneities.

The signal/contrast characteristics of b-SSFP are, however, quite interesting from a clinical point of view. In the following simplification, the magnetic field inhomogeneities will be considered to be

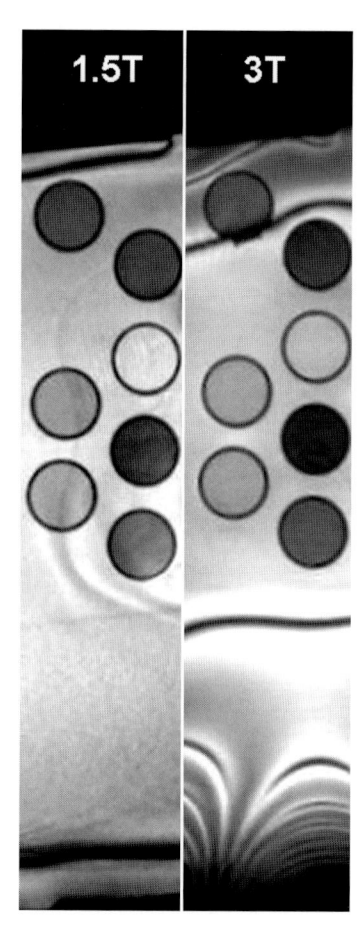

Fig. 2.3. Phantom images obtained with b-SSFP sequences at 1.5 T and 3 T: the image contrast and resolution are identical, whereas the banding artifact is different (*TR/TE/FA* = 5/2.5/60). At 3 T, the area at the center of magnet free of bands is about twice as small as at 1.5 T

small so that in the case of RF phase alternation, β can be considered to be equal to 180°. In this case, (2.4) simplifies to:

$$M_{SS} = \frac{M_0(1-E_1)E_2\sin\theta}{1-(E_1-E_2)\cos\theta - E_1E_2}. \quad (2.6)$$

In the short *TR* limit, i.e. when $TR \ll T2, T1$, (2.6) can be further simplified to:

$$M_{SS} \approx \frac{M_0 \sin\theta}{\left(\frac{T1}{T2}+1\right) - \cos\theta\left(\frac{T1}{T2}-1\right)}. \quad (2.7)$$

Thus, in the short *TR* limit ($TR \leq 10$ ms), the contrast of b-SSFP is weighted by the *T1/T2* ratio. From the

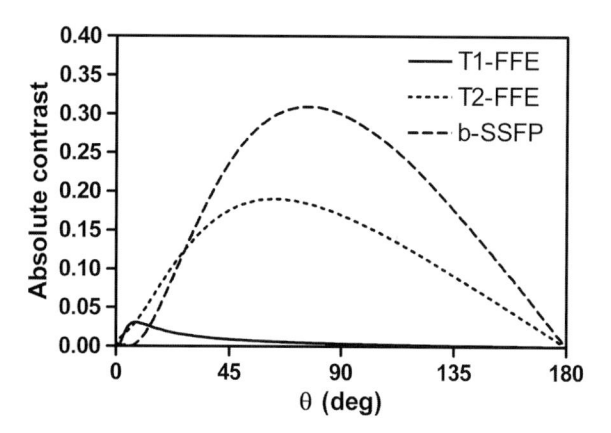

Fig. 2.4. Plot of the absolute contrast between bowel wall and water-filled lumen as a function of flip angle *theta* for *T1*-FFE, *T2*-FFE, and b-SSFP sequences. Simulation parameters are $TR = 5$ ms, $TE = 2.5$ ms

clinical practice point of view, this is an interesting contrast because it can provide "*T2*-weighted" images with very short imaging times. Another advantage of b-SSFP is related to maximum signal amplitude when the optimal flip angle is applied. The latter, derived from (2.6) and considering the short *TR* limit, is given by:

$$\theta = \arcos\left(\frac{\frac{T1}{T2}-1}{\frac{T1}{T2}+1}\right) \quad (2.8)$$

and the corresponding magnetization is then given by:

$$M_{SS} \approx \frac{1}{2}M_0\sqrt{\frac{T2}{T1}}. \quad (2.9)$$

The expression in (2.9) shows that when the optimal flip angle is applied, the signal that is obtained can approach half of the maximum possible signal for tissues with a large *T2/T1* ratio. This is very particular to b-SSFP and shows that large signal/contrast can be obtained with very short *TR*s, contrary to what happens with *T1*-FFE and *T2*-FFE as illustrated in Fig. 2.4 where the absolute contrast between bowel wall and water filled lumen was simulated for three different SSFP sequences. At 1.5 T, this enhanced contrast is of clinical relevance in, for example, imaging of Crohn's disease (Prassopoulos et al. 2001) where it is important to have a good contrast between bowel wall and lumen. The drawback, however, is that the optimal contrast for b-SSFP often occurs for larger flip angles which, at 3 T, can cause problems related to the SAR.

2.2 Changes to Accomodate These Problems

When imaging at 3 T, the changes in relaxation parameters, increased susceptibility, and chemical shift artifacts as well as increases in the SAR imply that several changes have to be made in pulse sequences to make them comply with high field strength imaging.

The increase in the $T1$ relaxation parameter causes a loss of contrast in $T1$-weigthed sequences. Thus, for a given set of sequence parameters and although at 3 T, an increase in the SNR by a factor of 2 is expected, the contrast of $T1$-weighted images obtained at 3 T can actually be worse than those obtained at 1.5 T (Soher et al. 2007). A possible change in pulse sequence design to overcome this problem is to increase the TR (and consequently the total scan time) to account for the increase in $T1$ relaxation rate. Another possibility is to apply magnetization inversion prepulses to increase $T1$ contrast without increasing TR. In the same way, the decrease in $T2$ ($T2^*$) relaxation parameter at 3 T may imply a shortening of the TE to keep the image contrast comparable with that obtained at 1.5 T. The increase in total scan time causes additional problems such as increased motion artifacts or less patient compliance. Also, the use of prepulses for magnetization preparation can also cause more problems related to SAR because of the additional power deposition. In certain circumstances, there are additional sequence parameters, such as number of signal averages, number of acquired k-lines, or number of acquired echoes, which can be adjusted to decrease the total scan time. However, these adjustments are often made at the expense of a decreased SNR and therefore alternative solutions that are able to keep SNR levels are desired.

2.2.1 Improvement Using Parallel and Fast Imaging Techniques

Additional solutions to decrease scan time without compromising SNR are the use of parallel imaging techniques (Larkman and Nunes 2007) or 3D fast imaging sequences that decrease scan time without compromising scan resolution. In parallel imaging, the independent signals recorded by a group of phased-array coils are combined to generate the image from the k-space, which is undersampled in the phase encoding direction. In other words, the undersampling of the k-space by each coil implies that the FOV of each coil is reduced. There are two categories of methods to reconstruct the image from coil signals: (1) image domain reconstruction; (2) frequency domain reconstruction. Methods such as SENSE (sensitivity encoding) (Pruessmann et al. 1999, Van Den Brink et al., 2003) reconstruct the image in the image domain by using the sensitivity profiles of each coil and combining the "intermediary images" obtained by each coil to obtain the final image. On the other hand, methods such as SMASH (simultaneous acquisition of spatial harmonics) (Blaimer et al. 2004) reconstruct the image in the k-space domain by computing a weighted average of the signals recorded by the different coils in this way reconstructing the missing k-lines. The weight corresponding to each coil takes into account the relative position of each coil. Finally, GRAPPA (generalized auto calibrating partially parallel acquisition) algorithms (Griswold et al. 2002) also reconstruct the image in the k-space domain, but in this case, some of the central k-space lines that would be skipped are acquired and used to calibrate the method in order to compute the remaining k-space lines that are skipped. This procedure lengthens the scan time, which however remains short. Parallel imaging might be especially useful in EPI sequences where the acquisition of multiple echoes make them very sensitive to motion and susceptibility artifacts and will therefore profit from reduced scan time. EPI, however, is nowadays seldomly applied in the abdomen except for diffusion weighted imaging where fast imaging is needed. Here, EPI is usually employed in the form of spin-echo ultra fast EPI. This is a hybrid sequence where after each 90° pulse and before each gradient echo readout, an additional 180° refocusing pulse is added. As a consequence, several gradient echoes with $T2$-weigthing, each corresponding to a different phase encoding step, are sampled in each readout.

The increased signal strength at 3 T make the use of higher gradient amplitudes and higher gradient switching speeds more beneficial when compared with 1.5 T, namely by allowing the acquisition of high-resolution images within short scan times. Thus, 3D fast imaging sequences take advantage of these possibilities to acquire data from an excited slab where phase encoding is also applied in the slice direction. In this way, there is an increase in SNR due to signal averaging during increased total scan time per slice. This is possible due to increased gradient performance at 3 T that allows for fast scan times comparable with those of 2D multislice imaging.

Both parallel and 3D imaging allow for the acquisition of high-resolution images with fast scan times but without having to make a trade-off with the SNR.

As mentioned before, SAR limitations are an important problem when imaging at 3 T. From (2.2), it is seen that if all sequence parameters remain the same, there is an increase by a factor of 4 when going from 1.5 to 3 T. Protocols such as TSE sequences that operate near the SAR limits have often to be modified by increasing the *TR* or decreasing the echo train length. However, additional solutions related to RF pulse design may be necessary to overcome SAR problems. Methods such as those described in Busse et al. (2004) and Hennig et al. (1988, 2001) are able to lower RF energy absorption by factors of 2.5–6 while keeping acceptable levels of SNR and contrast-to-noise ratio (CNR). The method described by Hargreaves et al. (2004), i.e. variable-rate selective excitation, is able to lower energy deposition without the need to decrease the flip angle.

In general, body imaging at 3 T is quite affected by SAR limitations because many imaging protocols that are used operate close to allowed SAR limits. Although the above-mentioned methods can be used to minimize this problem, often the advantages of imaging at 3 T such as increased SNR, temporal and spatial resolution have to compromise in order to overcome SAR limitations.

An illustration of a 3D *T1*-weighted spoiled gradient echo sequence is given for MR enterography in Fig. 2.5. Here, wall thickening after gadolinium injection at the level of the terminal ileum is clearly visible and one can expect that the theoretical signal benefit of imaging at high field strength can be obtained in clinical practice for these sequences. Fat suppression at the border of the images may, however, be problematic due the field inhomogeneities at these locations. Insufficient fat suppression can be observed in Fig. 2.5 near the borders of the images as indicated by the arrows.

Figure 2.6 shows a HASTE acquisition in MR colonography, showing great anatomical detail that will be beneficial for colon cancer detection. Both parallel imaging and decreased refocussing angles were employed in this acquition in order to limit SAR deposition while retaining high image resolution.

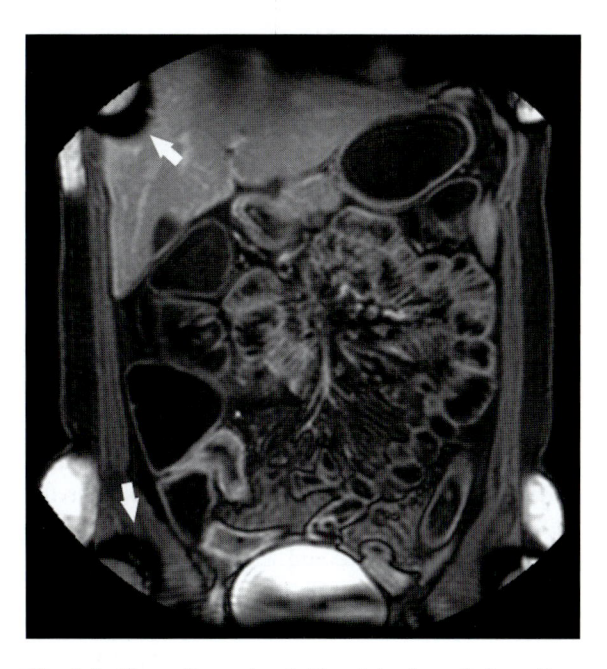

Fig. 2.5. Three-dimensional *T1*-weighted spoiled gradient echo sequence for MR enterography (*TR/TE*/FA = 2.1/1.0/10) and parallel imaging factor 2 (SENSE). Artifacts due to insufficient fat suppression resulting from magnetic field inhomogeneities are present at the borders and indicated by *arrows*

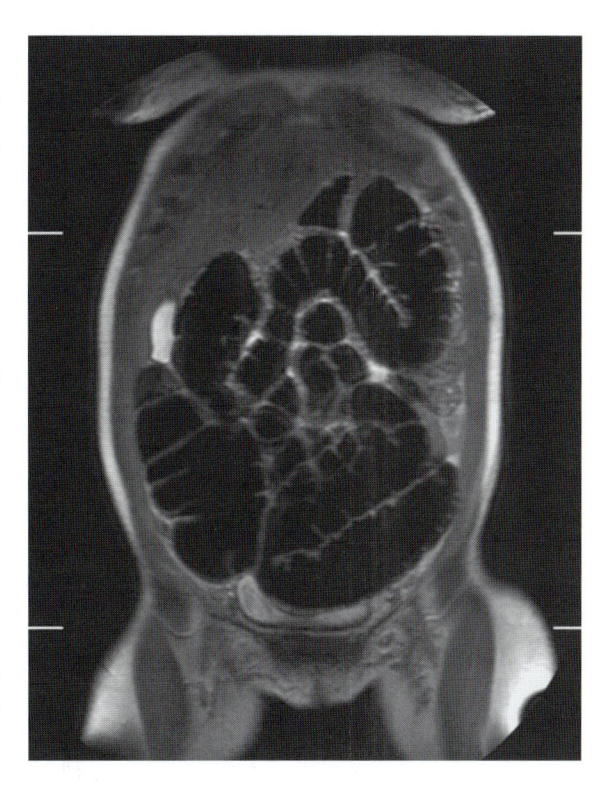

Fig. 2.6. HASTE acquisition in MR colonography (*TR/TE* = 500/65) using and parallel imaging factor 2 (SENSE)

2.2.2
Solving the Banding Artifact at 3T

The banding artifact that characterizes b-SSFP sequences also becomes quite prominent at 3 T and particularly when imaging the abdomen, where susceptibility artifacts are quite intense, it is often very difficult to use these type of sequences despite its clinical interest in imaging the abdomen (Gourtsoyiannis et al. 2001). As mentioned before, the effectiveness of shimming at 3 T is limited and therefore additional methods have to be used to minimize banding artifacts. Banding artifacts appear due to the periodicity of the spectral response of b-SSFP sequences as displayed in Fig 2.2. If phase alternation is applied to the RF pulse, the passband of the spectral response is centered on resonance and the stopband coincides with a phase offset of ±180°, as displayed in Fig. 2.2. In steady state, the phase offset is periodic with a period equal to TR and therefore it is equivalent to say that the stopband occurs at frequencies of $\pm 1/(2TR)$ Hz. Thus, a possible solution to avoid banding artifacts is to decrease the TR so that the nulls in the spectral response fall outside the distribution of frequency offsets (Duerk et al. 1998) present in the sample. Figure 2.7 displays the maximum phase offset as a function of TR for both 1.5 and 3 T field strength when the field inhomogeneities are of the order of 3 ppm. As expected, the phase offset shows a periodic behavior where the period T is such that $\gamma \delta B_0 T$ equals 2π. Note that this is the periodicity of the *maximum* phase offset. This implies that for $TR > T$, even if spins experiencing the maximum frequency offset have completed one period thus having again phase offsets well below 180°, other spins experiencing a smaller frequency offset may still show phase offsets in the neighborhood of the null of the spectral response. Thus, to guarantee that the null of the spectral response lies completely outside the distribution of phase offsets in the sample, TR should be kept well below T. From Fig. 2.7, it can be concluded that at 3 T, TR of a b-SSFP sequence should be kept well below 1 ms. Methods to solve banding artifacts by designing sequences with short TRs have been used at 1.5 T (Lu et al. 2004). However, though the hardware at 3 T allows for faster scan times, it can still be difficult to obtain such small TR values due to SAR limitations, gradient heating, high acoustic noise, and reduced contrast and SNR. Thus, other solutions to the banding artifact, which do not require such short scan times, may be more desirable. At 1.5 T, the banding artifact problem has been solved by averaging sets of complex image data sets obtained at different equally spaced offsets to obtain a uniform spectral response (Zur et al. 1990). More recently, an extension to this method has been proposed by Foxall (2002) where the RF phase is constantly increased during the entire duration of the experiment. This phase cycling scheme creates a frequency modulation of the spectral response. It is shown that if the images corresponding to the different RF phases are averaged then good banding artifact cancellation can be obtained without the need to have very short TR spacings. In conclusion, several methods exist to reduce the banding artifact, but a satisfactory solution has not been proposed so far.

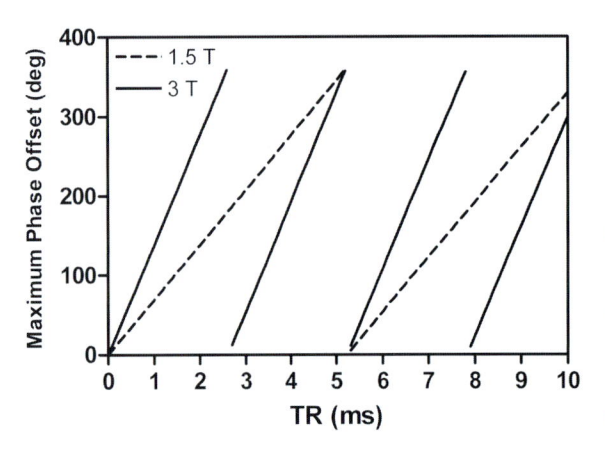

Fig. 2.7. Plot of the maximum phase offset as a function of TR when B0 field inhomogeneities are of the order of 3 ppm for both 1.5 and 3 T field strengths

References

Alsop DC, Connick TJ, Mizsei G, (1998) A spiral volume coil for improved RF field homogeneity at higher static magnetic field strength. Magn Reson Med 40(1): 49–54

Barth MM, Smith MP, Pedrosa I, Lenkinski RE, Rofsky NM (2007) Body MR Imaging at 3.0 T: Understanding the opportunities and challenges. Radiographics 27: 1445–1464

Bazelaire CMJ, Duhamel GD, Rofsky NM, Alsop DC (2004) MR Imaging relaxation times of abdominal and pelvic tissues measured in vivo at 3.0 T: Preliminary results. Radiology 230:652–659

Bernstein MA, Huston III J, Ward HA (2006) Imaging artifacts at 3.0 T. J Magn Reson Imaging 24:735–746

Blaimer M, Breuer F, Mueller M, Heidemann RM, Griswold MA, Jakob PM (2004) SMASH, SENSE, PILS, GRAPPA: how to choose the optimal method. Top Magn Reson Imaging 15(4):223–36

Bottomley PA, Foster TH, Argersinger RE, Pfeifer LM (1984) A review of normal tissue hydrogen NMR relaxation times and relaxation mechanisms from 1–100 MHz: dependence on tissue type, NMR frequency, temperature, species, excision, and age. Med Phys 11:1184–1197

Bulte JWM, Kraitchman DL (2004) Iron oxide MR contrast agents for molecular and cellular imaging. NMR Biomed 17: 484–499

Busse RF (2004) Reduced RF power without blurring: correcting for modulation of refocusing flip angle in FSE sequences. Magn Res Med 51(5): 1031–1037

Carr HY (1958) Steady-state free precession in nuclear magnetic resonance. Phys Rev 112: 1693–1701

Chavhan GB, Babyn PS, Bhavin G, Jankharia BG, Cheng HLM, Shroff MM (2008) Steady-state MR imaging sequences: Physics, classification, and clinical applications. Radiographics 28: 1147–1160

Corot C, Robert P, Idée JM, Port M (2006) Recent advances in iron oxide nanocrystal technology for medical imaging. Adv Drug Deliv Rev 58: 1471–1504

Duensing R, Fitzsimmons J (2006) 3.0 T versus 1.5 T: Coil design similarities and differences. Neuroimaging Clin N Am 16(2): 249–257

Duerk J, Lewin JS, Wendt M, Petersilge C (1998) Remember true FISP? A high SNR, near 1-second imaging method for T_2-like contrast in interventional MRI at .2 T. J Mag Res Imaging 8:203–208

Foxall DL (2002) Frequency-modulated steady-state free precession imaging. Magn Reson Med 48:502–508

Gourtsoyiannis N, Papanikolaou N, Grammatikakis J, Maris T, Prassopoulos P (2001) MR eneteroclysis between 3D FLASH with fat saturation after intravenous gadolinium injection and true FISP sequences. Eur Radiol 11: 908–913

Griswold MA, Jakob PM, Heidemann RM, Nittka M, Jellus V, Wang J, Kiefer B, Haase A (2002) Generalized autocalibrating partially parallel acquisitions (GRAPPA). Magn Reson Med 47(6):1202–1210

Haacke EM, Brown RW, Thompson MR, Venkatesan R (1999) Magnetic resonance imaging: Physical principles and sequence design. John Wiley & Sons, New York

Hargreaves BA, Cunningham CH, Nishimura DG, Conolly SM (2004) Variable-rate selective excitation for rapid MRI sequences. Magn Reson Med 52:590–597

Hennig J (1988) Multiecho imaging sequences with low refocusing flip angles. J Magn reson 78: 397–407

Hennig J, Scheffler K (2001) Hyperechoes. Magn Reson Med 46: 6–12

Hussain SM, Wieloplski PA, Martin DR (2005) Abdominal magnetic resonance imaging at 3.0 T: Problem or a promise for the future? Top Magn Reson Imaging 16: 325–335

Katscher U, Boernert P, (2006) Parallel RF transmission in MRI. NMR Biomed 19: 393–400

Larkman DJ, Nunes RG (2007) Parallel magnetic resonance imaging. Phys Med Biol 52(7): R15–55

Lu A, Barger AV, Grist TM, Block WF (2004) Improved spectral selectivity and reduced susceptibility in SSFP using a near zero TE undersampled three-dimensional PR sequence. J Magn Reson Imaging 19:117–123

Merkle EM, Dale BM, Paulson EK (2006) Abdominal MR imaging at 3T. Magn Reson Imaging Clin N Am 17–26

Merkle EM, Dale BM (2006) Abdominal MRI at 3.0 T: The basics revisited. AJR 186: 1525–1532

Patak MA, von Weymarn C, Froehlich JM (2007) Small bowel MR imaging: 1.5T vs 3T. Magn Reson Imaging Clin N Am 15: 383–393

Prassapoulos P, Papanikolaou, Grammatikakis J, Rousomoustakaki M, Maris T, Goutsoyiannis N (2001) MR enteroclysis imaging of crohn disease. Radiographics 21: S161–S172

Pruessmann KP, Weiger M, Scheidegger MB, Boesiger P (1999) SENSE: Sensitivity encoding for Fast MRI. Magn Reson Med 42: 952–962

Schick F (2005) Whole-body MRI at high field: technical limits and clinical potential. Eur Radiol 15: 946–959

Stanisz GJ, Odrobina EE, Pun J, Escaravage M, Graham SJ, Bronskill MJ, Henkelman RM (2005) T_1, T_2 Relaxation and magnetization transfer in tissue at 3T. Magn Reson Med 54: 507–512

Scheffler K, Lehnhardt S (2003) Principles and applications of balanced SSFP techniques. Eur Radiol 13: 2409–2418

Schindera ST, Merkle EM, Dale BM, DeLong DM, Nelson RC (2006) Abdominal magnetic resonance imaging at 3.0 T: What is the ultimate gain in signal-to-noise ratio?. Acad Radiol 13: 1236–1243

Schmitt M, Feiweier T, Voellmecke E, Lazar R, Krueger G, Reykowski A (2005) B1-homogenization in abdominal imaging at 3T by means of coupling coils. Proc Intl Soc Mag reson Med 13

Soher BJ, Dale BM, Merkle EM (2007) A review of MR physics: 3T versus 1.5T. Magn Reson Imaging Clin N Am 15: 277–290

Thensen S, Krueger G, Mueller E (2003) Compensation of dielectric resonance effects by means of composite excitation pulses. Proc Intl Soc Mag Reson Med 11.

Tomanek B, Ryner L, Hoult DI, Kozlowski P, Saunders JK (1997) Dual surface coil with high-B1 homogeneity for deep organ MR imaging. Magn Res Imaging 15(10): 1199–1204

Van den Brink JS, Watanabe Y, Kuhl CK, Chung T, Muthupillai R, Van Cauteren M, Yamada K, Dymarkowski S, Bogaert J, Maki JH, Mato C, Casselman JW, Hoogeveen RM (2003) Implications of SENSE MR in routine clinical practice. EJR 46: 3–27.

Vlaardingerbroek MT, Den Boer JA (1999) Magnetic resonance imaging: Theory and practice, 2nd edition. Springer-Verlag, Berlin

Vaughan JT, Adriany G, Snyder CJ, Tian J, Thiel T, Bolinger L, Liu H, DelaBarre L, Ugurbil K (2004) Efficient high-frequency body coil for high-field MRI. Magn Reson Med 52: 851–859

Zur Y, Wood M, Neuringer L (1990) Motion-insensitive, steady-state free precession imaging. Mag Res Med 16(3): 444–459

Contrast Media for MRI of the Gastrointestinal Tract

Arne S. Borthne and Claude Pierre-Jerome

CONTENTS

3.1 Introduction 33

3.2 **Contrast Agents, General Concepts** 34
3.2.1 Historical Overview 34
3.2.2 Contrast Resolution 35
3.2.3 Magnetic Properties and Relaxation 36
3.2.4 T1 and T2 Agents 36
3.2.5 General Requirements for Contrast Agents 36
3.2.6 Relaxivity 37
3.2.7 Future Aspects 38

3.3 **Bowel Contrast Agents** 38
3.3.1 Positive Agents: Bright Lumen 38
3.3.1.1 Mechanism of Action 39
3.3.1.2 Positive Bowel Agents 39
3.3.2 Negative Agents: Dark Lumen 39
3.3.2.1 Mechanism of Action 39
3.3.2.2 Negative Bowel Agents 40
3.3.3 Biphasic Agents: MR Hydrography 40
3.3.3.1 Osmosis 41
3.3.3.2 Water Balance 41
3.3.3.3 Osmolarity: A Decisive Parameter for Bowel Distension 41
3.3.3.4 Biphasic Agents and Additives 42

3.4 **Application of Bowel Agents** 43

3.5 **Gadolinium-Based Agents for Intravenous Use** 44
3.5.1 Mechanism of Action 44
3.5.2 Classification of Gadolinium Agents 44
3.5.3 Stability and Transmetallation 46

3.6 Conclusions 46

References 47

Arne S. Borthne, MD, PhD
Diagnostic Imaging Center,
Akershus University Hospital, Sykehusveien 25, 1478 Lørenskog, Norway
Claude Pierre-Jerome, MD, PhD
Department of Radiology,
Emory University Hospital, 1365 Clifton Road, Atlanta GA 30329, USA

KEY POINTS

MR contrast media catalytically improve the inherent image contrast between normal and pathologic tissues. This is achieved by mechanisms that increase the relaxation rates of water protons in areas where these agents are distributed. The first generations of systemic, intravenous contrast media are unspecific in action owing to their distribution in the extracellular compartments. The newer agents are more specific and are limited to anatomic target tissues. But in the future, contrast media are expected to act on processes even at the cellular level. Gastrointestinal MR agents have two main purposes: to improve the signals and contrast resolution between the bowel lumen and wall and to distend the gut. Water or watery solutions are the media most frequently used in this concept owing to the favorable signal characteristics, excellent distribution, and good tolerance. But to avoid absorption of water and the subsequent "collapse" of the gut, nonabsorbable particles need to be dissolved in the solution. By increasing the osmolarity, the distension of the intestine increases linearly as a consequence of the dose–response relationship that exists between these two parameters. The oral application of contrast is usually preferred for most of the gastrointestinal MR examinations except for the imaging of the large bowel, although the best degree of small bowel distension is obtained with enteroclysis.

3.1
Introduction

For years, magnetic resonance imaging (MRI) of the gastrointestinal tract was an unexplored field of application due to the technical inadequacy of the scanners. After the introduction of stronger gradients, multichannel coils, and the fast and ultrafast sequences, it became possible to perform motion-free examinations during breath-holding. As a result, since 1998 the number of publications started to increase (Zhu et al. 2008).

MRI has several advantages when compared with other methods. Among the more obvious of these are the excellent contrast resolution, flexible scan orientation, and lack of ionizing radiation. Abnormalities of the gastrointestinal tract such as in Crohn's disease: mucosal ulcers, wall thickening, bowel stenosis, prestenotic dilatation, fibro fatty proliferation, mesenteric hypervascularity, lymph nodes, fistula, phlegmone, abscess, and ascites can be visualized (Maglinte et al. 2003). In addition, the disease activity may be determined by the degree and pattern of gadolinium wall enhancement and the peristalsis can be visualized with dynamic cine imaging (Maccioni et al. 2000; Röttgen et al. 2006; Horsthuis et al. 2005). The two major challenges in gastrointestinal MR imaging are (a) to obtain high-quality images without motion artifacts, and (b) to achieve adequate distension of the entire bowel with homogeneous signals from the lumen. The former issue depends to a major degree on MR technology and software engineering, the latter is related to the kind of contrast chosen and the application of this agent.

The potential of MRI seems almost unlimited and the method has proven to be sensitive and efficient for gastrointestinal imaging. But there is a fast developing evolution in other fields of imaging as well (Maglinte 2006). The recent innovations within CT technology have realized an ultrafast scanning of the patient with advanced postprocessing of data for virtual endoscopy and colonography. Push-and-pull enteroscopy and the wireless capsule endoscopy give very detailed inspection of the entire gut and also biopsy procedures (Hartmann et al. 2004; Yamamoto and Kita 2005; Gay et al. 2006). To choose the most adequate diagnostic method for a certain clinical setting, an updated evaluation of the different methods available should be continuously performed.

3.2
Contrast Agents, General Concepts

In the earlier years of clinical MRI, it was believed that the images provided enough inherent contrast to exclude the need for exogenous contrast media. However, things turned out differently and during the recent 20 years, the application of MR contrast media have increased steadily to about 40–50% of all examinations performed (Bellin 2006). The first generation of contrast agents was intended for nonspecific distribution to the extracellular fluid compartments. They soon were followed by agents given orally to opacify the gut. Since then, several specific agents have currently been designed for selective enhancement of liver, lymph nodes, vascular system, etc., but efficient target agents have not yet been developed for use in the gastrointestinal tract. In this section is introduced the most important background information related to the physical and chemical basis of MR contrast media and the process of signal enhancement.

3.2.1
Historical Overview

In 1946, Felix Bloch managed to amplify the relaxation rate of water protons with ferric nitrate. In the mid-1950s, Bloembergen, Solomon, and Morgan described the accelerated magnetic relaxation of water protons in solutions of paramagnetic metal ions, and Eisinger and colleagues in 1961 showed that the effect of a metal ion on water proton relaxation depended on what kind of metal ion was used and the chemical environment the ion was in.

Paul Lauterbur produced in 1971 a description of MRI, and followed up with numerous contributions, which extended to human imaging in 1977. In 1978, he and his coworkers exploited the influence of a manganese (Mn)-(II)-solution administered into the left ventricle of a dog's heart, in which they already had produced a myocardial infarction by clamping a coronary artery. Their experiment showed that the paramagnetic ions altered the MR-parameters in vivo and enhanced the discrimination between the relaxation rates in normal heart muscle and the infarction area. The animal experiment was later repeated by Goldman, Brady, and colleagues who confirmed with true MR imaging that the signals in the normal myocardium increased with increasing manganese concentrations whereas the poorly perfused infarction area had low signals (Caravan and Lauffer 2006).

The first contrast-enhanced study in man was performed by Young et al. in 1981 as they used orally administered ferric chloride to "reduce the spin-lattice relaxation time in the fundus of the stomach" (Young et al. 1981). The morbidity caused by the absorption of iron precluded the application of this agent. In 1983, Runge et al. performed promising animal experiments with oral and rectal application of chromium ion chelates (Runge et al. 1983). The low toxicity of this agent was put forward as an advantage, but the contrast agent was not carried on to humans.

In the brief period from 1981 to 1982, some decisive and fascinating processes evolved with major future implications. Through the innovative cooperation between academic centers and pharmaceutical industries, two types of MR contrast agents were conceived: (a) the soluble paramagnetic gadolinium-based chelates and (b) the colloidal solutions of suitable-sized magnetic particles (De Haën 2001). The first trials with gadolinium-diethylenetriamine pentacetic acid (Gd-DTPA-H$_2$O) in human volunteers took place in Berlin in November 1983. Shortly thereafter, Carr and colleagues documented the first diagnostic examinations with intravenous Gd-based contrast media as they examined 20 patients with cerebral and hepatic tumors (Carr et al. 1984). Contrast enhancement was visualized with all tumors, particularly in the region of capillary breakdown and no short-term side effects were encountered. Four years later, the pharmaceutical product Gd-DTPA (Magnevist®, Schering AG) appeared in the market. It was well accepted and to date remains the market leader.

The first images with a colloidal solution of albumin-coated magnetic nanoparticles were obtained in 1982 and the results led to immediate optimism. As was expected, the contrast agent was taken up by the reticuloendothelial system and induced a reduction of the signals in the liver and spleen. But the path from idea to commercial product was more twisted for this new order of contrast than for Gd-DTPA. It appeared difficult and time-consuming to generate industrial interest for the production and also to gain patent protection for the inventions. Thus, it was not until 1995 that AM125 or ferumoxides first was distributed under the license as Endorem® (Berlex Laboratories Inc., USA; Tanabe Seiyaku Co., Japan).

The MR imaging of the gastrointestinal tract received little attention for many years, being limited to advanced and selected research centers (Schneider et al. 2005). The examinations had often limited clinical impact and were hampered by several technical barriers until the late-1990s as the quality of images was reduced by excessive movement artifacts from respiration, intestinal peristalsis, and cardiac motions. Throughout the years, numerous extrinsic contrast media were investigated as potential bowel agents: barium sulfate, fluids, food materials, gases, and agents based on gadolinium, iron, and manganese as well as pharmaceutical products such as methyl cellulose, mannitol, and polyethylene glycol preparations. The agents were originally designed to be taken orally, but some were later also applied rectally or as enteroclysis. The apparent insufficient imaging results obtained with these agents justified the statement by Jeffrey Brown in 1996: "At present, no oral MR contrast agent has achieved widespread clinical acceptance" (Brown 1996).

3.2.2
Contrast Resolution

MRI enables the acquisition of high-resolution, three-dimensional images of the distribution of water in vivo. The inherent contrast of an MR image refers to the relative difference in signal intensities between adjacent tissues as based on the numerical signal difference between voxels or pixels. When the body is exposed to an external magnetic field, a magnetization builds up within the soft tissue voxels. The protons align in the low-energy state with the majority of spins parallel with the external magnetic field. The larger the magnetization, the stronger the induced signals of the tilted magnetization. The stronger the induced signal of the magnetization, the brighter the pixel intensity displayed on the monitor (Nitz and Reimer 1999). Many factors determine the signal intensity of any tissue, including the proton spin density, the longitudinal relaxation time (T1), the transverse relaxation time (T2), as well as the inherent resonant frequency, chemical shift, magnetic susceptibility, associated flow, perfusion, and diffusion (Debatin and Patak 1999). The contrast resolution of the image can be widely modulated by changing the different parameters, thus the soft tissue characterization with MRI is more varied and precise than with any other imaging methods.

Though the inherent contrast resolution of MR images is high, it may be required to use extrinsic contrast media to enhance the differences between normal and pathologic tissue. MR contrast agents have a different mechanism of action than the radiographic agents or scintigraphic imaging media, which both can be traced directly on the film (Paley and Ros 1997). The concentrations of barium or iodinated contrast determine the degree of X-ray absorption and the radiation emitted by radioactive isotopes is proportionate to the local concentration of the radioisotope. MR contrast media are not visible by themselves but act indirectly by catalytically modulating the magnetic properties of nearby water molecules, thereby enhancing the contrast with background tissues.

3.2.3
Magnetic Properties and Relaxation

Most of the substances in nature are diamagnetic such as water, fat, or proteins. The molecules have no net electron spin in the outer orbital as the pairs of electrons have opposite spins and cancel each other. Paramagnetic agents, like metal ions, have several orbitals at similar or identical energies. If there are more orbitals than electron pairs, only one single electron is present per orbital (Burtea et al. 2008). These electrons all have parallel spins resulting in a net electron spin. An odd number of electrons can also cause a net electron spin. Molecules that are tumbling in the presence of an external magnetic field generate tiny, local magnetic fields that induce relaxation. But the magnetic field created by the paramagnetic unpaired electrons is far more potent than the sparse magnetism produced by the diamagnetic substances. The most usual paramagnetic species in nature are the small, isolated metal ions manganese and gadolinium. They possess from one to seven unpaired electrons that create an increase of the magnetic moments from 1.7 to 10.6 Bohr magnetons. The magnetic moment is the most important parameter to determine the effect on nuclear relaxation enhancement, and the magnitude of the magnetic moment is roughly proportionate to the number of unpaired electrons. Gadolinium has seven unpaired electrons and a magnetic moment of 8.0 Bohr magnetons, why gadolinium is very efficient as a contrast agent (Caravan and Lauffer 2006).

Materials that exhibit ferromagnetism like iron oxides or ferrites are built up as crystals of irons where each iron acts as a micro-magnet with an individual spin. The total crystal spin is a function of the number of spins. For ferrites, the total spin is very large and the magnetic susceptibility may be 2,500 times higher than the susceptibility of paramagnetic metal complexes. Superparamagnetic particles include the superparamagnetic iron oxides (SPIO) and the ultra small superparamagnetic iron oxides (USPIO). Both have an inner core of iron oxides that is covered by a membrane of either dextran or carbodextran to prevent aggregation. The susceptibility effect of superparamagnetic particles is very high, though the level is approximately 1/5 of the effect obtained with the ferromagnetic crystals (Caravan and Lauffer 2006).

3.2.4
T1 and T2 Agents

All contrast agents shorten both the longitudinal relaxation time T1 and the transverse relaxation time T2, but they do so to different degrees. It is therefore usual to categorize contrast media into two major groups:

Agents that increase both T1 relaxation rate (1/T1) and T2 relaxation rate (1/T2) to roughly the same amount are called T1 agents. Their dominant effect is a shortening of the T1 relaxation time (longitudinal relaxation – in simple terms, the time taken for the protons to realign with the external magnetic field) with most pulse sequences. Paramagnetic agents are mainly positive enhancers with increased signals on T1-weighted images. The paramagnetic contrast agents are built up with gadolinium ion as the active constituent. These agents dominate among the intravenous contrast media, but their use is limited for bowel application (Bottrill et al. 2006; Burtea et al. 2008).

Media that increase the transverse relaxation rate (1/T2) to a greater extent than the longitudinal relaxation rate (1/T1) are categorized as T2 agents. The transverse relaxation, T2, can simply be explained as the time taken for the protons to exchange energy with other nuclei. The T2 agents cause a marked reduction in signal intensity on T2 and T2*-weighted images. They also have a signal reducing effect on T1-weighted images, but to a lesser degree. So, they are called negative contrast agents. USPIOs may, however, produce "dual signals," e.g., increased signals on T1-weighted images and decreased on T2-weighted images. SPIOs are approved for liver imaging while USPIOs seems to be particularly useful for MR lymphography. Superparamagnetic agents have been used for intraluminal bowel opacification, but within limited scales (Bellin 2009a, b).

There is an important difference between gadolinium-based agents and the ferromagnetic agents: the signals increase with increasing concentration of gadolinium up to a certain level. Above this concentration, the tissue signals start to decrease both for T1-weighted and T2-weighted images. But large iron particles always cause decreased signals – at all concentrations.

3.2.5
General Requirements for Contrast Agents

MRI contrast agents are chemical compounds that are able to markedly increase the relaxation rates of water protons in tissues where they are distributed and thereby improve the image contrast. It follows that the contrast agent must enhance the target tissue rather than the surrounding tissue. The efficiency of an agent to improve the contrast resolution is referred to as the relaxivity.

The agent should localize for a period of time in the target tissue in preference to nontarget tissues to be of diagnostic value. Although the enhancement of the relaxation rates is determined by several parameters, the detection of an agent is usually a simple function of its tissue concentration.

Safety is an absolute requirement for MR contrast agents. In general, gadolinium-based contrast agents produce few acute adverse events. Allergy-like reactions occur with less than 1% of the administrations, the large majority of these are mild including headache, nausea, vomiting, hives, and altered taste (Heinz-Peer 2009). Severe anaphylactoid reactions have only sporadically been reported and occur significantly less frequent than with the iodine-based contrast agents, a fact that may partly be explained by the lower dose in clinical use.

The safety of the gadolinium-based contrast agents is related to their stability in vivo and the clearance behavior (Morcos 2009). Dechelation of the gadolinium complex with release of the free metal ion in different tissues of the body appears to be a key factor for the development of nephrogenic systemic fibrosis (NSF) in patients with impaired renal function (Grobner 2006; Sieber et al. 2008; Thomsen 2009).

NSF is a rare but potentially lethal disorder that is characterized by fibrosis of the skin and connective tissues. It was first described in 2000, although the cutanous manifestations were reported for the first time in 1997 (Cowper et al. 2000). To date, the number of NSF cases registered worldwide has reached about 250 (Sieber et al. 2008). To reduce the risk of NSF, the Food an Drug Administration (FDA) in 2007 requested a "black box" warning on all the five FDA-approved gadolinium-based MR contrast agents marketed in the USA (U.S. Food and Drug Administration 2007), although data suggest that low stability agents, particularly gadodiamide, possess a seemingly greater risk for precipitating NSF (Kanal et al. 2008).

3.2.6 Relaxivity

MR contrast agents contain paramagnetic or superparamagnetic metal ions, which affect the signal properties of the surrounding water molecules and lead to improved image contrast. The capability of a contrast agent to enhance the tissue is directly proportional to the increase of the longitudinal ($1/T1$) or transverse ($1/T2$) relaxation rate of the proton spins. Relaxivity is defined as the amount of increase of the relaxation rate $r1 = 1/T1$ and $r2 = 1/T2$, respectively, produced by 1 mmol/L of contrast agent. The values of $r1$ and $r2$ are used to determine the efficiency of a contrast agent, and they consist of contributions from both inner sphere and outer sphere relaxation mechanisms (Lowe 2002). The relaxivity must be sufficiently high to enable a detectable enhancement of the tissue, and the relaxation rates of the target tissue should be more affected than the relaxation rates of the adjacent nontarget tissues (Burtea et al. 2008).

Many mechanisms contribute to the efficiency of signal enhancement. In the simplest cases, the rate of relaxation increases proportional to the concentration of the contrast media in the tissue. Though the contrast has to stay for a period of time in the target tissue or compartment as toxic concentrations have to be avoided, the tissue concentration is not the only parameter that contributes to its efficiency. The distribution of contrast within each image voxel, the proton density, and the diffusion and chemical environment are also important contributors.

The relaxivity of gadolinium complexes has been explained with quantitative theoretical models. We forward a simplified version:

The gadolinium molecule is built up with a central metal ion of gadolinium ($Gd\,3+$) surrounded by a ligand that is directly bonded through atom sites to the metal core. Ligands with more than one binding site to the ion are termed chelates. The very high in vivo toxicity of gadolinium requires that the metal be complexed by strong and protective organic chelators. The ligands that are directly bonded to the metal, usually through the sharing of electrons, are called "inner sphere" ligands. "Outer-sphere" ligands are not directly attached to the metal, but are weakly bonded to the first coordination shell. The complex of the metal ion with the inner sphere ligands is called a coordination complex (Caravan and Lauffer 2006).

The efficiency of the contrast agents, the paramagnetic relaxation, is explained by "the inner sphere" and "outer sphere" mechanism, according to the theory of Solomon–Bloembergen–Morgan as described in the 1950s. The principle of the "inner sphere" relaxation rests on the chemical exchange when one or more water molecules leave the first coordination sphere of the paramagnetic center and then is replaced

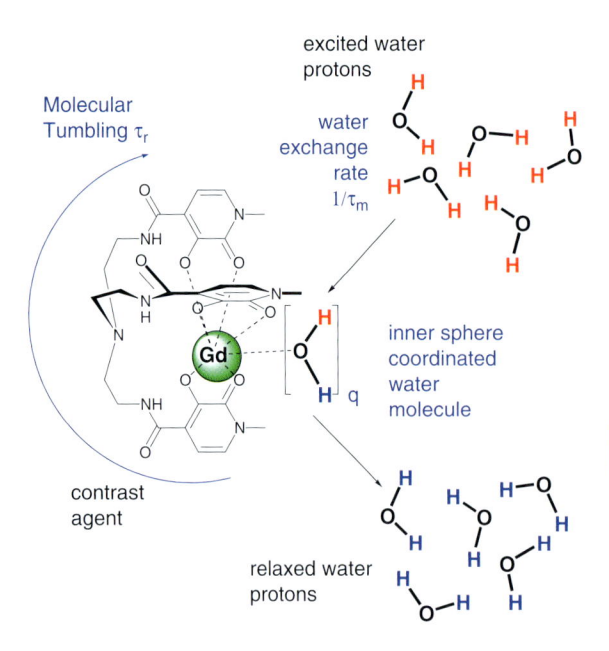

Fig. 3.1. Parameters influencing relaxivity

by other molecules. The mechanism allows a transmission of the paramagnetic effect to the entire solvent surrounding the paramagnetic complex, since water molecules may change sites from the center to the bulk water (Burtea et al. 2008) (Fig. 3.1).

3.2.7
Future Aspects

Nonspecific paramagnetic agents may enhance both normal and diseased tissue. The enhancement of specific tissues, structures, and organs are highly preferred, but the process of developing agents that are directed to inflammation, degeneration, tumor, or gene expression of disease is challenging. Among the most thoroughly investigated specific tissue agents are the high-relaxivity gadolinium-based agents and the USPIOs; most of them are particularly selected for hepatic imaging (Reimer et al. 2006). Agents selected for enhancement of diseased bowel tissue have not yet been approved.

Improved relaxivity of the gadolinium-based agents may be obtained by changing the design of the ligand as to (a) enable more water molecules to "visit" the inner sphere of the gadolinium complex, (b) shorten the water residence time to an optimal level, (c) slow down the tumbling rate of the complex, and (d) maintain the thermodynamic stability. It has already been shown that a slower molecular tumbling of the complex increases the relaxivity. But improved water residence time appears to be the most influential single parameter to improve the relaxivity of these agents (Raymond and Pierre 2005).

In the future, it is expected that MR contrast agents will not be limited to anatomic regions alone but will expand into cellular processes. This paradigm of imaging may involve the determination of cell membrane enzyme activities, measurement of receptor densities, and the evaluation of cell cycling for optimal selection and timing of drug therapies (Kruskal 2006).

3.3
Bowel Contrast Agents

The gastrointestinal tract extends from the mouth to the anus, a distance of 6–9 m. The small bowel accounts for 70–90% of the total length. A major advantage of MRI is the ability to visualize the wall and surroundings as mural involvement and extraluminal complications are the common denominators for inflammatory, infectious, ischemic, and malignant diseases (Lomas 2003). The imaging of the gastrointestinal tract is challenging for several reasons. The thin wall and steady peristaltic motion necessitate MR acquisitions with good temporal and spatial resolution. But adequate distension of this hollow and elastic tube is a prerequisite for diagnostic imaging. The contrast agent should be nontoxic, inert with homogeneous signals, well distributed, well tolerated, and not expensive. The ideal techniques and contrast agents are probably not yet found, although several centers are able to present their excellent imaging results. The following section is divided into three parts reflecting the usual classification of bowel agents according to signal characteristics.

3.3.1
Positive Agents: Bright Lumen

These agents have been almost neglected since they were introduced in the market. The main reason is presumably the signal characteristics, which reduce the contrast resolution between the lumen and the enhanced wall at T1-weighted sequences. The administration of positive contrast media in the gut means high signal intensity from the lumen on both T1-weigthed and T2-weighted images and high signals even from the bowel wall after intravenous contrast. The diffuse inflammatory diseases may thus be difficult to detect, as the alterations of tissue contrast may be the only means for detection. The structural changes are less pronounced with inflammation than with tumors. To obtain adequate distension of the intestine, mannitol was added to the paramagnetic solution to increase the osmolarity and avoid absorption. Another disadvantage is the price level as these agents are regarded to be relatively expensive. Besides the gadolinium chelates, this category of agents include even the ultra small ferrous particles. Their use is limited in the bowel.

3.3.1.1
Mechanism of Action

The positive gadolinium-based paramagnetic agents result in a reduction of both T1 and T2 relaxation times. Within "normal" gadolinium concentrations, the T1-shortening effects predominate with little effect on T2-weighted images. High signals from the watery contents are thus produced on both T1-weighted and T2-weighted images. At much higher gadolinium concentrations, the T2-shortening effect predominates, resulting in signal intensity loss with all sequences. T2-weighted images are more sensitive to this "negative enhancement" phenomenon and the signal loss occurs at lower concentrations on T2-weighted images than on the T1-weighted (May and Pennington 2000).

The signals from the lumen appear heterogeneous because of the variable concentrations of the positive contrast media throughout the entire gut. It may therefore be difficult to interpret the image findings.

But paramagnetic agents may have been underestimated as bowel agents. It is well known that the permeability of the mucosal wall is pathologically increased in inflammatory bowel disease, ischemia, or obstruction (Stordahl et al. 1988; Stordahl and Laerum 1988). The increased permeation of contrast material from the gut lumen to the vascular system could be detected by the enhanced urinary opacification of iodinated contrast agent in urine (Laerum et al. 1991). To our knowledge, similar experiments have not been performed with MRI. In theory, the amount of excreted gadolinium in the urine could be regarded as a quantitative measure of the mucosal disruption in the bowel.

3.3.1.2
Positive Bowel Agents

Gd-DOTA (Dotarem®, Guerbet, France) seems well suited as an oral MR gastrointestinal contrast agent.

It has an excellent safety profile and it has been shown to remain stable even in highly acidic environments, as may be encountered in the stomach. Furthermore, it is not absorbed in the intestines and has no measurable influence on bowel motion (Schwizer et al. 1994). Applied both orally and rectally, it has been used as a marker for gastric emptying as well as the basis of a T1-shortening enema for virtual endoscopy (Luboldt et al. 1997).

Gd-DTPA (Magnevist Enteral®, Bayer Schering Pharma, Germany) is well documented oral contrast agent. It is administered in conjunction with Mannitol to increase the osmolarity of the solution and thus obtain a better distension of the bowel. It can be given orally or rectally, usually as a 1.0-mmol/L solution. The agent is well tolerated, with an excellent safety profile (Laniado et al. 1988). Side effects are associated with the accompanying antiperistaltic agents used.

3.3.2
Negative Agents: Dark Lumen

The use of dark lumen bowel contrast agents has apparently passed the top of popularity since the 1990s (Hahn et al. 1990; Rubin et al. 1993; Vlahos et al. 1994; Low and Francis 1997; Burton et al. 1997; Small et al. 1998; Holzknecht et al. 1998; Rieber et al. 1999; Maccioni et al. 2002). The use of negative iron-based bowel agents today is limited, in spite of their favourable signal characteristics. Dark lumen on T1-weighted and T2-weighted images improves the contrast discrimination between lumen and wall, particularly after enhancement and inflammatory changes and structural abnormalities can easily be depicted. Negative agents are well distributed in the gut with relatively uniform drop of signals. An alternative path to the dark lumen is obtained by the production or insufflations of gas. This has recently been recommended for dark-lumen MR colonography although the opinions differ on this matter (Ajaj et al. 2004b; Gomez et al. 2008).

3.3.2.1
Mechanism of Action

Negative substances induce local inhomogeneity in the magnetic field that affects T1 and T2 relaxation time. The result is a marked signal drop on T1 and particularly T2-weighted images due to the dephasing of spins.

Superparamagnetic media made of iron oxide covered with dextran differ in their size from ultrasmall nanoparticles to aggregated large crystals. The susceptibility effects are stronger for the larger crystals. But the longitudinal relaxivity may be quite high for the smaller USPIO particles with concomitant signal enhancement on T1-weighted images. USPIOs may therefore act as biphasic agents with differing signals on T1 and T2-weighted images. Superparamagnetic contrast agents are built up of particles, not molecules, so there are no electron-bonding of inner-sphere water molecules within these particles. The outer-sphere relaxation of protons is exerted by the strong magnetic particles as the water molecules diffuse in the neighborhood. The net magnetization increases with the strength of the external magnetic field.

3.3.2.2
Negative Bowel Agents

Gas, in the form of air, carbon dioxide or perfluoroctyl bromide, can be introduced into the stomach or rectum to distend the bowel and create a negative contrast effect (MATTREY et al. 1994). Alternatively, gas can be produced with effervescent granule powder or liquids. The negative contrast effect is related to the reduced proton density in the intestinal lumen. Gas tends to stimulate peristalsis and may therefore cause significant motion artifacts. Although additional use of antiperistaltic agents is obligate, the clinical impact has been limited due to the prokinetic action of gas on peristalsis. There are further limitations like increased susceptibility artifacts and difficulty in controlling the distribution within the gut (DEBATIN and PATAK 1999).

Iron oxide particles. Several superparamagnetic iron-based substances have been investigated, some of which are available for clinical use. These agents are miscible with water and relatively uniformly distributed in the bowel producing homogeneous dark signals from the lumen. They are fairly well tolerated without serious adverse events. A potential advantage of this group of agents is the reduced motion artifacts because of decreased intraluminal signal. But the magnetic susceptibility on gradient echo sequences may alter image quality on breath-hold T1-weighted images (ZHU et al. 2008). After intravenous gadolinium, maximum contrast is achieved between the dark lumen and the bright, enhanced wall. If the use of intravenous contrast agents is excluded, the hyperintense signals from the bowel wall on T2-weighted sequences are favorable to visualize the signs of acute inflammatory disease.

Ferumoxsil (GastroMark®, Lumirem®) contains iron particles coated with silicon. The diameter of the average particle amounts 300 nm and the particles are in a low-viscosity suspension. The iron content of Lumirem is 175 mg/L (DEBATIN and PATAK 1999).

Barium sulfate has been the most widely evaluated negative contrast agent. It is cheap, widely available, with a known safety and tolerance record. The mechanism of action is a combination of T2 shortening due to diamagnetic susceptibility effects and replacement of intraluminal water by barium suspension, thus decreasing the proton density. It can be given both orally and rectally, and the best results are achieved with a relatively high concentration. Lower concentration of barium have been shown to exhibit positive contrast effects, probably due to the return of proton signals from water (PALEY and ROS 1997).

3.3.3
Biphasic Agents: MR Hydrography

The term "biphasic" was introduced to define those substances that show different signal intensities on T1-weighted and T2-weighted images. The first group includes manganese, manganese-containing substances, and gadolinium chelates at high concentrations (RIEBER et al. 2000). These agents may induce hyperintense signal on T1-weighted images and hypointense signal on T2-weighted images. The second group of agents includes water, hyperosmolar, and iso osmolar watery solutions and barium sulfate (ZHU et al. 2008). They follow the signal profile of water: low on T1-weighted images and high on T2-weighted images. In practice, these are the kind of agents we are referring to as biphasic agents.

Schunk et al. early realized the importance of using mannitol as an oral bowel agent. Already in 1995, he stated: "Aqueous mannitol solution is a safe bowel contrast agent and improves the diagnostic value of pelvic MRI, but in some cases delineation between marked bowel and cystic pelvic lesions may be uncertain" (SCHUNK et al. 1995). He later called this imaging technique for MR hydrography, thus focusing on the essential issue: water itself constitutes the "contrast" media, being attracted by different osmotic solvents (SCHUNK et al. 2000).

Water is ideal as contrast media in many ways, being the safest and cheapest agent with favorable signals. But unfortunately enough (in this concept) water absorbs and leaves the bowel inadequately distended distally. "Dark lumen" MR colonography as well is performed with water. One may therefore reintroduce the designation MR hydrography to include the large quantity of examinations of the entire gut from mouth to anus.

3.3.3.1
Osmosis

Water diffuses freely through a semi-permeable membrane so that equal concentration for water is achieved on both sides. Normally, zero net movement of water occurs. Under certain conditions, a concentration difference can develop across a membrane, leading to a net movement of water called osmosis. The osmotic pressure is equal to the amount of pressure required to stop osmosis. The osmotic pressure is exerted by molecules or ions in the solution. The average kinetic energies (k) of each individual particle in the solution are equal, as determined by the equation: $k = mv^2/2$.

Particles with smaller mass (m) move with higher Brownian velocity (v) than the larger and slower particles; each particle therefore exerts the same average amount of pressure against the membrane. The osmotic pressure of a solution is determined by the number of particles per unit volume of fluid (the molar concentration if the molecule is not dissociated) and not by the mass of the solute.

The unit osmole expresses the concentration of a solution in terms of number of particles. One osmole is 1 g molecular weight of an osmotically active solute. A solution that has 1 osmole of solute dissolved in each kilogram of water is said to have an osmolality of 1 osmole per kilogram water. The normal osmolality of the extracellular and intracellular fluids is about 300 milliosmoles per kilogram of water. For practical reasons, the osmolar concentration is expressed as osmolarity, which is the number of osmoles per liter of solution. For dilute solutions, as those in the body, the difference between osmolality and osmolarity is less than 1% (Guyton and Hall 2006).

3.3.3.2
Water Balance

Normally, water diffuses into and out of the intestine until the intraluminal osmotic pressure equals that of plasma (Field 2003). The osmolarity of the duodenal contents may be hypertonic or hypotonic depending on the kind of meal ingested, but by the time the meal enters the jejunum the chyme is close to isotonic and remains so throughout the rest of the bowel (Hoad et al. 2007). Osmotic active particles produced by digestion are removed by absorption in the small intestine making water passively diffuse out along the osmotic gradient thus generated. In the colon, Na+ is actively pumped out of the gut followed by water, so normally 98% of the approximately 9 L of fluid ingested or secreted are reabsorbed, leaving a fluid loss of about 200 mL in the stools per day.

Nonabsorbable substances like sorbitol, mannitol, and others have a direct effect on the transportation of water as their intraluminal presence provokes an influx from the extracellular compartments. The resulting increase of fluid in the bowel is induced by the osmotic active solutes. Laxatives made of poorly absorbable ions like magnesium, sulfate, or phosphate citrate are examples of such osmotic agents. But electrolytic absorption from the bowel is not impaired; the concentrations and losses of electrolytes in the stool water may consequently be quite low. Although the osmotic diarrhea may be profuse, it stops as soon as the intestine is emptied (Schiller and Sellin 2002).

3.3.3.3
Osmolarity: A Decisive Parameter for Bowel Distension

Owing to the absorption in the bowel, pure water is useless as an oral agent for the gastrointestinal tract, in spite of the very favorable signal characteristics. Thus, additives are needed to prevent a "collapse" of the distal small bowel. The oral administration of osmotic solutions results in far better bowel distension when compared with water alone (Schunk et al. 1999; Patak et al. 2001). It has been shown that the level of osmolarity seems to be a key factor as for the degree of luminal distension, presumably more important than the physico-chemical characteristics of the dissolved agent (Ajaj et al. 2005; Borthne et al 2006b). A linear dose–response correlation appears to exist between the osmolarity and the degree of bowel distension. This implies that by increasing the osmolarity of the solution, the volume given may be markedly reduced, thus allowing an easier administration. It is possible to achieve excellent distension of the bowel by administering a volume of approximately

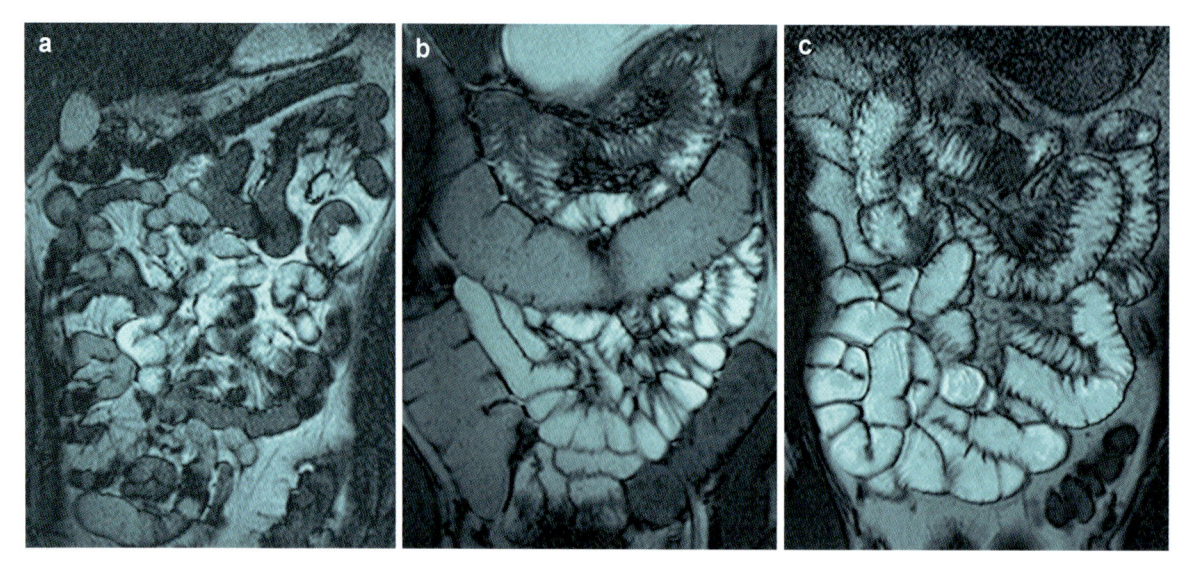

Fig. 3.2. There is a dose–response relationship between the level of osmolarity of a solution and the degree of bowel distension. This is illustrated by the administration of three different solutions with increasing osmolarities: (**a**) water (2 mOsm/L), (**b**) iohexol (189 mOsm/L), and (**c**) mannitol (325 mOsm/L)

300 mL of sorbitol to the patient about 45 min prior to examination (Borthne unpublished data; Kinner et al. 2008). Another advantage related to the reduced absorption is the reduced filling of the urinary bladder. Children may therefore go through a prolonged MR examination without interruptions as avoiding the tensions from a full bladder (Borthne et al. 2006a, b). There is also a well-documented dose–response relationship between the osmolarity and the level of side effects such as diarrhea and abdominal pain. Thus, a balance needs to be found satisfying both needs: an osmolarity as high as possible allowing for bowel distension and delineation, but also as low as possible to reduce side effects (Kinner et al. 2008) (Fig. 3.2).

3.3.3.4
Biphasic Agents and Additives

Water renders the bowel lumen bright on T2-weighted images and dark on T1-weighted MR images. Theoretically, it would be a perfect biphasic contrast medium for the small bowel, but the water is reabsorbed before it reaches the terminal ileum, so the intestine remains insufficiently distended (Lomas and Graves 1999). For "dark lumen" MR colonography, tempered water may be administered rectally using hydrostatic pressure (Lauenstein et al. 2001; Ajaj et al. 2004a).

Mannitol is an organic sugar alcohol. Aqueous solutions of Mannitol are available in concentrations of 5, 10, 15, 20, and 25%; osmolalities ranging from 274 to 1,372 mOsmol/L. It is not absorbed and not modified in the bowel. It is excreted by glomerular filtration after intravenous administration and not resorbed from the renal tubules. Mannitol is highly appreciated as volume expander in emergency situations and used as MR bowel agent, either as single contrast or as an additive (Schunk 2002; Lauenstein et al. 2003; Negaard et al. 2007). A disadvantage is the degradation to potentially explosive methane and hydrogen in the gut (Bigard et al. 1979).

Sorbitol is a sugar alcohol. It occurs naturally in many stone fruits and berries and is often used in diet foods and drinks, ice cream, as a nutritive sweetener, sugar-free chewing gum, mints and cough syrups, mouthwash, and toothpaste. It may be used as a laxative owing to the osmotic effect and has a prokinetic effect. Sorbitol's safety use is supported by the U.S. Food and Drug Administration and the Scientific Committee for Food of the European Union (FDA professional drug information database). Sorbitol is easily prepared and administered for bowel MR imaging (Ajaj et al. 2004c). A hydro solution containing a mixture of sorbitol 2.0% and 2.1% barium sulfate is also commercially available (Kuehle et al. 2006).

Polyethylene glycol (PEG) is a flexible, water-soluble polymer used in a variety of products including laxatives, skin creams, lubricants, toothpaste, and pharmaceutical products. PEG has been proposed by several authors as a suitable, well-tolerated biphasic contrast medium. It may be administered to adults or children, either orally or as enteroclysis (Gourtsoyiannis et al. 2000; Laghi et al. 2001; Papanikolaou et al. 2002; Magnano et al. 2003; Masselli et al. 2004). For enteric administration, the solution usually contains additional electrolytes. PEG is isosmolar, unabsorbable, remains unmodified in the small bowel, and is easily prepared and administered. The transit time is fast, allowing for small bowel distension within 30 min (32). Because of the prokinetic action of the solution, undesirable side effects as motion artifacts or severe diarrhea can occur.

Methyl cellulose is a synthetically produced chemical compound derived from vegetable cellulose. In pure form, it appears as a hydrophilic white powder that dissolves in cold water, forming a clear viscous solution or gel. It occurs as an additive in several products: hair shampoos, tooth pastes, liquid soaps, thickener, and emulsifier in various food, cosmetic products, ice cream, substitute for tears and saliva. Like cellulose, it is not digestible, not toxic or allergenic, and not absorbed by the intestines. It is used as a treatment of constipation, but since it absorbs water and increases viscosity, it may even be used to treat diarrhoea. Methyl cellulose has been administered as enteroclysis, either diluted or in combination with positive or negative contrast agents (Umschaden et al. 2000; Wiarda et al. 2005; Rieber et al. 2002).

Isphagula/Psyllium husk fiber (Metamucil, Procter and Gamble, Phoenix, Arizona, USA) is a natural fiber product derived from the plant genus plantago. The seeds are used for the commercial production of mucilage, a white fibrous material of clear, colorless, gelling agents. The milled seed is hydrophilic and increases in volume by tenfold when absorbing water. As a thickener, it has been used in ice cream and frozen desserts. Because of the water-holding capacity of the undigested fibers, it is used as a laxative. Isphagula has been given with good results as an oral distending additive in MR small bowel imaging (Patak et al. 2001).

Locust bean gum is a vegetable gum extracted from the seeds of the Carob tree. It is used as a thickening and gelling agent in food technology. It is soluble in hot water. Locust Bean Gum occurs as a white to yellow–white powder. It consists chiefly of high molecular weight hydrocolloidal polysaccharide. It is dispersible in either hot or cold water as forming a sol having a pH between 5.4 and 7.0. Locust bean gum may be proposed as a hydrogel additive to the osmotic solution to increase the quality of the MR examination (Lauenstein et al. 2003; Ajaj et al. 2004c).

Barium sulfate preparations consist of a suspension with insoluble barium sulfate particles that are not absorbed from the gut. The agent is inexpensive, has an excellent safety profile and is administered orally or rectally (Debatin and Patak 1999). The signal intensity can vary depending on the degree of dilution of barium sulfate. Generally, the signal intensity on T1-weighted images will be low. On T2-weighted images, the signal intensity may vary between intermediate to bright.

Pineapple and blueberry juice. These solutions contain manganese, which may suppress the disturbing signals from the stomach and duodenum on extreme T2-weighted images. The value of fruit juice, in this concept, is thus particularly related to the MRCP examinations (Hiraishi et al. 1995; Karantanas et al. 2000; Coppens et al. 2005).

3.4
Application of Bowel Agents

The contrast media can be administered orally, rectally, or as enteroclysis. The examination of the colon is normally performed with retrograde installation of contrast. Starting 48 h prior to examination, the patient uses a preparation of barium sulfate solution to modify the signals of fecal matter and thus make it be virtually invisible (Kinner et al. 2007). Water-based colonic distension is commonly administered by passively infusing 1.5–2.5 L of warm water using hydrostatic pressure. The dark-lumen technique can also be obtained if air is used instead of water to expand the large bowel (Ajaj et al. 2004b).

All the remaining examinations of the gastrointestinal tract are performed by administering the contrast media in antegrade direction. Contrast application by drinking is the simplest and best accepted method from the patient's point of view. It is possible to achieve excellent visualization of the entire gut, including the large bowel, with this technique. Studies comparing the oral method and enteroclysis document that both methods produce high-quality images with comparable diagnostic accuracy although better distension usually are obtained with enteroclysis (Gourtsoyiannis et al. 2006; Negaard et al. 2007).

Enteroclysis is an emerging technique for evaluation of the small bowel as the administration of an iso-osmotic water solution through a nasojejunal catheter can practically guarantee adequate luminal distension (Gourtsoyiannis and Papanikolaou 2005). Disadvantages connected to this method are the need of ionizing radiation, traumatizing intubation, and the relatively more complicated procedure and logistics with two different labs. These arguments are particularly relevant for young patients and children suffering with inflammatory bowel disease.

3.5
Gadolinium-Based Agents for Intravenous Use

There is good documentation of the improved assessment of disease on enhanced T1-weighted images. The combination of dark lumen and suppression of fat signals amplify the contrast resolution between normal and pathologic tissue. The nonspecific gadolinium-based complexes have a small molecular size, which makes them diffuse freely from the capillaries to the interstitial compartments. After contrast injection, the inflamed bowel segments or the infiltrating tumor light up against a dark background and the nature and boundaries of the diseased area are easier to define. The grade of disease activity can be determined by assessment of the degree of enhancement; the more severely inflamed, the more the bowel wall enhances. This correlation is explained by the increased perfusion and increased capillary permeability of the diseased areas (Horsthuis et al. 2005; Horsthuis et al. 2009). The gadolinium-based agents are safe in use. But these agents must be avoided in patients with acute and chronic severe renal insufficiency or acute renal insufficiency due to the risk for developing NSF.

3.5.1
Mechanism of Action

Most of the paramagnetic agents have gadolinium as the metal constituent. The different gadolinium-based compounds are positive agents that enhance the local water proton relaxation by shortening the T1 relaxation time in tissues. Shortly after the intravenous administration of the standard dose of 0.1 mmol/kg, a marked increase of signal intensity is observed in the target tissue. T1 relaxivity profiles are almost identical for the commercially available extracellular Gd-complexes. At normal concentrations, the contrast increases with increasing tissue concentration. At high concentrations of gadolinium though, which can be seen in the normal urinary tract, the T2 effect predominate and produce decreased signal intensity on both T1- and T2-weighted images.

The favorable magnetic properties of the lanthanide-metal are due to the large magnetic moment of gadolinium with seven unpaired electrons and the relatively slow electronic relaxation time (Burtea et al. 2008). The configuration of the ligand molecules and the number of attachments from the ligand to the central metal has an impact on the number of water molecules that are coordinated directly to the inner sphere of the paramagnetic complex.

Free gadolinium is toxic in vivo, why it is imperative to bind the metal ion to a ligand. The chelated, inert complex is excreted 550 times faster than the time for renal excretion of the free gadolinium (Bellin 2006). Nonspecific, extracellular agents are hydrophilic and are rapidly excreted by passive renal filtration, with >95% excreted by 1 day. These agents are not metabolized; they have a low molecular weight, do not cross the intact blood–brain barrier, and are rapidly distributed from the vascular space to the interstitial compartments.

The pharmacokinetics of the specific gadolinium agents differ from the nonspecific compounds, as they are transiently and reversibly attached to a protein molecule. They persist in the target tissue for a longer time. As a result of the increased relaxivity, prolonged imaging is allowed. These agents behave similarly to the extracellular agents immediately after intravascular injection, but are not distributed in the same way to the extracellular space. Because of their protein binding, they are excreted partly renal and partly biliary (Aspelin et al. 2009).

3.5.2
Classification of Gadolinium Agents

The two main categories of gadolinium agents are: (a) the nonspecific, extracellular compounds and (b) the new generation specific, high relaxivity agents that are attached to a protein and excreted both renal and biliary.

According to architecture of the ligand, gadolinium-based agents are classified as linear and macrocyclic chelates (Fig 3.3). Further subdivision groups

Ionic, linear

Gd-DTPA (gadopentetate dimeglumine)

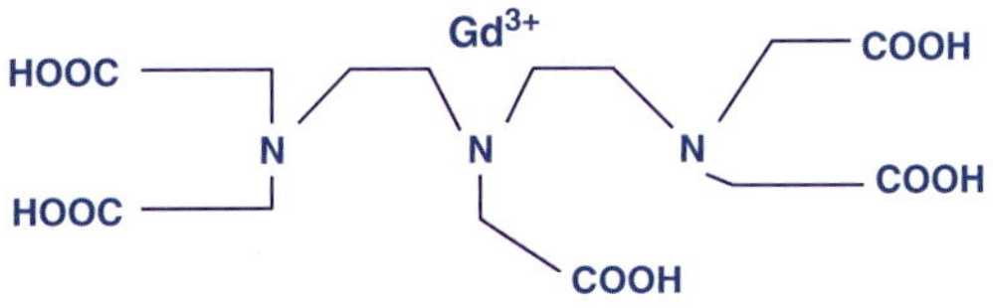

Nonionic, linear

Gd-DTPA-BMA (gadodiamide)

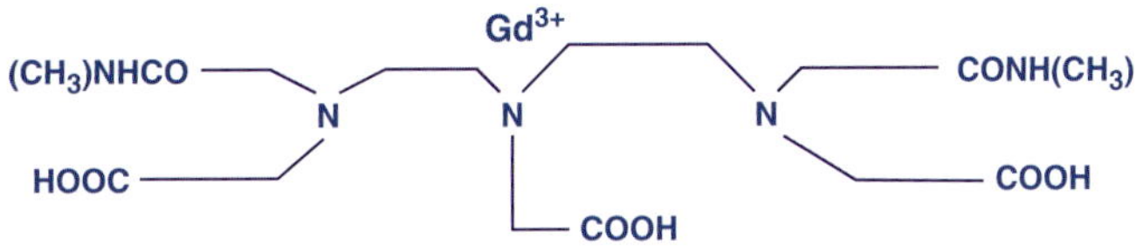

Gd-DTPA-BMEA (gadoversetamide)

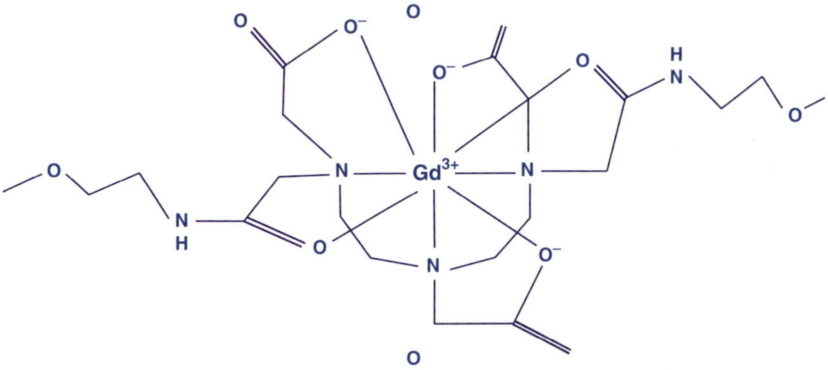

Ionic, cyclic

Gd-DOTA (gadoterate meglumine)

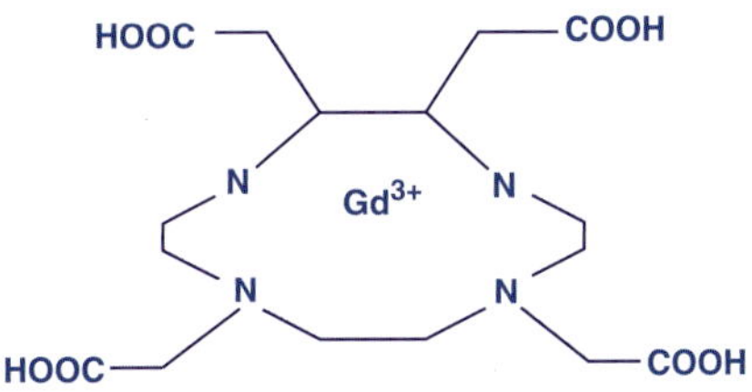

Nonionic, cyclic

Gd-HP-DO3A (gadoteridol)

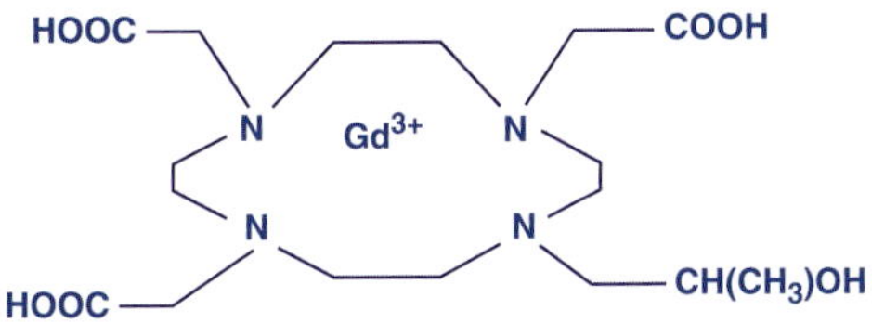

Gd-BT-DO3A (gadobutrol)

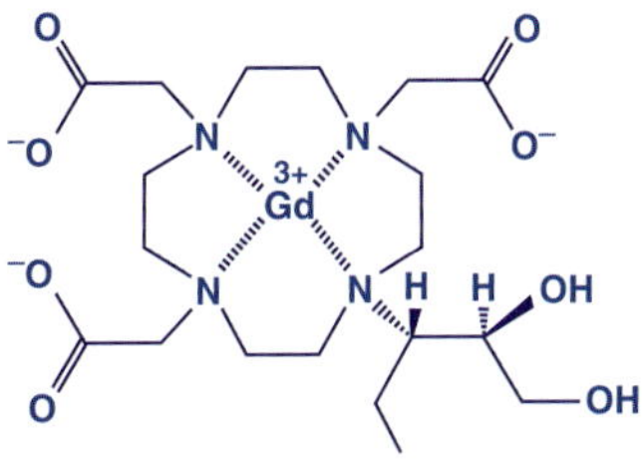

Fig. 3.3. Extracellular gadolinium-based contrast agents. From: P. Aspelin, M.-F. Bellini, J.A. Jakobsen, J.A. Webb (2009) Classification and Terminology. In: Thomsen/Webb: Contrast Media (Medical Radiology)

are ionic and nonionic agents, depending on whether they have a charge in solution or not. The macrocyclic ligands are derived from the tetraazacyclododecane ring system, which forms a rigid cage to fit the coordination sphere of the Gd3+ ion (Frenzel et al. 2008). The linear ligands DTPA support and twine around the Gd3+ ion but are not encaging the metal. The linear chelates thus appear more open and flexible than the rigid macrocyclic agents. The gadolinium contrast agents commercially available to date are:

1. Nonspecific extracellular gadolinium chelates:
   (a) Linear; ionic ligand
       Gadopentetate dimeglumine (Magnevist®, Bayer Schering Pharma, Germany)
   (b) Linear; nonionic ligands
       Gadodiamide (Omniscan®, GE Healthcare, USA)
       Gadoversetamide (Optimark®, Covidien, USA
   (c) Macrocyclic; ionic ligand
       Gadoterate meglumine (Dotarem®, Guerbet, France)
   (d) Macrocyclic; nonionic ligands
       Gadobutrol (Gadovist, Bayer Schering Pharma, Germany)
       Gadoteridol (ProHance®, Bracco, Italy)

2. High relaxivity agents. Linear and ionic ligands
   Gadobenate dimeglumine (MultiHance®, Bracco, Italy)
   Gadofoveset trisodium (Vasovist™, Bayer Schering Pharma, Germany; EPIX Pharmaceuticals Inc., USA)
   Gadotexetate disodium (Primovist™, Bayer Schering Pharma, Germany)

In clinical practice, the T1 relaxivity profiles appear as identical for the nonspecific, extracellular agents (Van Der Molen and Bellin 2008). The T1 relaxivity is increased for the more specific gadolinium-based agents as a result of the transient interaction with serum albumin (Bellin 2006). Gadobenate (MultiHance) is partly excreted biliary and is introduced for liver and CNS imaging. In practice, this contrast is mainly used as an extracellular agent. Gadofoveset (Vasovist) has been introduced for MR angiography as a blood-pool agent. Imaging is possible for a prolonged period of time after injection (from 5 to 50 min). Gadotexetate (Primovist; former Eovist) is intended for liver conditions as taken up by the hepatocytes. It is equally excreted renal and biliary (Fig. 3.3).

3.5.3
Stability and Transmetallation

Gadolinium-based MR agents are among the safest compounds in medical imaging. Minor adverse effects associated with these agents occur infrequently and include nausea, headache, and taste perversion. The gadolinium agents cannot be differentiated on the basis of these mild adverse effects. But recent studies have brought to light the issue of chelate stability, particularly following the observations associated with the least stable of these agents (Kirchin and Runge 2003). Strong evidences indicate that the safety is closely related to the stability of the gadolinium-complex not to release the free gadolinium ions to the environment, so-called transmetallation. The stability of the complexes depends to a major degree on the molecular structure of the ligand. Cyclic agents are generally more stable than their linear counterparts.

The dissociation of Gd3+ from its ligand is an equilibrium process, defined by two independent parameters, kinetics and thermodynamic stability. In vivo, the Gd complex is surrounded by several competitors to act with either the ligand or the Gd3+ ion. Proteins, inorganic ions, or organic ligands are ready to accept the Gd3+ ion, whereas metal ions like copper or zinc may compete with gadolinium and displace Gd3+ from the chelate. This competition may destabilize the complex and shift the dissociation equilibrium toward its free components for further binding to other partners. The process of exchange is called transmetallation. Transmetallation of Gd3+ has been discussed as one of the major factors associated with the development of NSF, as observed in patients with severe renal impairment or acute renal insufficiency.

3.6
Conclusions

MR imaging with modern equipment enables detailed morphologic information and functional data of the gastrointestinal tract. The optimal study is debatable, but the oral administration of contrast is faster, easier to perform, better tolerated by the patients, and less expensive. The oral method can be used to visualize the entire gut. But the preferred method for the imaging of the large bowel is the rectal administration of contrast. MR enteroclysis might be reserved for selected cases as a second-line study of the small bowel.

The dominating contrast agent in gastrointestinal imaging is water or water-based solutions. The signal characteristics are equal to the signals of water; it is therefore correct to use the designation MR hydrography for examinations based on watery solutions. But adequate distension of the small intestine is hardly achieved with oral agents unless a nonabsorbable solute is admixed in the solution. The level of osmolarity depends on the number of osmotic particles and a small volume of a concentrated agent has therefore the exact same distending effect as a larger volume of a more diluted agent.

The intravenous paramagnetic agents are based on gadolinium-chelates for the most. The majority of these media have a nonspecific action as being distributed in the extracellular space. But research centers worldwide are focusing on the innovation of tissue-specific agents with higher relaxivity and agents designed for molecular imaging. The improved and more precise enhancement of the pathologic target tissues in the near future will certainly have a tremendous impact on the quality of MR imaging.

References

Ajaj W, Debatin JF, Lauenstein T (2004a) Dark-lumen MR colonography. Abdom Imaging 29:429–433
Ajaj W, Lauenstein TC, Pelster G, et al (2004b) MR colonography: how does air compare to water for colonic distention? J Magn Reson Imaging 19:216–221
Ajaj W, Goehde SC, Schneemann H, et al (2004c) Oral contrast agents for small bowel MRI: comparison of different additives to optimize bowel distension. Eur Radiol 14:458–464
Ajaj W, Goyen M, Schneemann H, et al (2005) Oral contrast agents for small bowel distension in MRI: influence of the osmolarity for small bowel dis tension. Eur Radiol 15:1400–1406
Aspelin P, Bellin M-F, Jakobsen JÅ, et al (2009) General issues. Classification and terminology. In: Thomsen HS, Webb JAW (eds) Contrast media. Safety issues and ESUR guidelines, 2nd edn. Springer, Berlin. ISBN: 978-3.540-72783-5
Bellin M-F (2006) MR contrast agents, the old and the new. Eur J Radiol 60:314–323
Bellin M-F (2009a) Gadolinium-based contrast agents. In: Thomsen HS, Webb JAW (eds) Contrast media. Safety issues and ESUR guidelines, 2nd edn. Springer, Berlin. ISBN: 978-3.540-72783-5
Bellin M-F (2009b) Non-gadolinium-based contrast agents. In: Thomsen HS, Webb JAW (eds) Contrast media. Safety issues and ESUR guidelines, 2nd edn. Springer, Berlin. ISBN: 978-3.540-72783-5
Bigard M, Gaucher P, Lasalle C (1979) Fatal colonic explosion during colono scopic polypectomy. Gastroenterology 77:1307–1310.
Borthne AS, Abdelnoor M, Rugtveit J, et al (2006) Bowel magnetic resonance imaging of pediatric patients with oral mannitol. MRI compared with endoscopy and intestinal ultrasound. Eur Radiol 16:207–214
Borthne AS, Abdelnoor M, Storaas T, et al (2006a) Osmolarity: a decisive parameter of bowel agents in intestinal magnetic resonance imaging. Eur Radio 16:1331–1336
Bottrill M, Kwok L, Long NJ (2006b) Lanthanides in magnetic resonance imaging. Chem Soc Rev 35:557–571
Brown JJ (1996) Gastrointestinal contrast agents for MR imaging. MRI Clin North Am 4(1):25–35.
Burtea C, Laurent S, van der Elst L, et al (2008) Contrast agents: magnetic resonance. In: Semmler W, Schwaiger M (eds) Molecular Imaging I. Springer, Berlin. ISBN 978-3-540-72717-0
Burton SS, Liebig T, Frazier SD, et al (1997) High-density oral barium sulfate in abdominal MRI: efficacy and tolerance in a clinical setting. Magn Reson Imaging 15(2):147–153.
Caravan P, Lauffer RB (2006) Contrast agents: basic principles. In: Edelman RR, Hesselink JR, Zlatkin MB, Crues III JV (eds) Clinical magnetic resonance imaging, 3rd edn. Saunders, Philadelphia. ISBN 0-7216-0306-8
Carr DH, Brown J, Bydder GM, et al (1984) Gadolinium-DTPA as acontrast agent in MRI. Initial clinical experience in 20 patients. AJR Am J Roentgenol 143:215–224
Coppens E, Metens T, Winant C, et al (2005) Pineapple juice labeled with gadolinium: a convenient oral contrast for magnetic resonance cholan giopancreatography. Eur Radiol 15:2122–2129
Cowper SE, Robin HS, Steinberg SM, et al (2000) Scleromyxoedema-like cutaneous diseases in renal-dialysis patients. Lancet 356:1000–1001
Debatin JF, Patak MA (1999) MRI of the small and large bowel. Eur Radiol 9:1523–1534.
De Haën C (2001) Conception of the first magnetic resonance imaging contrast agent: a brief history. Top Magn Res Imaging 12:221–230
FDA Professional Drug information. http://www.drugs.com/pro/
Field M (2003) Intestinal ion transport and the pathophysiology of diarrhea. J Clin Invest 111:931–943
Frenzel T, Lengsfeld P, Schirmer H, et al (2008) Stability of gadolinium-based magnetic resonance imaging contrast agents in human serum at 37°C. Invest Radiol 43(12): 817–828
Gay G, Delvaux M, Fassler I (2006) Outcome of capsule endoscopy in determine ing indication and route for push-and-pull enteroscopy. Endoscopy 38(1):49–58
Gomez SR, Llinas MP, Garangou AC, et al (2008) Dark-lumen MR colonography with fecal tagging: a comparison of water enema and air methods of colonic dis tension for detecting colonic neoplasms. Eur Radiol 18:1396–1405
Gourtsoyiannis N, Papanikolaou N, Grammatikakis J, et al (2000) MR imaging of the small bowel with a True-FISP sequence after enteroclysis with water solution. Invest Radiol 35(12):707–711
Gourtsoyiannis NC, Papanikolaou N (2005) Magnetic resonance enteroclysis. Semin Ultrasound CT MRI 26:237–246
Gourtsoyiannis NC, Grammatikakis J, Papamastorakis G, et al (2006) Imaging of small intestinal Crohn's disease: comparison between MR enteroclysis and conventional enteroclysis. Eur Radiol 16:1915–1925

Grobner T (2006) Gadolinium – a specific trigger for the development of nephro genic fibrosing dermopathy and nephrogenic systemic fibrosis? Nephrol Dial Transplant 21:1104–1108

Guyton AC, Hall JE (2006) Textbook of medical physiology, 11th edn. Elsevier, Saunders, Amsterdam, Philadelphia. ISBN 0-7216-0240-1

Hahn PF, Stark DD, Lewis JM, et al (1990) First clinical trial of a new super paramagnetic iron oxide for use as an oral gastrointestinal contrast agent in MR imaging. Radiology 175(3):695–700

Hartmann D, Schilling D, Bolz G, et al (2004) Capsule endoscopy, technical impact, benefits and limitations. Langenbechs Arch Surg 389:225–233

Heintz-Peer G. MR contrast media. Gadolinium-based contrast media. Acute adverse reactions. In: Thomsen HS, Webb JAW (Eds) Contrast media. Safety issues and ESUR guidelines. 2nd edn. Springer Verlag, Berlin. ISBN: 978-3. 540-72783-5

Hiraishi K, Narabayashi I, Fujita O, et al (1995) Blueberry juice: preliminary evaluation as an oral contrast agent in gastrointestinal MR imaging. Radiology 194:119–123

Hoad CL, Marciani L, Foley S, et al (2007) Non-invasive quantification of small bowel water content by MRI: a validation study. Phys Med Biol 52:6909–6922

Holzknecht N, Helmberger T, Ritter C von, et al (1998) MRI of the small intestine with rapid MRI sequences in Crohn's disease after enteroclysis with oral iron particles. Radiologe 38(1):29–36

Horsthuis K, Lavini C, Stoker J (2005) MRI in Crohn's disease. J Magn Reson Imaging 22:1–12

Horsthuis K, Nederveen AJ, de Feiter M-W, et al (2009) Mapping of T1-values and gadolinium-concentrations in MRI as indicator of disease activity in luminal Crohn's disease: a feasibility study. J Magn Reson Imaging 29:488–493

Kanal E, Broome DR, Martin DR, et al (2008) Response to the FDA's May 23, 2007, nephrogenic systemic fibrosis update. Radiology 246:11–14

Karantanas AH, Papanikolaou N, Kalef-Ezra J, et al (2000) Blueberry juice used per os in upper abdominal MR imaging: composition and initial clinical data. Eur Radiol 10: 909–913

Kinner S, Kuehle CA, Langhorst J, et al (2007) MR colonography with fecal tagging: do patient characteris tics influence image quality? J Magn Reson Imaging 25:1007–1012

Kinner S, Kuehle CA, Herbig S, et al (2008) MRI of the small bowel: can sufficient bowel distension be achieved with small volumes of oral contrast? Eur Radiol 18:2542–2548

Kirchin MA, Runge VM (2003) Contrast agents for magnetic resonance imaging: safety update. Topics Magn Reson Imaging 14:426–435

Kruskal JB (2006) Molecular and cellular imaging. In: Edelman RR, Hesselink JR, Zlatkin MB, Crues III JV (eds) Clinical magnetic resonance imaging, 3rd ed. Saunders, Philadelphia. ISBN 0-7216-0306-8

Kuehle CA, Ajaj W, Ladd SC, et al (2006) Hydro-MRI of the small bowel: effect of contrast volume, timing of contrast administration, and data acquisition on bowel distension. AJR Am J Roentgenol 187:375–385

Lærum F, Stordahl A, Solheim KE, et al (1991) Intestinal follow-through examinations with iohexol and iopentol. Permeability alterations and efficacy in patients with small bowel ob struction. Invest Radiol 26:S177–S181

Laghi A, Carbone I, Catalano C, et al (2001) Polyethylene glycol solution as an oral contrast agent for MR imaging of the small bowel. AJR Am J Roentgenol 177:1333–1334

Laniado M, Kornmesser W, Hamm B, et al (1988) MR imaging of the gastrointestinal tract: value of Gd-DTPA. AJR J Roentgenol 150:817–821

Lauenstein TC, Herborn CU, Vogt FM, et al (2001) Dark lumen MR-colonography: initial experience. Fortschr Röntgenstr 173:785–789

Lauenstein TC, Schneemann H, Vogt FM, et al (2003) Optimization of oral contrast agents for MR imaging of the small bowel. Radiology 228:279–283

Lomas DJ, Graves MJ (1999) Small bowel MRI using water as a contrast medium. Br J Radiol 72:994–997

Lomas DJ (2003) Technical developments in bowel MRI. Eur Radiol 13:1058–1071

Low RN, Francis IR (1997) MR imaging of the gastrointestinal tract with iv Gadolinium and diluted barium oral contrast media compared with unenhanced MR imaging and CT. AJR Am J Roentgenol 169:1051–1059

Lowe MP (2002) MRI contrast agents: the next generation. Aust J Chem 55:551–556

Luboldt W, Bauerfeind P, Steiner P, et al (1997) Preliminary assessment of three-dimensional magnetic resonance imaging for various colonic disorders. Lancet 349:1288–1291

Maccioni F, Viscido A, Broglia L, et al (2000) Evaluation of Crohn disease activity with magnetic resonance imaging. Abdom Imaging 25:219–228

Maccioni F, Viscido A, Marini M, et al (2002) MRI evaluation of Crohn's disease of the small and large bowel with the use of negative superpara magnetic oral contrast agents. Abdom Imaging 27:384–393

Maglinte DDT, Goutsoyiannis N, Rex D, et al (2003) Classification of small bowel Crohn's subtypes based on multimodality imaging. Radiol Clin N Am 41:285–303

Maglinte DDT (2006) Small bowel imaging – a rapidly changing field and a challenge to radiology. Eur Radiol 16: 967–971

Magnano G, Granata C, Barabino A (2003) Polyethylene glycol and contrast- enhanced MRI of Crohn's disease in children: preliminary experience. Pediatr Radiol 33(6):385–391

Masselli G, Brizi GM, Parrella A, et al (2004) Crohn disease: magnetic resonance enteroclysis. Abdom Imaging 29: 326–334

Mattrey RF, Trambert MA, Brown JJ, et al (1994) Perflubron as an oral contrast agent for MR imaging: results of a phase III clinical trial. Radiology 191(3):841–848

May DA, Pennington DJ (2000) Effect of gadolinium concentration on renal signal intensity: an in vitro study with a saline bag model. Radiology 216:232–236

Morcos SK (2009) Chelates and stability. In: Thomsen HS, Webb JAW (eds) Contrast media. Safety issues and ESUR guidelines, 2nd edn. Springer, Berlin. ISBN: 978-3.540-72783-5

Nitz WR, Reimer P (1999) Contrast mechanisms in MR imaging. Eur Radiol 9:1032–1046

Negaard A, Paulsen V, Sandvik L, et al (2007) A prospective randomized comparison between two MRI studies of the small bowel in Crohn's disease, the oral contrast method and MR enteroclysis. Eur Radiol 17:2294–2301

Paley MR, Ros PR (1997) MRI of the gastrointestinal tract. Eur Radio 7:1387–1397

Papanikolaou N, Prassopoulos P, Grammatikakis J, et al (2002) Optimization of a contrast medium suitable for conventional enteroclysis, MR enteroclysis, and virtual MR enteroscopy. Abdom Imaging 27:517–522

Patak MA, Froehlich JM, Weymarn C von et al (2001) Non-invasive distension of the small bowel for magnetic-resonance imaging. Lancet 358:987–988

Raymond KN, Pierre VC (2005) Next generation, high relaxivity gadolinium MRI agents. Bioconjugate Chem 16:3–8

Reimer P, Helmberger T, Schima W (2006) Tissue-specific contrast agents. In: Edelman RR, Hesselink JR, Zlatkin MB, Crues III JV (eds) Clinical magnetic resonance imaging, 3rd edn. Saunders, Philadelphia. ISBN 0-7216-0306-8

Rieber A, Aschoff A, Nüssle K, et al (1999) MRI in the diagnosis of small bowel disease: use of positive and negative oral contrast media in combination with enteroclysis. Eur Radiol 10:1377–1382

Rieber A, Wruk D, Potthast S, et al (2000) Diagnostic imaging in Crohn's disease: comparison of magnetic resonance imaging and conventional imaging methods. Int J Colorectal Dis 15:176–181

Rieber A, Nüssle K, Reinshagen M, et al (2002) MRI of the abdomen with positive oral contrast agents for the diagnosis of inflammatory bowel disease. Abdom Imaging 27:394–399

Rubin DL, Muller HH, Sidhu MK et al (1993) Liquid oral magnetic particles as a gastrointestinal contrast agent for MR imaging: efficiency in vivo. JMRI 3:113–118

Runge VM, Clanton JA, Lukehart CM, et al (1983) Paramagnetic agents for contrast-enhanced NMR imaging: a review. AJR Am J Roentgenol 141:1209–1215

Röttgen R, Herzog H, Lopez-Hänninen E, et al (2006) Bowel wall enhancement in magnetic resonance colonography for assessing activity in Crohn's disease. J Clin Imaging 30:27–31

Schiller LR, Sellin JH (2002) Diarrhoea. In: Gastrointestinal and liver disease. Pa thophysiology/ Diagnosis/ Management, 7th edn. Sauders, Philadelphia. ISBN 0-7216-8973-6

Schneider G, Reimer P, Massmann A, et al (2005) Contrast agents in abdominal imaging. Current and future directions. Top Magn Reson Imaging 16(1):107–124

Schunk K, Kersjes W, Schadmand-Fischer S, et al (1995) A mannitol solution as an oral contrast medium in pelvic MRT. Rofo 163:60–66

Schunk K, Kern A, Heussel CP et al (1999) Hydro-MRI with fast sequences in Crohn's disease: a comparison with fractionated gastrointestinal passage. Rofo Fortschr Geb Rontgenstr Neuen Bildgeb Verfahr 170 (4):338–346

Schunk K, Kern A, Oberholzer K, et al (2000) Hydro-MRI in Crohn's disease: appraisal of disease activity. Invest Radiol 35(7):431–437

Schunk K (2002) Small bowel magnetic resonance imaging for inflammatory bowel disease. Top Magn Reson Imaging 13(6):406–425

Schwizer W, Fraser R, Maecke H, et al (1994) Gd-DOTA as a gastrointestinal contrast agent for gastric emptying measurements with MRI. Magn Reson Med 31:388–393

Sieber MA, Lengfeld P, Frenzel T, et al (2008) Preclinical investigation to compare different gadolinium-based contrast agents regarding their propensity to release gadolinium in vivo and to trigger nephrogenic systemic fibrosis-like le sions. Eur Radiol 18:2164–2173

Small WC, Macchi DD, Parker JR, et al (1998) Multisite study of the safety and efficacy of LumenHance, a new gastrointestinal contrast agent for MRI of the abdomen and pelvis. Acad Radiol 5(suppl):S147–S150

Stordahl A, Lærum F, Gjoelberg T, et al (1988) Water-soluble contrast media in radiography of small bowel obstruction. Comparison of ionic and non-ionic contrast media. Acta Radiol 29:53–56

Stordahl A, Lærum F (1988) Water-soluble contrast media compared with barium in enteric follow-through. Urinary excretion and radiographic efficacy in rats with intestinal ischemia. Invest Radiol 23:471–477

Thomsen HS (2009) Delayed reactions: nephrogenic systemic fibrosis. In: Thomsen HS, Webb JAW (eds) Contrast media. Safety issues and ESUR guidelines, 2nd edn. Springer Verlag, Berlin. ISBN: 978-3.540-72783-5

Umschaden HW, Szolar D, Gasser J, et al (2000) Small-bowel disease: comparison of MR enteroclysis images with conventional enteroclysis and surgical findings. Radiology 215:717–725

U.S. Food and Drug Administration (2007) FDA news: FDA requests boxed warning for contrast agents used to improve MRI images. Food and Drug Administration Web site. http://www.fda.gov/bbs/topics/NEWS/2007/NEW01638.html. Published 23 May 2007. Accessed 19 June 2007

Van der Molen AJ, Bellin M-F (2008) Extracellular gadolinium-based contrast media: differences in diagnostic efficacy. Eur J Radiol 66:168–174

Vlahos L, Gouliamos A, Athanasopoulou A, et al (1994) A comparative study be tween Gd-DTPA and oral magnetic particles (OMP) as gastrointestinal (GI) contrast agents for MRI of the abdomen. Magn Reson Imaging 12 (5): 719–726

Wiarda BM, Kuipers EJ, Houdijk LPJ, et al (2005) MR enteroclysis: imaging technique of choice in diagnosis of small bowel diseases. Dig Dis Sci 50(6):1036–1040

Yamamoto H, Kita H (2005) Enteroscopy. J Gastroenterol 40: 555–562

Young IR, Clarke GJ, Pennock JM, et al (1981) Enhancement of relaxation rate with paramagnetic contrast agents in NMR imaging. J Comput Tomogr 5:543–547

Zhu J, Xu J-R, Gong H-X, et al (2008) Updating magnetic resonance imaging of small bowel: imaging protocols and clinical indications. World J Gastroenterol 14:3403–3409

Dynamic Contrast-Enhanced and Diffusion-Weighted MRI of the Gastrointestinal Tract

VICKY GOH and N. JANE TAYLOR

CONTENTS

4.1 Introduction 51
4.2 Dynamic Contrast-Enhanced MRI (DCE-MRI) 52
4.2.1 Technical Parameters 52
4.2.2 Kinetic Modeling 53
4.2.2.1 Experiments Using T1-Weighted Sequences 53
4.2.2.2 Experiments Using T2*-Weighted Sequences 55
4.2.3 Histopathological Validation 55
4.2.4 Measurement Reproducibility 56
4.2.5 Clinical Studies 56
4.3 Diffusion-Weighted MRI (DW-MRI) 56
4.3.1 Technical Parameters 57
4.4 Image Analysis 58
4.5 Diffusion Tensor Imaging 58
4.6 Reproducibility and Histological Validation 59
4.7 Clinical Studies 60
4.7.1 Challenges for Bowel Imaging 60
References 61

KEY POINTS

Dynamic contrast-enhanced (DCE) MRI and diffusion-weighted (DW) MRI provide valuable information on tissue perfusion, vascular leakage, and water diffusion. DCE-MRI has yet to be integrated into mainstream clinical practice, but it has a role in oncological practice, drug development, and therapeutic assessment by providing evidence of an anti-vascular effect. DW-MRI is being integrated increasingly into oncological practice as it provides information on tissue cellularity, and it may aid tissue characterization, tumor detection, and therapeutic assessment. While these techniques remain challenging for bowel imaging, they are gaining favor in abdominal imaging.

This chapter reviews the pathophysiological basis of these imaging techniques, technical issues and challenges, and potential clinical applications for gastrointestinal imaging. Present experience primarily concerns colorectal cancer and some initial studies in Crohn's disease.

4.1 Introduction

The ability of MRI to assess tissue perfusion, vascular leakage, and water diffusion provides unique in vivo information on underlying physiology, and also perhaps on disease. In clinical practice, these techniques are gaining favor as biomarkers, particularly in the oncological setting, for example, for tumor detection, characterization, and therapeutic assessment. MRI techniques to assess tissue vascularity include intrinsic-contrast (blood oxygenation level dependent, BOLD) and extrinsic contrast-enhanced (dynamic contrast-enhanced MRI, DCE-MRI) techniques.

VICKY GOH, MD
N. JANE TAYLOR, PhD
Paul Strickland Scanner Centre, Mount Vernon Hospital, Northwood, London, UK

BOLD-MRI is sensitive to paramagnetic deoxyhemoglobin within red blood cells in perfused vessels and the induced microscopic magnetic field changes in adjacent surrounding tissue. Deoxyhemoglobin increases the apparent transverse relaxation rate of water in blood (R_2^*), thus BOLD-MRI may provide information on red cell delivery and the level of blood oxygenation, the "hypoxic blood volume." BOLD-MRI is challenging: the signal-to-noise ratio is low, and the relationship between R_2^* and tissue pO_2 is nonlinear. Furthermore, as tissue perfusion is required to gain information on oxygenation status, chronic hypoxia is less likely to be reflected by BOLD-MRI. There have been a few human studies mainly on prostate (Alonzi et al. 2009; Hoskin et al. 2007; Taylor et al. 2001), and this technique will not be discussed further in this chapter.

Contrast-enhanced techniques may inform on tissue perfusion, blood volume, and vascular leakage. Kinetic modeling of the contrast agent concentration–time curve following intravenous administration of low molecular weight gadolinium-based contrast agent allows these parameters to be quantified, for example, K^{trans}, which reflects perfusion and vascular leakage using a generalized kinetic model of dynamic contrast-enhanced T1 GRE data. As a biomarker of angiogenesis, DCE-MRI techniques have been used predominantly in the oncological setting for novel drug evaluation (Morgan et al. 2003; Thomas et al. 2005), but have also been performed to evaluate the effects of radiotherapy, for example, in colorectal cancer (De Lussanet et al. 2005; De Vries et al. 2000, 2001). Outside of this setting, there have been few bowel studies. For example, small studies have evaluated the use of DCE-MRI in Crohn's disease (Taylor et al. 2009; Horsthuis et al. 2009).

Diffusion-weighted MRI (DW-MRI) assesses the motion of water molecules in the body, providing information on cellular density and tissue composition. As a potential biomarker of cellularity, this technique is showing promise in the oncological setting, for example, tumor detection (Rao et al. 2008; Hosonuma et al. 2006) and therapeutic assessment (De Vries et al. 2003; Dzik-Jurasz et al. 2002; Hein et al. 2003). Data remain limited and currently there are little published data of the bowel per se (Kiryu et al. 2009).

4.2
Dynamic Contrast-Enhanced MRI (DCE-MRI)

The administration of an intravenous contrast agent and subsequent kinetic modeling of its behavior in the tissue of interest allows quantification of several parameters which provide insight into the macro and microcirculation. The most commonly used contrast agents are micromolecular or "low molecular weight" agents (typically <1 kDa), which are predominantly gadolinium-based and effectively diffuse freely between the intra and extra-vascular extracellular compartments. The rate at which low molecular weight contrast agents pass from the intravascular space to the extravascular–extracellular space, and return to the intravascular space over time following bolus injection differs for normal tissue, inflamed tissue, and tumor. This can be exploited to provide lesion-tissue-specific information. A number of factors influence this process: the rate of tissue delivery, vessel surface area, and the leakiness of the underlying vessels.

Transfer constant (K^{trans}), rate constant (k_{ep}), leakage space (v_e), and plasma volume (v_p) are parameters that may be quantified from dynamic T1-weighted imaging while *relative* perfusion, blood volume, and mean transit time may be assessed from T2*-weighted imaging. T1 parameters are favored in practice as T2* DCE-MRI parameters are challenging to quantify outside of the cranial circulation. This is due to the high first-pass extraction of contrast agent and the need for high-time resolution imaging, which precludes the use of navigator and breath-hold techniques that usually facilitate imaging in areas susceptible to motion. What T1 parameters reflect in vivo depends on the tissue and contrast agent studied. K^{trans}, the rate of extraction of contrast from the intravascular compartment, is the most commonly applied parameter in tumor assessment. It is influenced predominantly by inflow in the majority of extracranial tumors. k_{ep}, the backflow of contrast into the intravascular compartment, is influenced by inflow, vascular permeability, and interstitial pressure. Both provide an indirect measure of angiogenesis but K^{trans} has a greater dynamic range. Plasma volume reflects the functioning vascular volume, which is increased with angiogenesis. The leakage space reflects the volume of the extravascular–extracellular space or interstitium.

4.2.1
Technical Parameters

Different MR sequences may be applied to characterize the tissue vasculature (Table 4.1 and Table 4.2). T1-weighted sequences are sensitive predominantly to contrast in the extravascular–extracellular space (EES), although there is also a relatively small vascular contribution to the signal. Tissue enhancement occurs via shortening of the T1 relaxation time (Fig. 4.1) and can be better observed with T1-w images. T2*-weighted sequences are more suited to monitor the passage of contrast medium in the vascular bed, i.e., a bolus tracking technique. Decrease in signal intensity (susceptibility effects) occurs because of the magnetic susceptibility difference between the intravascular space, owing to the presence of highly concentrated contrast medium, and the surrounding environment (Fig. 4.1). The dose of contrast agent and method of administration is dependent on the MRI protocol performed (Table 4.1).

In general, MRI has a good intrinsic signal-to-noise ratio, but the relationship between signal intensity change and contrast agent concentration is not simple. Many factors influence MR signal intensity including sequence type, echo times (TE), repetition times (TR), flip angle of the nuclear spins, proton density, the T1 and T2 relaxation times of the tissue under investigation, and the concentration and type of contrast agent present. Paramagnetic contrast agents shorten the characteristic T1 relaxation times of tissues by allowing the magnetic moments of the hydrogen nuclei to return faster to their equilibrium-state after the application of an RF pulse, influencing signal intensity in an exponential fashion. However, other factors, e.g., the concentration of hydrogen nuclei (proton density), affect signal intensity; thus quantification is complex.

T1 at a time t after contrast administration is given by:

$$\frac{1}{T1(t)} = \frac{1}{T1(0)} + R_1 C_t$$

Where: $T1(0)$ is the initial T1 of the tissue, R_1 the T1 relaxivity and C_t the contrast at time t.

If the initial T1 values and the relaxivity are known, and the T1 at time t can be calculated from the DCE-MRI sequence, the contrast agent concentration at time t can be calculated. In practice, acquiring T1 measurements at the speed needed for accurate quantification requires either (1) the use of image ratios and calibration curves for a given sequence (Parker et al. 1998); (2) optimization of sequence parameters to ensure that signal intensity is as linear as possible with contrast concentration over the probable range of T1 values (Wang et al. 1987); or (3) measurement of T1 directly at high temporal resolution using EPI (Gowland and Mansfield 1993).

4.2.2
Kinetic Modeling

4.2.2.1
Experiments Using T1-Weighted Sequences

During a T1-weighted experiment, an increase in tissue signal intensity occurs due to the T1 shortening effects of gadolinium (see previous section). This

Table 4.1. Comparison of the characteristics of T1- and T2*-weighted experiments

DCE-MRI	T1W 2D or 3D	T2*W 2D
Contrast dose	0.1 mmol/kg	≥0.2 mmol/kg
Typical volume	10–15 mL	25–35 mL
Injection rate	3–5 mL/s bolus	4–6 mL/s bolus
Acquisition type	Single level/volume	Single level
Slice thickness (mm)	2–8	2–8
Data sampling	3–12 s for 5–7 min	1–2 s for 1–2 min
SNR of technique	Very high	Low
Signal change observed/magnitude of effect	Increase/large	Decrease/small
Kinetic analysis	General multi-compartment model	Gamma variate fitting
		Central volume theorem

Table 4.2. Typical acquisition parameters for T1- and T2*-weighted sequences for abdomino-pelvic DCE-MRI

Sequence	TR (ms)	TE (ms)	FA	NEX	Slice no/thickness (mm)	FOV (mm)	Matrix
Proton density (T1 mapping)	3–6	1–2	2°	4	20/5	200–350	256 × 256
T1 (3D GRE)	3–6	1–2	24°	1	20/5	200–350	256 × 256
T2* (2D GRE)	30–35	20	40	1	3/8	200–350	64 × 128

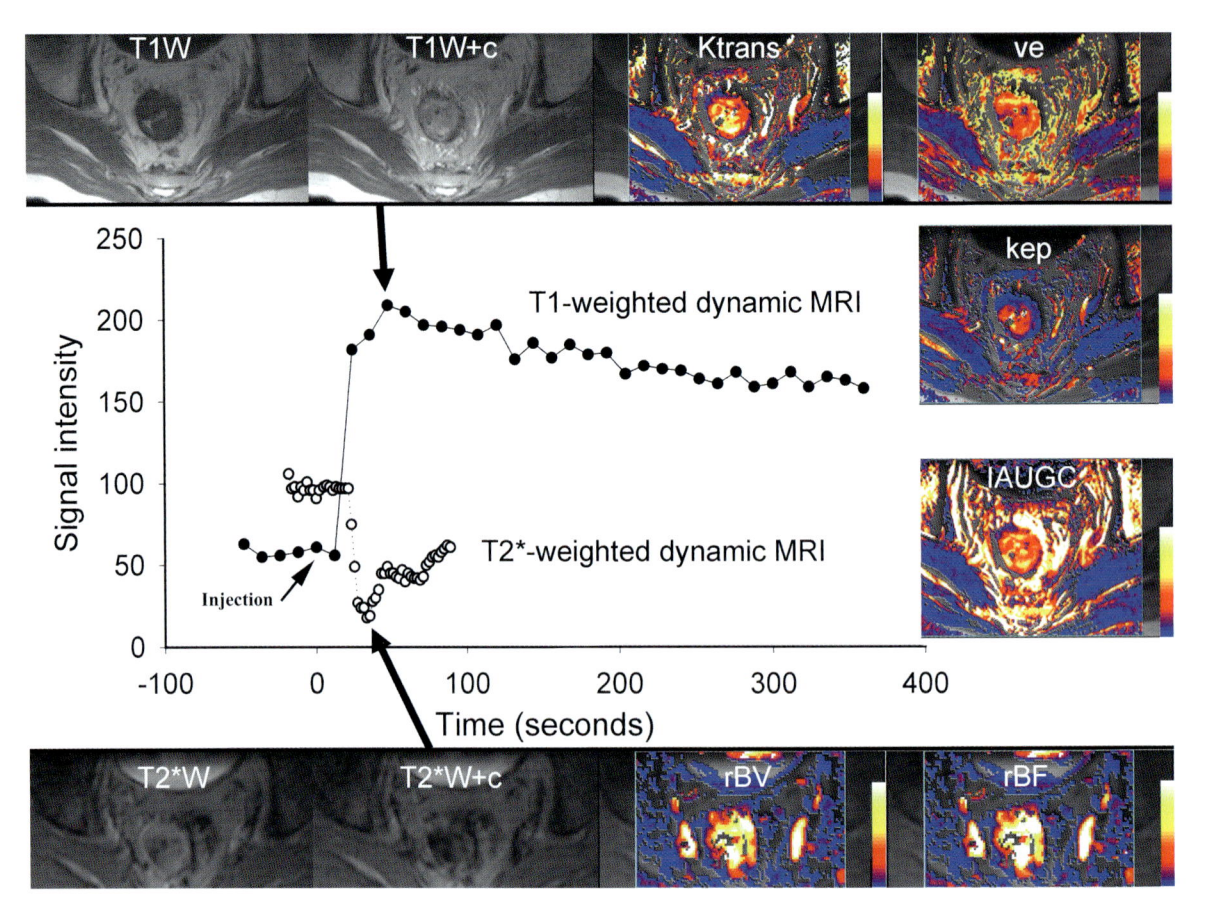

Fig. 4.1. Dynamic contrast-enhanced MRI parametric maps for a rectal cancer at staging. The typical signal intensity time curves for a T1 and T2* GRE sequence, transfer constant (K^{trans}), and extracellular leakage space (v_e) maps (*top row*) and relative blood volume (rBV) and relative blood flow (rBF) maps (*bottom row*) are shown with areas of high value color coded *white* and low value *blue*. The K^{trans} and v_e color maps demonstrate the heterogeneity within tumors. Inflammation at the luminal surface often results in an increase in K^{trans} (reproduced with permission from Elsevier; GOH et al. 2007)

change in signal intensity over time can be plotted as a graph and assessed qualitatively. Maximal enhancement, slope of the enhancement curve, and area under the enhancement curve are qualitative parameters that can be obtained. Alternatively, quantitative parameters may be obtained by converting signal intensity to contrast agent concentration values for each time point, and kinetic modeling. Given the dependency of signal intensity on acquisition factors (see previous section), conversion of signal intensity to gadolinium concentration is necessary for quantification. The most widely used model is the general kinetic model modified from the Kety model (KETY 1951; TOFTS 1997; TOFTS et al. 1999). This model provides information of the rate of contrast extraction (transfer constant, K^{trans}; units/min), fractional extracellular leakage space (v_e; units %), and rate of contrast return from the extravascular–extracellular compartment to the vascular compartment (rate constant, k_{ep}; units/min). These parameters are evaluated most commonly in clinical practice (LEACH et al. 2005).

The contribution of intravascular contrast to tissue contrast often is assumed to be negligible. With this assumption, the change in tissue contrast concentration over time is denoted by the following equation:

$$\frac{dC_t}{dt} = K^{trans}C_p - k_{ep}C_t,$$

where C_t = tissue extravascular–extracellular compartment contrast concentration; C_p = blood plasma contrast concentration; K^{trans} = transfer constant; k_{ep} = rate constant; or K^{trans}/v_e. where v_e = fraction of tissue volume occupied by the EES (KETY 1951; TOFTS 1997; TOFTS et al. 1999).

This may also be extended to provide information of the fractional plasma volume (v_p; units %) (PARKER et al. 1998). By using the following equation:

$$C_t = v_p C_p + v_e C_e$$

Together with the rate equation above, we obtain the solution to the tissue concentration $C_t(t)$

$$C_t(t) = v_p C_p(t) + K^{trans} \int_o^t C_p(t') \times \exp\left[\frac{-K^{trans}(t-t')}{v_e}\right] dt',$$

where C_t = tissue extravascular–extracellular compartment contrast concentration; C_p = blood plasma contrast concentration; K^{trans} = transfer constant; k_{ep} = rate constant; v_e = fraction of tissue volume occupied by the EES; v_p = fractional plasma volume.

Depending on the balance between flow and permeability in the tissue of interest, K^{trans} may reflect predominantly flow, permeability, or both:

$$K^{trans} = (1 - e^{-PS/F(1-Hct)})\, F\rho\, (1-Hct),$$

where F = flow; PS = permeability surface area product; ρ = tissue density; Hct = hematocrit.

If vessel permeability is high (PS>>F), then this approximates to the blood plasma flow per unit volume of tissue, i.e., $K^{trans} = F\rho (1-Hct)$. If vessel permeability is low (PS<<F), this approximates to permeability surface area product, i.e., $K^{trans} = PS\rho$. In untreated extracranial tumors, there is an overall tendency for the influence of flow to outweigh that of permeability surface area product. K^{trans} is heterogeneously distributed in primary colorectal cancer. At regions where the permeability surface area product is high compared with flow, such as at the peripheral highly angiogenic rims of tumors, K^{trans} estimates are dominated by plasma flow. At regions where permeability is low compared with flow, usually within the tumor center, K^{trans} predominantly reflects permeability surface area product. The "mixed situation" occurs most commonly where neither flow nor permeability surface area product predominates. Further modeling approaches have attempted to separate the contributions of blood flow, blood volume, and permeability surface area product to the signal intensity change with DCE-MRI, but these approaches are currently too demanding for routine clinical use. Other publications provide in-depth detail of such approaches (TOFTS 1997; TOFTS et al. 1999; PARKER et al. 2006).

4.2.2.2
Experiments Using T2*-Weighted Sequences

Relative perfusion and blood volume may be estimated from T2* experiments via gamma variate fitting of the contrast agent concentration–time curve. The gamma variate is a mathematical function used to describe probability distributions (DAVENPORT 1983). The least-squares method is commonly employed for curve-fitting to correct for effects of recirculation so that only the first pass is modeled. Direct quantification outside the brain is technically challenging due to artifacts from nonlaminar vascular flow, high vascular permeability resulting in loss of compartmentalization, and the subsequent competition with signal-enhancement effects caused by contrast media leakage (the T1 effects as described above). Nevertheless, semiquantitative values may be obtained outside the cranial circulation: relative transit time from the full-width-half-maximum of the fitted curve and relative blood volume to be obtained from the integral of the curve. Relative blood flow can be determined from these measurements as defined by the central volume theorem:

$$BF = \frac{BV}{MTT},$$

where BF = blood flow; BV = blood volume; MTT = mean transit time.

4.2.3
Histopathological Validation

Qualitative and quantitative colorectal cancer T1 kinetic parameters have been correlated with histological markers of angiogenesis. Tunckbilek et al. noted a negative correlation between time to peak enhancement and microvessel density (TUNCKBILEK et al. 2004), corroborated by Zhang et al., who also noted that time to peak was shorter in VEGF expressing tumors (ZHANG et al. 2008). George et al. noted a positive correlation between serum vascular endothelial growth factor and K^{trans} (GEORGE et al. 2001); however, another study has found no relationship between K^{trans} and serum/tumor vascular endothelial growth factor or microvessel density (ATKIN et al. 2006). Positive correlations between T1 kinetic parameters and microvessel density have been found in other cancers including prostate (SCHLEMMER et al. 2004), breast (TEIFKE et al. 2006; TURETSCHEK et al. 2001; BUCKLEY et al. 1997), and cervix (HAWIGHORST et al.

1998). Qualitative T1 kinetic parameters such as maximal enhancement and slope of the enhancement curve have been correlated positively with tumor grade in colorectal cancers (Tunckbilek et al. 2004), but negatively in renal cancers reflecting the degree of necrosis (Yabuki et al. 2003).

4.2.4
Measurement Reproducibility

For any quantitative technique to be useful on an individual patient basis, good measurement reproducibility is essential. While there are no data specific for colorectal cancer or the large bowel, both qualitative and quantitative MRI measurements have been shown to be reproducible in cancer, e.g., a coefficient of variation $\leq 20\%$ for K^{trans} (Morgan et al. 2006; Lankester et al. 2005, 2007). This variability is lower than the expected vascular effect of many antivascular therapies in current use and undergoing clinical evaluation.

4.2.5
Clinical Studies

Within the field of oncology, the main role of DCE-MRI has been in novel drug development. In early-phase clinical studies, DCE-MRI may define a biologically active dose that is lower than the traditional maximum-tolerated dose, provide early evidence of drug activity (Morgan et al. 2003; Thomas et al. 2005; Galbraith et al. 2003), and aid scheduling, which is pertinent for antivascular drugs that have a biological effect but minimal effect on tumor size. For example, in a Phase 1 study of PTK787/ZK 222584 (Vatalanib), a multiple vascular endothelial growth factor receptor inhibitor, in 26 metastatic colorectal cancers, DCE-MRI demonstrated drug activity with a 43% decrease in bidirectional transfer constant within 33 h of single drug dose; and a sustained reduction with dose increase to >1,000 mg on day 28 (Morgan et al. 2003). However, it is recognized that the relationship between biological effect and long-term outcome is complex (Jain et al. 2006). Bevacizumab has been one of the success stories in colorectal cancer: a 40–60% reduction in vascularity within 2 weeks of single dosing in early-phase studies (Willett et al. 2004), was followed by improvement in disease-free survival in Phase III studies (Hurwitz et al. 2004), but other novel drugs that have shown marked antivascular effect in early-phase trials have been ultimately disappointing in larger Phase III trials where progression-free or overall survival have been the end point (Jain et al. 2006).

DCE-MRI has also been performed in primary colorectal cancer to assess the vascular effect of radiotherapy. With the increasing use of antivascular/antiproliferative drugs in combination with radiation or chemoradiation, a better understanding of the in vivo acute and chronic vascular effects of radiation is necessary to facilitate treatment scheduling. Acutely, an increase in vascular permeability and perfusion may occur as a consequence of endothelial cell damage and inflammation, and possibly due to further new vessel formation. In the longer term, a decrease in vascular permeability is always seen due to basement membrane thickening, extracapillary fibrosis, and endothelial damage. Reduction in microvessel function from thrombosis and obliteration of the vessel lumen also occurs. This has been shown in a study of the weekly changes in vascularity during chemoradiation. A substantial increase in mean perfusion index in the first 2 weeks of treatment (from 100 to 125; $p < 0.01$), but reduction in mean perfusion index by week 4 of treatment occurred (DeVries et al. 2000). Other studies have demonstrated a reduction in rectal cancer vascularity following chemoradiation, e.g., mean transfer constant, K^{trans} of 6.5 vs. 26.5 in treated vs. untreated patients (De Lussanet et al. 2006), and reduction in mean ln K^{trans} from −0.46 to 0.86 (George et al. 2001).

Few bowel DCE-MRI studies have been published outside of the field of oncology because of the challenges of bowel imaging posed by a small target volume, peristaltic and respiratory movement, and susceptibility at the air–tissue interface. Small studies have performed DCE-MRI in Crohn's disease where slope of enhancement, a semi-quantitative parameter, has correlated negatively with microvessel density ($r = -0.86$ $p = <0.001$) and positively with disease chronicity suggesting that chronic low perfusion may stimulate new vessel formation (Taylor et al. 2009). Semi-quantitative parameters such as curve shape have also been found to correlate with disease score in perianal Crohn's disease (Horsthuis et al. 2009).

4.3
Diffusion-Weighted MRI (DW-MRI)

Diffusion-weighted MRI provides information of the diffusion of water molecules within the body. In vivo, the movement of water molecules is not random but restricted by a high cellular density, interaction with cell membranes, intracellular elements, and macromolecules (STEJSKAL and TANNER 1965; LE BIHAN et al. 1988; CHENEVERT et al. 1990), and thus is much less than pure water. On current standard MRI scanners, the diffusion interval is in the order of 40–80 ms; thus at body temperature the average diffusion distance is in the order of 30 μm (NORRIS 2001), making DW-MRI sensitive to changes at a cellular level.

Diffusion in vivo is affected by water exchange between the intravascular and extravascular–extracellular space and the characteristics of the extravascular–extracellular space. In clinical practice, this can be exploited to provide indirect assessment of tumor cellularity. Although diffusion-weighted imaging has potential as a cancer biomarker, technical issues such as standardization, reproducibility, and histological validation still require further evaluation (PADHANI et al. 2009).

4.3.1
Technical Parameters

The motion of the water molecules within the intravascular space, extravascular–extracellular space, and intracellular space is detected as a reduction in signal intensity. The sensitivity to water motion can be altered by changing "*b*-values," which predominantly reflect the amplitude of gradient pulses applied during MRI. Water molecules with a large degree of motion will show signal attenuation at low "*b*-values," while slow-moving molecules will only show gradual signal attenuation with increasing "*b*-values" (Fig. 4.2). For example, blood flow signal is rapidly attenuated at low *b*-values (0–150 s/mm^2). In a diffusion experiment, the optimal *b*-value for a tissue is such that the *b*-value multiplied by the apparent diffusion coefficient is equal to 1. The diffusion equation is given by:

$$\frac{S}{S_0} = e^{-\gamma^2 G^2 \delta^2 (\Delta - \delta/3) D} = e^{-bD},$$

where S_0 is the signal without diffusion gradients, S is the signal with diffusion gradients, γ is the gyromagnetic ratio, G is the diffusion gradient strength, δ is the gradient duration, Δ is the interval between the two diffusion gradients, and D is the diffusion coefficient.

Rearranging the above for *D*, the diffusion within a given voxel can be calculated and this is termed the apparent diffusion coefficient (ADC), which can be displayed as a parametric image.

This Stejskal and Tanner approach to DW-MRI is the basis of many sequences (single-shot echo planar imaging) in clinical use today (Table 4.3) (STEJSKAL and TANNER. 1965). It is important during image acquisition to optimize signal-to-noise ratio (SNR), fat suppression, and to reduce artifacts, e.g., from motion,

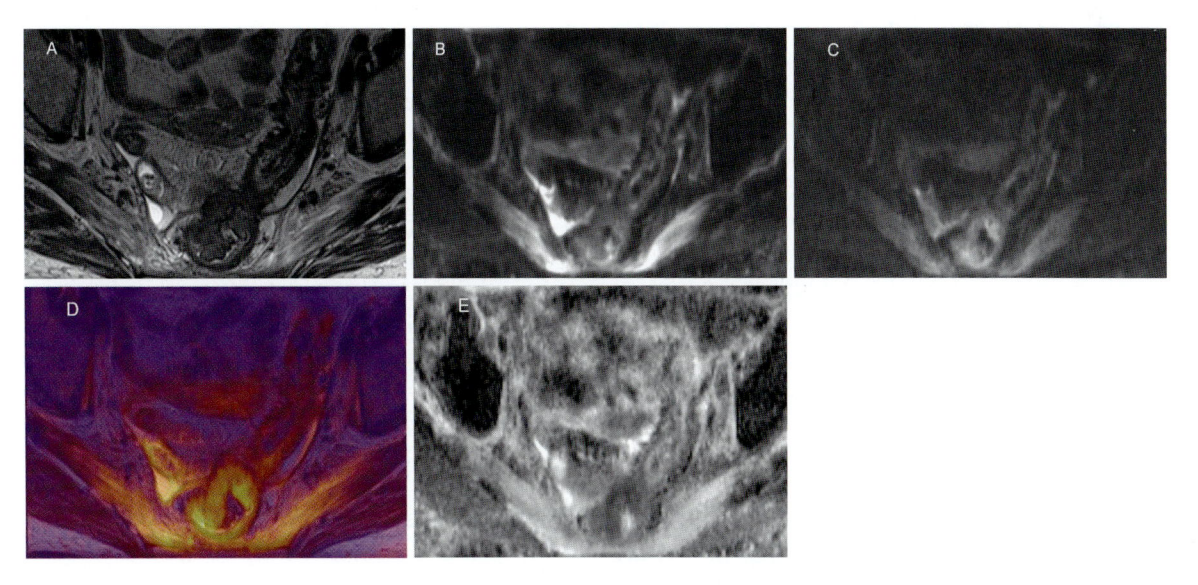

Fig. 4.2. Rectosigmoid cancer coexisting with diverticular disease: axial T2 GRE image (**a**), DWI EPI image (*b* = 0 and 800 s/mm^2; **b**, **c**), fused T2 and DWI image (**d**) and ADC map (**e**) shown. The cancer appears of high signal intensity on the high *b*-value DWI image and of low signal intensity on the ADC maps reflecting restriction of diffusion

Table 4.3. Typical acquisition parameters for DW-MRI

1.5-T protocols	Abdomen	Pelvis
Sequence type	Single-shot echo planar imaging	Single-shot echo planar imaging
TR (ms)	2,500	2,900
TE (ms)	60–90	80–100
FOV (mm)	300	300
Matrix	128 × 128	128 × 128
Fat suppression	Y	Y
Parallel imaging factor	2	2
EPI factor	128	128
Signal averages	4	4
Section thickness (mm)/total	5/20	5/20
Directions of MPGs	3	3
b-values (s/mm^2)	0, 100, 250, 500, 750	0, 100, 500, 800
Pixel bandwidth (Hz)	1,500	1,500
Breathing	Respiratory-triggered	Free-breathing

incomplete fat suppression, eddy currents induced by diffusion gradients, and EPI techniques. Signal to noise and artifacts can be improved by using as short a TE as possible (e.g., 60–90 ms at 1.5 T); performing multiple averaging, particularly at higher b-values, to compensate for the reduction in SNR; applying parallel imaging to reduce the echo train length, acquisition time, and also susceptibility and field inhomogeneity artifacts. Motion artifacts can be reduced in the upper abdomen by using respiratory/cardiac-gated techniques, and in the pelvis by the use of antispasmolytics to reduce peristalsis. Good fat suppression is necessary to reduce ghosting artifacts.

4.4
Image Analysis

A qualitative or quantitative approach may be taken to image analysis. For qualitative imaging (i.e., visual assessment of the relative attenuation of signal intensity), adequate suppression of the background signal from normal tissue is essential for lesion detection and characterization, and a sufficient degree of diffusion weighting is necessary. On high b-value images, cellular tissues appear of high signal intensity. The disadvantage of using a qualitative approach for tumor detection, tumor characterization, and therapeutic response is that tissue T2 relaxation time also affects DW-MRI signal intensity. An area with a long T2 relaxation time may remain at high signal on high b-value images and be mistaken for an area of restricted diffusion, an effect known as "T2 shine-through," e.g., peripheral zone of the prostate.

In clinical practice, quantitative analysis by plotting the logarithm of the relative signal intensity (y-axis) vs. b-value (x-axis) allows calculation of the apparent diffusion coefficient (ADC) from the slope of the fitted line (monoexponential decay model; Fig. 4.2). Multiple b-values are necessary to calculate the ADC. In practice, three or more b-values improve ADC quantification, e.g., $b = 0$, ≥ 150 s/mm^2 and ≥ 500 s/mm^2. The TR should be sufficiently long to avoid T1 saturation effects (predisposing to ADC underestimation). The experimental setup will determine whether the ADC is dominated by macroscopic or microscopic water motion. At low b-values (<150 s/mm^2), bulk water motion (intravoxel incoherent motion) is the predominant factor determining ADC. At higher b-values (500–1,000 s/mm^2), ADC predominantly reflects extracellular space water diffusion. Flow-insensitive ADC values (fitting of high b-values only, e.g., b-values >150 s/mm^2) may provide a more accurate estimate of the tumor microenvironment by minimizing the intravascular contribution, though in highly vascular tissues, perfusion will impart significant signal attenuation over the low b-value range leading to ADC overestimation.

Region of interest analysis allows mean or median ADC values to be determined for the tissue of interest. Delineation should include the entire volume of interest. The region of interest is best contoured using images with the highest lesion to background signal. Diffusion-weighted images can be used in which case the b0 (T2-weighted) DW-MRI images may be appropriate. However, lesion heterogeneity is not addressed by such ROI analysis.

4.5
Diffusion Tensor Imaging

Diffusion in some tissues is directionally dependent, e.g., CNS and muscle. To measure this directional dependency, multiple different gradient directions

Fig. 4.3. Diffusion tensor imaging of the anal canal using a multidirectional EPI sequence. T2-weighted (a) B0 (b), fractional anisotropy (c), and ADC (d) maps are shown. Color coding of the fractional anisotropy map demonstrates the directionality of diffusion: *red*-medial/lateral; *green*-anterior/posterior; *blue* cranial/caudal

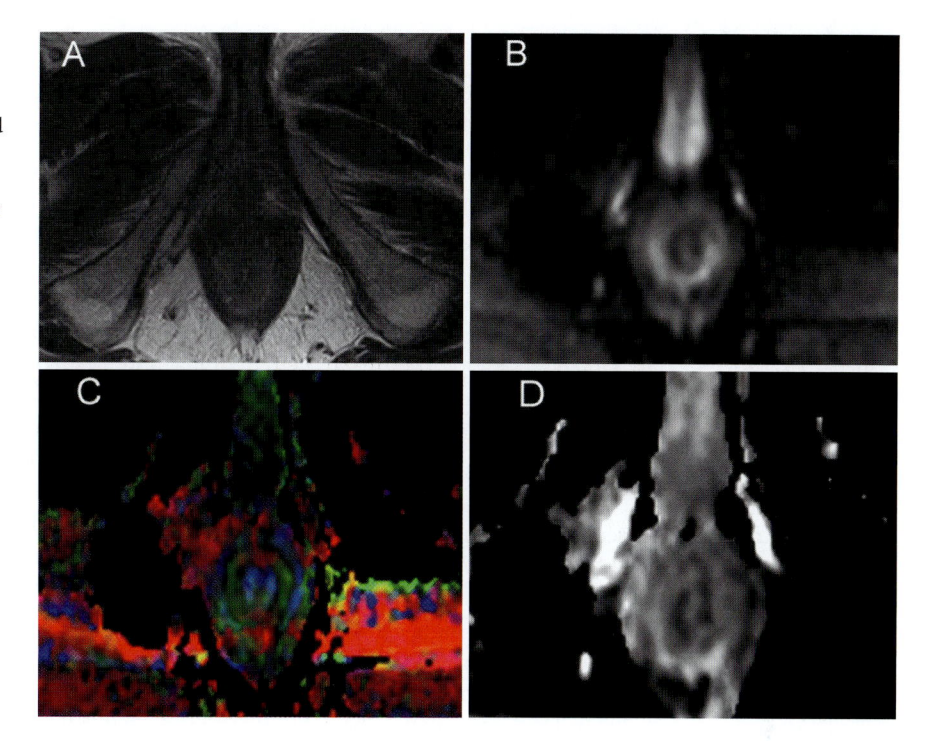

are needed, with a minimum of six directions, though the greater the number (up to 32), the better the quality. Measures include

(1) Fractional anisotropy (FA), the ratio of the anisotropic component to the whole diffusion tensor defined as follows (Basser and Pierpaoli 1996):

$$\text{FA}(D) = \sqrt{\frac{3}{2}} \frac{\sqrt{(\lambda_1 - \langle D \rangle)^2 + (\lambda_2 - \langle D \rangle)^2 + (\lambda_3 - \langle D \rangle)^2}}{\sqrt{\lambda_1^2 + \lambda_2^2 + \lambda_3^2}},$$

where $\langle D \rangle = 1/3\,(\lambda_1 + \lambda_2 + \lambda_3)$, the mean diffusivity (apparent diffusion coefficient, ADC)

(2) Relative anisotropy (RA), the ratio of the variance of the computed eigenvalues to their mean, defined as follows (Basser and Pierpaoli 1996):

$$\text{RA}(D) = \sqrt{\frac{1}{3}} \frac{\sqrt{(\lambda_1 - \langle D \rangle)^2 + (\lambda_2 - \langle D \rangle)^2 + (\lambda_3 - \langle D \rangle)^2}}{\langle D \rangle},$$

where $\langle D \rangle = 1/3\,(\lambda_1 + \lambda_2 + \lambda_3)$, the mean diffusivity (apparent diffusion coefficient, ADC).

Fractional anisotropy may be less susceptible to noise than relative anisotropy.

In the brain, diffusion tensor imaging (DTI) may be applied to assess the relationship between tumor and adjacent white matter tracts, i.e., infiltration vs. displacement; likewise in the prostate where the peripheral gland demonstrates anisotropy. This technique has clinical potential in the evaluation of the anal canal where anisotropy is demonstrated (Fig. 4.3). For example, this technique might provide additional information to physiological studies in postpartum sphincter dysfunction, while in the oncological setting anal cancer infiltration vs. displacement might be distinguished.

4.6
Reproducibility and Histological Validation

At the time of writing, no reproducibility or histological validation studies of DW-MRI of the large bowel have been performed. Several studies in human cancers have noted a negative correlation between cellularity and ADC (Humphries et al. 2007; Squillaci et al. 2004; Yoshikawa et al. 2008). One study incorporating assessment of observer agreement noted that agreement in the detection of rectal cancer was good with a kappa value of >0.8 (Ichikawa et al. 2006).

4.7
Clinical Studies

To date, few bowel studies have been performed. Studies have focussed primarily on cancer, though a study of DW-MRI of Crohn's disease has been published (Kiryu et al. 2009). Studies remain exploratory; nonetheless, initial studies show that DW-MRI has promise as a clinical tool. DW-MRI may improve lesion conspicuity and aid detection of colorectal cancer (Rao et al. 2008; Hosonuma et al. 2006; Ichikawa et al. 2006) (Fig. 4.2). In one study, the sensitivity increased from 82–84% to 93–95% with the addition of DW-MRI to standard T2-weighted imaging (Rao et al. 2008). Another study reported a mean sensitivity of 90.9% and specificity of 100% for DW-MRI in 33 patients with colorectal adenocarcinoma (Ichikawa et al. 2006). Cellular tumors appear of high signal intensity on DW-MRI and of low ADC (mean ADC in the order of $1.19–1.41 \times 10^{-3}$ mm^2/s (Hosonuma et al. 2006; Dzik-Jurasz et al. 2002). This is thought to be related to increased cellularity, tissue disorganization, and tortuosity of the extracellular, extravascular space. False-positive results may occur with abscesses on DW-MRI although ADC values are typically higher than for cancer (Fig. 4.4), false-negatives with cystic, necrotic lesions and well-differentiated tumors. Not all studies have demonstrated clinical benefit. In a whole body DWI study of 24 patients with esophageal cancer, the primary tumor detection rate was only 49.4%. When applied to nodal assessment, the ADC was higher in metastatic than normal nodes (1.46 vs. 1.15 mm^2/s), but the degree of overlap precluded differentiation on an individual basis (Sakurada et al. 2009). A study in 15 patients with advanced gastric cancer showed no additional benefit of DWI compared with contrast-enhanced CT staging (Shinya et al. 2007). A study of 31 patients with Crohn's disease of the small or large bowel has demonstrated that the ADC value in the disease-active areas is significantly lower than disease-inactive areas (Kiryu et al. 2009). Reference standard was either conventional barium examination or surgery.

An abdominal area where DW-MRI has been shown to have value is in liver imaging. DW-MRI may aid in lesion detection as well as lesion characterization in the liver. Studies have shown that ADC values are higher in benign lesions vs. metastases: ADC: 2.95×10^{-3} mm^2/s and 3.63×10^{-3} mm^2/s for hemangioma and cyst, respectively, vs. 0.94×10^{-3} mm^2/s for metastases (Taouli et al. 2003). From data of 136 malignant and 75 benign focal liver lesions, a threshold value of 1.60×10^{-3} mm^2/s or less has a sensitivity and specificity of 74.2% and 75.3% for malignant disease (Parikh et al. 2008). DW-MRI has been shown to be feasible as an early marker of treatment response as cell death and vascular alterations occur prior to size change. An increase in ADC following treatment is a marker of response (Dzik-Jurasz et al. 2002) (Fig. 4.5), though it should be noted that areas of fibrosis may manifest as areas of low ADC. Baseline tumor ADC values may be predictive of response: a higher fraction of ADC values are associated with poorer response to chemoradiation in rectal cancer, which has been ascribed to the presence of necrosis (De Vries et al. 2003). Similarly, in colorectal metastases higher baseline ADC: 2.21×10^{-3} vs. 1.63×10^{-3} mm^2/s for nonresponders and responders to standard chemotherapy (Koh et al. 2007). A transient decrease in ADC may occur early in treatment related to cellular swelling, reduction in blood flow, or reduction in the extravascular extracellular space.

4.7.1
Challenges for Bowel Imaging

Outside of the field of oncology, DCE-MRI and DW-MRI assessment of the bowel remains technically

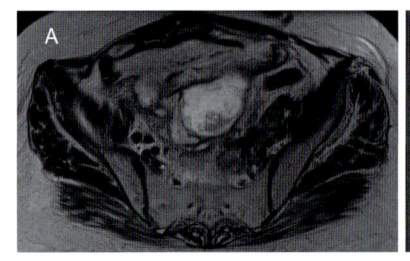

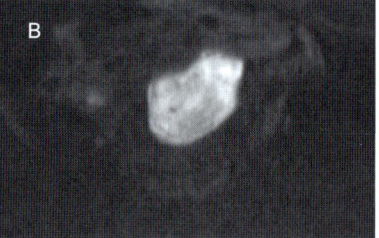

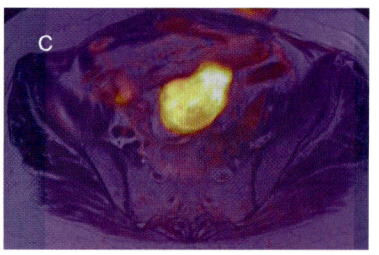

Fig. 4.4. Pelvic abscess in a patient with rectal cancer undergoing neoadjuvant chemoradiation: axial T2 GRE image (**a**), DWI EPI image (*b*-value = 800 s/mm^2; **b**), and fused T2 and DWI (*b*-value = 800 s/mm^2) images (**c**) demonstrate the high signal abscess

Fig. 4.5. Rectal cancer pre (**a**) and post (**b**) neoadjuvant chemoradiation: T2 GRE and fused T2 GRE and DWI EPI (b-value = 800 mm^2/s) images are shown. The tumor demonstrates a reduction in size and signal intensity on the high b-value diffusion-weighted image following treatment

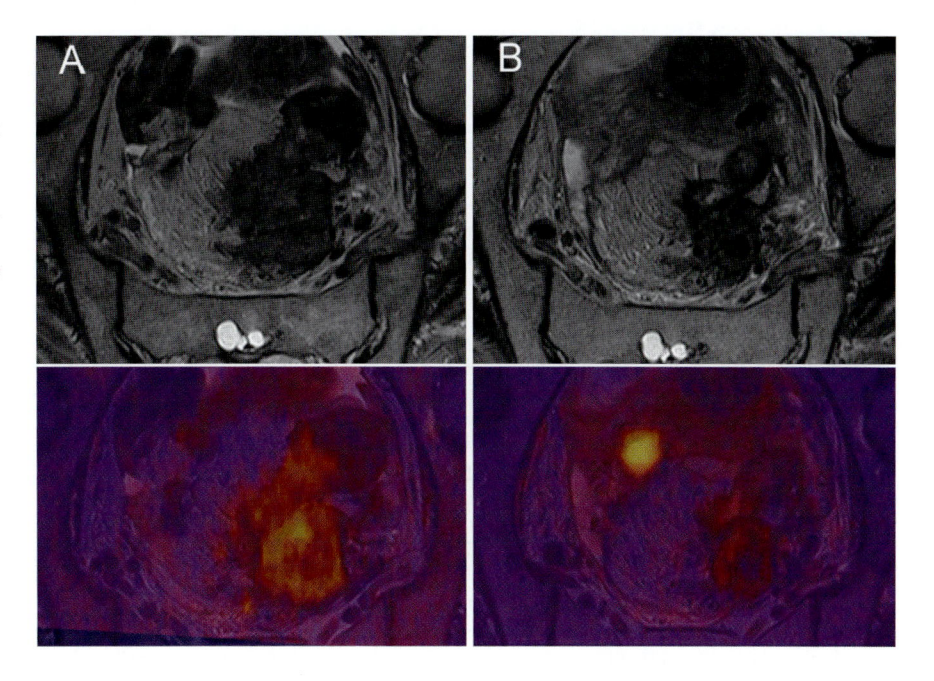

challenging contributing to the paucity of data to date with little published outside the context of Crohn's disease (Taylor et al. 2009; Horsthuis et al. 2009; Kiryu et al. 2009). Peristalsis, respiratory motion, presence of bowel gas, and signal-to-noise issues affect both techniques. Peristalsis and respiratory motion result in blurring, phase artifacts, and partial volume effects from motion in and out of plane. Susceptibility artifact from the presence of bowel gas at the air–tissue boundary may be marked on susceptibility-weighted imaging, e.g., T2* sequences and DW-MRI resulting in considerable distortion. For DCE-MRI, direct estimation of the arterial input function remains a challenge because of inflow artifact and turbulent arterial flow within abdomino-pelvic vessels. Nevertheless, steps are being taken to surmount this with dual bolus 3D slab techniques explored to provide direct arterial input estimation (Kostler et al. 2004; Risse et al. 2006). For DW-MRI field, inhomogeneities remain problematic causing distortion, particularly on high b-value images.

To optimize imaging, several procedures may be helpful. Evacuation prior to imaging, oral or rectal contrast agents can reduce the susceptibility from bowel gas; antiperistaltics to reduce blurring artifact can be given, but the beneficial effect remains controversial. Dedicated coils and parallel imaging techniques are essential to improve the signal-to-noise ratio, temporal or spatial resolution, and reduce artifacts. Careful shimming (making the magnetic field uniform) will improve central field homogeneity (having second-order shims added at installation and using them for auto shimming during acquisition) for DW-MRI.

Standardization of the techniques, image analysis, and quantification remains an issue requiring consensus (Leach et al. 2005; Padhani et al. 2009). Nevertheless, these techniques are being applied increasingly in clinical practice as multiparametric imaging is increasingly recognized as a clinically valuable, comprehensive approach to tumor characterization and response assessment.

Acknowledgments

We thank Dr. Anwar Padhani, Mr. J. James Stirling, and Mr. Ian Simcock for their input.

References

Alonzi R, Padhani AR, Maxwell RJ, et al (2009) Carbogen breathing increases prostate cancer oxygenation: a translational MRI study in murine xenografts and humans. Br J Cancer 100:644–648

Atkin G, Taylor NJ, Daley FM, et al (2006) Dynamic contrast enhanced magnetic resonance imaging is a poor measure of angiogenesis. Br J Surg 93:992–1000

Basser PF, Pierpaoli C (1996) Microstructural and physiological features of tissues elucidated by quantitative-diffusion-tensor MRI. J Magn Reson B 111:209–219

Buckley DL, Drew PJ, Mussurakis S, et al (1997) Microvessel density of invasive breast cancer assessed by dynamic Gd-DTPA enhanced MRI. J Magn Reson Imaging 7:461–464

Chenevert TL, Brunberg JA, Pipe JG (1990) Anisotropic diffusion in human white matter:demonstration of MR techniques in vivo. Radiology 177:401–405

Davenport R (1983) The derivation of the gamma-variate relationship for tracer dilution curves. J Nucl Med 24:945–948

De Lussanet QG, Backes WH, Griffioen AW, et al (2005) Dynamic contrast-enhanced magnetic resonance imaging of radiation therapy-induced microcirculation changes in rectal cancer. Int J Radiat Oncol Biol Phys 63:1309–1315

De Vries A, Griebel J, Kremser C, et al (2000) Monitoring of tumor microcirculation during fractionated radiation therapy in patients with rectal carcinoma: preliminary results and implications for therapy. Radiology 217:385–391

DeVries AF, Griebel J, Kremser C, et al (2001) Tumor microcirculation evaluated by dynamic contrast enhanced magnetic resonance imaging predicts therapy outcome for primary rectal carcinoma. Cancer Res 61:2513–2516

DeVries AF, Kremser C, Hein PA, et al (2003) Tumor microcirculation and diffusion predict therapy outcome for primary rectal carcinoma. Int J Radiat Oncol Biol Phys 56:958–965

Dzik-Jurasz A, Domenig C, George M, et al (2002) Diffusion MRI for prediction of response of rectal cancer to chemoradiation. Lancet 360:307–308

Galbraith SM, Maxwell RJ, Lodge MA, et al (2003) Combretastatin A4 phosphate has tumor antivascular activity in rat and man as demonstrated by dynamic magnetic resonance imaging. J Clin Oncol 21:2831–2842

George ML, Dzik-Jurasz AS, Padhani AR, et al (2001) Non-invasive methods of assessing angiogenesis and their value in predicting response to treatment in colorectal cancer. Br J Surg 88:1628–1636

Goh V et al (2007)Functional imaging of colorectal cancer angiogenesis. Lancet Oncol 8:245–255

Gowland P, Mansfield P (1993) Accurate measurement of T1 in vivo in less than 3 seconds using echo-planar imaging. Magn Reson Med 30:351–354

Hawighorst H, Weikel W, Knapstein PG, et al (1998) Angiogenic activity of cervical carcinoma: assessment by functional magnetic resonance imaging-based parameters and a histomorphological approach in correlation with disease outcome. Clin Cancer Res 4:2305–2312

Hein PA, Kremser C, Judmaier W, et al (2003). Diffusion-weighted magnetic resonance imaging for monitoring diffusion changes in rectal carcinoma during combined, preoperative chemoradiation: preliminary results of a prospective study. Eur J Radiol 45:214–222

Hoskin PJ, Carnell DM, Taylor NJ, et al (2007) Hypoxia in prostate cancer: correlation of BOLD-MRI with pimonidazole immunohistochemistry-initial observations. Int J Radiat Oncol Biol Phys 68:1065–1071

Horsthuis K, Lavini C, Bipat S, et al (2009). Perianal Crohn disease: evaluation of dynamic contrast-enhanced MR imaging as an indicator of disease activity. Radiology 251:380–387

Hosonuma T, Tozaki M, Ichiba N, et al (2006) Clinical usefulness of diffusion-weighted imaging using low and high b-values to detect rectal cancer. Magn Reson Med Sci 5:173–177

Humphries PD, Sebire NJ, Siegel MJ, et al (2007) Tumors in pediatric patients at diffusion weighted MR imaging: apparent diffusion coefficient and tumor cellularity. Radiology 245:848–854

Hurwitz H, Fehrenbacher L, Novotny W, et al (2004) Bevacizumab plus irinotecan, fluorouracil, and leucovorin for metastatic colorectal cancer. N Engl J Med 350:2335–2342

Ichikawa T, Erturk SM, Motosugi U, et al (2006) High B value diffusion MRI in rectal cancer. AJR Am J Roentgenol 187:181–184

Jain RK, Duda DG, Clark JW, et al (2006) Lessons from phase III clinical trials on anti-VEGF therapy for cancer. Nat Clin Pract Oncol 3:24–30

Kety SS (1951) The theory and applications of the exchange of inert gas at the lungs and tissues. Pharmacol Rev 3:1–41

Kiryu S, Dodanuki K, Takao H, et al (2009) Free breathing diffusion weighted imaging for the assessment of inflammatory activity in Crohns disease. J Magn Reson Imaging 29:880–886

Koh DM, Scurr E, Collins D, et al (2007) Predicting response of colorectal hepatic metastasis value of pretreatment apparent diffusion coefficients. AJR Am J Roentgenol 188:1001–1008

Köstler H, Ritter C, Lipp M, et al (2004) Prebolus quantitative MR heart perfusion imaging. Magn Reson Med 52:296–299

Lankester KJ, Taylor NJ, Stirling JJ, et al (2005) Effects of platinum/taxane based chemotherapy on acute perfusion in human pelvic tumours measured by dynamic MRI. Br J Cancer 93:979–985

Lankester KJ, Taylor JN, Stirling JJ, et al (2007) Dynamic MRI for imaging tumor microvasculature: comparison of susceptibility and relaxivity techniques in pelvic tumors. J Magn Reson Imaging 25:796–805

Leach MO, Brindle KM, Evelhoch JL, et al; Pharmacodynamic/Pharmacokinetic Technologies Advisory Committee, Drug Development Office, Cancer Research UK (2005) The assessment of antiangiogenic and antivascular therapies in early stage clinical trials using magnetic resonance imaging: issues and recommendations. Br J Cancer 92:1599–1610

Le Bihan D, Breton E, Lallemand D, et al (1988) Separation of diffusion and perfusion in intravoxel incoherent motion MR imaging. Radiology 168:497–505

Morgan B, Thomas AL, Drevs J, et al (2003) Dynamic contrast enhanced magnetic resonance imaging as a biomarker for the pharmacological response of PTK787/ZK 222584, an inhibitor of the vascular endothelial growth factor receptor tyrosine kinases, in patients with advanced colorectal cancer and liver metastases: results from two phase I studies. J Clin Oncol 21:3955–3964

Morgan B, Utting JF, Higginson A, et al (2006) A simple, reproducible method for monitoring the treatment of tumours using dynamic contrast-enhanced MR imaging. Br J Cancer 94:1420–1427

Norris DG (2001) The effects of microscopic tissue parameters on the diffusion weighted magnetic resonance experiment. NMR Biomed 14:77–93

Padhani AR, Liu G, Koh DM, et al (2009) Diffusion weighted magnetic resonance imaging as a cancer biomarker: consensus and recommendation. Neoplasia 11:102–125

Parikh T, Drew SJ, Lee VS, et al (2008) Focal liver lesion detection and characterization with diffusion weighted MR imaging: comparison with standard breathhold imaging. Radiology 246:812–822

Parker GJ, Suckling J, Tanner SF, et al (1998) MRIW: parametric analysis software for contrast-enhanced dynamic MR imaging in cancer. Radiographics 18:497–506

Parker GJ, Roberts C, Macdonald A, et al (2006) Experimentally-derived functional form for a population-averaged high-temporal-resolution arterial input function for dynamic contrast-enhanced MRI. Magn Reson Med 56:993–1000

Rao SX, Zeng MS, Chen CZ, et al (2008) The value of diffusion-weighted imaging in combination with T2-weighted imaging for rectal cancer detection. Eur J Radiol 65:299–303

Risse F, Semmler W, Kauczor HU, et al (2006) Dual-bolus approach to quantitative measurement of pulmonary perfusion by contrast-enhanced MRI J. Magn. Reson Imaging 24:1284–1290

Sakurada A, Takahara T, Kwee TC, et al (2009) Diagnostic performance of diffusion magnetic resonance imaging in esophageal cancer. Eur Radiol 19:1461–1469

Schlemmer HP, Merkle J, Grobholz R, et al (2004) Can pre-operative contrast-enhanced dynamic MR imaging for prostate cancer predict microvessel density in prostatectomy specimens? Eur Radiol 14:309–317

Shinya S, Sasaki T, Nakagawa Y, et al (2007) The usefulness of diffusion-weighted imaging (DWI) for the detection of gastric cancer. Hepatogastroenterology 54:1378–1381

Squillaci E, Manenti G, Cova M, et al (2004) Correlation of diffusion weighted MR imaging with cellularity of renal tumours. Anticancer Res 24:4175–4179

Stejskal EO, Tanner JE (1965) Spin diffusion measurements: spin echoes in the presence of a time dependent field gradient. J Chem Phys 42:288–292

Taouli B, Vilgrain V, Dumont E, et al (2003) Evaluation of liver diffusion isotropy and characterization of focal hepatic lesions with two single shot echo planar MR imaging sequences: prospective study in 66 patients. Radiology 226:71–78

Taylor NJ, Baddeley H, Goodchild KA, et al (2001) BOLD-MRI of human tumor oxygenation during carbogen breathing. J Magn Reson Imaging 14:156–163

Taylor SA, Punwani S, Rodriguez-Justo M, et al (2009) Mural Crohn disease: correlation of dynamic contrast-enhanced MR imaging findings with angiogenesis and inflammation at histologic examination–pilot study. Radiology 251: 369–379

Teifke A, Behr O, Schmidt M, et al (2006) Dynamic MR imaging of breast lesions: correlation with microvessel distribution pattern and histologic characteristics of prognosis. Radiology 239:351–360

Thomas AL, Morgan B, Horsfield MA, et al (2005) Phase I study of the safety, tolerability, pharmacokinetics, and pharmacodynamics of PTK787/ZK 222584 administered twice daily in patients with advanced cancer. J Clin Oncol 23: 4162–4171

Tofts PS (1997) Modelling tracer kinetics in dynamic Gd-DTPA MR imaging. J Magn Reson Imaging 7:91–101

Tofts PS, Brix G, Buckley DL, et al (1999) Estimating kinetic parameters from dynamic contrast enhanced T(1)-weighted MRI of a diffusible tracer: standardized quantitities and symbols. J Magn Reson Imaging 10:223–232

Tuncbilek N, Karakas HM, Altaner S (2004) Dynamic MRI in indirect estimation of microvessel density, histologic grade, and prognosis in colorectal adenocarcinomas. Abdom Imaging 29:166–172

Turetschek K, Huber S, Floyd E, et al (2001) MR imaging characterization of microvessels in experimental breast tumors by using a particulate contrast agent with histopathologic correlation. Radiology 218:562–569

Wang HZ, Riederer SJ, Lee JN (1987) Optimizing the precision in T1 relaxation estimation using limited flip angles. Magn Res Med 5:399–416

Willett CG, Boucher Y, di Tomaso E, et al (2004) Direct evidence that the VEGF-specific antibody bevacizumab has antivascular effects in human rectal cancer. Nat Med 10: 145–147

Yabuki T, Togami I, Kitagawa T, et al (2003) MR imaging of renal cell carcinoma: associations among signal intensity, tumor enhancement and pathologic findings. Acta Med Okayama 57:179–186

Yoshikawa MI, Ohsumi S, Sugata S, et al (2008) Relation between cancer cellularity and apparent diffusion coefficient values using diffusion weighted magnetic resonance imaging in breast cancer. Radiat Med 26:222–226

Zhang XM, Yu D, Zhang HL, et al (2008) 3D dynamic contrast-enhanced MRI of rectal carcinoma at 3T: correlation with microvascular density and vascular endothelial growth factor markers of tumor angiogenesis. J Magn Reson Imaging 27:1309–1316

Clinical Application

MRI of the Esophagus and Stomach

Angela M. Riddell

CONTENTS

5.1 Introduction 67
5.2 Techniques 69

5.2.1 Patient Preparation 69
5.2.2 Conventional MRI 69
5.2.3 High Resolution MRI 69
5.2.3.1 External Surface Coil 69
5.2.3.2 Endoluminal: Endoscopic and Expandable surface coils 70

5.3 Normal Anatomy on MRI 71
5.3.1 Wall Layers 71
5.3.2 Surrounding Structures 72

5.4 Clinical Application: Staging Malignant Disease 72
5.4.1 T Staging 72
5.4.1.1 Conventional MRI 72
5.4.1.2 High Resolution MRI 73
5.4.2 N Staging 76
5.4.3 Metastatic Disease 77

5.5 Conclusion 78

References 78

KEY POINTS

Advances in MRI technology in recent years with the development of surface coils and faster sequence acquisition times now makes it possible to acquire images at high spatial resolution (small voxel size and field of view) with good signal-to-noise ratio. Different techniques are available for imaging the upper GI tract using either an external surface coil or a modified endoscope with a receiver coil mounted on the tip of the scope. The improved spatial resolution enables visualization of the individual layers of the esophageal and stomach wall, which is not possible when using conventional MRI techniques.

The superior soft tissue contrast of MRI enables identification of tumor separate from the individual wall layers and thus offers an additional method for the local staging of patients with esophageal and gastric cancer. There are some recognized limitations of the current staging techniques, CT, and endoscopic ultrasound (EUS), and it is very likely that these new MRI techniques will play a greater role in the staging of patients with esophageal and gastric cancer in the future.

5.1 Introduction

The role of MRI in the assessment of diseases of the esophagus and stomach continues to evolve. Faster sequences incorporating the use of parallel imaging techniques and improvements in coil technology have overcome some of the initial difficulties encountered due to poor signal-to-noise ratio and motion artifact from peristalsis, heart and respiration. High spatial resolution MRI techniques using either an endoluminal coil or an external surface coil have

Angela M. Riddell, MD FRCS FRCR
The Royal Marsden Hospital NHS Foundation Trust, Fulham Road, London SW3 6JJ, UK

been shown to be able to delineate the individual wall layers, indicating that the technique would be of value in the staging of both esophageal and gastric tumors (Marcos and Semelka 1999; Palmowski et al., 2006; Riddell et al., 2006). The majority of endoluminal work has been performed ex vivo and all techniques are yet to be validated in a large series. Current experience with esophageal and gastric MRI is relatively limited and has mainly focused on local staging of cancer. Some work has also been performed assessing the role of MRI for the assessment of esophageal motility disorders (Panebianco et al. 2006) (see Chap. 6). The focus of this chapter is the development of MRI in the staging of upper GI malignancy. The technique currently remains within the realm of clinical research rather than forming part of the established staging algorithm.

The principal requirements for imaging tumors of the esophagus and stomach are to establish the extent of tumor invasion into the wall, determine tumor resectability by establishing the relationship of the tumor to surrounding anatomical structures (T stage), and to assess nodal involvement (N Stage), Endoscopic ultrasound (EUS) is able to demonstrate the individual esophageal and gastric wall layers. It is currently the investigation of choice for local staging of esophageal cancer enabling definition of the craniocaudal extent of the tumor together with the depth of tumor spread through the wall. The depth of tumor spread is one of the criteria used to determine the need for multimodality therapy; with T1 and T2 tumors mainly being treated with primary surgery and patients with T3 and T4 tumors given pre-operative chemotherapy or chemoradiotherapy. A recent multi-centre study comparing EUS staging in esophageal cancer with CT staging alone demonstrated that EUS provided additional information that changed patient management in one-third of cases. For the majority of cases (85%), EUS up-staged the patients and resulted in less radical treatment (Mortensen et al. 2007). The technique, however, does have some limitations in that there is a limited sonographic range, restricting assessment of the surrounding structures; it is operator-dependent and is unable to differentiate inflammatory change from tumor infiltration. Computed tomography (CT) has limited soft tissue contrast and is not able to demonstrate individual wall layers reliably. Given the limitations of the current local staging techniques and the speed of advancement in MRI technology, it is quite likely that MRI will play a greater role in the work-up of carcinoma of the esophagus and stomach in the future.

For those individuals considered likely to benefit from neoadjuvant therapy prior to surgery (i.e. stage T2N1, T3N0, T3N1), the assessment of treatment response assists in planning the most appropriate future treatment and also provides prognostic information. It has been shown that patients who achieve downstaging or complete response have significantly improved long-term survival (Donahue et al. 2009). CT and EUS rely on a reduction in size to demonstrate response, which clearly occurs over time. PET-CT offers a method of assessing response much more rapidly, as alterations in tumor metabolic activity can occur soon after the commencement of treatment (Mamede et al. 2007; Chuang and Macapinlac 2009). Standard MRI sequences demonstrate a response to treatment both in alteration in tumor size and also changes in signal intensity. Replacement of tumor with fibrosis causes a drop in signal intensity. However, both these features take time to manifest and in order to optimize treatment management ideally, response assessment should be performed at an early stage allowing for swift alterations in therapeutic regimes in patients who are clearly not responding. Dynamic contrast enhanced MRI offers a method of measuring alterations in blood flow and vascular permeability. A pilot study involving five patients with esophageal adenocarcinoma and two controls showed a reduction in the tumor vascular permeability (kTrans) after chemoradiation, suggesting that this may provide a method for assessing early treatment response in the future (Chang et al. 2008).

Between 20 and 30% of patients have metastatic disease at the time of presentation. Multidetector CT has been shown to be highly sensitive for the identification of hepatic and pulmonary metastatic disease (Kuszyk et al. 1996). More recently 2-[fluorine-18] fluoro-2-deoxy-D-glucose positron emission tomography (^{18}FDG-PET) and PET-CT have been evaluated and shown to increase the sensitivity for detecting metastatic disease; this is discussed in more detail in Sect. 5.4.3. The technique is undoubtedly of value in patient selection for radical surgery, where the morbidity from surgery is not insubstantial and it is essential that only those patients who are likely to achieve long-term survival are selected for surgical intervention. The metabolic activity of gastric cancers is variable. The diffuse histological subtype is generally associated with lower FDG avidity and therefore the utility of PET and PET-CT for assessment of gastric cancer is less well established than for esophageal cancer (Mukai et al. 2006).

Staging laparoscopy is advocated for all gastric cancer patients being considered for surgery and for those patients with esophageal cancer that extends below the diaphragm. The microscopic peritoneal deposits are often beyond the resolution of CT and unless the metabolic activity is significantly increased, will not be identified on PET-CT. The presence of ascites on conventional CT has been shown to have a specificity of 97% and sensitivity of 51% for peritoneal dissemination (Yajima et al. 2006). The absence of peritoneal disease determined by a lack of ascites on CT, however, has been shown to have a sensitivity of only 30%, evidence that supports the need for direct inspection of the peritoneum (D'Elia et al. 2000).

Identification of supraclavicular lymph nodes on ultrasound has also been shown to be of value in detecting occult metastatic disease. The addition of a cervical ultrasound to conventional CT staging has been shown to be the most cost-effective method of detecting metastatic disease in patients with esophageal and gastric carcinoma using "decision tree analysis" (van Vliet et al. 2007).

The role of MRI in evaluation of metastatic disease is reserved essentially for the characterization of indeterminate liver lesions detected on CT. The MRI techniques used for local staging of esophageal and gastric cancer use a small field of view and therefore would be restricted to detecting metastatic spread close to the site of primary disease.

5.2
Techniques

5.2.1
Patient Preparation

Patients with tumors confined to the esophagus require no special preparation. Prior to imaging the stomach, patients are starved for 4–6 h, to ensure the stomach is empty. For patients with tumors that extend into the gastro-esophageal junction or arise within the stomach, imaging is optimized by the administration of 500–1,000 mL water to distend the stomach and the administration of an antiperistaltic agent, such as hyoscine bromide, prior to scanning. Dependent upon the location of the tumor within the stomach, the patient will either be positioned prone or supine, to improve tumor visualization.

To reduce cardiac motion artifact when imaging the esophagus and gastro-esophageal junction, ECG gating is often used. The R wave on the ECG is used to trigger each RF pulse. The system can be set to trigger an RF pulse at every second or third R wave, enabling manipulation of the 'effective TR' allowing for both T1- and T2-weighted imaging to be performed.

Particular attention is needed to position the coil when using an external surface coil. The center of the coil must be placed over the tumor to maximize the signal-to-noise ratio achieved. Fast sequences such as single shot T2-weighted sequences reduce the impact of artifact related to respiration, swallowing, and cardiac motion, which can degrade the image achieved using a turbo spin-echo T2-weighted sequence. However, delineation of tumor with respect to the surrounding layers of the esophageal wall is less clearly defined than when using a TSE T2-weighted sequence. Therefore, it is often necessary to use a combination of both types of sequence to optimize the images acquired.

5.2.2
Conventional MRI

Initial studies investigating the use of MRI for the assessment of esophageal cancer used a variety of magnetic field strengths (0.35–1.5 T) with a slice thickness of 3–10 mm. The studies used T1- and T2-weighted images, acquiring images in the axial and sagittal plane with ECG-gating (Quint et al. 1985; Nakashima et al. 1997). MR imaging of the stomach most often uses a combination of T1-weighted spoiled gradient echo with and without contrast enhancement and T2-weighted single shot turbo spin-echo sequences using breath-hold techniques to avoid misregistration errors. The field of view (FOV) used is 400 × 400 mm with a matrix size of 192 × 256 mm and a slice thickness between 8 and 10 mm, giving a voxel size of between 25.96 and 32.45 mm^3. Images are acquired in the axial plane together with sequences perpendicular to the plane of the tumor to asses for resectability (Matsushita et al. 1994; Marcos and Semelka 1999).

5.2.3
High-Resolution MRI

5.2.3.1
External Surface Coil

The advent of multichannel receiver coils has improved the signal-to-noise ratio achieved from structures further removed from the receiver coil.

Table 5.1. Sequence parameters used for High-Resolution MRI using an external surface coil

Parameter	Sagittal TSE T2W	Axial TSE T2W	Axial TSE T2W with cardiac gating	Single shot coronal T2W
FOV (mm)	400	225	250	375
Matrix (mm^2)	263 × 1,024	224 × 256	296 × 512	144 × 256
Slice thickness / gap (mm)	3/0.4	3/0.3	4/0.4	5/1.0
TSE Factorfactor	35	16	24	91
TR (ms)	3,500	3,620	3,000	830
TE (ms)	120	80	90	80
NSA	4	6	8	1

High-resolution images of the esophagus (voxel size between 1.62 and 2.65 mm^3) can be achieved using an external 5-channel cardiac coil and a 1.5-T system (Riddell et al. 2006). The technique uses T2-weighted sequences, the parameters of which are illustrated in Table 5.1. The sagittal sequence enables planning of high-resolution axial images perpendicular to the long axis of the tumor. As a consequence, the depth of extramural extension of disease can be accurately measured and correlated with the corresponding pathology section. The image acquired also depicts the true relationship of tumor to surrounding anatomical structures within the posterior mediastinum.

For tumors at the gastro-esophageal junction, a single-shot coronal T2-weighted sequence is also acquired, which demonstrates the cranio-caudal extent of the tumor and establishes the extension of disease above and below the diaphragmatic hiatus. The distribution of tumor above and below this landmark effectively corresponds to the Siewert and Stein Classification of gastro-esophageal junction (GOJ) tumors (Siewert and Stein 1998): with Type I GOJ tumors located above the hiatus, Type II straddling the hiatus and Type III tumors primarily involving the gastric cardia but extending up to the hiatus. The distinction into subtypes has implications for operative planning, with Type I tumors requiring a thoraco-abdominal approach to achieve an adequate margin on the tumor and mediastinal nodal clearance. Type III tumors are resected from the abdomen alone and generally require a total gastrectomy. The treatment of Type II tumors is variable, but the consensus view is that their biological profile is more akin to Type III tumors and as such that they should be treated in a similar fashion (Siewert et al. 2005). As such, MRI should in the future be able to assist in surgical planning for these patients.

Diffusion-weighted imaging shows some early promise in locally advanced (T3/T4) tumors, showing restricted diffusion (Sakurada et al. 2009). However, this pilot study was not able to detect early tumors. It is hoped that the technique may help to differentiate benign from malignant lymph nodes. It is widely acknowledged that the use of size as a criterion for distinguishing nodal involvement is inadequate, with microscopic foci of disease often being present within nodes considered to be within normal limits for size. Malignant nodes show more restricted diffusion than reactive nodes. However, the results from this pilot study showed overlap between the two groups. Clearly, further research is required to establish the future role of this emerging technique in the evaluation of upper GI malignancy.

5.2.3.2
Endoluminal: Endoscopic and Expandable surface coils

Endoscopic MRI is performed with a receive-only coil mounted on the tip of a standard endoscope. The endoscope contains light and fibreoptic bundles and can be manipulated in multiple directions to allow for precise placement of the coil adjacent to the tumor. In the esophagus, axial images are acquired using a body coil to localize the tip of the MRI endoscope. Once in an optimum position, a balloon attached to the tip of the endoscope is inflated to prevent movement of the endoscope during scanning, due to the action of peristalsis and swallowing.

The inflated balloon also serves to separate the coil from the mucosa by a few millimetres, which improves image quality. The proximity of the coil to the esophagus increases signal-to-noise ratio, enabling a small FOV and thin slice acquisition to be employed, resulting in improved in-plane resolution (voxel size: 0.92–1.46 mm³). As a consequence, the individual layers of the esophageal wall can be identified. Inui et al. were the first to describe the technique in the esophagus and stomach. They were able to depict the three main wall layers (INUI et al. 1995). Further studies have shown that disruption of the wall layers due to the presence of tumor correlates with pathological T stage (FELDMAN et al. 1997; KULLING et al. 1998; DAVE et al. 2004). The endoscopic technique has recognized limitations, namely the inability of the coil to traverse strictures, limiting the use for the evaluation of esophageal cancers; a short radius for receiving signal (3–4 cm), which necessitates repositioning of the endoscope for evaluation of long tumors, increasing the overall scan time; and the action of peristalsis resulting in motion artifact within the images acquired and possible coil migration.

There are limited studies investigating MR endoscopy of the stomach in vivo, Inui et al. assessed 24 patients with gastric disorders, using spoiled gradient echo breath-hold sequences and spin-echo T1- and T2-weighted sequences without breath holding, achieving adequate images is 14 (58%) patients (INUI et al. 1995). Subsequent studies have focused on in vitro assessment, which allows for optimum coil positioning close to the site of the tumor and clearly overcomes the difficulty of motion artifact (KULLING et al. 1997).

The most recent in vitro work has focused on a self-expanding loop coil. The coil consists of a foldable and self-expanding receiver loop and is composed of nitinol, a flexible "memory wire", which passes through a specifically designed MR compatible endoscope. It is covered with silicone, to prevent direct contact of the metal with the stomach wall. The coil enables high-resolution imaging of the primary tumor because of its location adjacent to the tumor and since the diameter of the coil (8 cm) is much larger than the endoscopic MR increasing the radius for receiving signal from 3–4 cm to 8 cm. This allows for both detailed analysis of the depth of tumor invasion through the layers of the stomach wall and assessment of involvement of the gastric serosa and surrounding tissues (HEYE et al. 2006). A combination of T1- and T2-weighted TSE and gradient sequences were used with a 220-mm FOV, 3–4 mm slice thickness, and a voxel size between 0.13 and 2.2 mm³.

5.3
Normal Anatomy on MRI

5.3.1
Wall Layers

The individual layers of the esophageal wall are only visualized when high spatial resolution techniques are employed using small FOV, thin slice imaging with either an endoluminal coil or an external surface coil. Ex vivo and in vivo studies of the esophagus have demonstrated that spin-echo T2-weighted sequences provide optimum visualization of the esophageal wall layers. The ex vivo studies by Yamada et al. demonstrated up to 8 layers of the esophageal wall with a spin-echo T2-weighted sequence (YAMADA et al. 2001). This study was performed using a 1.5-T system and an external surface coil, with a sequence acquisition time of 34 minutes. where as three layers corresponding to the mucosa (intermediate signal), submucosa (high signal) and muscularis propria (intermediate to low signal) have been demonstrated by in vivo studies, again using a T2-weighted sequence (Fig. 5.1) (RIDDELL et al. 2006).

The spatial resolution achieved using conventional MRI with a phased array body coil is insufficient to consistently demonstrate individual stomach wall layers on either T1- or T2-weighted imaging. In vivo studies employing a high-resolution technique using an endoluminal coil have been able to demonstrate the main component layers of the stomach wall: the mucosa (low signal intensity), submucosa (low or high signal intensity, dependent on the sequence parameters), and muscularis propria (low signal intensity) on both T1- and T2-weighted sequences (INUI et al. 1995). Experimental work on ex vivo specimens using either endoluminal or external surface coil techniques have consistently shown three to five stomach wall layers on T1- and T2-weighted sequences (YAMADA et al. 2001; HEYE et al. 2006). The muscularis propria layer is either depicted as a single low signal intensity layer or can appear as three distinct layers: the inner circular muscle (low signal intensity), high signal interposed connective tissue and the outer longitudinal muscle layer (low signal intensity). As with esophageal imaging, further development is necessary to be able to achieve such high spatial resolution in vivo, particularly as the sequence acquisition time would need to be reduced from the 20 min used in these studies to between 6 and 7 min for realistic clinical application.

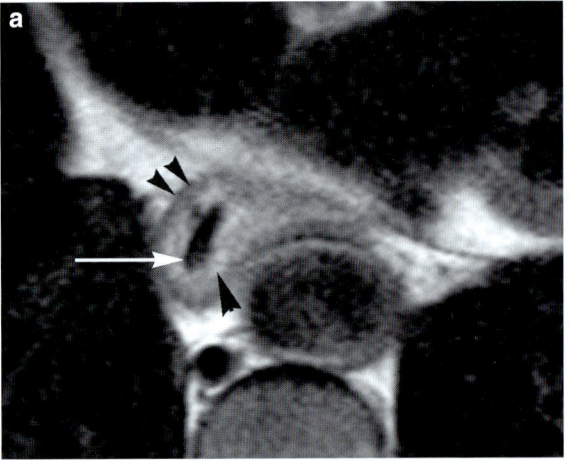

Fig. 5.1. The appearance of normal esophageal wall layers. The axial T2-weighted MRI image, (**a**) using an external surface cardiac coil demonstrates the individual layers of the esophageal wall: the intermediate signal mucosa (*arrow*), the high signal submucosa (*single arrow head*) and the outer muscularis propria layer (*double arrow heads*). The individual layers are confirmed on the corresponding histology section (**b**)

5.3.2
Surrounding Structures

The multiplanar capability of MRI allows assessment of the relationship of tumors within esophagus and stomach to the surrounding anatomical structures, enabling assessment of tumor resectability. Multidetector CT (MDCT) also allows for the reformatting of images in multiplanes and has improved the prediction of tumor resectability (ONBAS et al. 2006). However, the superior soft tissue contrast achieved using MRI would suggest that MRI is very likely to be able to depict the individual soft tissues structures with more clarity than CT, particularly when structures lie in direct contact with no interposing fat plane.

The high-resolution MRI appearances of structures within the posterior mediastinum surrounding the esophagus have been described. The right pleural reflection which, for part of its length, lies in direct contact with the esophagus has been demonstrated on both in vivo and ex vivo studies (RIDDELL et al. 2006; RIDDELL et al. 2007). Other anatomical structures that are of importance in the assessment of resectability have been clearly demonstrated on high-resolution MRI and correlated with the corresponding histological wholemount sections. Figure 5.2 demonstrates the normal esophagus and its relationship to the thoracic duct, azygos vein, right pleura, and the fascial attachment extending from the esophagus to the descending thoracic aorta on MRI.

Similarly for the stomach, the multi-planar capability enables assessment of the relationship of the stomach to the pancreas, left lobe of the liver, and transverse colon.

5.4
Clinical Application: Staging Malignant Disease

5.4.1
T Staging

5.4.1.1
Conventional MRI

The majority of early studies comparing conventional MRI with CT have shown no advantage to using MRI for the local staging of esophageal or gastric carcinoma. This is mainly because the studies used low spatial resolution techniques, which were unable to delineate the individual wall layers and used similar criteria for T staging and assessment of resectability as used for CT (LEHR et al. 1988; TAKASHIMA et al. 1991; WU et al. 2003). The accuracy for predicting resectability based on detection of tumor invasion of the aorta, tracheobronchial tree, pericardium, or the presence of metastatic disease has been reported to be 87% for MRI when compared with 84% for CT (TAKASHIMA et al. 1991). The overall T staging accuracy for EUS is between 80 and 90%, but is lower for

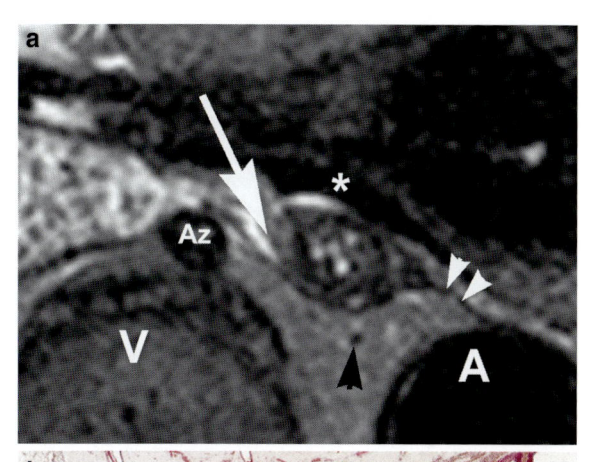

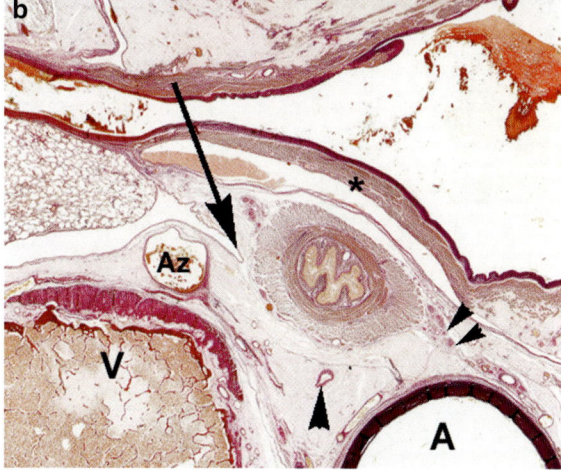

Fig. 5.2. The relationship of the lower esophagus to surrounding structures The axial T2-weighted MR image, (**a**) demonstrates the close relationship of the lower esophagus to the right parietal pleura (*arrow*). On the left side, a fine fascial layer attaches the lower esophagus and is attached to the anterior aspect of the aortic adventitia (*double arrow heads*). The *asterisk* denotes part of the posterior myocardium of the left atrium, the oblique sinus of the pericardium is interposed between this and the esophagus. The thoracic duct is located posterior to the esophagus (*single arrow head*). The descending thoracic aorta (*A*), the vertebral body (*V*), and azygos vein (*Az*) are also marked. The structures are confirmed on the corresponding histology wholemount section (**b**). Images reprinted with kind permission from AJR (Riddell et al 2007)

tumors greater than 5 cm in length. The larger tumors are most often understaged, possibly due to poor visualization of the most stenotic part of the tumor, as the endoscope is pulled through the stenosis and suddenly passes through the stenotic area preventing full interrogation (HEEREN et al. 2004).

In the case of evaluation of gastric carcinoma, the individual layers of the gastric wall, like the esophageal wall, cannot be depicted using conventional MRI techniques. Attention has been focused on the potential of conventional MRI to differentiate disease confined within the serosa (T2) and extraserosal (T3) disease. Studies have used a contrast-enhanced spoiled gradient recalled acquisition (GRASS) to detect extraserosal extension of disease. Classification of the degree of serosal invasion has been based on the presence or absence of a low-signal-intensity band around the tumor. The low signal-intensity band disappears or shows irregularity in an area of extraserosal invasion. Using this criterion, studies with 48 and 37 patients have reported an overall accuracy of 88–93% for predicting the presence of extra-serosal disease (MATSUSHITA et al. 1994; OI et al. 1997). A further prospective study of 26 patients with biopsy-proven advanced gastric cancer has shown a slight superiority of MRI for T staging over helical CT: with a T staging accuracy 81% compared with 73%; $p < 0.05$. This was mainly due to the superior soft tissue contrast of MRI being able to differentiate contact with surrounding structures (T3) from direct invasion (T4) (KIM et al. 2000).

5.4.1.2
High-Resolution MRI

The use of high-resolution techniques using either an external surface coil or an endoluminal coil enables more detailed staging of both esophageal and gastric cancer. The technique enables delineation of the individual layers of the wall allowing for detection and staging of early tumors that are confined to the wall.

T Staging Using an External Surface Coil

An external surface coil overcomes the difficulty of traversing bulky esophageal tumors encountered with endoscopic techniques (EUS and endoluminal MRI). The inability to traverse bulky tumors prevents full assessment of the potential radial margin and distal extent of disease in up to 20% of tumors, using a standard EUS probe (WAKELIN et al. 2002).

Using a fast spin-echo T2-weighted sequence, tumor returns intermediate signal intensity, which can be differentiated from the adjacent normal layers of the esophageal wall (RIDDELL et al. 2007). Figures 5.3 and 5.4 illustrate the appearance of T2 and T3 tumors on MRI using this technique with pathological correlation. This allows for the staging of tumors confined to the wall (stages T1 and T2) as well as those

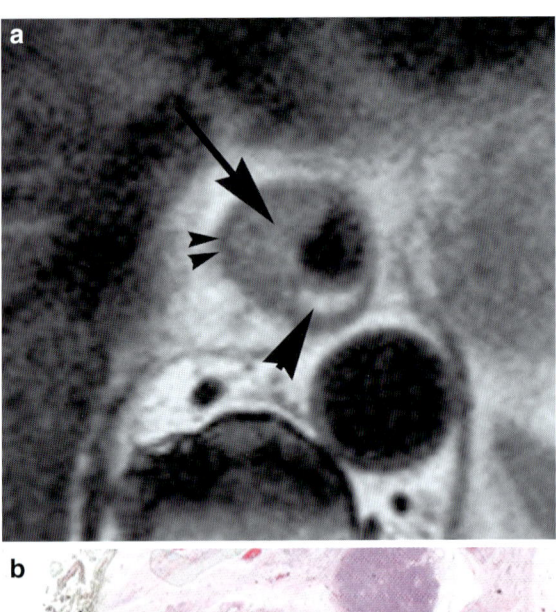

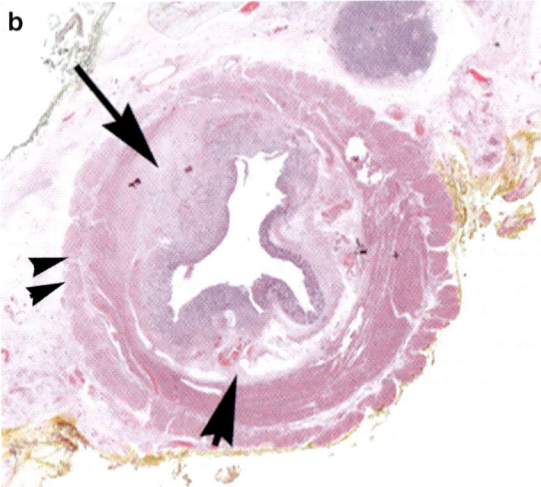

Fig. 5.3. Stage T2 esophageal cancer. The axial T2-weighted MR image (**a**) which demonstrates tumor (*arrow*) involving the right side of the esophageal wall. The outer margin of the muscularis propria layer remains in tact (*double arrow heads*) indicating that tumor is confined to the esophageal wall and is therefore staged as T2. The normal layers of the esophageal wall are preserved on the left side (*arrow head*). The findings are confirmed on the corresponding histology section (**b**)

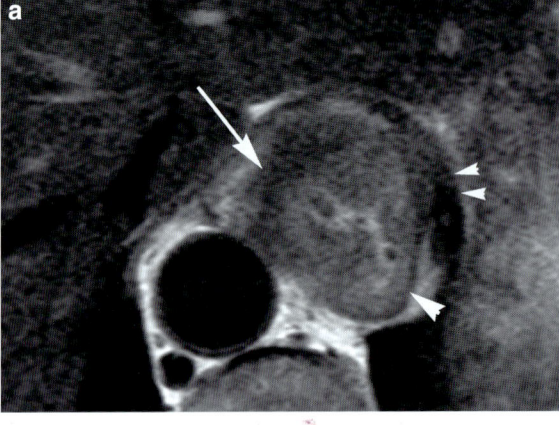

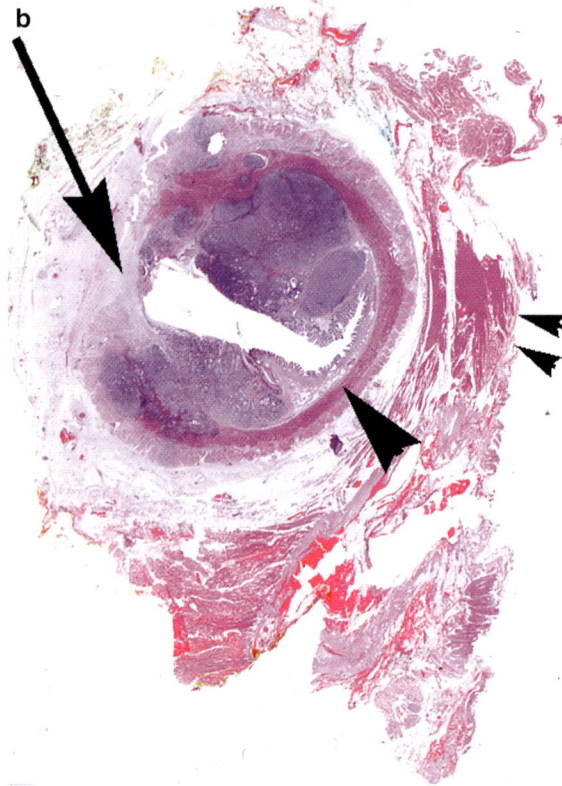

Fig. 5.4. Stage T3 esophageal cancer. The axial T2-weighted MR image (**a**) demonstrates irregularity of the outer margin of the esophageal wall on the right side with extension of intermediate signal tumor beyond the wall into the periesophageal tissues (*arrow*). The normal layers of the esophageal wall are preserved on the left side (*single arrow head*). Part of the diaphragmatic crus is seen anterior to the esophagus and was removed en bloc with the esophagus (*double arrow heads*). Tumor lies close to the aortic adventitia posteriorly and reflection of the right parietal pleura and in this case is of similar signal intensity. Dynamic evaluation of this area on the workstation indicated that there was not direct invasion. The corresponding histology section confirms the findings (**b**)

extending through the wall into the periesophageal tissues (T3 disease). The accuracy of preoperative T staging with EUS has been documented between 80 and 90% (VICKERS and ALDERSON 1998). Currently, there are no published data directly comparing the accuracy of T staging using this high-resolution technique when compared with EUS.

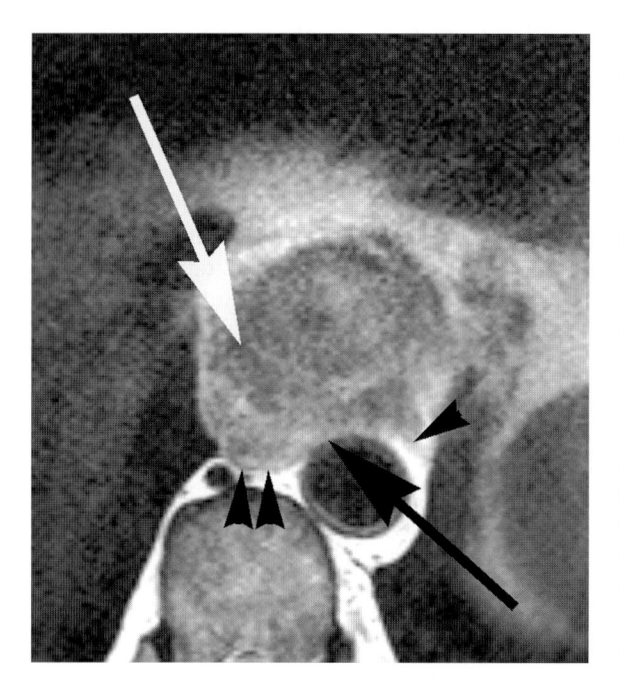

Fig. 5.5. Unresectable T4 tumor. The axial T2-weighted image demonstrates extensive tumor within the periesophageal fat (*white arrow*), beyond the outer margin of the muscularis propria. Posteriorly, the tumor infiltrates the right and left pleural reflections (*double and single arrow heads*, respectively) and the aortic adventitia (*black arrow*)

Assessment of Resectability

Using an FOV 225–250 mm, the periesophageal tissues are clearly demonstrated, enabling assessment of the relationship of the tumor to surrounding structures. Tumor has been shown to return different signal intensities to the surrounding structures and therefore differentiation can be made between tumor lying in contact with a surrounding structure (T3 disease) and actual direct invasion of the structure (T4 disease). As such, MRI is very likely to be able to be more accurate in determining the resectability of tumor than CT, which has limited soft tissue contrast. Figure 5.5 demonstrates the appearance of a locally advanced esophageal tumor on MRI, which demonstrates infiltration into the aortic adventitia. The criteria used to determine resectability using MRI is that there should be a margin of greater than or equal to 1 mm between the tumor and a surrounding structure not resected at the time of surgery. This correlates with the pathological definition of an R0 resection: tumor greater than 1 mm from the surgical resection margin.

Although it remains a challenge to differentiate infiltration of tumor into surrounding structures when compared with simple contact, the superior soft tissue contrast of MRI allows clearer definition of tissue planes. Tumor obliterating tissue planes, such as the aortic adventitia (as in Fig. 5.5), the pericardium or pleura is highly suggestive of tumor infiltration.

The ultrasound frequencies used for EUS in general are 7.5 and 12 MHz, giving a maximum depth of view of 7 and 3 cm, respectively. However, studies have shown that there are shortcomings in the ability of EUS to evaluate the relationship of tumor to the surrounding structures and as such predict resectability. A tumor is considered resectable based on achieving an R0 resection (that is tumor greater than 1 mm away from the circumferential surgical resection margin), using EUS the rate of a positive circumferential resection margin is between 31 and 47% (DEXTER et al. 2001; DAVIES et al. 2006; SUJENDRAN et al. 2008). This may in part be due to tumor extending beyond the sonographic range of EUS or alternatively due to assessment of the outer margin of the tumor being made at a tangential rather than perpendicular view leading to inaccuracies in interpretation. High-resolution MRI may in the future offer a more robust, reproducible method for assessment of the outer margin of the tumor, although further evaluation of the technique is required to establish its role in clinical practice. The high resolution MRI technique using an external surface coil has not as yet been used to evaluate gastric carcinoma.

T Staging Using an Endoluminal Surface Coil

The majority of studies assessing both esophageal and gastric carcinoma using endoluminal MRI have been ex vivo. In vivo work is limited: one pilot study showed accurate T stage correlation with pathology in 6/7 patients with esophageal cancer (DAVE et al. 2004). Another study showed correct T stage with endoluminal MRI in eight of the nine tumors. One Tis tumor was staged as T1 tumor because of submucosal edema (STOKER et al. 1999). Further studies have confirmed that disruption of the wall layers correlates with T stage, although again the study groups were small in size with limited pathological correlation (FELDMAN et al. 1997; KULLING et al. 1998). The endoscopic technique has recognized limitations, namely the inability of the coil to traverse strictures, limiting the use for the evaluation of esophageal cancers; a short radius for receiving signal (3–4 cm), which necessitates repositioning of the endoscope for evaluation of long tumors, increasing the overall scan time; and the action of peristalsis resulting in motion artifact within the images acquired and possible coil migration. The short radius for receiving signal also prevents full evaluation of the perioesophageal tissues using the endoluminal coil. Assessment of resectability can only be made with sequences using a body coil and a large FOV, reducing the achievable spatial resolution. Potentially, in the future the endoluminal technique could be combined with high-resolution MR imaging using an external surface coil. Although in practice the endoluminal technique offers little advantage over the external surface coil, which clearly has the benefit of being noninvasive.

Ex vivo studies using surface coils have been able to achieve high levels of accuracy for T staging esophageal and gastric cancer – both early and advanced types. Yamada et al. demonstrated a T staging accuracy of 94% when assessing 67 esophageal specimens containing 70 squamous cell carcinomas using a 4-cm surface coil in a 4.7-T system (Yamada et al. 1997). Further work by the same group using a 1.5-T system has confirmed the potential for the technique to accurately stage early oesophageal cancer ex vivo. Using a T2-weighted high-resolution sequence, the depth of tumor invasion on MRI was shown to correlate with histology in 39/41 cases (accuracy 95%), including 11 cases of early esophageal cancer where the tumor was confined to the mucosal or submucosal layer (Yamada et al. 2001). The high spatial resolution enables demonstration of up to eight layers of the esophageal wall but this reduces the range for receiving signal, limiting assessment to tumor confined to the esophageal wall.

For gastric carcinoma, the in vivo experience using endoscopic MRI is limited. It has proved challenging to achieve adequate visualization of the tumor consistently, as it is difficult to maintain the coil in the correct position to image the tumor. In 15 patients with gastric cancer investigated using the technique (mainly T3 and T4 tumors), 9 (60%) were adequately visualized (Inui et al. 1995). The images obtained using MRI were not considered to be as clear as the corresponding EUS images, with the MR images being degraded by motion artifact. The technique also involved long acquisition times (8 min to obtain a T2-weighted sequence with 8–12 images) and the coil has a short signal range limiting assessment of tumor resectability. The main advantage of the technique is its ability to obtain images in multipleplanes. Given the fact that multiplanar reformats are now achievable using multidetector CT, the technique will require further development before it has a confirmed role in clinical practice.

Ex vivo studies using endoluminal surface coils to stage gastric cancer have shown good correlation with pathology and the spatial resolution achieved enables staging of both early and advanced gastric tumors (Dux et al. 1997). A recent development has been the design of an expandable surface coil in an attempt to overcome the difficulty of imaging large tumors in their entirety, due to limitation in the FOV with small surface coils. The expandable coils have a diameter of 8 cm and as such have a larger FOV (10 cm) at maintained high spatial resolution. The initial study using this technology in 28 surgical specimens using T1-weighted, T2-weighted, and opposed phased sequences demonstrated 75% accuracy for T staging with 80% sensitivity for detecting serosal involvement (Heye et al. 2006).

5.4.2
N Staging

The presence of involved lymph nodes in both esophageal and gastric carcinoma is acknowledged to be an independent predictor of poor prognosis. It has been shown that for esophageal cancer that the survival rate is significantly reduced if greater than 10% of the lymph nodes harvested are involved (Hagen et al. 2001; Eloubeidi et al. 2002). The proportion of lymph nodes involved for gastric cancer already forms part of the TNM staging classification, with patients with greater than six nodes involved being staged as N2 (AJCC 2002). Therefore, to stratify patients into high-risk groups in the pre-operative setting, imaging must be able to identify involved lymph nodes with a high degree of accuracy.

In general, periesophageal and subdiaphragmatic lymph nodes greater than 10 mm are considered pathological (>8 mm in the gastro-hepatic ligament). Using these criteria, the specificity for nodal detection is high, but the sensitivity is low as it is recognized that metastatic infiltration occurs in smaller-sized lymph nodes. As a consequence, overall accuracy for nodal staging using CT ranges from 45 to 88% (Gore et al. 2004; Castillo and Lawler 2005). Similar rates of accuracy have been quoted for conventional MRI for N staging of both esophageal and gastric cancers (Sohn et al. 2000; Wu et al. 2003), which is unsurprising as the same imaging criteria were applied to MRI assessment as for CT. FDG-PET has a variable accuracy for detecting nodal involvement ranging from 24 to 82%, due to the difficulty differentiating malignant from inflammatory nodes. The spatial resolution has improved with the incorporation of FDG-PET-CT fusion, but still differentiating periesophageal lymph nodes lying in proximity to the primary tumor remains problematic (Rasanen et al. 2003; Chowdhury et al. 2008).

The accuracy for preoperative lymph node staging with EUS is 60–80% (Vickers and Alderson 1998). EUS uses the morphology of lymph nodes for classification rather than basing the evaluation on size criteria. Hyperechoic, heterogeneous, flat, or oval lymph nodes on EUS are considered benign. Malignant lymph nodes are round, hypoechoic, homogeneous masses, which are more clearly defined than benign nodes (Richards et al. 2000). It is also possible using specific EUS probes (curved linear array) to obtain fine-needle aspiration (FNA) samples from suspicious lymph nodes. One large series demonstrated EUS-FNA sensitivity, specificity, and accuracy for the evaluation of malignant lymph nodes to be 92, 93, and 92%, respectively (Wiersema et al. 1997). The procedure, however, is time-consuming and the ultrasound probe used is regarded as being less suited to staging than the convention endoscopes with radial ultrasound probes. Therefore, patients require an initial staging EUS with a radial probe and a repeat EUS using a linear array probe for the FNA, adding time and complexity to the procedure. This technique is also limited to nodes somewhat removed from the primary tumor, to prevent sample contamination if the needle passes through the primary tumor prior to needle puncture of the lymph node.

Using high spatial resolution MRI techniques ex vivo, the sensitivity and specificity for detecting involved lymph nodes in the perigastric tissues have been shown to be 87% and 60%, respectively. T1-weighted sequences were best able to detect the lymph nodes. Malignant nodes were oval in shape and had similar signal intensity (low signal) to the primary tumor, although the signal intensity did vary (Dux et al. 1997). Using endoscopic MRI limits assessment of lymph nodes to those within 3 cm of the primary tumor, due to the limited signal range using this technique (Inui et al. 1995). For patients with esophageal cancer, there has been no formal comparison of N staging using an external surface coil with EUS and CT. An initial study suggests that there is an increased likelihood of node positive disease in patients with nodular densities greater than 2 mm within the periosophageal fat, although specific nodal mapping has not been performed in the study (Riddell et al. 2007). In an ex vivo study of nine specimen, endoluminal MRI with a 10-mm receive only coil detected 35 of 91 lymph nodes (Stoker et al. 1999). Using a 5-mm cut-off, 14 were true-positives, 5 were false-positives, 1 was a false-negative, and 15 were true-negatives. The majority of the 56 missed lymph nodes (including seven nodes with metastatic involvement) were outside the FOV. TN classification was correct in six specimens (67%).

Some recent work has focused on the use of ultrasmall iron oxide particles with MRI in an attempt to help characterize lymph nodes in the preoperative setting. Ultrasmall particles of iron oxide (USPIO) are taken up by macrophages within normal lymph nodes and return low signal intensity on T2-weighted imaging. Lymph nodes infiltrated with tumor do not take up the iron oxide and return high signal. For upper gastrointestinal cancer, there is limited published research in the use of USPIOs. Small group studies have illustrated its potential for predicting lymph node involvement and its ability to estimate the extent of nodal spread, although the results will need confirmation in larger studies (Imano et al. 2004; Ishiyama et al. 2006; Nishimura et al. 2006).

5.4.3
Metastatic Disease

The role of MRI in the detection of metastatic disease from both esophageal and gastric carcinoma is mainly confined to the characterization of focal liver lesions detected on CT (Namasivayam et al. 2007). MRI has been shown to be superior to CT in both detection and characterization of small liver lesions (0.5–1.5 mm) (Reimer et al. 2000; Rappeport and Loft 2007). The importance of characterizing these lesions has been emphasized by research showing that only 50% liver lesions less than 1.5 cm will be malignant (Jones et al. 1992). Full characterization of these lesions with dynamic gadolinium-enhanced MRI and delayed phase imaging helps one to ensure that patients are not denied radical, potentially curative treatment on the basis of an indeterminate liver lesion identified on CT being considered malignant.

[18]FDG-PET-CT has been shown to detect occult metastases in approximately 14–20% of patients considered potentially resectable by conventional CT and EUS staging (Heeren et al. 2004; Kato et al. 2005). The early reported studies involved small patient numbers or limited pathological correlation and a recently published prospective multicenter trial, which evaluated 189 patients considered operable by conventional staging demonstrated only 9 patients (4.8%) to be upstaged

by PET (Meyers et al. 2007). There were 18 other patients who were considered to have M1b disease, which was not confirmed with pathology. In addition, the study highlighted some limitations of the technique, with 7/145 (5%) false-negative predictions with patients identified with metastatic disease at surgery; and 5/189 (2.6%) patients were confirmed to have a false-positive PET. In spite of these limitations, there is likely to be an increase in the use of PET-CT for the identification of metastatic disease.

The detection of peritoneal spread is a challenge for all imaging modalities, with small volume disease often being beyond the spatial resolution of even the most advanced multidetector CT. It is possible to identify peritoneal infiltration using MRI. Sequences using fat suppression and dynamic gadolinium show enhancement and nodularity of the peritoneum (see Chap. 15). The most sensitive method for detecting peritoneal disease, however, is under direct vision at laparoscopy.

5.5 Conclusion

Currently, the role of MRI in the work of patients diagnosed with upper GI cancer remains limited and within the realm of clinical research. In the future, it is likely to play a more pivotal role, particularly in the local staging of patients with esophageal cancer. Further sequence development for both T2-weighted sequences and diffusion are likely to result in improved image quality. MRI will offer an accurate method for local staging and also demonstrating the cranio-caudal extent of disease, which aids planning for either radiotherapy or surgery. Future developments may also target methods of assessing treatment response either by monitoring alterations in dynamic contrast enhancement parameters or the apparent diffusion coefficient (ADC) values. The ultimate aim being to use MRI to improve the work-up of these patients, to individualize treatment strategies, optimize chemotherapeutic regimes, and ensure that radical surgery is reserved for patients who are likely to achieve long-term survival.

References

AJCC (2002) Cancer staging handbook. TNM classification of malignant tumours. Springer, Berlin
Castillo E, Lawler LP (2005) Diagnostic radiology and nuclear medicine. J Surg Oncol 92(3):191–202
Chang EY, Li X, et al (2008) The evaluation of esophageal adenocarcinoma using dynamic contrast-enhanced magnetic resonance imaging. J Gastrointest Surg 12(1):166–175
Chowdhury FU, Bradley KM, et al (2008) The role of 18F-FDG PET/CT in the evaluation of oesophageal carcinoma. Clin Radiol 63(12):1297–1309
Chuang HH, Macapinlac HA (2009) The evolving role of PET-CT in the management of esophageal cancer. Q J Nucl Med Mol Imaging 53(2):201–209
D'Elia F, Zingarelli A, et al (2000) Hydro-dynamic CT preoperative staging of gastric cancer: correlation with pathological findings. A prospective study of 107 cases. Eur Radiol 10(12):1877–1885
Dave UR, Williams AD, et al (2004) Esophageal cancer staging with endoscopic MR imaging: pilot study. Radiology 230(1):281–286
Davies AR, Deans DA, et al (2006) The multidisciplinary team meeting improves staging accuracy and treatment selection for gastro-esophageal cancer. Dis Esophagus 19(6):496–503
Dexter SP, Sue-Ling H, et al (2001) Circumferential resection margin involvement: an independent predictor of survival following surgery for oesophageal cancer. Gut 48(5):667–670
Donahue JM, Nichols FC, et al (2009) Complete pathologic response after neoadjuvant chemoradiotherapy for esophageal cancer is associated with enhanced survival. Ann Thorac Surg 87(2):392–398; discussion 398–399
Dux M, Roeren T, et al (1997) MRI for staging of gastric carcinoma: first results of an experimental prospective study. J Comput Assist Tomogr 21(1):66–72
Eloubeidi MA, Desmond R, et al (2002) Prognostic factors for the survival of patients with esophageal carcinoma in the U.S.: the importance of tumor length and lymph node status. Cancer 95(7):1434–1443
Feldman DR, Kulling DP, et al (1997) MR endoscopy: preliminary experience in human trials. Radiology 202(3):868–870
Gore R, Yaghami V, et al (2004). Oesophageal cancer. In: Husband JE, Reznek R (eds) Imaging in oncology, vol 1. Taylor and Francis, London, pp 159–187
Hagen JA, DeMeester SR, et al (2001) Curative resection for esophageal adenocarcinoma: analysis of 100 en bloc esophagectomies. Ann Surg 234(4):520–530; discussion 530–531
Heeren PA, Jager PL, et al (2004) Detection of distant metastases in esophageal cancer with (18)F-FDG PET. J Nucl Med 45(6):980–987
Heeren PA, van Westreenen HL, et al (2004) Influence of tumor characteristics on the accuracy of endoscopic ultrasonography in staging cancer of the esophagus and esophagogastric junction. Endoscopy 36(11):966–971
Heye T, Kuntz C, et al (2006) New coil concept for endoluminal MR imaging: initial results in staging of gastric carcinoma in correlation with histopathology. Eur Radiol 16(11):2401–2409
Imano H, Motoyama S, et al (2004) Superior mediastinal and neck lymphatic mapping in mid- and lower-thoracic esophageal cancer as defined by ferumoxides-enhanced magnetic resonance imaging. Jpn J Thorac Cardiovasc Surg 52(10):445–450
Inui K, Nakazawa S, et al (1995) Endoscopic MRI: preliminary results of a new technique for visualization and staging of gastrointestinal tumors. Endoscopy 27(7):480–485.

Ishiyama K, Motoyama S, et al (2006) Visualization of lymphatic basin from the tumor using magnetic resonance lymphography with superparamagnetic iron oxide in patients with thoracic esophageal cancer. J Comput Assist Tomogr 30(2):270–275

Jones EC, Chezmar JL, et al (1992) The frequency and significance of small (less than or equal to 15 mm) hepatic lesions detected by CT. AJR Am J Roentgenol 158(3):535–539

Kato H, Miyazaki T, et al (2005) The incremental effect of positron emission tomography on diagnostic accuracy in the initial staging of esophageal carcinoma. Cancer 103(1):148–156

Kim AY, Han JK, et al (2000) MRI in staging advanced gastric cancer: is it useful compared with spiral CT? J Comput Assist Tomogr 24(3):389–394

Kulling D, Bohning DE, et al (1997) Histological correlates to pig gastrointestinal wall layers imaged in vitro with the magnetic resonance endoscope. Gastroenterology 112(5):1568–1574

Kulling D, Feldman DR, et al (1998) Local staging of esophageal cancer using endoscopic magnetic resonance imaging: prospective comparison with endoscopic ultrasound. Endoscopy 30(9):745–749

Kuszyk BS, Bluemke DA, et al (1996) Portal-phase contrast-enhanced helical CT for the detection of malignant hepatic tumors: sensitivity based on comparison with intraoperative and pathologic findings. AJR Am J Roentgenol 166(1):91–95

Lehr L, Rupp N, et al (1988) Assessment of resectability of esophageal cancer by computed tomography and magnetic resonance imaging. Surgery 103(3):344–350

Mamede M, Abreu ELP, et al (2007) FDG-PET/CT tumor segmentation-derived indices of metabolic activity to assess response to neoadjuvant therapy and progression-free survival in esophageal cancer: correlation with histopathology results. Am J Clin Oncol 30(4):377–388

Marcos HB, Semelka RC (1999) Stomach diseases: MR evaluation using combined t2-weighted single-shot echo train spin-echo and gadolinium-enhanced spoiled gradient-echo sequences. J Magn Reson Imaging 10(6):950–960

Matsushita M, Oi H, et al (1994) Extraserosal invasion in advanced gastric cancer: evaluation with MR imaging. Radiology 192(1):87–91.

Meyers BF, Downey RJ, et al (2007) The utility of positron emission tomography in staging of potentially operable carcinoma of the thoracic esophagus: results of the American College of Surgeons Oncology Group Z0060 trial. J Thorac Cardiovasc Surg 133(3):738–745

Mortensen MB, Edwin B, et al (2007) Impact of endoscopic ultrasonography (EUS) on surgical decision-making in upper gastrointestinal tract cancer: an international multicenter study. Surg Endosc 21(3):431–438

Mukai K, Ishida Y, et al (2006) Usefulness of preoperative FDG-PET for detection of gastric cancer. Gastric Cancer 9(3):192–196

Nakashima A, Nakashima K, et al (1997) Thoracic esophageal carcinoma: evaluation in the sagittal section with magnetic resonance imaging. Abdom Imaging 22(1):20–23

Namasivayam S, Martin DR, et al (2007) Imaging of liver metastases: MRI. Cancer Imaging 7:2–9

Nishimura H, Tanigawa N, et al (2006) Preoperative esophageal cancer staging: magnetic resonance imaging of lymph node with ferumoxtran-10, an ultrasmall superparamagnetic iron oxide. J Am Coll Surg 202(4):604–611

Oi H, Matsushita M, et al (1997) Dynamic MR imaging for extraserosal invasion of advanced gastric cancer. Abdom Imaging 22(1):35–40

Onbas O, Eroglu A, et al (2006) Preoperative staging of esophageal carcinoma with multidetector CT and virtual endoscopy. Eur J Radiol 57(1):90–95

Palmowski M, Grenacher L, et al (2006) Magnetic resonance imaging for local staging of gastric carcinoma: results of an in vitro study. J Comput Assist Tomogr 30(6):896–902

Panebianco V, Tomei E, et al (2006) Functional MRI in the evaluation of oesophageal motility: feasibility, MRI patterns of normality, and preliminary experience in subjects with motility disorders. Radiol Med 111(7):881–889

Quint LE, Glazer GM, et al (1985) Esophageal imaging by MR and CT: study of normal anatomy and neoplasms. Radiology 156(3):727–731

Rappeport ED, Loft A (2007) Liver metastases from colorectal cancer: imaging with superparamagnetic iron oxide (SPIO)-enhanced MR imaging, computed tomography and positron emission tomography. Abdom Imaging 32(5):624–634

Rasanen JV, Sihvo EI, et al (2003) Prospective analysis of accuracy of positron emission tomography, computed tomography, and endoscopic ultrasonography in staging of adenocarcinoma of the esophagus and the esophagogastric junction. Ann Surg Oncol 10(8):954–960

Reimer P, Jahnke N, et al (2000) Hepatic lesion detection and characterization: value of nonenhanced MR imaging, superparamagnetic iron oxide-enhanced MR imaging, and spiral CT-ROC analysis. Radiology 217(1):152–158

Richards DG, Brown TH, et al (2000) Endoscopic ultrasound in the staging of tumours of the oesophagus and gastro-oesophageal junction. Ann R Coll Surg Engl 82(5):311–317

Riddell AM, Allum WH, et al (2007) The appearances of oesophageal carcinoma demonstrated on high-resolution, T2-weighted MRI, with histopathological correlation. Eur Radiol 17(2):391–399

Riddell AM, Davies DC, et al (2007) High-resolution MRI in evaluation of the surgical anatomy of the esophagus and posterior mediastinum. AJR Am J Roentgenol 188(1):W37–W43

Riddell AM, Hillier J, et al (2006) Potential of surface-coil MRI for staging of esophageal cancer. AJR Am J Roentgenol 187(5):1280–1287

Riddell AM, Richardson C, et al (2006) The development and optimization of high spatial resolution MRI for imaging the oesophagus using an external surface coil. Br J Radiol 79(947):873–879

Sakurada A, Takahara T, et al (2009) Diagnostic performance of diffusion-weighted magnetic resonance imaging in esophageal cancer. Eur Radiol 19(6):1461–1469

Siewert JR, Feith M, et al (2005) Biologic and clinical variations of adenocarcinoma at the esophago-gastric junction: relevance of a topographic-anatomic subclassification. J Surg Oncol 90(3):139–146; discussion 146

Siewert JR, Stein HJ (1998) Classification of adenocarcinoma of the oesophagogastric junction. Br J Surg 85(11):1457–1459

Sohn KM, Lee JM, et al (2000) Comparing MR imaging and CT in the staging of gastric carcinoma. AJR Am J Roentgenol 174(6):1551–1557

Stoker J, van Velthuysen ML, van Overhagen H, van Kempen D, Tilanus HW, Laméris JS (1999) Esophageal carcinoma. Ex vivo endoluminal magnetic resonance imaging. Invest Radiol 34:58–64

Sujendran V, Wheeler J, et al (2008) Effect of neoadjuvant chemotherapy on circumferential margin positivity and its impact on prognosis in patients with resectable oesophageal cancer. Br J Surg 95(2):191–194

Takashima S, Takeuchi N, et al (1991) Carcinoma of the esophagus: CT vs MR imaging in determining resectability. AJR Am J Roentgenol 156(2):297–302

van Vliet EP, Steyerberg EW, et al (2007) Detection of distant metastases in patients with oesophageal or gastric cardia cancer: a diagnostic decision analysis. Br J Cancer 97(7):868–876

Vickers J, Alderson D (1998) Oesophageal cancer staging using endoscopic ultrasonography. Br J Surg 85(7):994–998

Wakelin SJ, Deans C, et al (2002) A comparison of computerised tomography, laparoscopic ultrasound and endoscopic ultrasound in the preoperative staging of oesophago-gastric carcinoma. Eur J Radiol 41(2):161–167

Wiersema MJ, Vilmann P, et al (1997) Endosonography-guided fine-needle aspiration biopsy: diagnostic accuracy and complication assessment. Gastroenterology 112(4):1087–1095

Wu LF, Wang BZ, et al (2003) Preoperative TN staging of esophageal cancer: comparison of miniprobe ultrasonography, spiral CT and MRI. World J Gastroenterol 9(2):219–224

Yajima K, Kanda T, et al (2006) Clinical and diagnostic significance of preoperative computed tomography findings of ascites in patients with advanced gastric cancer. Am J Surg 192(2):185–190

Yamada I, Izumi Y, et al (2001) Superficial esophageal carcinoma: an in vitro study of high-resolution MR imaging at 1.5T. J Magn Reson Imaging 13(2):225–231

Yamada I, Murata Y, et al (1997) Staging of esophageal carcinoma in vitro with 4.7-T MR imaging. Radiology 204(2):521–526

Yamada I, Saito N, et al (2001) Early gastric carcinoma: evaluation with high-spatial-resolution MR imaging in vitro. Radiology 220(1):115–121

MRI of Upper GI Tract Motility

Valeria Panebianco, Giuseppe Pelle and Andrea Laghi

CONTENTS

6.1 Introduction 81
6.2 Physiology of Deglutition 82
6.3 MR-Fluoroscopy: Technique and Protocols 83
6.3.1 Background 83
6.3.2 Oral Contrast Agent 84
6.3.3 Oro-Pharyngeal Motility 84
6.3.4 Esophageal Motility 85

6.4 MR Patterns 87
6.4.1 Normal Findings 87
6.4.2 Abnormal Findings 87
6.4.2.1 Oro-Pharyngeal Motility 87
6.4.2.2 Esophageal Motility 87

6.5 MR Evaluation of Gastric Motility 88

6.6 Discussion 89
6.6.1 Advantages and Drawbacks 89

6.7 Conclusion 90

References 90

KEY POINTS

The evaluation of upper gastrointestinal motility requires either invasive techniques or ionizing radiation. Videofluoroscopy offers the opportunity to examine the oropharynx and cervical esophagus in patients who are at risk for aspiration due to swallowing difficulty. Because of the drawback of ionizing radiation exposure, repeated evaluation, especially in children, can be problematic.

Endoscopy is limited to the evaluation of the superficial mucosa, while radiographic examinations offer indirect information on motility based on the dynamics of swallowed contrast medium.

Dynamic magnetic resonance imaging of the esophagus and stomach has represented one of the major challenges in MRI. With the introduction of ultra-fast MR sequences, which have pushed scan times to the subsecond domain, MR fluoroscopic evaluation of physiological activity of soft tissue has become a reality. This allows a new non-invasive approach for the visualization of most motility processes in the human body, including swallowing function and esophageal peristalsis.

Valeria Panebianco, MD
Giuseppe Pelle, MD
Department of Radiological Sciences, "Sapienza" University of Rome, ICOT Hospital, Polo Pontino, Latina, V.le Regina Elena, 324, 00161 Rome, Italy
Andrea Laghi, MD
Department of Radiological Sciences, University of Rome "La Sapienza", ICOT Hospital, Polo Pontino, Latina, Via Franco Faggiana 34, 04100 Latina, Italy

6.1 Introduction

Available clinical methods for the detailed evaluation of upper gastrointestinal motility require either invasive techniques or ionizing radiation. Invasive techniques include indirect laryngoscopy or, more recently, fiber-optic nasal endoscopy. Alternatively, radiographic techniques with contrast media, such as videofluoroscopy, offer the opportunity to examine the oropharynx and cervical esophagus in patients who are at risk for aspiration due to swallowing difficulty.

Because of invasiveness and exposure to ionizing radiation, repeated evaluation, especially in children, can be problematic. Endoscopy is limited to the evaluation of the superficial mucosa, while radiographic examinations offer indirect information of motility based on the dynamics of swallowed contrast medium.

The study of esophageal morphology and motility currently relies on a combined radiological and manometric approach. While esophageal morphology and its changes during physiological events are studied by performing a barium swallow (Fuller et al. 1999; Aly 2000), motility is investigated by manometry. This technique provides precise measurements of parameters not assessable with other methods, such as intensity of the single peristaltic wave or the opening pressure of the lower esophageal sphincter (Bathia et al. 1995; Caste et al. 1990).

An alternative study for functional evaluation of the upper gastrointestinal tract is radionuclide scintigraphy. This technique has shown excellent diagnostic performance in several function or motility disorders. Dynamic scintigraphy with a radioactive liquid or semisolid bolus gave important information on both the oropharyngeal and the esophageal phases of swallowing, representing a valid alternative to conventional invasive tests (such as esophageal manometry).

Despite the diagnostic usefulness of these techniques, scintigraphic assessment of esophageal transit has met with only moderate success probably due to the lack of protocols standardization (Mariani et al. 2004).

At present, no alternative imaging method has proved sufficiently reliable compared with conventional radiology.

Dynamic magnetic resonance imaging (dMRI) has represented one of the major challenges in MRI. Actually, the major field of application is cardiovascular imaging, where advanced state-of-the-art equipment is necessary. Conversely, dynamic gastrointestinal MR imaging is a relatively unexplored field: the assessment of gastrointestinal function needs high levels of spatial and temporal resolution, a prerogative of videofluoroscopic techniques.

With the introduction and wide diffusion of ultrafast MR sequences, which have pushed scan times to the sub-second domain, MR fluoroscopic evaluation of physiological activity of soft tissue has become a reality. This allows a new noninvasive approach for the visualization of most motility processes in the human body, including esophageal functionality.

Current experience with dMRI of the gastrointestinal tract is limited to some preliminary and clinical studies on deglutition and other more recent reports on the evaluation of esophageal and gastric motility. Only one group has investigated the use of dMRI for the evaluation of esophageal motility (MR-Fluoroscopy), introducing an optimized protocol based on T1-weighted fast-field-echo (FFE) sequences (Manabe et al. 2004).

In recent years, a growing effort has been made to investigate the upper gastrointestinal tract noninvasively by dynamic magnetic resonance imaging (MRI).

Advanced imaging protocols include various high-speed MRI sequences such as echo planar imaging, GRE (FLASH), and fast GRE (Turbo FLASH) techniques using commercial MR magnets (1.5-T).

6.2
Physiology of Deglutition

Deglutition is a neuromuscular act coordinated by neural centers located in the brainstem and controlled by a widespread network of cortical regions including the sensory-motor cortex, the insula, the cingulate gyrus, and the cerebellum. In the vertebrates, swallowing is sustained by structures of the oral cavity, pharynx, larynx, and esophagus.

Deglutition is a complex function coordinated by voluntary and involuntary muscles of the oropharynx, the larynx, and the upper digestive pathway. The motility of these structures is very rapid because the pharynx has to carry out many functions different from bolus deglutition; it is mandatory that the respiratory function is not compromised in favor of deglution.

The swallowing process is generally divided in three phases (Guyton 2001): (1) the *voluntary phase*, the onset of deglutition, (2) the *pharyngeal phase*, consisting of bolus passage from the mouth to the superior esophageal sphincter through the pharynx, (3) the *esophageal phase*, characterized by bolus progression to the stomach through the esophagus. The last two phases are involuntary.

The *voluntary phase* starts when the tongue moves backwards and upward against the palate, working as a piston driving the bolus into the oro-pharynx in a sequential propulsion.

When the bolus reaches the posterior oral cavity, the *pharyngeal phase* begins by activation of "triggering centers" located in the tonsil pillars and in the oro-pharyngeal mucosa, responsible for nervous reflexes directed to the encephalic trunk and activation of pharyngeal muscular automatic contractions.

Simultaneously, the soft palate moves upward to prevent bolus regurgitation in the nasopharynx. The larynx and the hyoid bone move upwards closing the superior laryngeal vestibule. The epiglottis is deflected preventing bolus aspiration in the upper airways. The bolus enters the esophagus by the opening of the superior esophageal sphincter. The entire process lasts for approximately 1–2 s.

The *esophageal phase* starts with the opening of the superior esophageal sphincter. The primary function of the esophagus is to transport and direct the bolus from the pharynx to the stomach. The sequence of the muscular contractions is known as *Peristalsis*.

In normal subjects, two types of peristaltic activity are described:

The *Primary peristalsis* is the continuation of the pharyngeal peristaltic wave along the entire esophagus. It lasts for approximately 15–18 s. In erected patients, the normal esophageal bolus progression time is shorter due to gravity forces effect. If the primary peristalsis is not sufficient to transport the entire bolus in the stomach, *secondary peristaltic waves* are generated by the esophageal enteric nervous system, activated by mechanical esophageal distension. Multiple secondary peristaltic waves are generated until the entire bolus is led into the stomach. The *secondary peristalsis* is supported by afferent and efferent nervous fibers located in the vagal nerves, which connect the esophagus with the encephalic bulb.

At the distal end of the esophagus, 2–5 cm above the esophagi-gastric junction, is located the *inferior esophageal sphincter*. This anatomical region, unlike the remaining esophagus, has continuous tonic contractions (intraluminal pressure: 30 mmHg). However, when a peristaltic wave descends along the esophagus, the inferior sphincter musculature releases in advance, allowing the bolus passage in the stomach (Guyton 2001).

6.3
MR-Fluoroscopy: Technique and Protocols

6.3.1
Background

The identification of the deglution phases has been described in dynamic MR studies using the different dynamic sequences such us turbo-FLASH, TrueFISP, and EPI combined with an oral positive-contrast agent. Turbo-FLASH and echo-planar (EPI) MRI sequences demonstrated a sufficient temporal resolution for dynamic imaging of the deglutition process. However, detailed analysis is still restricted, mainly by the significantly lower SNR of high-speed MRI compared with conventional MRI, and by the occurrence of shape distortions in regions of large susceptibility gradients. The temporal resolution provided by ultra-fast MRI is essential for the analysis of deglutition.

Hagen et al. obtained good-quality images using turbo-FLASH sequences for dynamic oro-pharyngeal evaluation with temporal resolution of 0.2 s/slice and 0.3 s/slice (Hagen et al. 1990).

A significant loss of image quality was described by Breyra et al. (2009), when temporal resolution was raised to 0.55 s/slices due to oro-pharyngeal motion related artifact. Others employed balanced steady-state free precession sequence (real-time TrueFISP) with ultrafast slice acquisition for the visualization of swallowing (Barkhausen et al. 2002). This sequence is based on very short repetition and echo times, allowing collection of up to 13 frames/s. Although such a temporal resolution is sufficient to resolve the different components of the swallowing process and to identify pharyngo-esophageal pathologies, improvement in spatial resolution of this real-time TrueFISP sequence is desirable. In this regard, the implementation of half Fourier acquisition, SENSE, SMASH, or projection reconstruction strategies into the TrueFISP sequence design should be valuable.

Recently, it was demonstrated that dynamic imaging of swallowing is possible using open-configuration MRI (0.5 T) carrying out image swallowing in a sitting position (Yasutoshi et al. 2007). The study suggests that open-configuration MRI is useful for evaluating the normal physiological motion of swallowing in a seated position. An opinion of these authors is that videofluorography, which is currently the standard method for diagnosing swallowing disorders, provides poor visualization motion of the posterior pharyngeal wall. Dynamic MRI is a useful addition to videofluorography in assessing the soft-tissue motion of swallowing, and can be a second-tier choice for diagnosing dysphagia. Significant changes in coordination of the swallowing function have been reported between upright and supine positions (Castell et al. 1990). In the supine position, the lack of gravity forces modifies the physiologic sequence of normal erected swallowing muscular contractions;

this situation creates some difficulties when pathologic patterns of deglution are studied with reference to a standard upright physiologic model of deglution. This limitation applies to the vast majority of MRI studies available in the literature, as these report data obtained in patients studied in the supine position. Although this may hamper comparison of findings at videofluoroscopy and MRI, it does not hamper comparison between MRI studies.

6.3.2
Oral Contrast Agent

Gd-based oral contrast agents are widely used for MRI evaluation of bolus transit along the pharyngeal and esophageal tract. A suitable contrast agent for the examination should have the physical properties of barium while ensuring that the MRI signal is good. Gd-DTPA-based contrast agent provides optimum signal intensity, while its combination with semi-fluid yoghurt (1:100) offered barium-like physical properties, improving at the same time patient comfort and granting good compliance during the examination (PANEBIANCO et al. 2006).

The bolus is injected in the patient's mouth by the doctor or technician before the start of the dynamic sequence by a syringe (20 mL) and oral silicone cannula.

6.3.3
Oro-Pharyngeal Motility

Velopharynx, tongue base, valleculae, piriform sinuses, pharyngeal walls, and larynx are examined during respiration and swallowing with morphologic and dynamic MRI with patient positioned supine; head and neck coils are placed to increase the SNR (Table 6.1).

At our institution, the standard protocol is divided in three phases:

- *Preliminary assessment* of the oral cavity, pharynx, and laryngeal structures. T2-weighted half-Fourier acquisition single-shot turbo spin-echo (HASTE) sequences are acquired in the axial, coronal, and sagittal projection (TR 4.4 ms; TE 20 ms; flip angle 150°) from the base of the skull to the superior esophageal sphincter.
- *Morphologic assessment*: all images are acquired in the axial, coronal, and sagittal planes. The main structures involved in deglutition are analyzed describing the main morphological features: Tongue, Soft Palate, Walls of the Pharynx, Epiglottis, Laryngeal-Hyoid bone.
- *Dynamic (MR-Fluoroscopy):* dynamic assessment is subdivided into three steps. All images are acquired in the axial, sagittal projections by T1-weighted dynamic turbo-FLASH sequences (see Table 6.1). The sagittal slice is positioned through the oral and pharyngeal lumen. The time resolution is 3–4 frames/s.

Phase 1: The first dynamic session is performed without any contrast media. The patients have to repeatedly swallow during the entire period of the sequences (15 s) in order to visualize the movements of the structures mentioned above (Figs. 6.1 and 6.2).

Phase 2: The second session is performed injecting 5 mL of oral contrast agent (yogurt + Gd-DTPA, see below) based contrast medium in the patient's mouth. The bolus should be maintained in the oral cavity during the entire scanning time (15 s). This step is designed in order to evaluate the oral contention function (no contrast should be found in the pharynx if the soft palate closed the oral cavity at the level of glosso-palatal junction correctly) (Fig. 6.3).

Phase 3: The patient has to swallow the bolus previously injected in PHASE 2 in a single act. The bolus is then followed through the oral and pharyngeal track, from the oral cavity to the superior esophageal sphincter. This session is repeated three times, acquiring dynamic images only in the sagittal projection, to better depict bolus transit and eventual contrast media residue. Transit time (s) is calculated (Fig. 6.4).

Table 6.1. Dynamic MR parameters at 1.5 T (Siemens)

Parameter	HASTE T2-weighted parameters	Modified dynamic turbo FLASH parameters
TR (ms)	704	416
TE eff. (ms)	20	1.2
Flip angle	150	8
No. of slices	20	1
Slice thickness (mm)	7	20
Field of view	360	350
Matrix	160 × 256	90 × 126
No. of acquisitions	0.5	45
Trigger	Off	Off

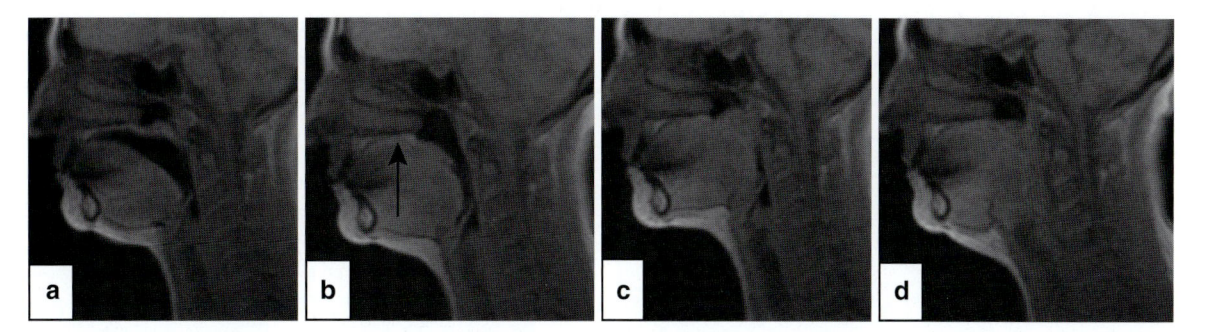

Fig. 6.1. Male patient, age 46, with aspecific swallowing disorders. Normal pattern: (**a**) Beginning of the oral phase of swallowing. The tongue moves away from the palate with the opening of the oral cavity (the soft palate transiently closes the nasopharynx), (**b**) Tongue contraction starts elevating the apex that touches the hard palate (*black arrow*); the nasopharynx is opened. (**c**) The progression of tongue contraction is characterized by an elevation/backwarding of the tongue radix (the soft palate, in contact with the tongue, closes the nasopharynx preventing bolus ingoing); the epiglottis is still erected. (**d**) The pharyngeal phase starts with the triggering of pharyngeal peristaltic wave that leads to the anterior displacement of the posterior pharyngeal wall that narrows the oro-pharyngeal cavity. The epiglottis is now oriented transversally closing the laryngeal vestibule and preventing the bolus aspiration

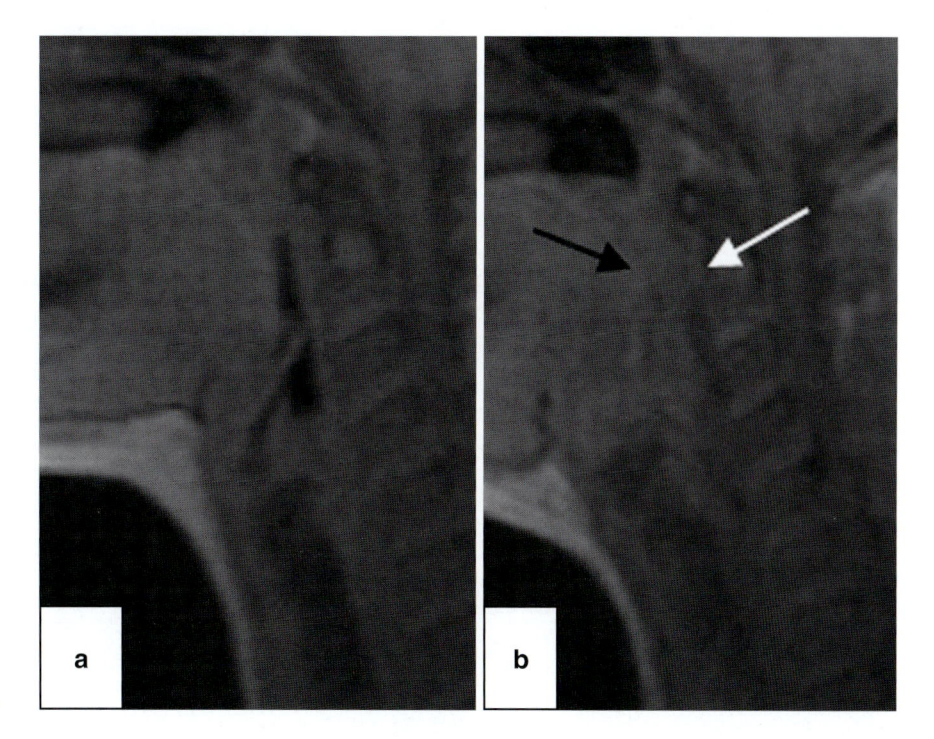

Fig. 6.2. Normal posterior pharyngeal wall: (**a**) normal appearance (**b**) peristaltic wave: posterior pharyngeal wall anterior displacement and thickening (*black arrow*); appearance of a hypointense rim (*white arrow*) between the pharyngeal wall and the cervical spine related to anterior spinal ligament and fascia

6.3.4
Esophageal Motility

Scans are acquired with the patients placed first in the prone position and then in the supine position. The imaging protocol (Table 6.1) is divided into two steps.

Phase 1: A breath-hold half-Fourier single-shot turbo-spin echo (HASTE) T2-weighted sequence orientated on coronal and axial planes is used to visualize the position of the esophagus and the gastro-esophageal junction.

Phase 2: Dynamic examination is performed with a single-slice sagittal slab (10 mm thickness) T1-weighted (turbo-FLASH) sequence. This slice is positioned at the centre of the esophageal lumen, in order to depict the transit of contrast agent boluses through the esophageal lumen. The parameters of the turbo-FLASH sequence are modified to obtain a temporal resolution of approximately 3–4

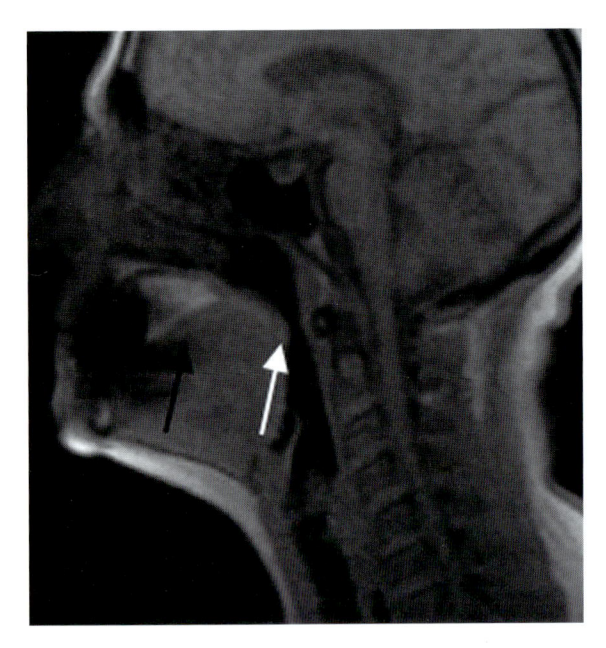

Fig. 6.3. The bolus is retained in the oral cavity without swallowing (*black arrow*); no contrast media should be visualized in the pharynx. The tongue and the velum platinum are the main structures configuring the glosso-palatal junction (*white arrow*)

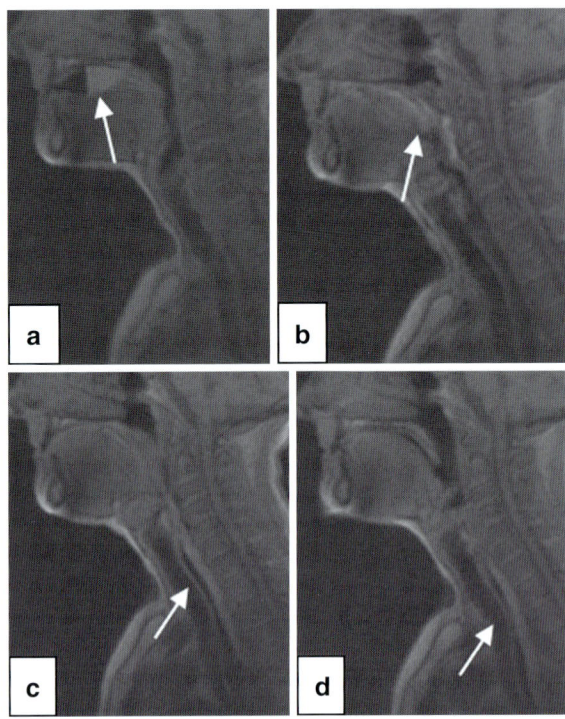

Fig. 6.4. Dynamic progression of the bolus through the oral (**a**) and the pharyngeal (**b–d**) phase. In normal subjects, the bolus (*arrows*) progression is very rapid (1 s)

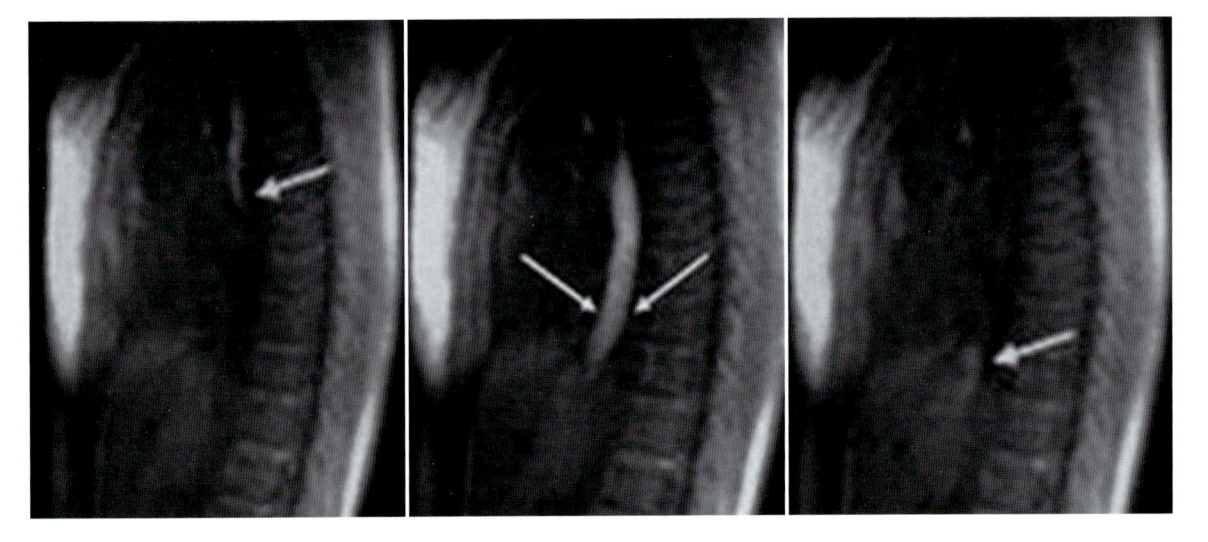

Fig. 6.5. Bolus progression on images obtained with dynamic T1-weighted turbo fast low-angle shot (FLASH) sequences

images/s. Immediately before the sequence starts, a small amount of contrast agent (10–15 mL) is administered directly into the oral cavity. Patients are instructed to swallow the entire bolus immediately after the onset of the gradient pulsations. Patients with severe deglution disorders are at high risk for airways aspiration of oral contrast agent; in such situations oral contrast media should not be used.

Five series of dynamic acquisitions are obtained: four acquired on the median sagittal and coronal plane to visualize esophageal motility and one on the oblique axial plane to depict gastro-esophageal junction functionality (Fig. 6.5).

6.4
MR Patterns

6.4.1
Normal Findings

The use of normal patterns for comparison is a fundamental condition for the diagnostic assessment of patients with motility disorders.

The spatial resolution of the sequence used allows the evaluation of morphologic parameters at MRI. Normal findings are:

- Esophageal length (mean 22.8 cm, SD = ±2.7 cm)
- Esophageal diameter (mean 21 mm, SD = ±1.8 mm)

The temporal resolution achieved with turbo FLASH sequences (2.5–4 frames/s), although substantially lower than that of a normal fluoroscopic examination (25–30 frames/s), allows for accurate assessment of main patterns of movement:

- Type of peristalsis: primary peristalsis (known as a homogeneous contraction of esophageal musculature with steady progression of the contrast bolus down to the stomach).
- Velocity of peristalsis: (mean = 2.34 cm/s, SD = ±0.2 cm/s).
- Bolus transit time: (mean = 9 s, SD = ±1.7 s).
- Gastro-esophageal junction function: continent and relaxing on passage of the bolus.

6.4.2
Abnormal Findings

6.4.2.1
Oro-Pharyngeal Motility

At present, the application of dynamic MRI protocols in the evaluation of pharyngeal motility is premature. To our knowledge, studies available in the literature are limited to the evaluation of physiologic pharyngeal deglution.

For the reasons mentioned above, this paragraph is centered on abnormal dynamic MRI patterns of esophageal disorders.

6.4.2.2
Esophageal Motility

According to the classification proposed by (SPECHLER et al. 2001), esophageal motility disorders can be categorized into four major patterns of alterations. Current dynamic MR protocols are able to detect pathological findings corresponding to those identified at conventional videofluoroscopy (e.g., early or advanced achalasia). In patients with achalasia, the main findings are the stenotic appearance of the distal esophagus with and/or without wall thickening and the dilatation of the segments above; poor relaxation of the gastro-esophageal junction; inefficient peristalsis replaced by "to-and-fro" movements (repeated upward/downward movement of the bolus in the esophageal lumen caused by abnormal peristalsis and unrelaxed gastro-esophageal junction) and the increased bolus transit time (up to 20 s). In advanced stages, the main findings is represented by a marked and widespread distension of the esophageal lumen (maximum caliber >60 mm) with tertiary peristalsis that is unable to activity and fully empty the organ (Fig. 6.6) (RICHTER et al. 2001; FIORENTINO et al. 2005; SCHIMA et al. 1998).

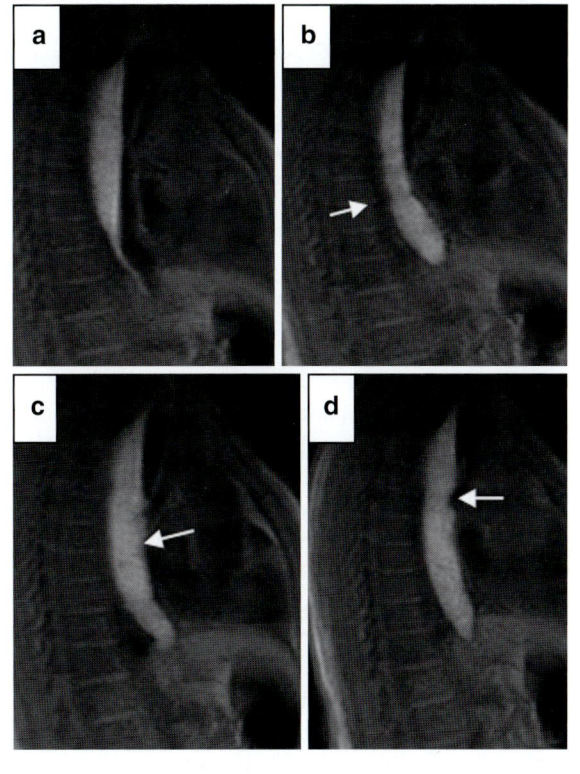

Fig. 6.6. Advanced achalasia. Images acquired at 5 s (**a**), 10 s (**b**), 15 s (**c**) and 20 s (**d**) after bolus administration show distension of the esophageal lumen (60 mm), narrowing of the distal esophagus, and replacement of the normal peristalsis by tertiary activity. The gastro-esophageal junction is closed and the bolus does not progress

Fig. 6.7. Esophageal spasm. The image after 4 s (**a**) shows rapid filling of the esophageal lumen; normal progression of the contrast medium is then interrupted by intermittent tertiary contractions (**b**), with typical corkscrew pattern (*arrow*)

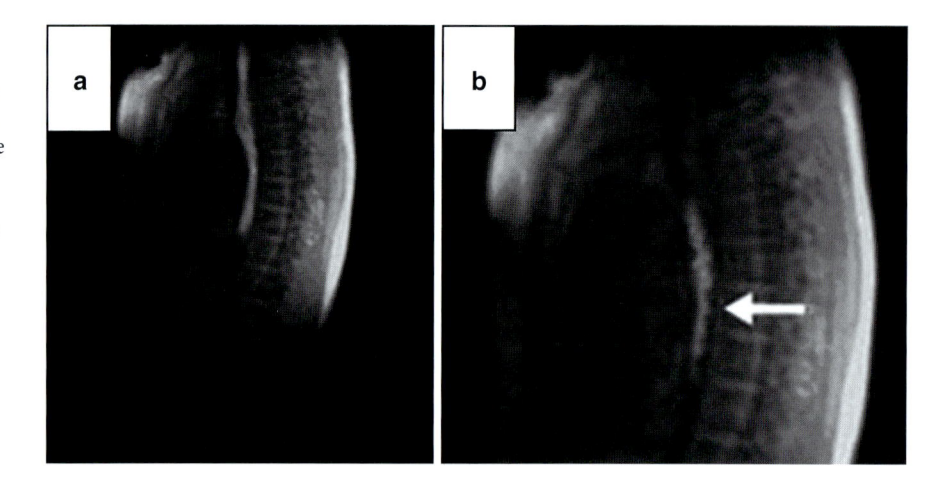

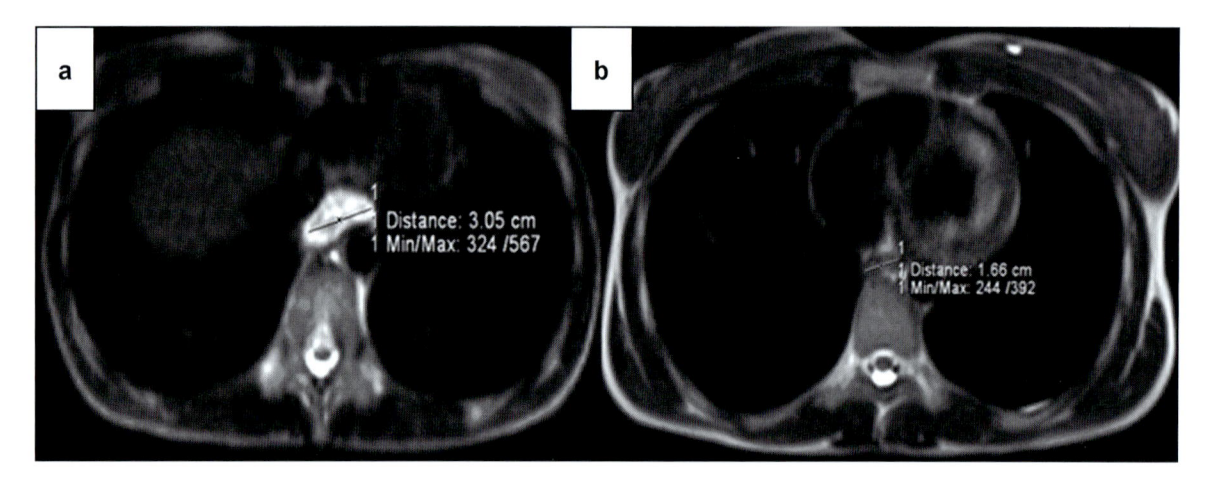

Fig. 6.8. Morphologic axial T2w sequences demonstrate a significant reduction of esophageal caliber after balloon dilatation of the distal esophagus (**a,b**)

MRI findings in patients with esophageal body motility uncoordination (EBMU) are intermittent progression of the contrast bolus along the lumen with tertiary peristalsis, increased transit time (12–15 s), and reduced with a "corkscrew" appearance (Fig. 6.7) (Prabhakar et al. 2004; Schima et al. 1992).

In ineffective esophageal motility (IEM)/scleroderma of the esophagus (SE), a weak peristaltic activity, enlarged diameter, mildly reduced esophageal clearance, are considered significant diagnostic features of gastro-esophageal junction incontinence with reflux and diminished clearance with delayed cleansing time (>18 s) (Nelson et al. 1988; Ipsen et al. 2000).

An additional application of MR-Fluoroscopy is the follow-up of patients affected by achalasia after conservative treatment such as balloon dilatation of the distal esophagus. In this patient, population dynamic MRI is also adequate in the post treatment follow-up to evaluate the efficacy therapy (Figs. 6.8 and 6.9) (Panebianco et al. 2009).

6.5
MR Evaluation of Gastric Motility

Functional gastrointestinal disorders have high prevalence but their diagnosis and follow-up are difficult because of the limitations of the diagnostic tools. Nuclear medicine is a widespread used technique for the gastric emptying evaluation, but is limited because of insufficient temporal and spatial resolution and isotopes radioactivity. Other tests for

Fig. 6.9. The same patient before (**a**) and after balloon dilatation (**b**): sagittal dynamic TFL sequencies confirm the caliber reduction, the prompt bolus transit, and the disappearance of residual alimentary material

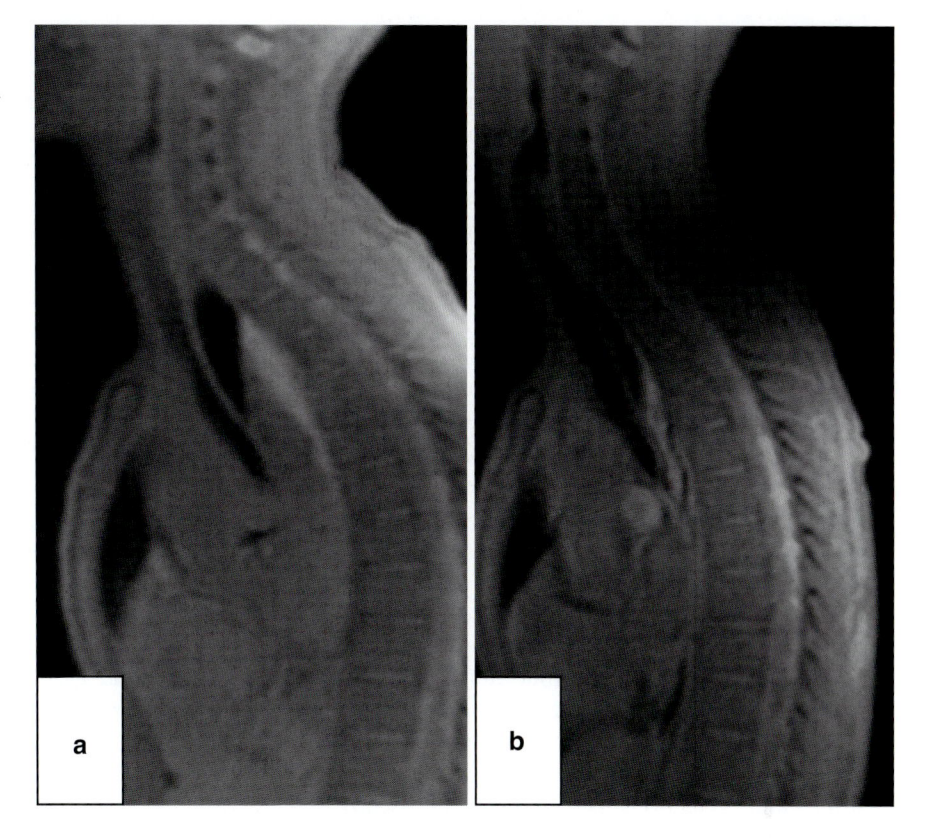

the evaluation of motility impairment are invasive, such as gastric manometry, or with a poor correlation with gastric activity, such as electrogastrography. The first application of MRI in the study of GI function was for the assessment of gastric emptying. MRI is also used for the measurement of gastric accommodation and gastric motility. The assessment of gastric emptying using MRI involves the repeated acquisition of axial image stacks covering the gastric region after a test meal. The most widely applied method uses a multislice turbo spin echo (TSE) technique. Imaging is performed during breath-holds to minimize movement artifacts. However, the evaluation of gastric motility and emptying disorders remains a difficult and somewhat inexact method. Gastric physiology is complex and depends on the appropriate interplay of different gastric functions (Schwizer et al. 2003). Increased or decreased gastric motion can be reliably distinguished with MRI; this imaging modality may be an attractive alternative to conventional invasive diagnostic tools for diagnosis of gastric motility disorders and consecutive therapeutic monitoring (Ajaj et al. 2004).

6.6
Discussion

6.6.1
Advantages and Drawbacks

Compared with conventional radiology, MRI fluoroscopy of the pharynx and esophagus has several major advantages: multiplanar imaging capabilities with visualization of the esophagus and intrathoracic soft tissues in different spatial planes, the possibility of making acquisitions with dedicated sequences at high contrast resolution. The greatest advantage is, however, the possibility of investigating esophageal function without the use of ionizing radiation. Despite the advent of digital equipment and considerable reduction in dose, radiation exposure (Mean mSv: 0.3) (Crawley et al. 2004) remains the main drawback of fluoroscopy.

Videofluoroscopy is a valuable and reasonably specific (79%) and sensitive (80%) technique for screening for esophageal motor disorders (Schima et al. 1992).

With MRI fluoroscopy, it would be possible to repeat examinations over time (for example, in the follow-up before and after dilatation and/or myotomy in patients with achalasia) and to study patients, such as pregnant women and younger subjects, in whom radiation exposure is contraindicated.

The MRI technique presented does, however, suffer some limitations:

First, the spatial resolution of the sequences used, although adequate for assessing esophageal function, is still too low to adequately visualize the pharyngeal wall profile, as can be done with videofluoroscopy. We should, however, add that MRI is often able to detect typical luminal "filling defect" and wall thickening at the level of the gastro-esophageal junction as in cases of pseudoachalasia due of advanced cardial gastric cancer.

Second, the maximum temporal resolution (2.5 frames/s (fps)) is still far below the standards currently obtainable with conventional radiology (25–30 fps). A further technical limitation is that with the actual commercially available techniques patients can be scanned only in the supine position; this is particularly true if we consider the wide range of positions and projections used in videofluoroscopy and manometry. However, we can state that even the information obtained with the patients in the supine position may be valuable for diagnosis of the motility disorders. The diagnostic performance of MR fluoroscopy was overall satisfactory with a sensitivity of 87.5% and specificity of 100% in the general depiction of motility alterations (Panebianco et al. 2006).

Another limitation is the relatively long time required to complete a dynamic MRI examination (20–30 min); videofluoroscopy is usually faster (8–10 min).

6.7 Conclusion

Based on the relative sparse literature until now, dynamic MRI technique seems a promising tool. It represents for the future a potential alternative to videofluoroscopy in the evaluation of upper gastrointestinal motility disorders. It has the advantage to be relatively noninvasive. There is no need of intravenous administration of contrast media and, compared to videofluoroscopy, no exposure to ionizing radiation.

However, more energy should be invested to optimize the spatial and temporal resolution dynamic sequences in order to obtain a better dynamic representation of a complex function such as deglutition. Further technical improvements are necessary taking into account the high incidence (18 million adults only in the USA) and social cost of dysphagia (Robbins 2005).

References

Ajaj W, Goehde SC, Papanikolaou N, et al (2004) Real time high resolution magnetic resonance imaging for the assessment of gastric motility disorders. Gut 53(9):1256–1261

Aly YA (2000) Digital radiography in the evaluation of oesophageal motility disorders. Clin Radiol 55:561–568

Barkhausen J, Goyen M, von Winterfeld F, et al (2002) Visualization of swallowing using real-time TrueFISP MR fluoroscopy. Eur Radiol 12:129–133

Bhatia SJ, Malkan GH, Ravi P, et al (1995) Correlation of manometric and radiographic diagnosis in esophageal motility disorders. Indian J Gastroenterol 14:124–127

Breyera T, Echternachc M, Arndtd S, et al (2009) Dynamic magnetic resonance imaging of swallowing and laryngeal motion using parallel imaging at 3 T. Magn Reson Imaging 27:48–54

Castell DJ, Dalton JB (1990) effect of body position and bolus consistency on the manometric parameter and coordination of the upper esophageal sphincter and pharyngx. Dysphagia 5:179–186

Crawley MT, Savage P, Oakley F (2004) Patient and operator dose during fluoroscopic examination of swallow mechanism. Br J Radiol 77:654–656

Fiorentino E, Barbiera F, Grassi N, et al (2005) Digital videofluorography and esophageal achalasia: from diagnosis to follow-up. Chir Ital 57:59–64

Fuller L, Huprich JE, Theisen J, et al (1999) Abnormal esophageal body function: radiographic–manometric correlation. Am Surg 65:911–914

Guyton AC, Hall JE (2001) Textbook of medical physiology. Saunders, Philadelphia

Hagen R, Haase A, Matthaei D, et al (1990) Oropharyngeale Funktionsdiagnostikmit der FLASH-MR-Tomographie. HNO 38:421–425

Ipsen P, Egekvist H, Aksglaede K, et al (2000) Oesophageal manometry and video-radiology in patients with sys-temic sclerosis: a retrospective study of its clinical value. Acta Derm Venereol 80:130–133

Manabe T, Kawamitsu H, Higashino T, et al (2004) Esophageal magnetic resonance fluoroscopy: optimization of the sequence. J Comput Assist Tomogr 28:697–703

Mariani G, Boni G, Barreca M, et al (2004) Radionuclide gastroesophageal motor studies. J Nucl Med 45:1004–1028

Nelson JB, Castell DO (1988) Esophageal motility disorders. Dis Mon 34:297–389

Panebianco V, Fortunee Irene H, Paolantonio ETP, et al (2006) Initial experience with magnetic resonance fluoroscopy in the evaluation of oesophageal motility disorders. Comparison with manometry and barium fluoroscopy. Eur Radiology 16(9):1926–1933

Panebianco V, Osimani M, Bernardo S, et al (2009) MR-fluoroscopy as follow-up examination in patients with achalasia after dilatation treatment Eur radiology 19(1):533–586

Prabhakar A, Levine MS, Rubesin S, et al (2004) Relationship between diffuse esophageal spasm and lower esophageal sphincter dysfunction in barium studies and manometry in 14 patients. AJR Am J Roentgenol 183:409–413

Richter JE (2001) Oesophageal motility disorders. Lancet 358 (9284): 823–828

Robbins J (2005) Swallowing disorders: interventions. Bulletin of US department of veterans affair. (http://aging.senate.gov/award/vet10.pdf)

Schima W, Ryan JM, Harisinghani M, et al (1998) Radiographic detection of achalasia: diagnostic accuracy of videofluoroscopy. Clin Radiol 53:372–375

Schima W, Stacher G, Pokieser P, et al (1992) Esophageal motor disorders: videofluoroscopic and manometric evaluation-prospective study in 88 symptomatic patients. Radiology 185:487–491

Schwizer W, Fox M, Steingötter A (2003) Non-invasive investigation of gastrointestinal functions with magnetic resonance imaging: towards an "ideal" investigation of gastrointestinal function. Gut 52(Suppl 4):iv34–iv39

Spechler SJ, Castell DO (2001) Classification of oesophageal motility abnormalities. Gut ; 49(1):145–51

Yasutoshi H, Nobuhiko H (2007) Dynamic imaging of swallowing in a seated position using open-configuration MRI. J Magn Reson Imaging 26(1):172–176

MRI of the Duodenum

Celso Matos and Martina Pezzullo

CONTENTS

7.1 Introduction 93
7.2 Examination Technique 94
7.2.1 General Considerations 94
7.2.2 Sequences 94

7.3 Magnetic Resonance Imaging Findings 96
7.3.1 General Considerations 96
7.3.2 Lesions of Duodenal Origin 96
7.3.2.1 Diverticula 96
7.3.2.2 Duodenal Duplication 96
7.3.2.3 Duodenal Lipoma 97
7.3.2.4 Duodenal Hematoma 98
7.3.2.5 Duodenal Stromal Tumors 98
7.3.2.6 Duodenal Adenocarcinoma 99
7.3.2.7 Duodenal Lymphoma 101
7.3.2.8 Duodenal Carcinoids 102
7.3.2.9 Duodenal Metastases 102
7.3.3 Lesions of Ampullary Origin 103
7.3.3.1 Choledococele 103
7.3.3.2 Ampullary Tumors 103
7.3.4 Lesions of Pancreatic Origin 105
7.3.4.1 Annular Pancreas 105
7.3.4.2 Paraduodenal Pancreatitis 105
7.3.5 MRI Compared to CT 107

References 114

Celso Matos, MD
Martina Pezzullo, MD
Department of Radiology, MR Imaging Division, Cliniques Universitaires de Bruxelles, Hôpital Erasme, Université Libre de Bruxelles, Route de Lennik 808, 1070 Brussels, Belgium

KEY POINTS

Magnetic resonance imaging (MRI) of the duodenum is indicated whenever common bile duct and main pancreatic duct involvement is suspected and when a duodenal stenosis is present. In these settings, it allows differentiating congenital disease and benign and malignant causes of ductal obstruction or of duodenal obstruction. In addition to conventional T1- and T2-weighted sequences, MRI of the duodenum should include magnetic resonance cholangiopancreatography (MRCP) sequences along with hormonal stimulation with secretin to improve the visualization of ductal anatomy and distend the duodenal lumen. Gadolinium chelates should be used whenever a tumor is suspected or if functional imaging of the biliary tree is indicated. Diffusion-weighted imaging might be included in the work-up of patients presenting with duodenal wall thickening or suspicion of a space-occupying lesion filling the groove between the duodenum and the head of the pancreas or involving the head of the pancreas.

Compared to computer tomography, the major role of MRI of the duodenum is related to its capabilities of providing noninvasively MRCP renderings and to its superior contrast resolution. This allows identifying the majority of duodenal disorders, especially congenital anomalies, cystic lesions, and inflammatory processes involving the duodenal groove.

7.1 Introduction

The duodenum is the proximal segment of the small intestine, is about 25–30 cm long, and is divided into four sections. The first portion of the duodenum extends from the pylorus to the neck of the gallbladder. The second portion extends from the neck of the gallbladder to the genu. The third portion of the duodenum extends from the fourth lumbar vertebra to the level of the aorta. The fourth portion extends from the level of the aorta to the ligament of Treitz. Therefore, a close and fixed anatomic relation with the liver, the gallbladder, and the extra hepatic bile ducts, the pancreas and the transverse mesocolon, as well as with the aorta and its collaterals and the portal and mesenteric veins is an important landmark when imaging the duodenum. The diagnosis of diseases of the duodenum involves primarily endoscopy, which allows a direct view of the mucosa, and endoscopic ultrasound (EUS), which allows investigating the entire duodenal wall and the area behind it. In addition, both techniques may be used to perform biopsies, and EUS may be used as a guide for interventional procedures. Because of both reasons (its location and the role of endoscopy and EUS), magnetic resonance imaging (MRI) of the duodenum is performed when a patient presents with symptoms that may be related to a lesion involving the liver, the pancreas, the gallbladder, and the bile ducts, to a lesion causing a duodenal stenosis that precludes endoscopic techniques and for the local staging of a tumor previously diagnosed by endoscopy or EUS. In this chapter we review the most frequent duodenal lesions diagnosed at MRI in the above-mentioned clinical settings.

7.2
Examination Technique

7.2.1
General Considerations

Abdominal MRI has undergone an important evolution owing to the improved performance of gradient and phased-array coils and to the use of parallel imaging techniques. These improvements allowed obtaining T1- and T2-weighted sequences faster, with increased spatial resolution and the ability to explore larger volumes. To specifically investigate the duodenum, the bile ducts, and the pancreas, magnetic resonance cholangiopancreatography (MRCP) will be added to the above-mentioned sequences. The MRCP will be optimally acquired after a fasting period of at least 4 h. If significant residual fluid is present in the stomach we may consider using a T2-negative oral contrast agent (iron oxide particles, pineapple juice or 1 mL of gadolinium mixed with 50 mL of water) to avoid overlap between residual gastric fluid and the pancreatic ducts. To improve the delineation of the pancreatic ducts, to detect outflow obstruction of the main or accessory pancreatic duct, and to fill and distend the duodenal lumen, hormonal stimulation with secretin should be used. When a duodenal wall mass is suspected, the use of gadolinium-based contrast agents to further characterize the lesion and to make vascular assessment will be considered. Finally, the more recent advancements in technology provided the possibility of acquiring high b-value diffusion-weighted imaging (DWI) (see also Chap. 4) with acceptable signal-to-noise ratio and spatial resolution. In DWI, signal intensity reflects the degree of restriction of microscopic water movements in tissues and is correlated to tissue cellularity, the integrity of cell membranes and the amount of tissue fibrosis, which make it a very sensitive sequence for the detection of tumors and inflammation (Koh and Collins 2007). In addition, the DWI sequence allows obtaining quantitative data when apparent diffusion coefficient (ADC) maps are generated. This noninvasive strategy that provides a complete assessment of the duodenum and of its environment can be performed in modern MR scanners in about 30 min.

7.2.2
Sequences (see Table 7.1)

(a) T2-weighted sections are acquired in the axial and coronal planes using a single-shot TSE sequence during free breathing with respiratory triggering or a navigator-echo, to minimize the need for patient cooperation. The field-of-view will include the whole liver, the pancreas, and the duodenum and section thickness is about 4–5 mm. Because it may decrease the delineation of duodenal and pancreatic contours fat suppression is not routinely applied. It may be used whenever a paraduodenal inflammatory process is suspected. This sequence provides a very good contrast between the duodenal lumen, the duodenal wall, and the pancreas parenchyma and depicts the bile ducts and the pancreatic ducts in cross-section. It is also used as a guide for MRCP acquisition and is generally acquired after secretin challenge when duodenal filling is complete in order to overcome pitfalls that may be related to a lack of duodenal distension. T2-weighted sequences are very sensitive for detecting cystic lesions.

Table 7.1. MR Imaging protocol

Sequence	Parameters
Axial and coronal T2-weighted single-shot TSE	Motion correction: respiratory triggering
	Echo time: 80 ms; echo train length: 72
	Parallel imaging: sense factor 2 in the phase-encoding direction
	Slice thickness: 4–5 mm
	FOV: 400 × 450
	Matrix size: 226 × 400
Axial 3D GRE T1-weighted	Selective fat saturation
	Motion correction: breath-hold (18 s)
	Repetition time/echo time: 3.9 ms/1.9 ms
	Parallel imaging: sense factor 2 in the phase-encoding direction
	Slice thickness: 2 mm
	FOV: 400 × 400
	Matrix size: 192 × 256
Coronal oblique T2-weighted thick slab single-shot TSE Dynamic MRCP	Selective fat saturation
	Echo time: 1,000 ms; echo train length: 256
	Slice thickness: 20–50 mm
	FOV: 250 × 250
	Matrix size: 256 × 256
Axial diffusion-weighted SE-EPI	STIR fat suppression (inversion time: 180 ms)
	Motion correction: respiratory triggering
	Repetition time/echo time: 2,000 ms/70 ms
	Parallel imaging: sense factor 2 in the phase-encoding direction
	b-values: 0.150, 1,000 s/mm^2
	Slice thickness: 5 mm
	FOV: 400 × 450
	Matrix size: 272 × 189

(b) T1-weighted sections are obtained with a breath-hold three-dimensional gradient echo (3D GRE) fat suppressed technique generally in the axial plane with nearly isotropic voxels. This sequence allows improved spatial resolution and multiplanar reformatting. However, patient cooperation is required. Fat suppression improves the delineation of the normal pancreas, which appears homogeneously bright compared to the surrounding low-intensity fat and with the duodenal wall, and provides further characterization of fat-containing lesions. To address the fat component of a lesion, 2D GRE sequences with a double echo time (in and out-of-phase) may also be used. If gadolinium administration is needed, the three-dimensional (3D) GRE sequence is repeated at least 3 times to obtain the information in the arterial, portal venous, and delayed phases. In order to optimize the arterial phase, fluoroscopic triggering of the contrast bolus will be used. Then multiphase angiographic renderings will be reconstructed from the source images. The 3D GRE sequence may also be used after the administration of a gadolinium-chelate with biliary excretion whenever functional imaging of the bile ducts is necessary (FAYAD et al. 2003).

(c) Imaging of the bile ducts and of the pancreatic ducts is obtained with a TSE T2-weighted sequence using a very long echo time (about 1 s). The routinely adopted sequence uses a single, 20–50-mm-thick section that can be obtained in any desired plane during a single short breath-hold (<3 s). At least two different planes (coronal and transversal) are usually acquired, providing selectively display of pancreatic and bile ducts with no respiratory artifact and a relatively good in-plane resolution. This acquisition scheme is preferred to a 3D sequence because it allows acquiring dynamic views of the Vaterian sphincter complex (Kim et al. 2002a) and of the pancreatic ducts along with hormonal stimulation with secretin. Once the appropriate MRCP projection has been identified (usually coronal oblique, displaying the full length of the pancreatic duct, the biliary tract, and the duodenum), the same scan is repeated every 30 s for 10 min after intravenous secretin administration at a dose of 1 mL/10 kg of body weight (Matos et al. 1997).

(d) DWI sections are obtained in the axial plane using a respiratory-triggered fat-saturated spin-echo echo-planar sequence (SE-EPI) with b-values of 0 and 1,000 s/mm^2 and the same geometry parameters (number of slices, slice thickness and field-of-view) as the TSE T2-weighted acquisition. This allows combining both datasets (T2-weighted and diffusion-weighted) in a fused image to increase the conspicuity of diffusion-positive lesions (Tsushima et al. 2007).

7.3
Magnetic Resonance Imaging Findings

7.3.1
General Considerations

MRI will generally be obtained when a space occupying lesion is suspected. To achieve a diagnosis we should determine the origin of the lesion (primary duodenal or from a surrounding organ, such as the pancreas), characterize its content (presence of fluid, blood, fat, or mainly solid components) and assess its extension (presence of a duodenal stricture, presence of dilated bile ducts, and of dilated main pancreatic duct, involvement of the groove between the duodenal wall and the head of the pancreas, involvement of the pancreas parenchyma, and of the vascular structures). The multiplanar imaging characteristics and the high-contrast resolution of MRI will allow identifying these imaging features in the majority of the patients. In this chapter we present the MRI findings of the most common duodenal lesions generally diagnosed in patients addressed for bile ducts and pancreas investigations.

7.3.2
Lesions of Duodenal Origin

7.3.2.1
Diverticula

The most frequent location of duodenal diverticula is along the medial wall of the second and third portions of the duodenum adjacent to the ampulla of Vater. They are generally incidentally discovered when performing MRCP studies. Rarely they may increase in size and become symptomatic because of bile duct obstruction or inflammatory changes (diverticulitis) that may be complicated by perforation. If the ampulla of Vater drains into the diverticulum, it can be a source of difficult cannulation at endoscopic retrograde cholangiopancreatography (ERCP). At MRI often they present a fluid–air interface easily recognizable on axial T2-weighted imaging. Coronal T2-weighted imaging (multisection and MRCP renderings) will better display the exact location and distance to the ampullary region and potential associated dilation of the bile ducts and of the pancreatic duct. Secretin injection may help in ruling out any functional pancreatic duct obstruction and will allow to better demonstrate the connection with the duodenal lumen and the filling of the diverticulum (Fig. 7.1a–c). In case of any suspicion of bile duct obstruction, it may be useful to use a gadolinium chelate with biliary excretion to rule out any functional impairment to bile excretion (Fig. 7.2a–c).

7.3.2.2
Duodenal Duplication

Duodenal duplications are rare and represent about 4–12% of gastrointestinal tract duplications (Guibaud et al. 1996). Most often they are located in the medial wall of the second and third portions of the duodenum. Although patients may present with

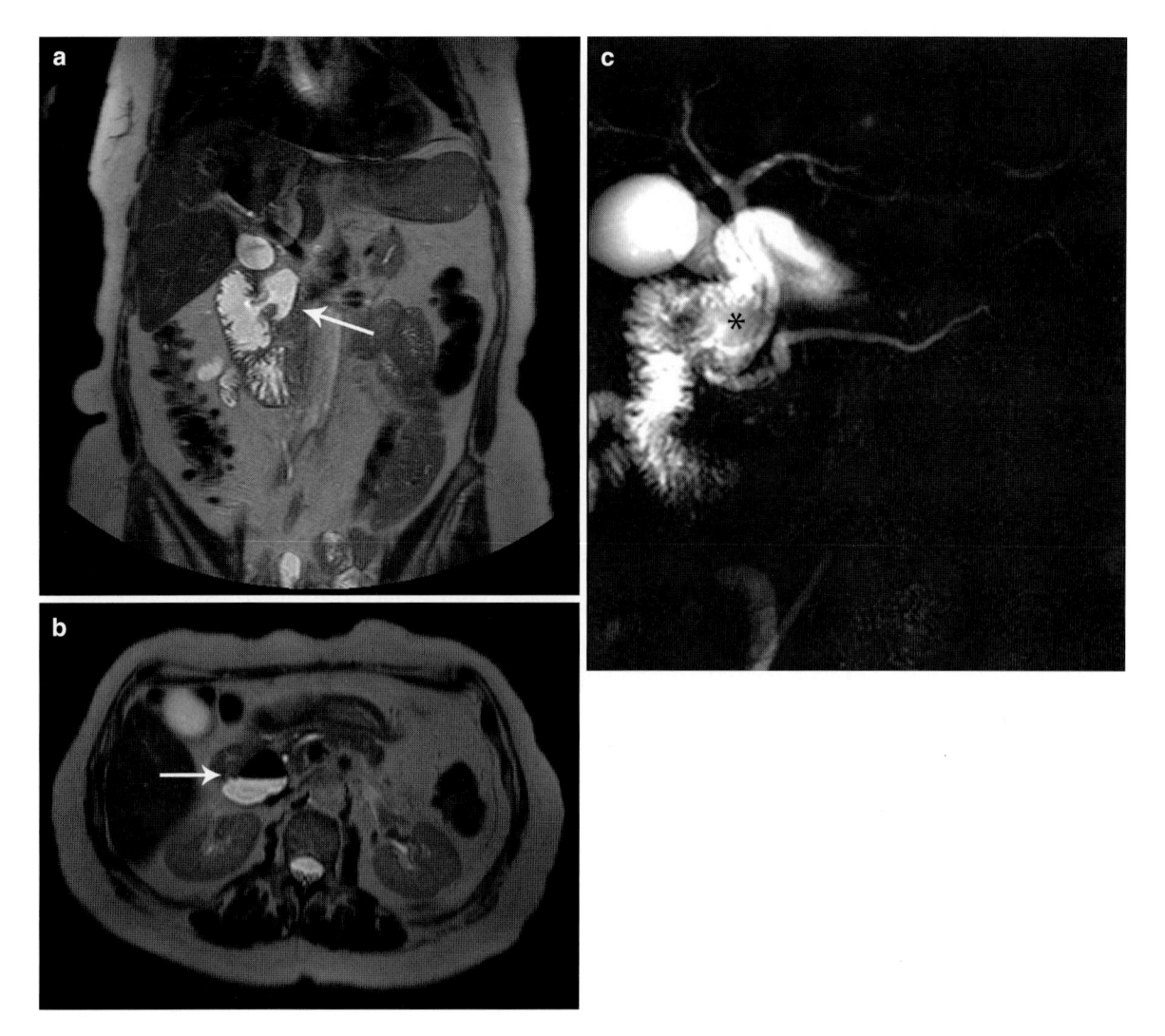

Fig. 7.1. Duodenal diverticulum. Coronal T2-weighted image (**a**) shows the presence of a diverticulum on the medial wall of the second duodenum (*arrow*). Axial T2-weighted images (**b**) show the air-fluid level (*arrow*) and in the MRCP images obtained after secretin stimulation (**c**) the duodenum and the diverticular pouch (*asterisk*) are filled with fluid and obstruction of the main pancreatic duct is depicted

abdominal pain or recurrent pancreatitis, most of the time these lesions are clinically silent. Typically they appear as a well-circumscribed cystic lesion lined by an epithelium and no communication with the duodenal lumen is observed. At MRI the lesion presents homogeneous high signal intensity and a thin and well-delineated hypointense peripheral rim on T2-weighted imaging. To better demonstrate the absence of communication with the duodenal lumen and rule out any communication with the bile ducts secretin administration along with MRCP will be helpful (Fig. 7.3a–c).

7.3.2.3
Duodenal Lipoma

Lipomas are slow-growing tumors, most of the time solitary, and can occur anywhere in the duodenum (Thompson 2005). They may appear submucosal or as intraluminal mass. Generally, the lesion is incidentally discovered or when imaging is obtained because of a compressive lesion in a patient with epigastric pain and bleeding secondary to mucosal erosions diagnosed at endoscopy. MRI shows a well-delineated hyperintense lesion on nonfat-saturated T1-weighted

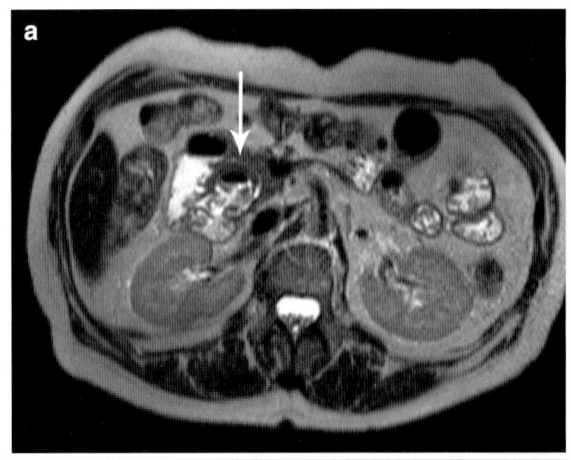

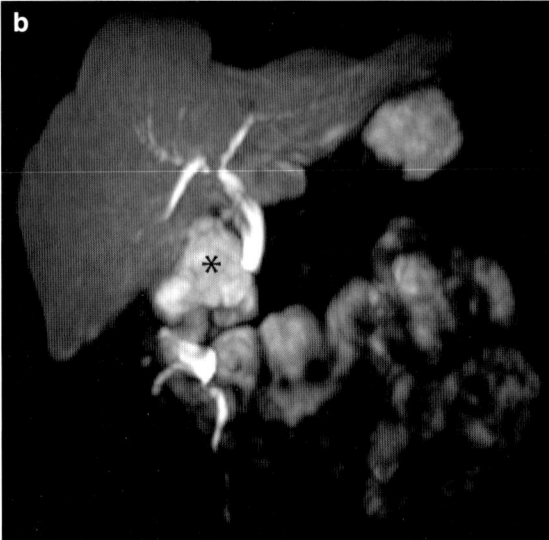

Fig. 7.2. Duodenal diverticulum. Axial T2-weighted image (**a**) shows a duodenal diverticulum in its typical location (*arrow*). T1-weighted coronal cholangiogram after administration of a gadolinium chelate with biliary excretion (**b**) clearly depicts the duodenal diverticulum filled with contrast (*asterisk*), with no evidence of biliary obstruction

sequences and a hypointense lesion surrounded by the hyperintense duodenal fluid on fat-saturated T2-weighted sequences or on MRCP which allows easy discrimination with a pancreatic pseudocyst (would be hyperintense on MRCP) (Fig. 7.4a, b).

7.3.2.4
Duodenal Hematoma

Duodenal hematomas are most commonly of traumatic origin or may be diagnosed in patients on anticoagulation therapy or with complicated acute pancreatitis. Location is generally subserosal and a duodenal stricture is commonly an associated finding. On MRI the diagnosis of a duodenal hematoma is generally easy to make when a space occupying lesion within or adjacent to the duodenal wall presents typical signal changes on T1-weighted imaging (heterogeneous lesion with hyperintense peripheral ring related to hemoglobin degradation products) (Fig. 7.5a, b).

7.3.2.5
Duodenal Stromal Tumors

These include leiomyomas, leiomyosarcomas, schwanommas, neurofibromas, and gastrointestinal stromal tumors (GISTs). GISTs are the most common mesenchymal neoplasms of the gastrointestinal tract and are defined by their expression of a tyrosine-kinase growth factor receptor (KIT/CD117). The expression of KIT is important to distinguish GISTs from the other stromal tumors and also to determine the appropriateness of KIT-inhibitor therapy (Levy et al. 2003). In a recent review of a series of 113 patients (Hong et al. 2006), 9% of GISTs were located in the duodenum. Most commonly they have an exophytic growth pattern and manifest as space-occupying lesions outside the duodenal lumen displacing the pancreatic ducts and adjacent vessels. When lesions are very large, it may be difficult to identify the organ of origin. The lesions may present areas of hemorrhage, necrosis, or cyst formation, and therefore on MRI the pattern of signal intensity is quite variable on both T1- and T2-weighted sequences (Fig. 7.6a, b). After intravenous gadolinium administration the tumor enhances more prominently in the venous phase in large lesions (Fig. 7.7a–d). Metastases (liver, peritoneum, soft tissue, lungs, and pleura) are found in nearly 50% of patients with GISTs (Nilsson et al. 2005). High *b*-value DWI may be used and will show a mixed pattern according to the proportion of solid and cystic components. Also, DWI has the potential to assess the response to treatment with imatinib. Indeed treatment with imatinib results in decreases in the size of GISTs, but this response typically takes several months (Hong et al. 2006). Measuring the ADC of the lesion may allow identifying early changes after imatinib treatment. An increase in ADC may be observed as a result of an initial decrease in tumor cellularity. Interestingly, these changes in ADC of the tumor may occur before any reduction in tumor size is observed (Fig. 7.8a, b) (Patterson et al. 2008).

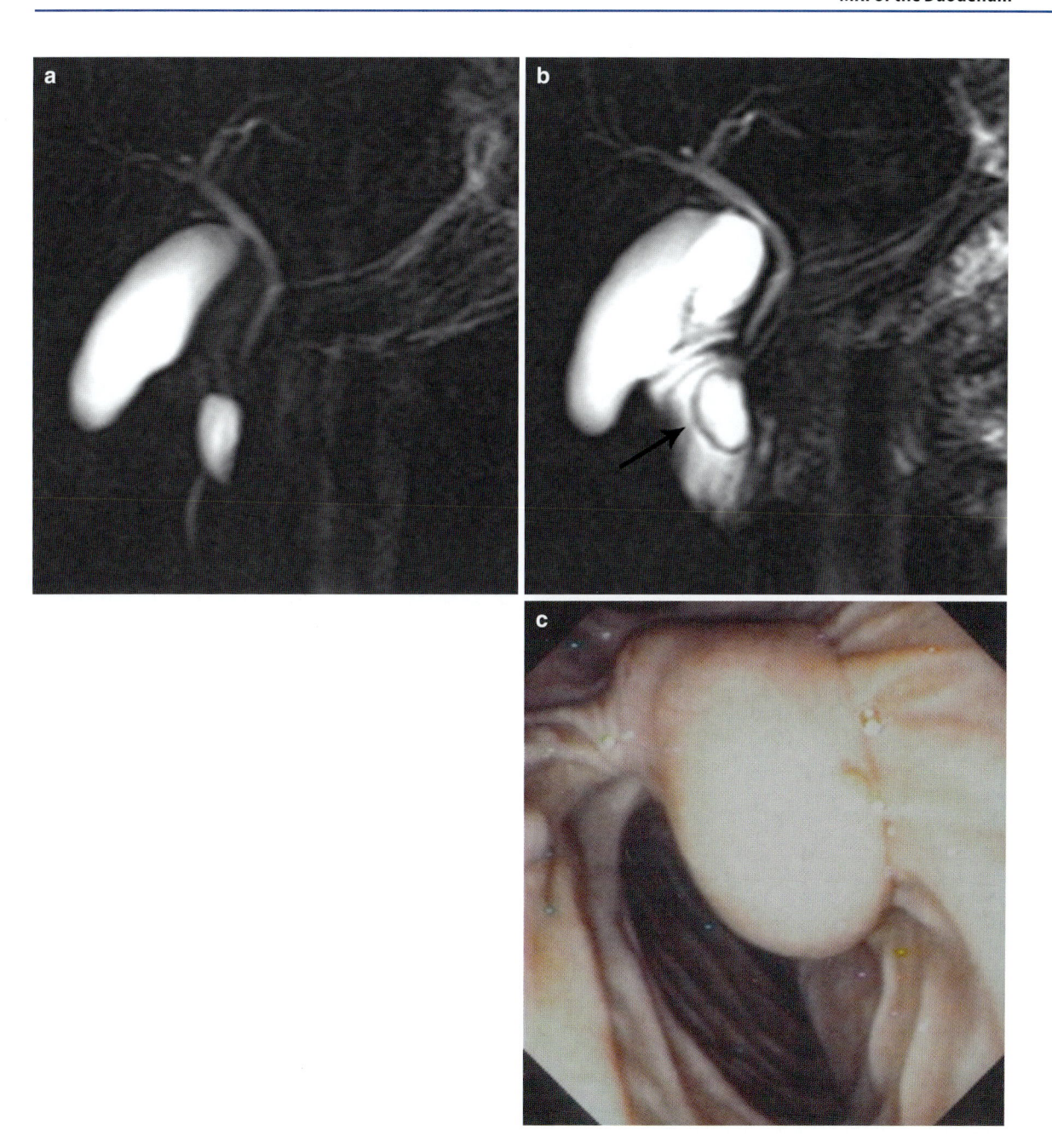

Fig. 7.3. Duodenal duplication. MRCP images before (**a**) and after (**b**) secretin stimulation shows the presence in the second portion of the duodenum of a well-circumscribed fluid-filled lesion with a thin wall (*arrow*) without communication with the common bile duct or the duodenal lumen, as confirmed by endoscopy (**c**)

7.3.2.6
Duodenal Adenocarcinoma

Malignant primary neoplasms of the duodenum and of the small bowel are rare and primary adenocarcinomas accounts for about 40–50%. About 50% of these are of duodenal origin (LACHACHI et al. 1996). The lesions are most commonly located in the second portion of the duodenum adjacent to the ampullary region, and in such cases the differential diagnosis with ampullary tumors may be impossible. Because the duodenum is not lined in its posterior portion by the peritoneum, invasion of the posterior fatty tissue is common. About 50% of the patients have metastases at the time of

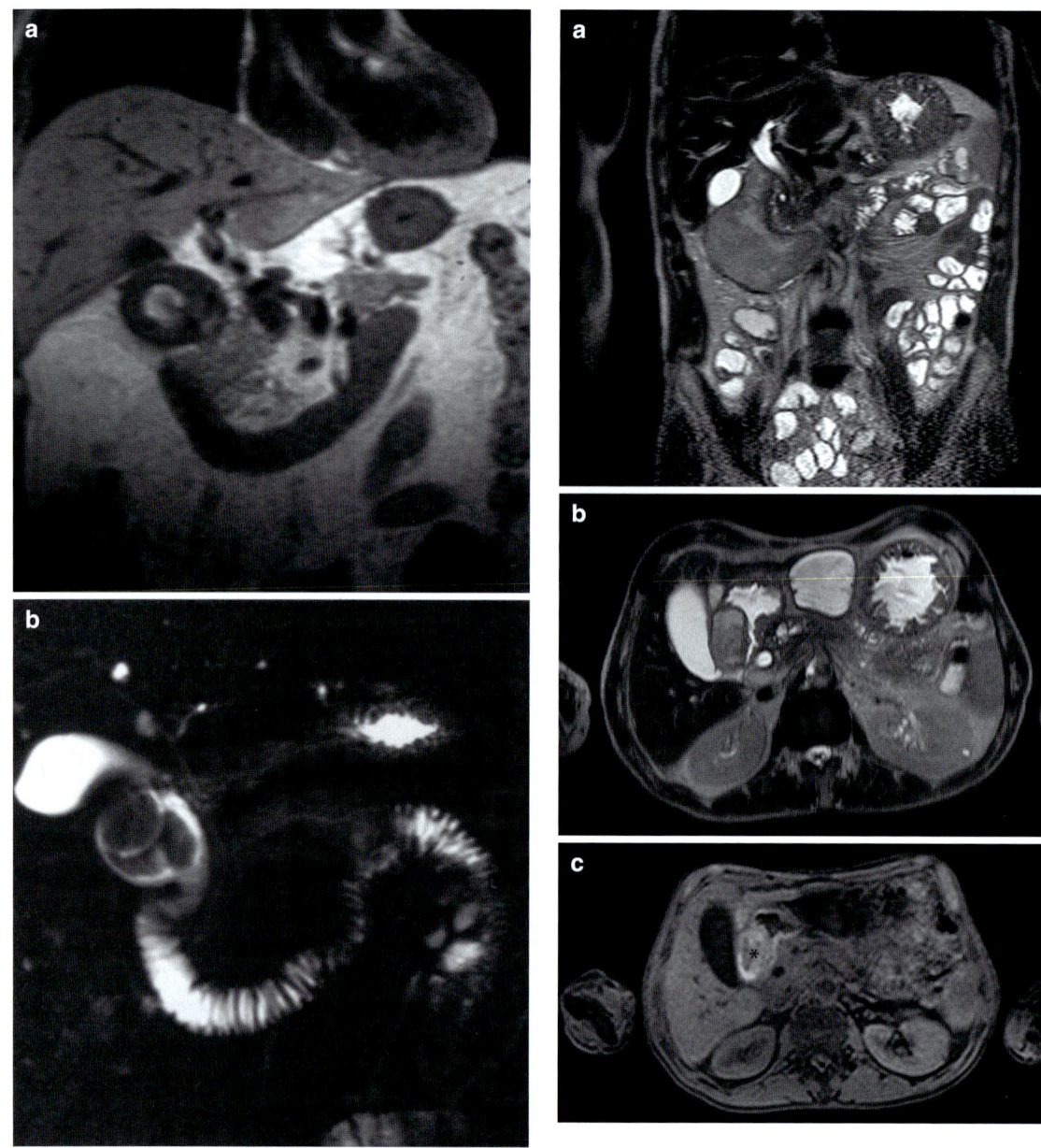

Fig. 7.4. Duodenal lipoma. Coronal T1-weighted image (**a**) shows the presence of a hyperintense round mass within the duodenal wall which appears as a hypointense area surrounded by fluid in the fat-saturated MRCP projection obtained after secretin administration (**b**)

Fig. 7.5. Duodenal hematoma. Coronal (**a**) and axial (**b**) T2-weighted images show a large and heterogeneous mass located in the lateral wall of the second duodenum and a stenosis of the lumen. On axial fat-saturated T1-weighted image the lesion has a peripheral hyperintense ring (*asterisk* in **c**) due to hemoglobin degradation products

diagnosis (Ashley et al. 1988). The peak prevalence is in the seventh decade. Symptoms are variable and generally related to associated complications (duodenal stenosis and/or common bile duct obstruction). At MRI the lesions are generally diagnosed when performing MRCP for distal common bile duct obstruction and are therefore associated to bile duct dilation. They may present as a polypoid intraluminal mass or as an intramural mass thickening the duodenal wall. Polypoid lesions in the duodenal lumen are easily identified on T2-weighted sequences when the lumen is distended with fluid after intravenous administration of secretin. They will appear as a soft tissue hypointense lesion outlined by hyperintense fluid. Polypoid lesions may

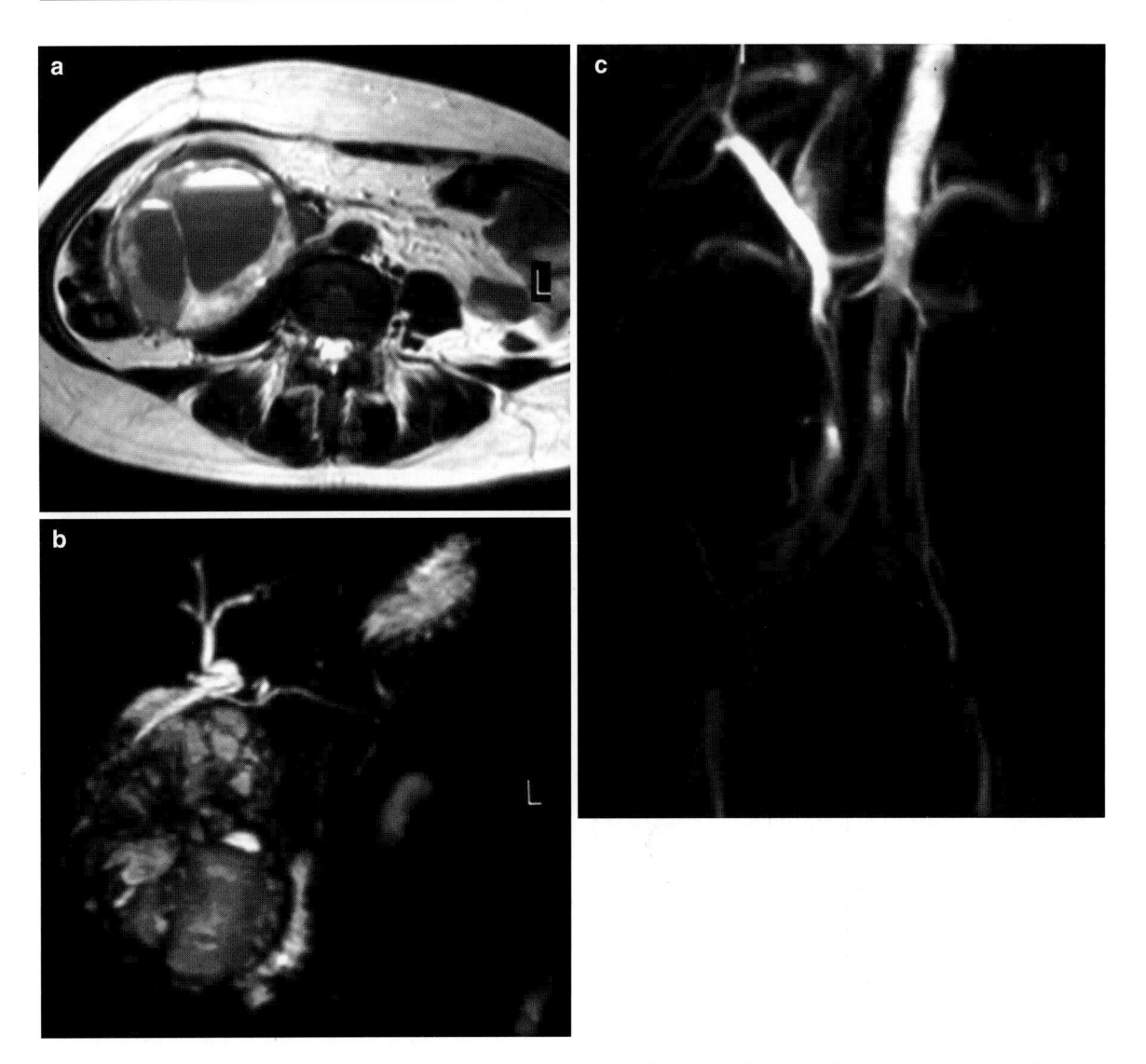

Fig. 7.6. GIST. Axial T2-weighted images (**a**) shows a huge lesion with inhomogeneous texture and fluid-fluid level related to intralesional hemorrhage and cystic components. MRCP (**b**) shows the extrinsic compression of the bile ducts. Coronal MR angiography renderings (**c**) shows the compression of the superior mesenteric vein and inferior vena cava

enhance after intravenous gadolinium administration (Fig. 7.9a–c). Intramural lesions not associated with duodenal or bile duct obstruction are more difficult to diagnose because they are nearly isointense to the normal duodenal wall on T2- and on T1-weighted imaging (Fig. 7.10a, b). Intravenous gadolinium administration may facilitate the diagnosis because the lesion generally enhances less than the normal duodenal wall. Although not yet widely used, DWI should be added to the conventional MRI protocol whenever the diagnosis is highly suspected, and no definite lesion is observed on T2-weighted and on gadolinium-enhanced T1-weighted sequences (Fig. 7.11a, b).

7.3.2.7
Duodenal Lymphoma

Lymphoid tissue is quite poor at the duodenal level, and therefore the involvement by lymphoma is rare. Lymphoma may be primary or more often secondary to systemic disease. Associated risk factors include *Helicobacter pylori* infection, immunosuppression after solid organ transplantation, celiac disease, inflammatory bowel disease, and human immunodeficiency virus infection. Imaging studies of lymphoma show a wide variety of appearances. Features that are strongly suggestive include a bulky mass or a diffuse bowel wall dilation of the duodenal lumen is highly suggestive of the diagnosis (Fig. 7.12a, b). Contrast enhancement after intravenous administration of gadolinium is generally mild.

7.3.2.8
Duodenal Carcinoids

Duodenal carcinoids may be discovered incidentally or may produce symptoms from hormonal or peptide production. They represent 2–3% of all gastrointestinal neuroendocrine tumors. G-cell tumors (one-third produce the clinical manifestations of Zollinger–Ellison syndrome) are the most frequent. Eighty-five percent of sporadic G-cell carcinoids associated with gastrin production (also called gastrinomas) are solitary lesions and occur in the "gastrinoma triangle," which is anatomically defined as the region limited by the confluence of the cystic and common bile ducts superiorly, the second and third portions of the duodenum inferiorly, and the neck and body of the pancreas medially (Stabille 1984). When associated to multiple endocrine neoplasia type 1 (MEN-1) gastrinomas are usually multiple, of small size (<5 mm) and located in the proximal duodenum. About one-fifth of duodenal carcinoids are somatostatin-producing (D-cell) tumors and occurs exclusively in and around the ampulla of Vater. D-cell carcinoids are associated with neurofibromatosis type 1 (NF-1) (Levy et al. 2007). At imaging around 50% of duodenal carcinoids manifest as polypoid masses and 40% as intramural masses. On MRI the lesions usually present variable signal intensity on T1- and on T2-weighted sequences and are easily recognizable when intraluminal (Fig. 7.13). After intravenous gadolinium administration they usually enhance in the arterial phase which may be a helpful distinguishing feature compared to duodenal adenomas and adenocarcinomas which typically do not show arterial enhancement.

7.3.2.9
Duodenal Metastases

Secondary involvement of the duodenum with other primary neoplasms can occur by means of local extension from a neighbor organ (pancreatic adenocarcinoma most often) (Fig. 7.14) or metastases from distant sites, such as the colon, stomach, melanoma, breast, ovary, and lung.

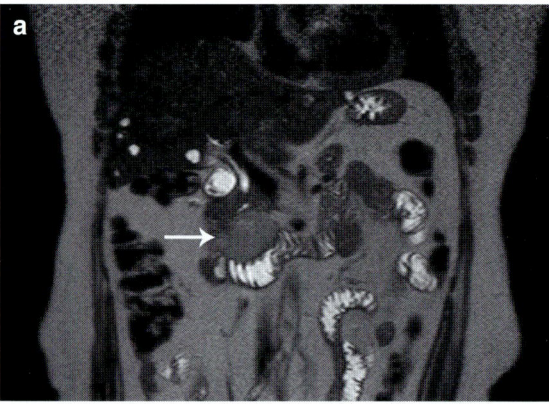

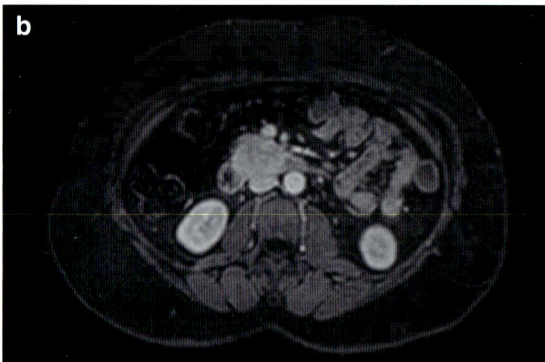

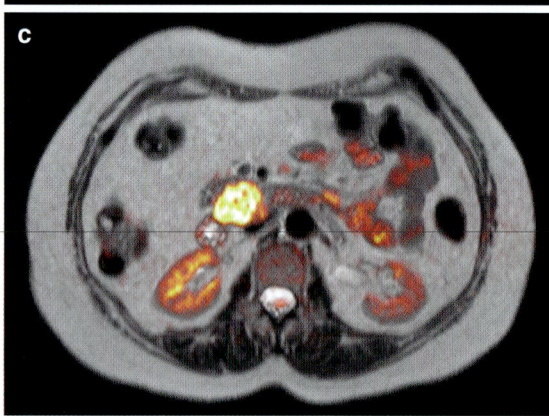

Fig. 7.7. GIST. Coronal (a) T2-weighted image show a heterogeneous mildly hyperintense mass (*arrow*) located in the duodenal genu under the head of the pancreas. Axial (b) gadolinium-enhanced fat-saturated T1-weighted images shows clear enhancement in the delayed venous phase. The fusion image (c) obtained from the T2-weighted images and the DWI set in the axial plane shows a clear restriction in water diffusion within the tumor

infiltration with preservation of fat planes and no obstruction, multiple site involvement and associated large size lymph nodes (Ghai et al. 2007). Bowel wall thickening is generally larger and better delineated than in adenocarcinoma. Associated "aneurismal"

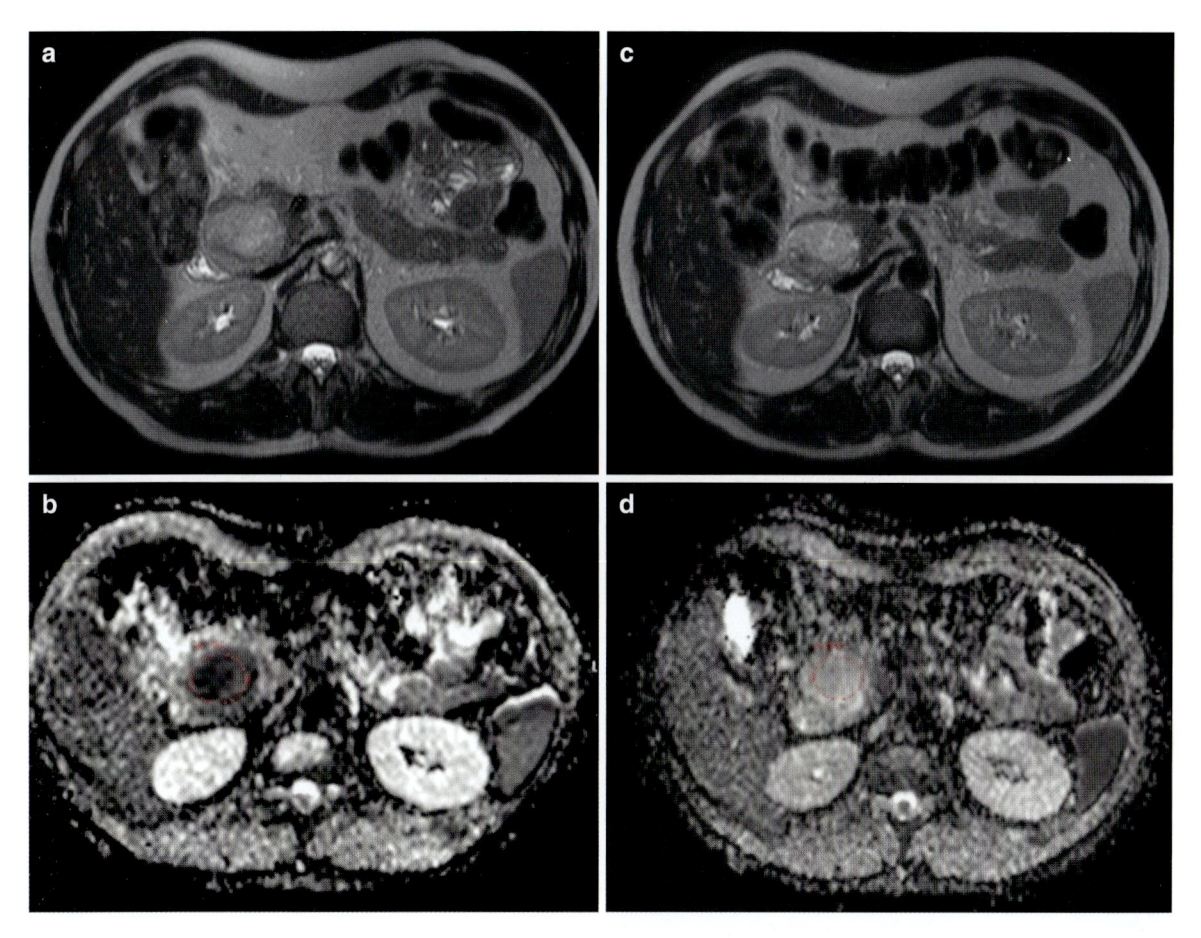

Fig. 7.8. GIST. Axial T2-weighted images (**a** and **c**) and ADC maps (**b** and **d**) of the same patient before (**a** and **c**) and after treatment (**b** and **d**) with imatinib show an increased ADC value after treatment (from 450 mm^2/s to 1,300 mm^2/s) that correlates with a good response in absence of any reduction in the size of the lesion

7.3.3
Lesions of Ampullary Origin

7.3.3.1
Choledococele

Choledococele is the less frequent type of choledochal cyst. It is located in the intramural segment of the common bile duct and presents as a cystic dilation that herniates into the duodenal lumen. Associated common bile duct stones are the most common complication and in such case patients may have recurrent abdominal pain and obstructive jaundice. Malignant transformation is rare and less frequent than with the other types of choledochal cysts. On MRCP the intramural segment of the common bile duct presents a clubbed appearance. T2-weighted cross-sectional MRI will display a focal, smooth, round, or ovoid fluid-filled "mass" protruding into the duodenal lumen at the major papilla (DE BACKER et al. 2000) (Fig. 7.15).

7.3.3.2
Ampullary Tumors

Benign lesions include adenoma, leiomyoma, neurofibroma, hemangioma, and hamartoma. Adenoma is considered a premalignant lesion (YAMAGUCHI et al. 1991), and its diagnosis is generally obtained at endoscopy. Ampullary carcinoma arise from the glandular epithelium of the ampulla of Vater and recent reports suggest that ampullary carcinoma should be classified as a duodenal cancer because ampullary and duodenal carcinoma share the same molecular development and the clinical outcomes of both are better than those of bile duct and pancreatic cancer. Jaundice is common and is generally the first

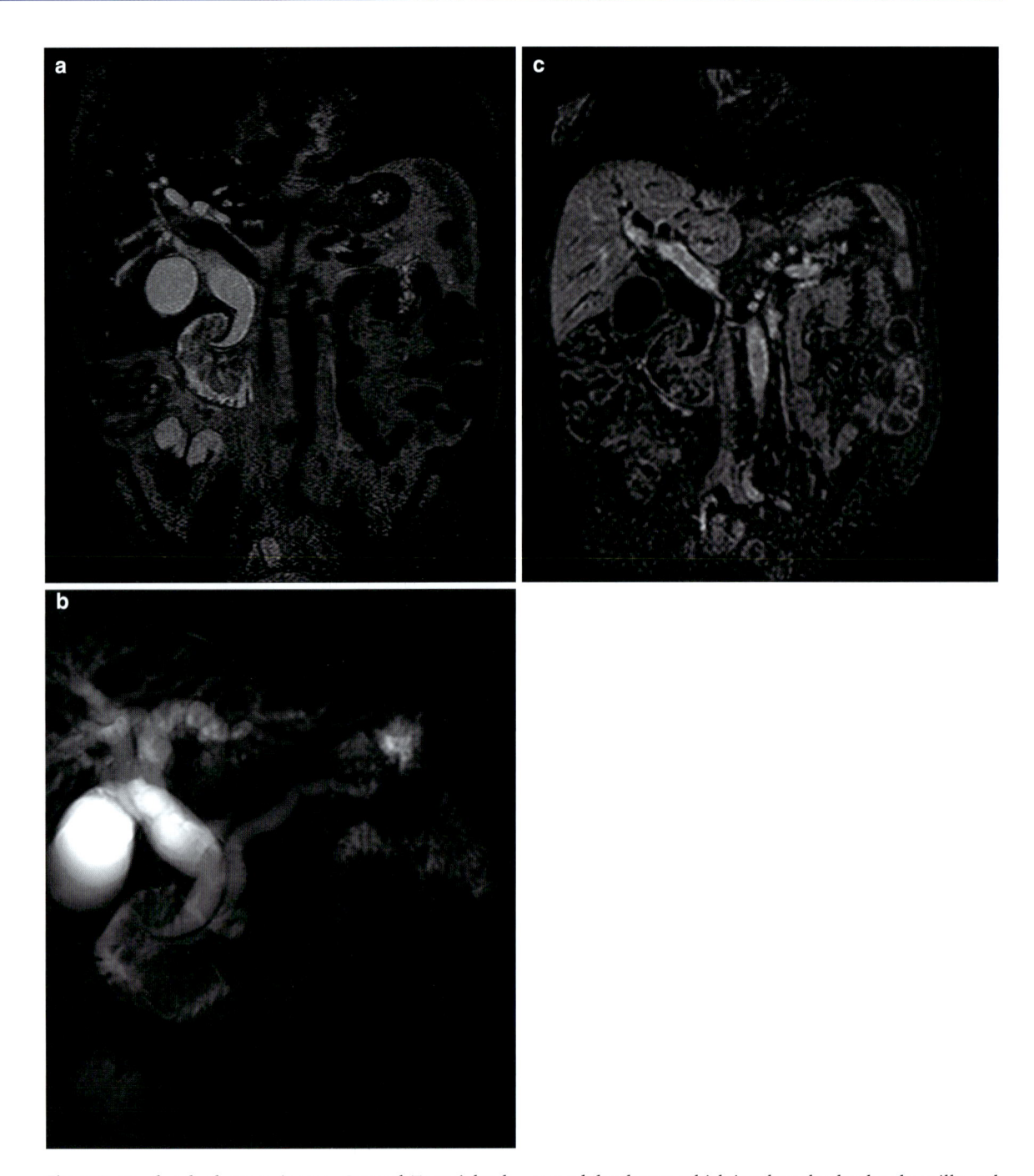

Fig. 7.9. Duodenal adenocarcinoma. Coronal T2-weighted image (**a**) secretin-enhanced MRCP (**b**) and gadolinium-enhanced coronal T1-weighted image (**c**) show the presence of a large polypoid lesion rising from the medial wall of the second duodenum which involves the duodenal papilla and determines obstruction of both the biliary and the pancreatic ducts. The mass is easily depictable as the lumen is filled with fluid (**a** and **b**) and enhances

symptom. Ampullary carcinomas may have a nodular appearance or manifest as irregular periductal thickening. Both forms may present as protruding mass into the duodenum (KIM et al. 2002b). On MRI an irregular inner margin of the distal common bile duct and/or of the main pancreatic duct allows differentiation with benign causes of ductal obstruction. As for other periampullary lesions MRI should

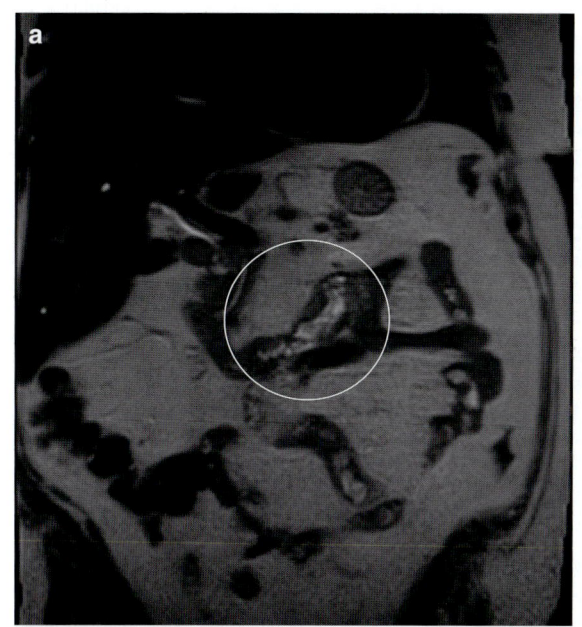

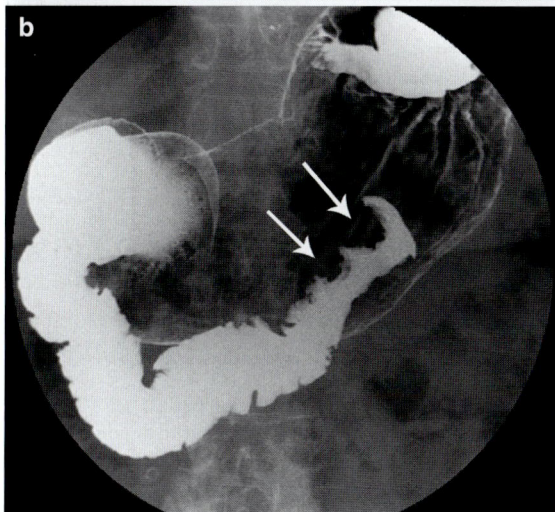

Fig. 7.10. Adenocarcinoma of the fourth portion of the duodenum. The lesion appears as an isointense intramural thickening (*circle*) visible in the coronal T2-weighted image (**a**) without signs of obstruction. Comparative barium follow-through examination (**b**) clearly depicts the duodenal stricture (*arrows*) and its irregular borders

7.3.4
Lesions of Pancreatic Origin

7.3.4.1
Annular Pancreas

Annular pancreas is a rare congenital variation in which pancreatic tissue in continuity with the head of the pancreas completely encircles the duodenum, usually in its second portion. In approximately 50% of the cases it is present in childhood with duodenal obstruction. This younger group frequently suffers from other associated abnormalities, such as Down's syndrome (Rizzo et al. 1995). In a review of 266 patients with symptoms, 48% were adults (Kiernan et al. 1980). Symptoms are usually nonspecific and include abdominal pain, nausea, and vomiting. If acute pancreatitis develops, duodenal obstruction may occur. On MRI fat-suppressed T1-weighted sequences are diagnostic by identifying a thickened and hyperintense duodenal wall tissue in continuity with the hyperintense head of the pancreas (Fig. 7.17). MRCP along with secretin stimulation may show the ventral component of the main pancreatic duct encircling the duodenum (Fig. 7.18).

7.3.4.2
Paraduodenal Pancreatitis

This entity is more and more diagnosed and represents a distinct form of chronic pancreatitis occurring predominantly in and around the duodenal wall (near the minor papilla). It has been reported under various names, including cystic dystrophy of heterotopic pancreas, pancreatic hamartoma of the duodenum, para-duodenal wall cyst, and groove pancreatitis, which reflect the different aspects of microscopic pathology (Adsay et al 2004). In typical cases, the duodenal wall in the vicinity of the minor papilla shows myofibroblastic proliferation and Brunner's gland hyperplasia is prominent and contributes to the thickening of the duodenal wall. When heterotopic pancreas is present cystically dilated pancreatic ducts can be identified (Triantopoulou et al. 2009). The disease affects mainly male patients with a history of heavy alcohol consumption. The exact prevalence is not known but ranges in between 2.7% and 24.5% in surgical series of patients affected by chronic pancreatitis (Triantopoulou et al. 2009). Predominant symptoms are upper abdominal pain, weight loss, and postprandial nausea and vomiting (due to

be performed with secretin to achieve good duodenal distension and increase the contrast between the intermediate signal of the tumor and the bright fluid in the duodenum. This strategy allows better assess the intraduodenal and the intraductal extension of the tumor (Fig. 7.16).

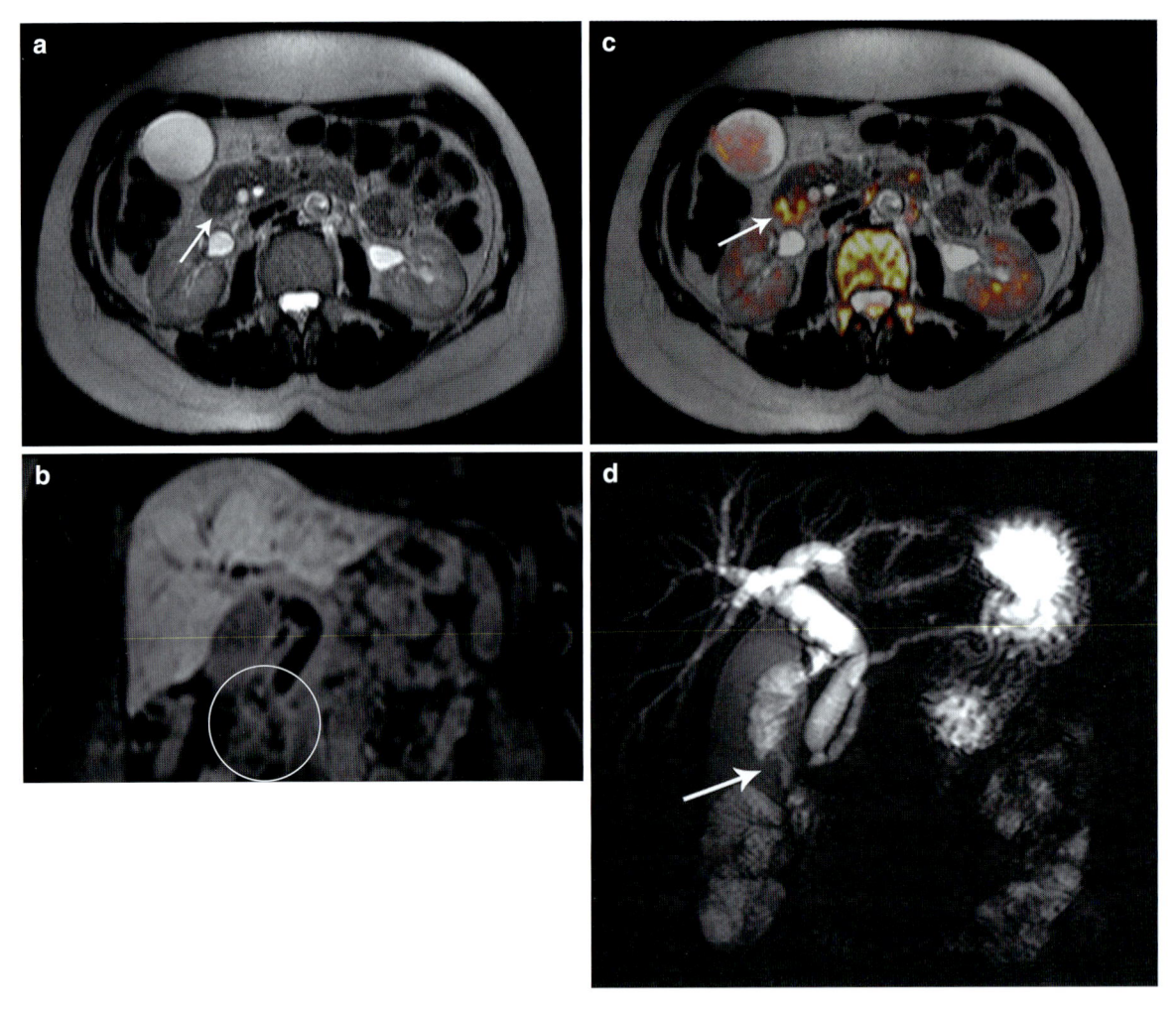

Fig. 7.11. Adenocarcinoma of the second portion of the duodenum. The tumor presents as a circumferential thickening of the wall that appears isointense in the axial T2-weighted image (*arrow* in **a**), hypovascular in the coronal T1-weighted image after gadolinium injection (*circle* in **b**) and strongly hypersignal in the axial images fused with the DWI set (*arrow* in **c**). The apple-core appearance of the duodenal lumen in the MRCP image (*arrow* in **d**) typically shows the associated duodenal stenosis)

stenosis of the duodenum). Paraduodenal pancreatitis has been divided into pure (the head of the pancreas is spared), segmental (the pancreatic head and the ducts are affected) and nonsegmental (secondary to established chronic pancreatitis) forms (Becker et al. 1991). On MRI the pure form appears as a sheet-like mass filling the groove between the head of the pancreas and the thickened duodenal wall. This mass appears hypointense to pancreatic parenchyma on fat-suppressed T1-weighted images and shows variable signal intensity on T2-weighted images according to the time of disease's onset, being higher in subacute phase (due to oedema) and lower in chronic (due to more prominent fibrosis) (Blasbalg et al. 2007). Cyst-like changes in the groove or the duodenal wall will be better displayed on T2-weighted sections. The cysts may be tiny or quite large. In case of heterotopic pancreas a dilated duct with pseudocysts may be identified. Additional findings include duodenal stenosis with or without associated gastric dilation. On MRCP the bile ducts and the main pancreatic duct will have a normal appearance (Fig. 7.19). In the segmental form the inflammatory process extends to the pancreatic head and associated stenosis of the common bile duct and of the main pancreatic duct will be seen on MRCP. The strictures are generally smooth, long, and incomplete and associated with mild upstream dilation. Involvement of the pancreas

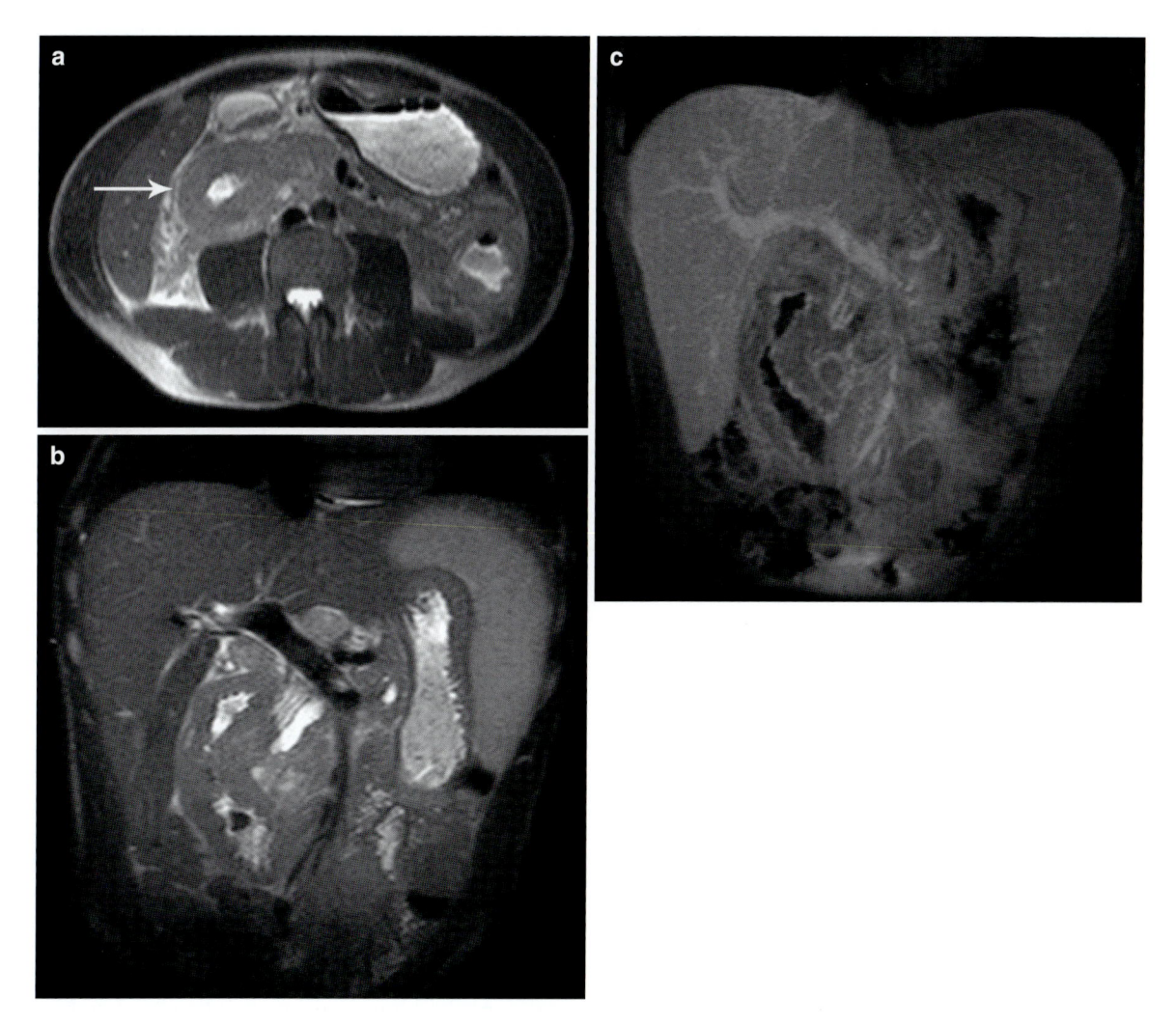

Fig. 7.12. AIDS related duodenal lymphoma. Axial (**a**) and coronal fat-saturated (**b**) T2-weighted images show a homogeneous well-defined duodenal wall thickening (*arrow* in **a**) with aneurismal dilation of the lumen and no extension to surrounding fatty tissues. Coronal gadolinium-enhanced T1-weighted image (**c**) shows mild enhancement of the lesion (courtesy of Drs Bart Op de Beeck and Anemie Snoeckx from the University Hospital of Antwerpen, Belgium)

parenchyma in the head is easier to identify on DWI compared to T2-weighted imaging (Fig. 7.20). Paraduodenal pancreatitis may also be complicated by classical changes of chronic pancreatitis or be a consequence of chronic pancreatitis when superimposed acute pancreatitis extends to the groove. In all cases, intravenous gadolinium should be administered to help differentiate pancreatitis and carcinoma. In a recent preliminary experience a patchy focal enhancement in the portal venous phase was more commonly observed in groove pancreatitis and peripheral enhancement was only observed in groove carcinomas (Ishigami et al. 2009). Another clue for the differential diagnosis consists in identifying the relationship between the groove lesion and the gastroduodenal artery. In carcinomas the gastroduodenal artery is located between the lesion and the duodenum while in pancreatitis it is displaced leftward (Ishigami et al. 2009). In any case the presence of marked pancreatic duct dilation should be considered as a suspicious feature for the presence of a carcinoma.

7.3.5
MRI Compared to CT

No comparative studies of both modalities have been produced. Multidetector computed tomography

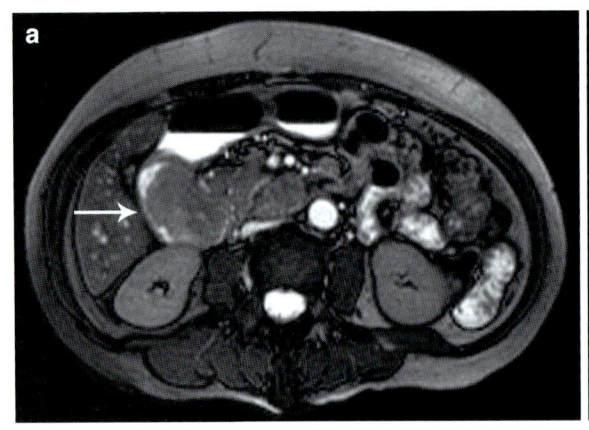

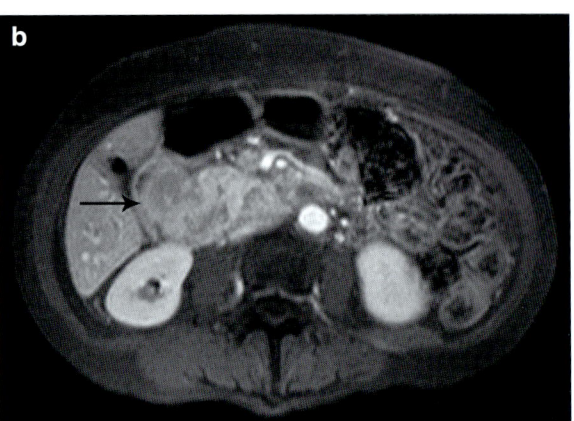

Fig. 7.13. Duodenal somatostatinoma. Axial TRUE-FISP (**a**) shows a well-defined intraluminal mass at the ampulla of Vater with no signs of obstruction. Gadolinium-enhanced fat-saturated T1-weighted image (**b**) shows an avid enhancement of the mass (*arrow*) (courtesy of Drs Bart Op de Beeck and Anemie Snoeckx from the University Hospital of Antwerpen, Belgium)

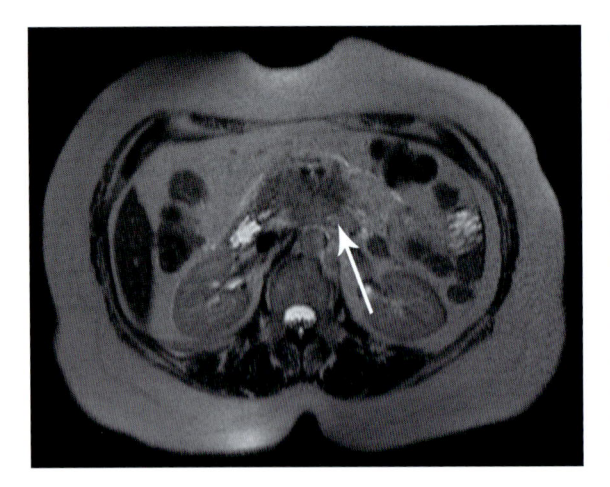

Fig. 7.14. Adenocarcinoma of the pancreas. Axial T2-weighted image shows a tumor in the body of the pancreas with irregular and spiculated contours that extends to the adjacent third portion of the duodenum determining a direct invasion (*arrow*)

(MDCT) is more available and image acquisition is standardized. Therefore it is considered the optimal cross-sectional imaging technique for evaluating duodenal disorders. Thin collimation and multiphase acquisition after iodine contrast administration allows obtaining high-quality off-axis scans, especially helpful in evaluating duodenal and paraduodenal space-occupying lesions and the surrounding vessels. MDCT plays a vital role in the diagnosis of traumatic injuries and is a reliable diagnostic method for evaluating inflammatory processes of the duodenum secondary to pancreatitis. In this context the major contribution of MRI is related to its capabilities of providing noninvasively MRCP renderings and to its superior contrast resolution which allows identifying the majority of duodenal disorders, especially congenital anomalies, cystic lesions, and inflammatory processes involving the duodenal groove.

MRI of the Duodenum 109

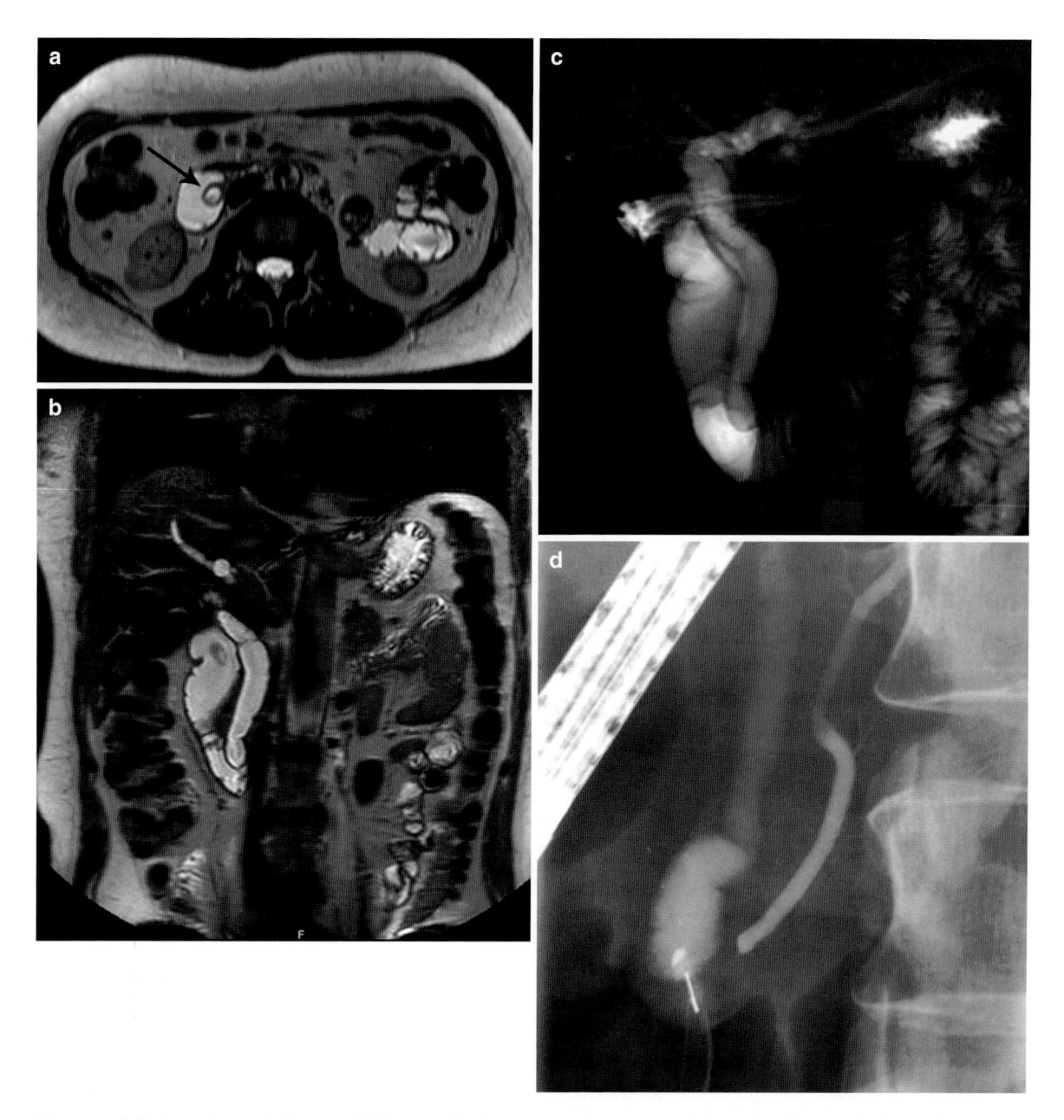

Fig. 7.15. Choledococele. Axial (**a**), coronal (**b**) T2-weighted images and MRCP (**c**) images depict a cystic fluid-filled dilation of the intramural segment of the common bile duct (*arrow*). Comparative ERCP (**d**) and endoscopic view (**e**) show the bulging intraluminal sacculation and the major papilla orifice (*arrow*)

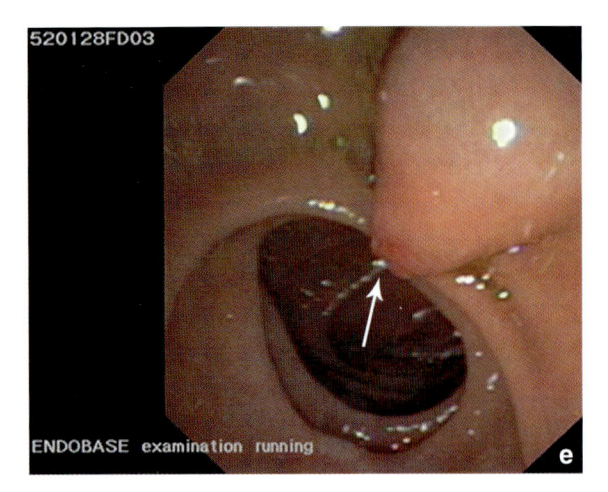

Fig. 7.15. continued

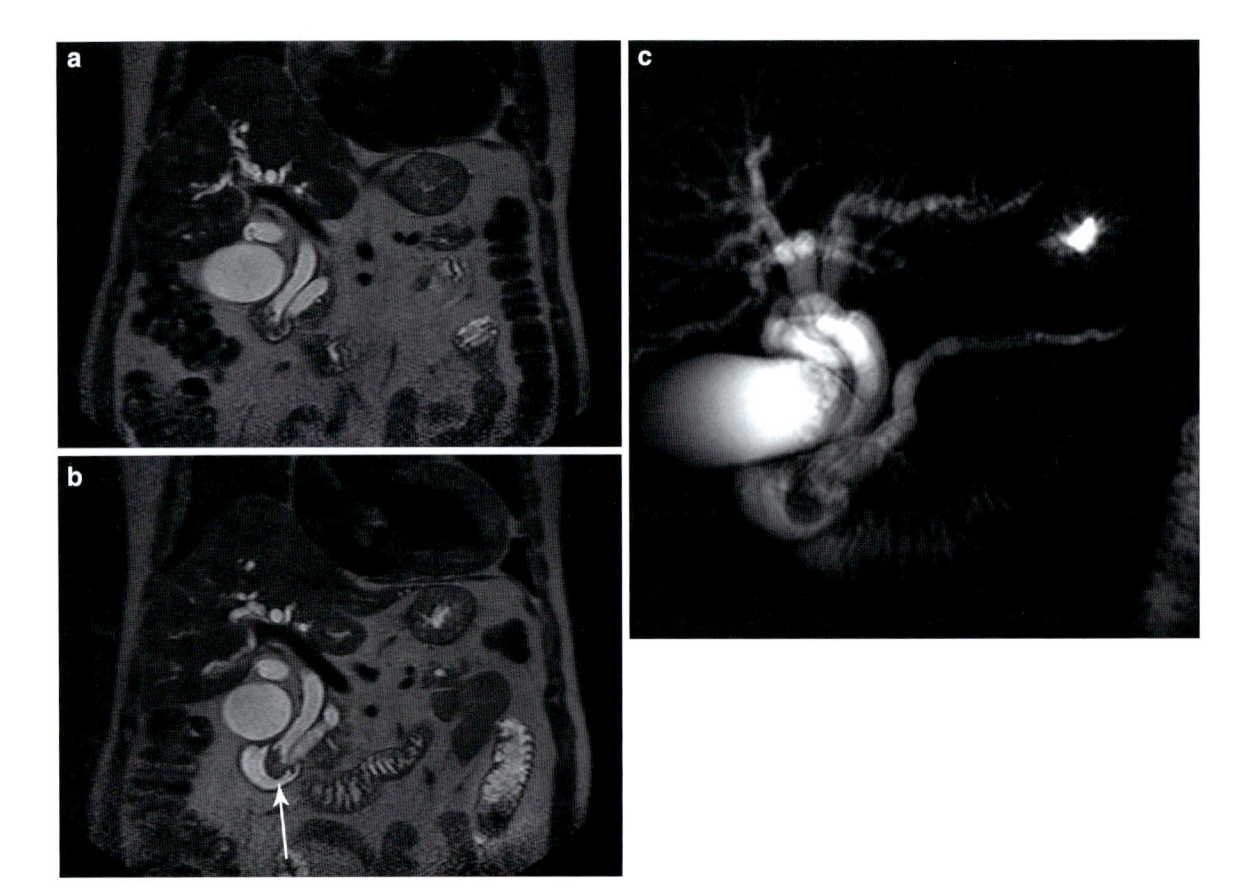

Fig. 7.16. Carcinoma of the ampulla. Coronal T2-weighted images before (**a**) and after (**b**) secretin injection demonstrate the presence of a nodular thickening of the duodenal papilla (*arrow*) that irregularly protrudes into the lumen and determines distal obstruction and dilation of both the common bile duct and the pancreatic duct as clearly showed on MRCP image (**c**)

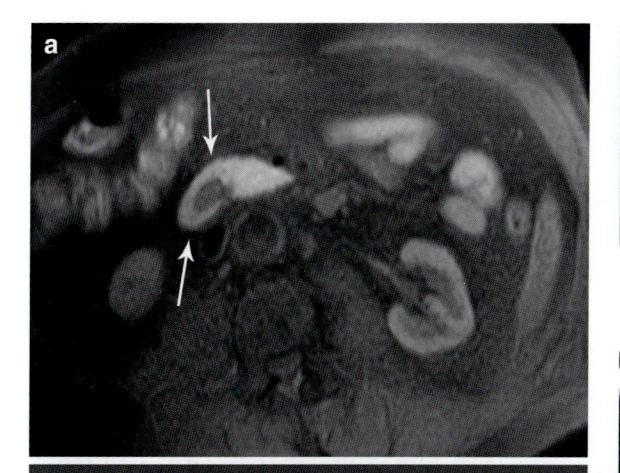

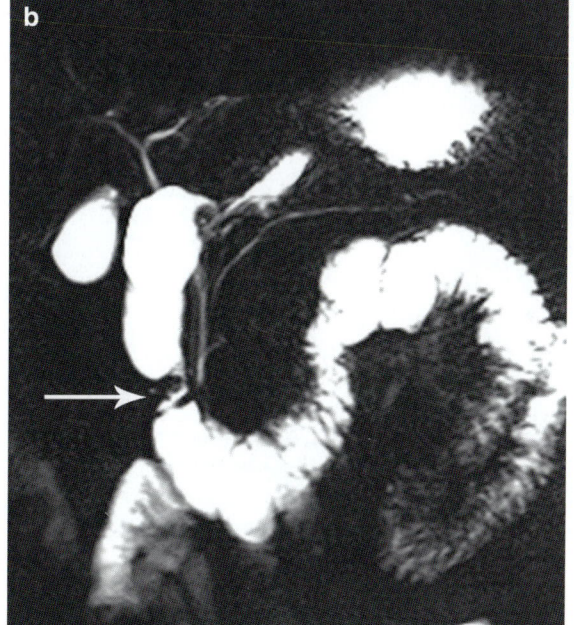

Fig. 7.17. Annular pancreas. Axial fat-saturated T1-weighted image (**a**) shows the presence of hyperintense ring of pancreatic tissue that completely encircles the second portion of the duodenum (*arrows*). The MRCP image (**b**) obtained after secretin injection shows the associated duodenal stenosis (*arrow*) but failed to demonstrate the ventral pancreatic duct

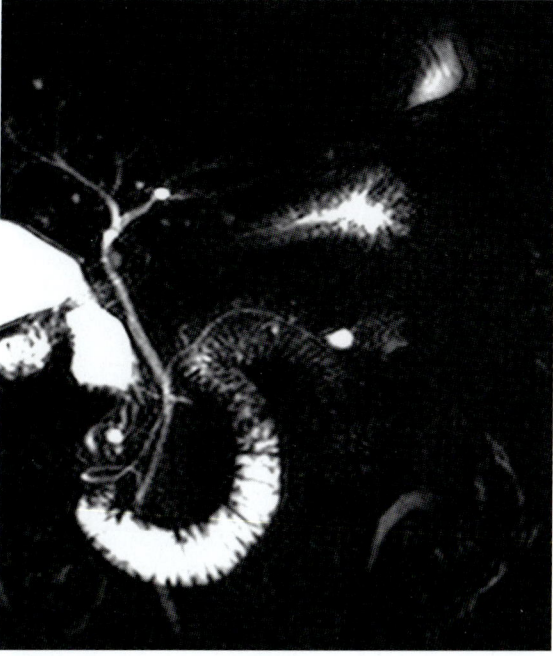

Fig. 7.18. Annular pancreas. MRCP image after secretin injection shows the ventral component of the main pancreatic duct encircling the duodenum

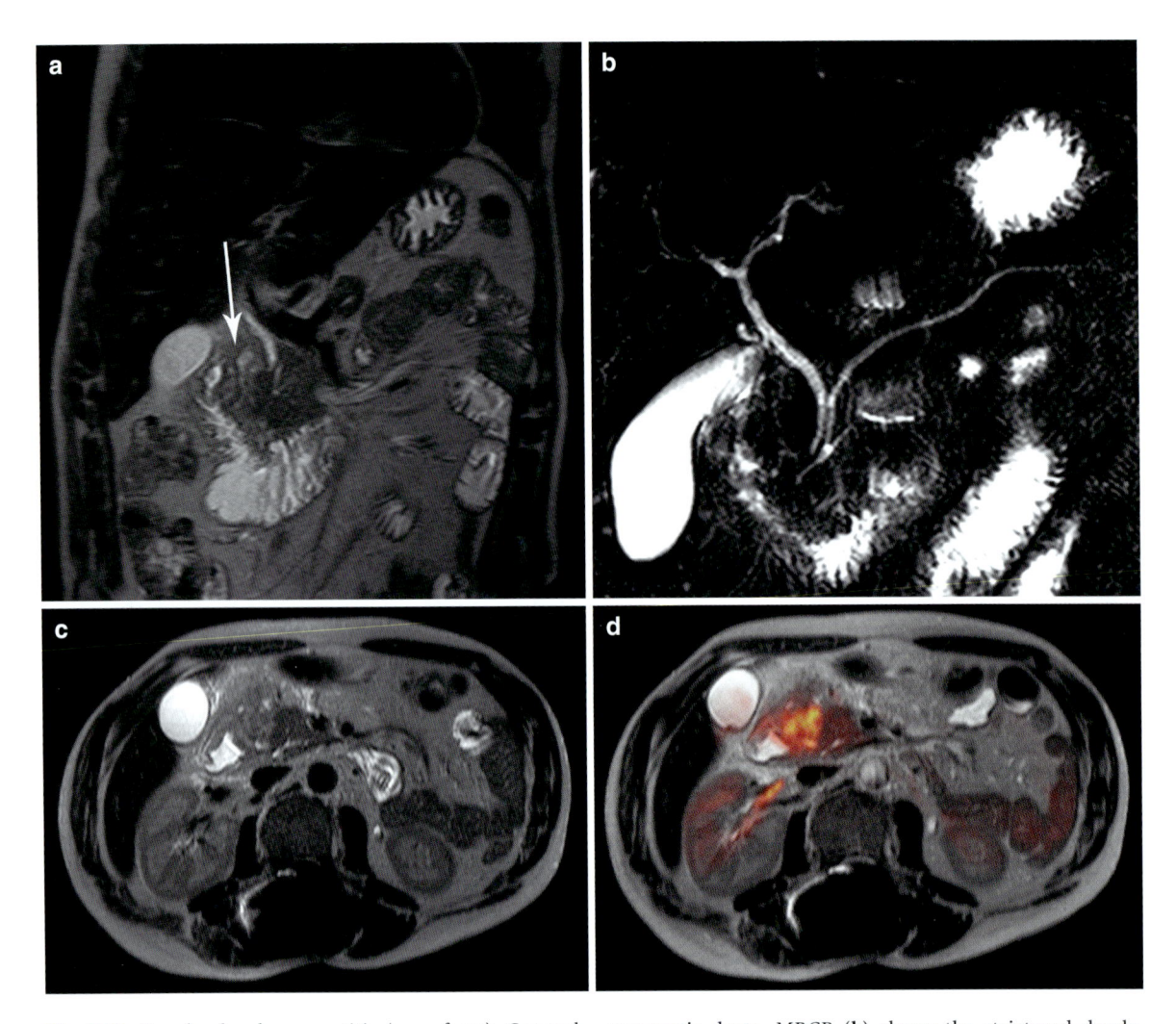

Fig. 7.19. Paraduodenal pancreatitis (pure form). Coronal (a) and axial (c) T2-weighted images shows the presence of an heterogeneous "mass" in the groove between the head of the pancreas and the duodenal wall, with evidence of linear fluid-filled structures (*arrow*) corresponding to heterotopic pancreatic ducts. MRCP (b) shows the strictured duodenal lumen and the normal caliber of the bile and pancreatic ducts. Fused T2-weighted and DWI images (d) shows restricted water diffusion within the groove, sparing the pancreatic head

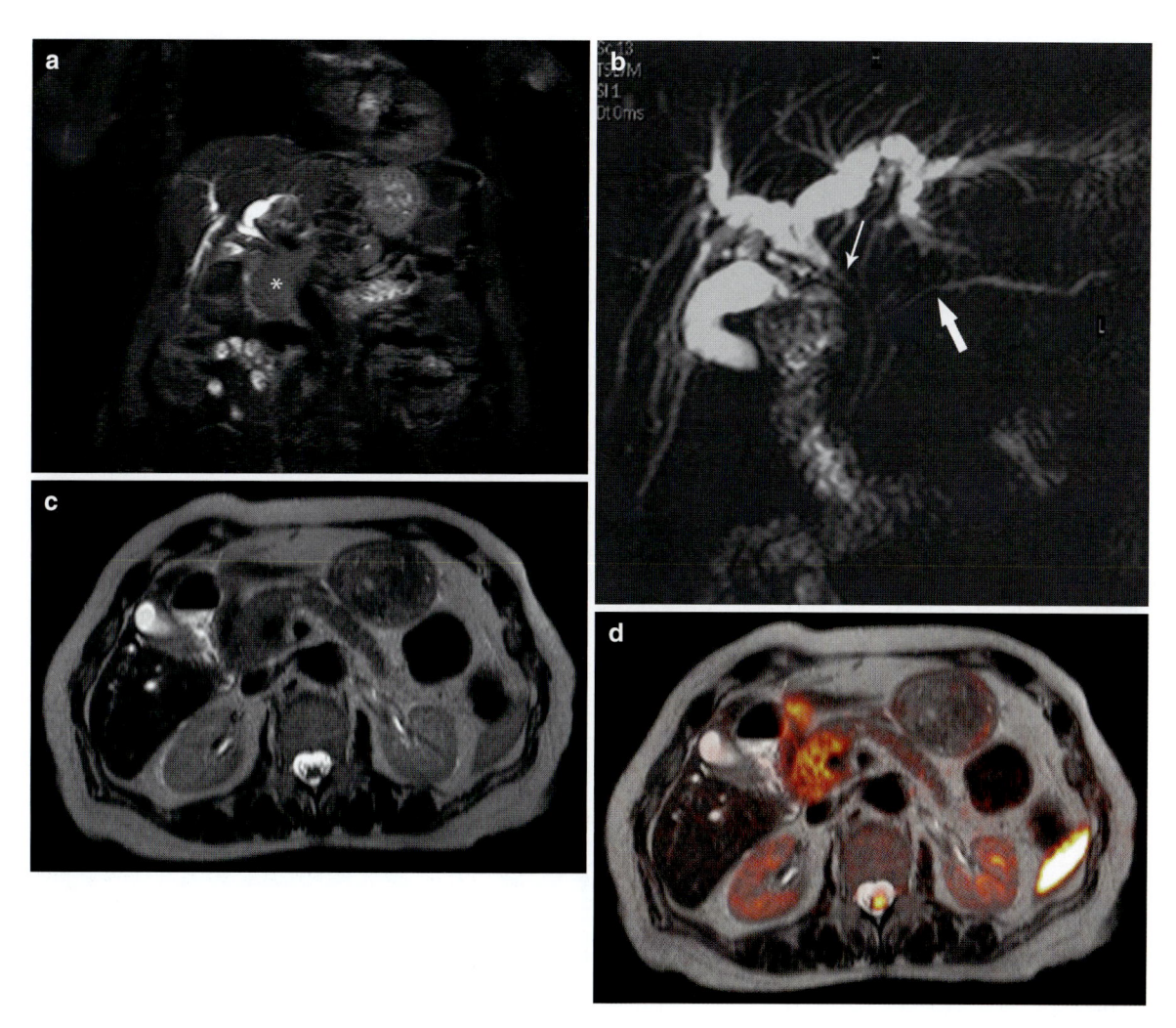

Fig. 7.20. Paraduodenal pancreatitis (segmental form). Coronal fat-saturated T2-weighted image (**a**) shows the presence of a pancreatic head pseudo-mass (*asterisk*) with peripancreatic edema and duodenal lumen narrowing. The common bile duct (*thin arrow*) and the main pancreatic duct have (*thick arrow*) a smooth and incomplete stenosis, associated to a dilation of the intrahepatic biliary tree, as shown on the MRCP image (**b**). The axial T2-weighted (**c**) and the fused T2-weighted and DWI images (**d**) clearly demonstrate the involvement of the pancreatic head that show restricted water diffusion

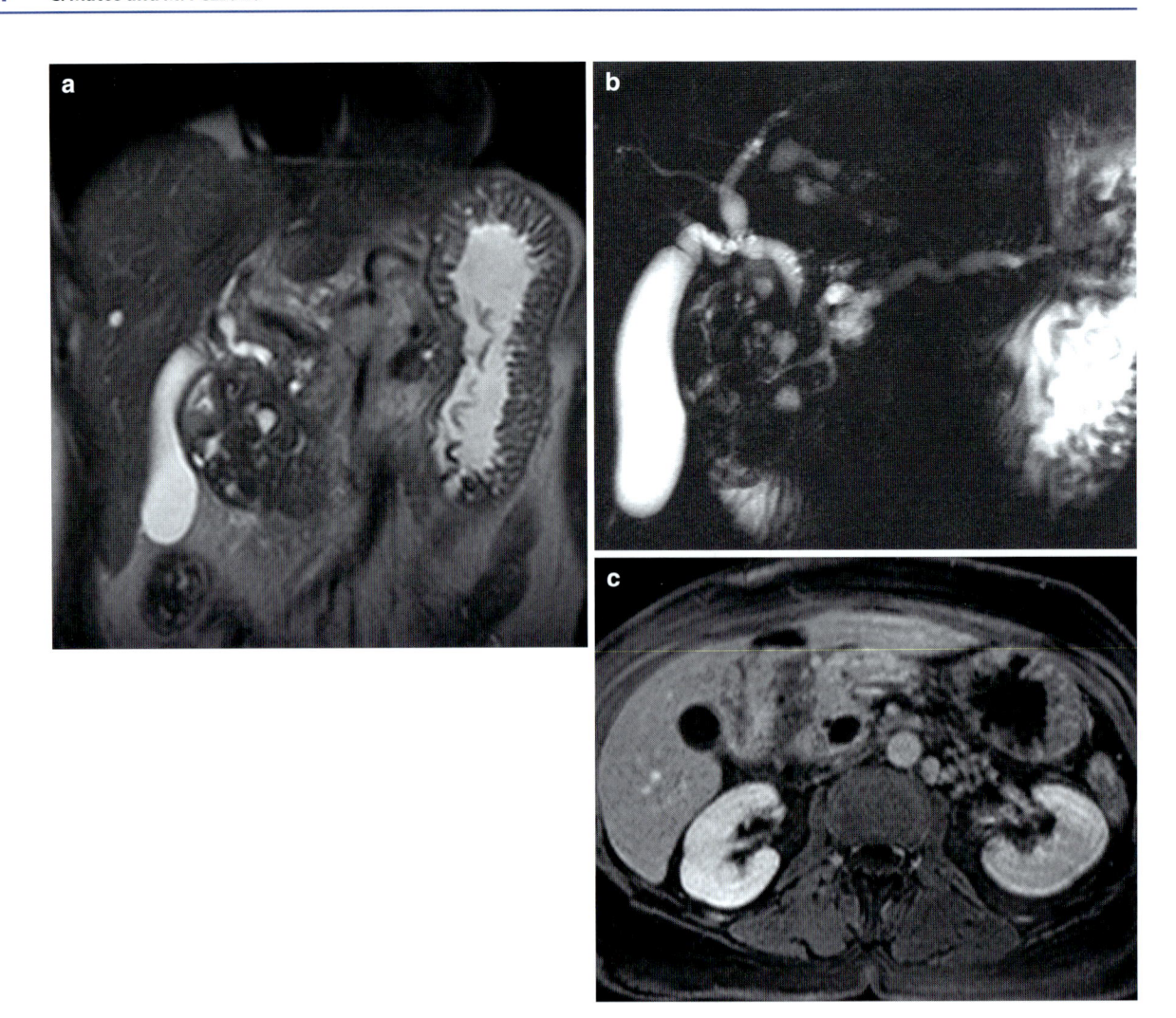

Fig. 7.21. Paraduodenal pancreatitis and chronic pancreatitis. Coronal T2-weighted section (**a**) and MRCP (**b**) show a duodenal stricture and a common bile duct and main pancreatic duct stricture. Tiny cystic lesions are depicted in the groove between the duodenal wall and the head of the pancreas. Axial gadolinium-enhanced fat-saturated T1-weighted image (**c**) shows peripheral enhancement of the lesion

References

Adsay NV, Zamboni G (2004) Paraduodenal pancreatitis: a clinico-pathologically distinct entity unifying "cystic dystrophy of heterotopic pancreas", "para-duodenal wall cyst" and "groove pancreatitis". Semin Diagn Pathol 21:247–254

Ashley SW, Wells SA (1988) Tumors of the small intestine. Semin Oncol 15:116–128

Becker V, Mischke U (1991) Groove pancreatitis. Int J Pancreatol 10:173–182

Blasbalg R, Baroni RH, Costa DN, et al (2007) MRI features of groove pancreatitis. AJR Am J Roentgenol 189:73–80

De Backer AI, Van den Abbeele K, De Schepper AM, et al (2000) Choledochocele: diagnosis by magnetic resonance imaging. Abdom Imaging 25:508–510

Fayad LM, Holland GA, Bergin D, et al (2003) Functional magnetic resonance cholangiography of the gallbladder end biliary tree with contrast-enhanced magnetic resonance cholangiography. JMRI 18:449–460

Ghai S, Pattison J, Ghai S, et al (2007) Primary gastrointestinal lymphoma: spectrum of imaging findings with pathologic correlation. Radiographics 27:1371–1388

Guibaud L, Fouque P, Genin G, et al (1996) CT and ultrasound of gastric and duodenal duplications. J Comput Assist Tomogr 20:382–385

Hong X, Choi H, Loyer EM, et al (2006) Gastrointestinal stromal tumor: Role of CT in diagnosis and in response evaluation and surveillance after treatment with imatinib. Radiographics 26:481–495

Ishigami K, Tajima T, Nishie A, et al (2009) Differential diagnosis of groove pancreatic carcinomas vs groove pancreatitis:

usefulness of the portal venous phase. Eur J Radiol doi: 10.1016/j.ejrad.200904.026

Kiernan PD, ReMine SG, Kiernan PC, et al (1980) Annular pancreas: mayo clinic experience from 1957 to 1976 with review of the literature. Arcg Surg 115:46–50

Kim JH, Kim MJ, Park SI, et al (2002a) Using kinematic MR cholangiopancreatography to evaluate biliary dilatation. AJR Am J Roentgenol 178:909–914

Kim JH, Kim MJ, Chung JJ, et al (2002b) Differential diagnosis of periampullary carcinomas at MR imaging. Radiographics 22:1335–1352

Koh DM, Collins DJ (2007) Diffusion-weighted MRI in the body: applications and challenges in oncology. AJR Am J Roentgenol 188:1622–1635

Lachachi F, Descottes B, Valleix D, et al (1996) Adénocarcinome primitif du duodénum. Ann Chir 50:333–339

Levy A, Remotti HE, Thompson WM, et al (2003) Gastrointestinal stromal tumors: radiologic features with pathologic correlation. Radiographics 23:283–304

Levy A, Sobin LH (2007) Gastrointestinal carcinoids: imaging features with clinicopathologic comparison. Radiographics 27:237–257

Matos C, Metens T, Devière J, et al (1997) Pancreatic duct: morphology and functional evaluation with dynamic MR pancreatography after secretin stimulation. Radiology 203:435–441

Nilsson B, Bumming P, Meis-Kindblom JM, et al (2005) Gastrointestinal stromal tumors: the incidence, prevalence, clinical course and prognostication in the preimatinib mesylate era: a population-based study in western Sweden. Cancer 103:821–829

Patterson DM, Padhani AR, Collons DJ (2008) technology insight: water diffusion MRI-a potential new biomarker of response to cancer therapy. Nat Clin Pract Oncol 5:220–233

Rizzo RJ, Szucs RA, Turner MA (1995) Congenital abnormalities of the pancreas and biliary tree in adults. Radiographics 15:49–68

Stabile BE, Morrow DJ, Passaro E Jr (1984) The gastrinoma triangle: operative implications. Am J Surg 147:25–31

Thompson WM (2005) Imaging and findings of lipomas of the gastrointestinal tract. Pictorial essay. AJR Am J Roentgenol 184:1163–1171

Triantopoulou C, Dervenis C, Giannakou N, et al (2009) Groove pancreatitis: a diagnostic challenge. Eur Radiol 19:1736–1743

Tsushima Y, Takano A, Taketomi-Takahashi A, et al. (2007) Body diffusion-weighted MR imaging using high b-value for malignant tumor screening: usefulness and necessity of referring to T2-weighted images and creating fusion images. Acad Radiol 14:643–650

Yamaguchi K, Enjoji M (1991) Adenoma of the ampulla of Vater: putative precancerous lesion. Gut 32:1558–1561

MRI of the Small Bowel: Enterography

Manon L.W. Ziech and Jaap Stoker

CONTENTS

8.1 Introduction 117
8.2 **Contrast Media Used for MR Enterography** 118
8.2.1 Positive Oral Contrast Agents 118
8.2.2 Negative Oral Contrast Agents 119
8.2.3 Biphasic Oral Contrast Agents 119
8.2.4 Intravenous Contrast Agents 120
8.2.5 Anti-Spasmolytic Agents 120
8.3 **Technique** 120
8.3.1 Sequences 121
8.3.1.1 Half-Fourier Single Shot RARE (HASTE) 121
8.3.1.2 Balanced Steady-State Free Precession 121
8.3.1.3 T1-Weighted Sequences 121
8.3.1.4 Diffusion-Weighted Imaging (DWI) 121
8.3.1.5 Cine Imaging 122
8.4 **Results** 123
8.4.1 Crohn's Disease 123
8.4.1.1 Bowel Wall Thickening 123
8.4.1.2 High Signal Intensity of the Bowel Wall on T2-Weighted Images 124
8.4.1.3 Enhancement After Intravenous Contrast Administration 124
8.4.1.4 Bowel Wall Stratification 124
8.4.1.5 Ulcerations 124
8.4.1.6 Comb Sign 125
8.4.1.7 Lymph Nodes 125
8.4.1.8 Fistula and Abscess 125
8.4.1.9 Stenosis 126
8.4.1.10 Creeping Fat 126
8.4.1.11 CD Disease Activity Assessment 126
8.4.1.12 CD Disease Severity Assessment 127
8.4.1.13 Place of MR Enterography in CD Patients 127
8.4.2 Celiac Disease 129
8.4.3 Benign Small Bowel Neoplasms 129
8.4.4 Malignant Small Bowel Neoplasms 130
8.4.5 Miscellaneous 131
8.5 **Future Prospects of MR Enterography** 132
References 132

Manon L.W. Ziech, MD
Jaap Stoker, MD PhD
Department of Radiology, Academic Medical Center, University of Amsterdam, Meibergdreef 9, 1105 AZ, The Netherlands

KEY POINTS

MR enterography has become an important technique for imaging of the small bowel. Technical advances, especially fast imaging techniques, were a major impetus for this development. Luminal distension is obtained by oral intake of a contrast agent; often a biphasic contrast agent is used. This has been shown to be sufficient to demonstrate pathologic findings. The major indication for MR enterography is follow-up of disease activity in Crohn's disease. It can also be used as an alternative for endoscopy and MR enteroclysis for the work-up of patients with symptoms most likely related to small bowel diseases and for specific conditions such as lymphoma and small bowel polyps. Patient acceptance of MR enterography is high when compared to MR enteroclysis and colonoscopy, which is important for frequent application of the technique for monitoring treatment. Thereby, the technique has logistical advantages over MR enteroclysis.

8.1 Introduction

In the last 15 years, imaging of the small bowel has improved with great steps. With endoscopic techniques, the stomach and colon can be easily reached, but the use of traditional endoscopy for evaluation of the small bowel is limited, owing to the length and location of the small bowel. Over the years, new methods have been developed for better visualization of the small bowel. Wireless video capsule, double-balloon enteroscopy, and imaging techniques have all been designed for this purpose. Traditionally, imaging of the small bowel was done by barium enteroclysis, the first technique to visualize the entire small bowel. The limitation of conventional enteroclysis is that only abnormalities of the luminal wall could be visualized. The development of cross-sectional imaging techniques cleared this void. Computed tomography (CT) can be used for this purpose; its only disadvantage is the use of radiation that is not favorable to younger patients. Ultrasound is not associated with ionizing radiation exposure and gives valuable information on bowel diseases. However, the field of view is limited by bowel gas and some areas of the GI tract are not assessable with abdominal ultrasound. Also, comparison between studies is hampered as only limited views are captured.

For a long time, high-quality MR imaging of the small bowel was not considered to be possible because of long acquisition times and therefore artifacts associated with respiration and bowel peristalsis. Since the development of rapid imaging techniques and the possibility to perform sequences in one breath-hold, small bowel imaging became possible. With MR enterography and enteroclysis, not only can luminal pathologies be visualized better, but it has also the possibility to look at extra-luminal pathologies, which is not possible with endoscopic techniques. The lack of ionizing radiation and better patient acceptance than MR enteroclysis (Negaard et al. 2008) make MR enterography (MR with oral contrast intake) a suitable technique for the assessment of small bowel diseases. A weakness of MR enterography when compared to MR enteroclysis is the suboptimal distension of the proximal jejunum, that is superior in MR enteroclysis (Negaard et al. 2007). Readers are referred to Chap. 9 for MR enteroclysis and Chap. 10 for the clinical role of MRI enterography in relation to other diagnostic techniques.

8.2
Contrast Media Used for MR Enterography

To adequately assess small bowel pathology, optimal luminal distension has to be achieved. The first MR enterography studies were performed without oral contrast (Shoenut et al. 1993, 1994). Side-by-side data comparison concerning MRI of the small bowel with and without oral contrast administration have not yet been performed. One study that compares MR enteroclysis with MRI without oral contrast has found that the reliability for luminal findings increases when luminal contrast is given (Wiarda et al. 2009).

In MR enterography, the patient drinks the contrast agent prior to the exam, as opposed to MR enteroclysis, where the luminal contrast is given through a naso-duodenal tube during the examination.

There are many contrast agents studied for small bowel MRI. Important features of a good contrast agent are a high contrast resolution between the bowel wall and the small bowel lumen and homogeneous signal intensity of the lumen.

Contrast media can be classified according to how they appear on T1- and T2-weighted images. Negative contrast agents give low signal intensity on T1- and T2-weighted images ("dark lumen"), whereas positive contrast agents produce high signal intensity on T1- and T2-weighted images ("bright lumen"). Biphasic contrast agents give high signal intensity on one sequence and low signal intensity on the opposite sequence. Here, a short description is given concerning contrast agents. Readers are referred to Chap. 3 for more details on contrast agents.

8.2.1
Positive Oral Contrast Agents

Most of the positive contrast agents used are paramagnetic substances based on gadolinium-chelate, ferrous or manganese ions. An increase in signal intensity at T1-weighted sequences (appearing as bright lumen) is caused by the paramagnetic effect that causes a reduction in the T1 relaxation time. There is no effect on T2 relaxation time in the concentrations used in clinical practice, so on T2-weighted images the signal intensity is also high because of the high water content of the contrast agent.

Wall thickening is demonstrated well by positive oral contrast agents. A limitation of positive oral contrast agents is that the luminal high signal intensity at T1-weighted sequences may interfere with the enhancement of the bowel wall after the administration of intravenous contrast.

Gadopentate dimeglumine (Magnevist Enteral, Schering AG, Berlin, Germany) is a commercially available positive oral contrast agent. It consists of 1.0 mmol/L gadolinium-DTPA with 15 g/L mannitol (to reduce water reabsorption in the bowel). The gadolinium-DTPA is absorbed only in trace amounts. Mild side effects (flatulence, diarrhea, and thin stools) occur in 11% of patients. These are caused by the addition of the mannitol (Kaminsky et al. 1991).

Ferric ammonium citrate is another example of a positive oral contrast agent. This oral contrast agent is a mixture of granular and crystalline powders based on iron salt with paramagnetic effects, and has to be dissolved in water (600–1,200 mg in 600 mL). Some patients (15%) report minor gastrointestinal side effects (Kivelitz et al. 1999).

Also, natural substances may act as positive contrast agents. Substances such as milk, green tea, and blueberry juice appear bright on MR because the contents of these substances shorten the T1 relaxation time (Giovagnoni et al. 2002). Limitation of these positive contrast agents is that their signal intensity is not constant through the gastrointestinal tract.

8.2.2
Negative Oral Contrast Agents

Negative oral contrast agents are superparamagnetic substances that are based on iron oxide particles. They act by inducing local field inhomogeneties, thus resulting in shortening T1 and T2 relaxation time. The signal intensity on both T1- and T2-weighted images is thus much lower ("dark lumen" appearance). This is especially true for T1-weighted images when using gradient echo sequences, as these are highly sensitive to local field inhomogeneity. These local field inhomogenities could hypothetically lead to an underestimation of bowel wall thickness. No studies have evaluated this potential drawback. The accuracy of detecting Crohn's disease (CD) lesions is similar on T1- and T2-weighted images (93% vs. 95%) (Maccioni et al. 2006). The hypointense bowel wall is visualized due to the negative contrast in the bowel lumen and the high signal intensity of the mesenteric fat. The administration of intravenous contrast gives additional tissue contrast between the intestinal wall and pathologic findings (inflammation or tumor). The pathologic bowel wall is hyperintense after contrast injection and the lumen remains hypointense. Fat suppression is recommended to suppress the high signal intensity of the mesenteric fat for optimal contrast after intravenous contrast injection.

Ferumoxsil (Lumirem; Laboratoires Guerbet, Paris, France) is a negative contrast agent, which contains superparamagnetic particles of iron oxide coated in a layer of silicone that prevents it from being absorbed by the small bowel. Side effects include mostly minor gastrointestinal symptoms (Maccioni et al. 2000).

8.2.3
Biphasic Oral Contrast Agents

Biphasic contrast agents are now the most widely used oral contrast agents for MR enterography. Most of the available biphasic agents have low signal intensity on T1-weighted images and high signal intensity on T2-weighted images. On T1-weighted images, the contrast between the enhancing bowel wall and the dark lumen is optimized.

Water has been used as a luminal contrast agent, as it has several advantages: it is widely available, cheap, and safe. A disadvantage is that it is rapidly absorbed, often before it reaches the terminal ileum (Lomas and Graves 1999). Therefore, various additives have been proposed to diminish intestinal absorption. Mannitol is an osmotic agent that can be added, but can also cause osmotic effects such as diarrhea and cramping (Lauenstein et al. 2003). Nonosmotic agents such as locust bean gum (a thickening agent extracted from the seeds of the European carob tree) can also be used or in combination with mannitol (Lauenstein et al. 2003).

Polyethylene glycol solution (PEG), often used as a bowel cleansing agent, is a poorly absorbed carbohydrate that retains fluid in the bowel lumen. As a secondary effect, it promotes peristalsis and leads to the evacuation of bowel contents several hours after ingestion. Good distension has been achieved with the administration of 600 mL; increasing the dosage did not improve distension (Laghi et al. 2001; Pallotta et al. 1999). Similar to mannitol, PEG can cause side effects such as cramping and diarrhea. We prefer mannitol over PEG, as PEG is less appreciated by patients because of its salty taste.

Barium sulfate, often used in conventional fluoroscopic exams, can be used as biphasic contrast agent. The signal intensity depends on the concentration. The advantage of barium sulfate is the high safety and low cost. It is also widely available. The taste is a drawback for the use of barium sulfate. Gastrointestinal side effects have been reported (Burton et al. 1997).

In our practice, we use 200 mL of mannitol 20% and 1,400 mL of tap water (2.5% mannitol solution) as this is well accepted and results in good distension. Patients refrain from eating and drinking 4 h before the exam, although drinking water is permitted. One hour prior to the exam, the patient starts with drinking the mannitol–water solution in aliquots of 1 cup per 5 min. Mannitol is a well-accepted oral contrast agent, with a neutral taste. For better acceptance, a sweetener such as syrup can be added. A precaution is that colonoscopy with electrocoagulation should not be performed directly after an MR enterography with a mannitol solution. This as methane and hydrogen are formed when mannitol dissociates.

8.2.4
Intravenous Contrast Agents

Detection of active inflammation can be improved by the administration of intravenous contrast, especially in patients with CD (Low et al. 2002; SCHUNK et al. 2000). The peak bowel wall enhancement is found in the portal venous phase at 60–70 s in normal patients without caloric intake (LAUENSTEIN et al. 2005). In patients with CD, the peak enhancement of the bowel wall may vary. A study with dynamic MRI has shown that the mean peak enhancement in patients with active CD is after 39 s (±19 s) (FLORIE et al. 2006). In our institution, we administer Gadolinium (0.1 mL/kg) and start with the postcontrast series after 60 s. In patients with renal impairment (low glomerular filtration rate) or pregnancy, the usage of intravenous contrast is contraindicated.

8.2.5
Anti-Spasmolytic Agents

To prevent blurring or artifacts due to peristalsis, antispasmolytic agents are often administered. This is especially important in fast gradient echo series (such as 3D T1w interpolated volume imaging series, see sequences) and to avoid intraluminal flow-void artifacts in Half-Fourier single shot RARE sequences. Either *N*-butyl scopolamine bromide (Buscopan, Boehringer, Ingelheim, Germany) or glucagon can be utilized for this purpose (in the USA, Buscopan is not approved for this use by the Federal Drug Administration). Although the aperistalsis has been reported to be significantly longer with glucagon (18.3 ± 7 min) than with buscopan (6.8 ± 5.3 min) (FROEHLICH et al. 2009), we use buscopan in our clinic because of lower costs and the fact that buscopan gives aperistalsis long enough to perform the necessary sequences. The dose of Buscopan is 20 mg intravenously just before the contrast-enhanced sequence.

8.3
Technique

The implementation of fast imaging techniques made it first possible to perform sequences in one breath-hold. All sequences in this chapter are performed in breath-holds. Breath-holds are usually between 15 and 25 s. For breath-holds over 15 s, hyperventilation directly prior to the sequence is advised. Good explanation of the procedure and length of the breath-hold is mandatory.

Most abdominal imaging is done on 1.5 T MR scanners. The sequences in this chapter can all be applied to these scanners, but in slightly adapted form applied to 1 T and 3 T scanners as well. For discussion of the technical challenges at 3 T, the reader is referred to Chap. 2.

Patient position

Most institutions will perform MR enterography in supine position. This is more comfortable, especially in older individuals. Prone imaging is advised by some researchers. This gives compression of the bowel loops resulting in better loop separation and can give some reduced scan coverage due to a smaller bowel cavity in the coronal plane. In a study that investigated this subject, prone scanning position did lead to improved small bowel distension but not to improved lesion detection (CRONIN et al. 2008). We perform MR enterography in supine position, as this is more comfortable.

Patient acceptance of MR enterography

MR enterography is generally tolerated well by patients. In a study that evaluated patient acceptance of MR enterography and MR enteroclysis in 38 patients, MR enterography was preferred by patients and these patients experienced less abdominal pain and discomfort associated with the procedure (NEGAARD et al. 2008). Also, more patients were willing to repeat the MR enterography than the MR enteroclysis.

Other advantages of MR enterography are the shorter image time when compared with MR enteroclysis (fixed protocol for MR enterography while the length of the MR enteroclysis is dictated by obtaining optimal distension) and favorable logistics (the nasoduodenal tube has to be placed under fluoroscopic guidance before the MR enteroclysis).

8.3.1
Sequences

For adequate assessment of the small bowel, multiple sequences have to be performed. This section gives an overview of sequences useful for MR enterography. For more details on sequences, the reader is referred to Chap. 1.

8.3.1.1
Half-Fourier Single Shot RARE (HASTE)

The Half-Fourier single shot RARE (Half Fourier Single Shot Turbo Spin-Echo, HASTE) sequence is often performed in the axial and coronal plane. This sequence generates images with a strong T2-weighting. Because of short acquisition times (less than 1 s per slice), breathing artifacts are minimal. Normal bowel wall has low signal intensity on HASTE sequences, an increased signal intensity can be seen in edematous lesions (inflammation). The HASTE sequence can be sensitive to intraluminal flow-void artifacts. These can occur because of peristaltic motion, but can be limited if spasmolytic drugs are given. The HASTE sequence can be used for measuring wall thickness, because it is not sensitive to the chemical shift artifact. HASTE images can be performed using fat suppression. Fat and edema (intramural edema of the bowel wall is indicative of inflammation) both have high signal intensity on T2-weighted images. To visualize the difference between both entities, a sequence with fat suppression is recommended.

For more functional information, a dynamic thick slab T2-weighted TSE hydrography sequence can be performed.

8.3.1.2
Balanced Steady-State Free Precession

The balanced steady-state free precession (true Fast Imaging with Steady-state Precession; True-FISP) sequence, although now often used in MR enterography, was first introduced for MR enteroclysis (Gourtsoyiannis et al. 2000). This sequence is more complex in generation of tissue contrast. This tissue contrast comes from both T1 and T2 in a ratio, namely the T2/T1 ratio. A higher ratio corresponds with higher signal intensity. At 1.5 T, the bowel wall has an intermediate to low signal intensity and fluids have a high signal intensity.

The true-FISP sequence is sensitive to susceptibility artifacts and magnetic field inhomogeneities. Flow-void artifacts in the bowel lumen are not common due to the balanced and symmetric design of the gradients, so the use of antiperistaltic drugs is not needed. The most common artifact in the true-FISP sequence is the black boundary artifact, due to chemical shift. This artifact is seen where both fat and water protons are present in a voxel. It is based on a phase-cancellation effect of the fat and water within the same voxel.

8.3.1.3
T1-Weighted Sequences

Contrast-enhanced T1-weighted gradient echo sequences with fat suppression are performed to assess whether there are areas of increased enhancement. These sequences are performed either two-dimensional (2D) or three-dimensional (3D). Commonly used is the 3D T1w interpolated volume imaging sequence (3D VIBE: Volumetric Interpolated Breath-Hold Examination or comparable sequences (see Chap. 1)). To reduce the acquisition time, small flip angles and short TR (repetition time) are used. The authors recommend a precontrast coronal series and coronal and axial postcontrast series to optimal assess the bowel wall enhancement. 3D ultrafast gradient echo sequences are sensitive to bowel peristalsis, so spasmolytic drugs are advised. We administer the spasmolytic agent directly prior to the intravenous contrast agent administration.

8.3.1.4
Diffusion-Weighted Imaging (DWI)

DWI at MR enterography has been researched recently in one small study of 11 patients for detection of active CD (Oto et al. 2009). DWI reflects the changes in water mobility caused by interactions with macromolecules and cell membranes. This is measured by the apparent diffusion coefficient (ADC) value. In patients with active CD, ADC values are decreased, indicating diffusion restriction. The sensitivity for detecting inflammation with DWI was 95% and specificity 82%. More studies have to be performed to test the reproducibility of these data and the relevance in comparison with other MR findings. For more technical details on DWI, readers are referred to Chaps. 1 and 4.

8.3.1.5
Cine Imaging

Additional cine MR imaging can be added to MR enterography to obtain information about peristalsis and bowel motion. The most common indication is the diagnosis of adhesions, which are visualized by fixation of bowel loops and lack of normal peristalsis (see Chap. 16). This is best seen on true-FISP images.

Alternately, information about bowel peristalsis can also be seen on the different MR sequences to assess the difference between bowel peristalsis and functional stenosis. Readers are referred to Chap. 15 for more information on bowel motility.

In our hospital, we perform HASTE, true-FISP, and 3D T1w interpolated volume imaging sequences (see Table 8.1). The HASTE and true-FISP images are performed in the coronal and axial plane. We perform one coronal precontrast 3D T1w interpolated volume imaging and a coronal and axial postcontrast 3D T1w interpolated volume imaging. All axial sequences are executed in 2 or 3 stacks, depending on the size of the patient. The antispasmolytic agent is given just before the postcontrast series. The total in room time of the examination is approximately 45 min.

Table 8.1. MR protocol for 1.5 T scanner with external phased array coil

Sequences	2	3	4	5	6	7	8
Sequence	True-FISP	HASTE	HASTE	True-FISP	VIBE	VIBE	VIBE
Generic sequence name	Balanced steady-state free precession	Half-Fourier single shot RARE	Half-Fourier single shot RARE	Balanced steady-state free precession	3D T1w interpolated volume imaging	3D T1w interpolated volume imaging	3D T1w interpolated volume imaging
Aquisition time	0:12	0:24	0:38	0:22	0:28	0:28	0:21
PAT (SENSE)	2	Off	Off	2	2	2	2
Voxel size	2.0 × 1.2	2.7 × 2.0	1.6 × 1.2	1.5 × 0.9	2.2 × 1.8	2.2 × 1.8	2.0 × 1.6
Plane	Coronal	Coronal	Transverse	Transverse	Coronal	Coronal	Transverse
Slices	23	40	40	40	80	80	120
Distance factor (%)	0	5	5	0	20	20	20
Phase encoding dir.	R>L	R>L	A>P	A>P	R>L	R>L	A>P
FOV read (mm)	450	400	360	350	450	450	400
FOV phase (%)	84.4	100	68.8	84.4	100	100	62.5
Slice thickness (mm)	5.0	6	6	5	2	2	3
TR (ms)	3.85	800	1200	4.11	3.23	3.23	3.23
TE1/TE2	1.93	81	81	2.06	1.12	1.12	1.14
Average	1	1	1	1	1	1	1
Flip angle (degrees)	70	150	150	70	12	12	12
Fat sat	Fat sat	None	None	Fat sat	Q-fat sat	Q-fat sat	Q-fat sat
Base resolution	384	256	256	384	256	256	256
Phase resolution (%)	60	76	76	60	80	80	80
Bandwidth (Hz/Px)	501	275	275	501	490	490	490
Turbofactor		195	195				

8.4 Results

8.4.1 Crohn's Disease

Diagnosis and therapy monitoring for CD is the major indication for performing MR enterography. CD is an inflammatory bowel disease that is most often located in the terminal ileum (MAGLINTE et al. 2003) and is often diagnosed in younger patients. The disease is chronic and often patients relapse and remit. Because clinical symptoms do not accurately represent CD disease activity, other methods have been researched. MRI is capable of diagnosing CD, evaluating severity and monitoring treatment response (KOH et al. 2001; SHOENUT et al. 1993, 1994). Several findings seen on MRI reflect active disease activity of CD.

In CD, pathological bowel segments are separated by normal bowel ("skip lesions") (Fig. 8.1). This pattern is typical for CD and is not found in ulcerative colitis, where a continuous region of inflammation starting in the rectum and up to the more proximal bowel is the common presentation.

8.4.1.1 Bowel Wall Thickening

Normal bowel wall thickness is 3 mm or less when the bowel is distended. In patients with active CD the bowel wall can be thickened, due to edema and infiltration or preexisting fibrosis. The bowel wall can be more than 10 mm thick (Fig. 8.2). Good correlation is found between bowel wall thickness seen on MRI and colonoscopy with biopsies and histology, where inflamed bowel wall had a greater bowel wall thickness than noninflamed bowel wall (PUNWANI et al. 2009; GIROMETTI et al. 2008). In a study of 18 patients, MR estimates of bowel thickness demonstrated

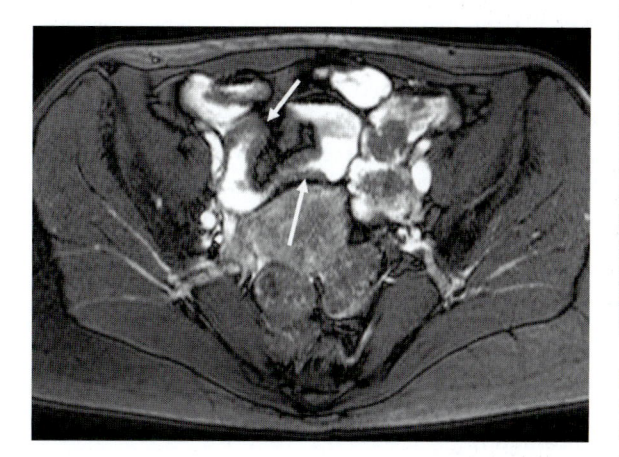

Fig. 8.1. Thirty-five-year-old patient with Crohn's disease. Transverse true-FISP image with fat saturation shows skip lesions in the ileum; multiple stenoses are visible (*arrows*)

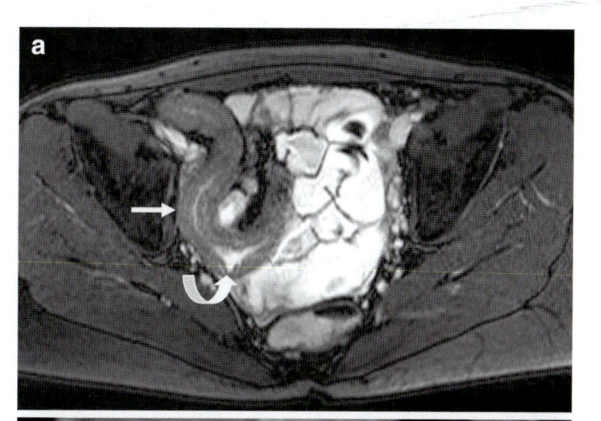

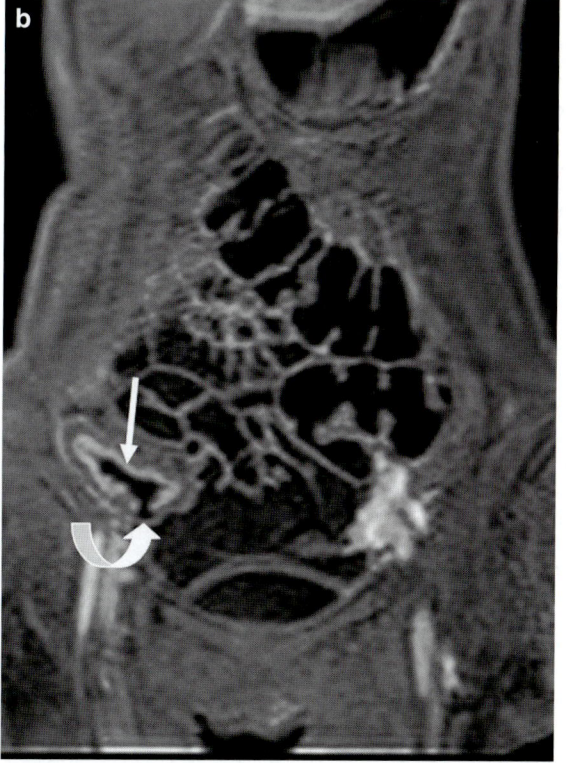

Fig. 8.2. (a) Twenty-three-year-old female patient with Crohn's disease. Transverse fat suppressed true-FISP image shows thickened ileal wall (*arrow*) with an ulceration (*curved arrow*). (b) Coronal T1w interpolated volume imaging image after intravenous contrast shows three-layered enhancement of the bowel wall (*arrow*) with ulceration (*curved arrow*)

strong association with bowel wall thickness of matched histological coupes and also with degree of inflammation (Punwani et al. 2009).

In patients with active CD, the mean maximum wall thickness is significantly greater than in patients with inactive disease (6.7 mm vs. 3.3 mm, $p < 0.01$) (Koh et al. 2001). For adequate measurement of bowel wall thickness, optimal bowel distension has to be achieved. Nonoptimal distension can lead to false-positive results because collapsed bowel wall can mimic bowel wall thickening. Therefore, the MR enterography sequences have to be scrutinized for the sequence with the most optimal distension of a certain bowel segment.

8.4.1.2
High Signal Intensity of the Bowel Wall on T2-Weighted Images

High signal intensity on T2-weighted images is often seen in tissues where edema/inflammation is present. In patients with active CD, the bowel wall has a higher signal intensity compared to non-affected bowel wall. High signal intensity on T2-weighted images has a good correlation with biological parameters such as Crohn's Disease Activity Index (CDAI) and laboratory values such as c-reactive protein and histology (Maccioni et al. 2000; Punwani et al. 2009). In a histology matched study, the mural signal intensity on T2-weighted images was compared with cerebro-spinal fluid (CSF) signal intensity. The ratio of these signal intensities (T2 mural/CSF) was positively correlated with histology (a higher ratio denotes a more inflamed bowel wall) (Punwani et al. 2009).

The use of fat suppression in T2-weighted sequences can be useful, to distinguish edema from fat (which also has a high signal intensity).

8.4.1.3
Enhancement After Intravenous Contrast Administration

Bowel wall enhancement seen on postcontrast T1-weighted images has long been one of the most important findings for active CD (Florie et al. 2006; Miao et al. 2002; Pupillo et al. 2007). In a study with 28 patients, the severity of CD was correctly depicted in 93% of patients using T1-weighted contrast-enhanced series vs. in 43% of patients at single-shot fast SE imaging (Low et al. 2002). Recently, in a study with histological matching, there was no correlation found between degree of inflammatory activity and degree of enhancement of the bowel wall (Punwani et al. 2009). A reason for this phenomenon could be that changes in the bowel wall in CD (e.g., presence of fibrosis, edema, neo-angiogenesis) are more complex to be seen as simple enhancement. Inter- and intraobserver variability of enhancement is reported to be poor, but improving after choosing fixed regions-of-interest (Sharman et al. 2009). New techniques, such as T1-mapping, are being developed to overcome these deficiencies, as this results in objective T1 measurements (Horsthuis et al. 2009b) (see future prospects of MR enterography).

8.4.1.4
Bowel Wall Stratification

Different patterns of bowel wall enhancement are described in CD at MRI similar to at CT where multilayered appearance of the bowel wall was associated with inflammatory activity (Choi et al. 2003). These results have also been reproduced with MR imaging (Del Vescovo et al. 2008; Miao et al. 2002). Different stratification patterns are described in the literature. Enhancement can be mucosal (innermost layer of bowel enhancing), homogeneous (all bowel wall enhancing equally), and layered (both mucosal and serosal bowel wall layers enhancing with a central band of relatively reduced enhancement). One study compared the pattern of wall enhancement with the CDAI (Best et al. 1976) and C-reactive protein and found that patients with clinically active CD had a pattern of enhancement where the mucosal layer first enhanced and the serosal layer followed, whereas clinically inactive patients tended to show homogeneous enhancement of the bowel wall (Del Vescovo et al. 2008).

When multilayered appearance after intravenous contrast administration was compared with histological findings, a correlation was found between inflammatory activity and multilayered enhancement (Fig. 8.3). This stratified enhancement was often seen in segments with fibrostenosis (Punwani et al. 2009). It is not yet clear what entity gives rise to this layered pattern (mural fibrosis, submucosal edema, or both).

8.4.1.5
Ulcerations

Ulcerations of the bowel wall are best seen on true-FISP images (Fig. 8.2) (Prassopoulos et al. 2001).

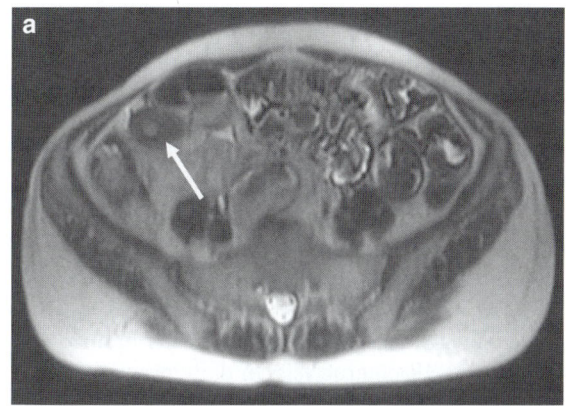

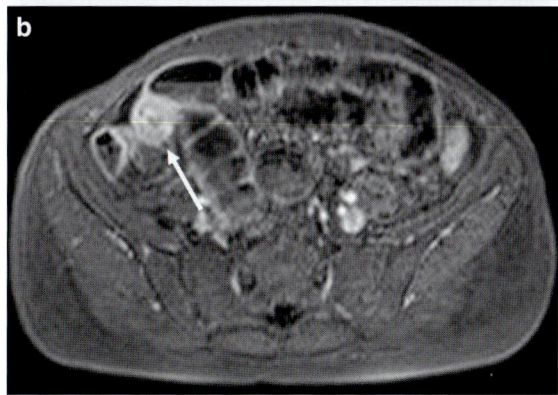

Fig. 8.3. (a) Fifty-three-year-old female patient with Crohn's disease who previously underwent an ileocecal resection. Transverse HASTE image shows a thickened bowel wall loop of the neo-terminal ileum (*arrow*). (b) Transverse 3D T1w interpolated volume imaging fat suppressed image shows three-layered enhancement (*arrow*) of the affected bowel loop

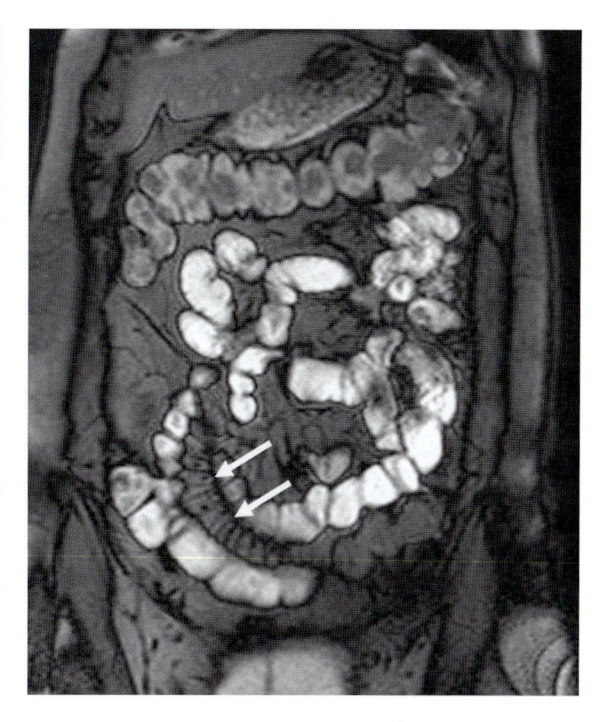

Fig. 8.4. Forty-year-old patient with suspected Crohn's disease. Coronal true-FISP image with fat saturation shows increased blood flow in the mesenteric vessels – comb sign (*arrows*)

Deep linear ulcers appear as thin lines of high signal intensity, longitudinally or transversely (fissure ulcers) orientated within the thickened bowel wall. True-FISP images are superior to HASTE in demonstrating linear ulcers. Ulcerations can develop into fistulas. For the detection of mural ulcerations, MR enterography has a sensitivity of 56% and a specificity of 96% when compared with conventional enteroclysis (MASSELLI et al. 2008).

8.4.1.6
Comb Sign

The comb sign (Fig. 8.4) indicates the presence of increased blood flow in the vasa recta of a bowel segment with active CD. The vasa recta are aligned like the teeth of a comb, hence the name comb sign. This sign is best seen on true-FISP series, but can be present on T1-weighted contrast-enhanced images. The comb sign is considered to indicate the presence of active disease.

8.4.1.7
Lymph Nodes

Enlarged lymph nodes (>1 cm) are often present in patients with CD. Mesenteric lymph nodes can best be seen on true-FISP series. Although some studies suggest that enhancing lymph nodes indicate active CD (GOURTSOYIANNIS et al. 2004), histological studies have not found a correlation (PUNWANI et al. 2009).

8.4.1.8
Fistula and Abscess

Extra intestinal manifestations such as fistulas and abscesses can be assessed on MRI. Fistulas are best visualized on T1-weighted postcontrast images, because of their inflammation and therefore high signal intensity after contrast agent administration (Fig. 8.5). Abscesses can best be seen on T1-weighted images after intravenous contrast administration as

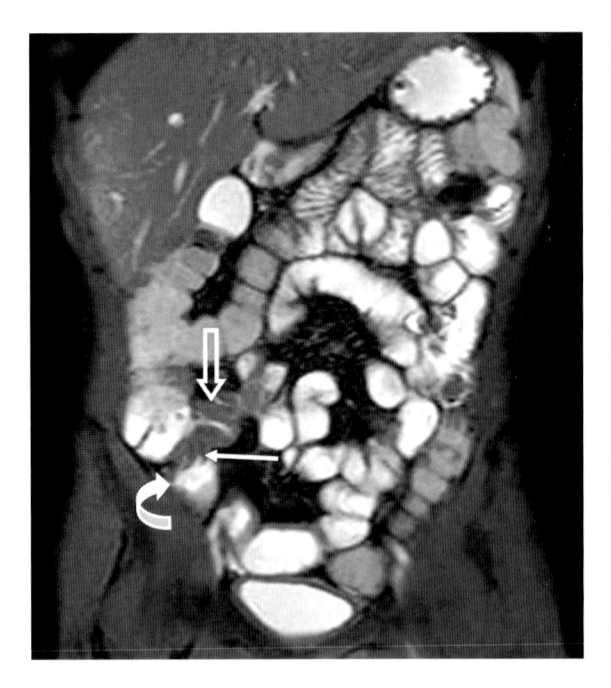

Fig. 8.5. Twenty-three-year-old male patient with Crohn's disease. Coronal fat suppressed true-FISP image shows a stenosis in the terminal ileum (*open arrow*) with a fistulous tract (*arrow*) to an abscess (*curved arrow*)

mation, it is important to differentiate between the two. Fibrotic stenoses do not enhance after intravenous contrast injection while active disease leads to enhancement (Figs. 8.7 and 8.8).

The accuracy for detecting stenosis of the terminal ileum in CD patients was assessed in a study by Negaard et al. (2007). The sensitivity of MR enterography was 86% vs. 100% for MR enteroclysis. The specificity was 93% vs. 100%. The higher diagnostic accuracy was not statistically significant ($p = 0.13$). This higher accuracy is due to the better luminal distension in MR enteroclysis. In daily practice, detection of stenoses at MR enterography does not pose difficulties. The thickened, nondistending bowel wall at a stenosis is readily appreciated while the obstructed flow of the enteral contrast medium gives rise to dilatation so the stenosis is easily visualized. Verification of the degree of obstruction on the different sequences performed during the MR enterography procedure gives important information on the degree of obstruction. Alternatively, a dedicated dynamic thick slab T2-weighted TSE hydrography sequence can be performed to evaluate the degree of obstruction.

the center will be low signal intensity due to their fluid content and the wall shows enhancement (Fig. 8.6). On T2-weighted sequences, both tracks and abscesses can have a relative thick fibrotic wall and will have central high signal intensity. The high signal intensity is caused either by fluid or granulation tissue. These can be differentiated by intravenous contrast agent administration when considered clinically relevant. The sensitivity for detecting fistulas at MR enterography is 78% and the specificity 100% (Masselli et al. 2008).

8.4.1.9
Stenosis

Stenosis of the bowel wall can be seen as luminal narrowing of more than 50% and can be assessed on all sequences. In the literature, there is no consensus about which gradation of luminal narrowing defines a stenosis; the authors define narrowing of 50% as a stenosis. Sometimes, a prestenotic dilatation of the proximal bowel is present, indicating (partial) obstruction (Fig. 8.7). Stenosis can be either due to inflammation or fibrosis. Because medical therapeutic options do exist if the stenosis is based on inflam-

8.4.1.10
Creeping Fat

Creeping fat or fibro fatty proliferation is the stranding and retracting of mesenteric fat around affected bowel segments. This separation of other bowel loops facilitates identification of these loops. This is often seen in patients with a past episode of active CD.

8.4.1.11
CD Disease Activity Assessment

There is currently no gold standard for assessment of disease activity of CD. Usually, a combination of clinical findings, laboratory findings, ileocolonoscopy, and MRI is used. Several studies have shown that the aforementioned MR parameters can be used to assess CD disease activity (Florie et al. 2005; Koh et al. 2001; Maccioni et al. 2000; Shoenut et al. 1994). The sensitivity of MR enterography is 91% on a per patient basis, the specificity is 71%. Per segment is the sensitivity 59% and the specificity 93% (Koh et al. 2001). The low sensitivity in this study of 23 patients was due to missed superficial ulcerations, which are known to be difficult to detect on MR.

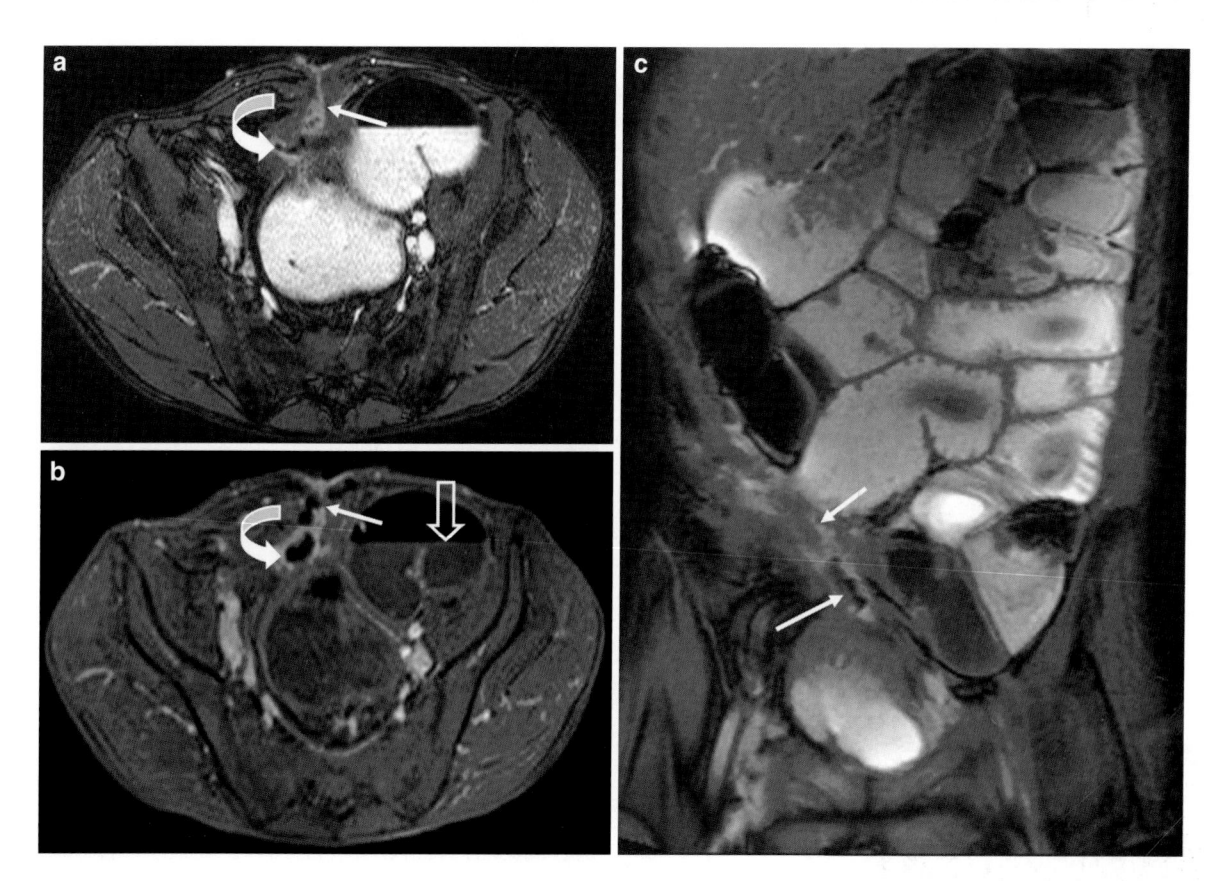

Fig. 8.6. (a) Forty-one-year-old patient with longstanding severe Crohn's disease who underwent four previous ileal bowel resections. Transverse true-FISP image with fat saturation shows an enterocutaneous fistula (*arrow*) and an intra-abdominal abscess (*curved arrow*), which contains air. (b) Transverse 3D T1w interpolated volume imaging image with fat saturation after intravenous contrast shows the enterocutaneous fistula (*arrow*) and the intra-abdominal abscess with enhancing rim (*curved arrow*). The bowel loops are dilated and a gas–fluid interface is visible (*open arrow*), the patient has a small bowel paralytic ileus. (c) Coronal true-FISP image with fat suppression shows multiple fistulous tracts and fibrosis (*arrows*). Distended bowel loops are well demonstrated

8.4.1.12
CD Disease Severity Assessment

Although there is no consensus based grading system on luminal CD, transmural inflammation (resulting in the formation of abscesses and fistulas) is indicative of severe disease activity. Also, the length of the affected bowel segment plays a part in assessing disease activity.

In a meta-analysis by Horsthuis et al. (2009a), the accuracy of grading CD disease activity was assessed. Seven studies (in total 140 patients) were included. Eighty-seven percent of patients with frank disease were correctly depicted by MRI, whereas it showed only 65% of patients with mild disease activity.

8.4.1.13
Place of MR Enterography in CD Patients

For diagnosing CD, there is no consensus on the place of MR enterography. This as CD can be present throughout the gastrointestinal tract and especially small bowel. Distension of the complete small bowel is thus mandatory to detect also relatively rare CD in the (proximal) jejunum and duodenum. MR enteroclysis gives better proximal distension than MR enterography. However, proximal small bowel lesions can be demonstrated at MR enterography (Fig. 8.7) as well and MR enteroclysis has not proven to be more accurate in the detection of CD lesions (Torkzad and Lauenstein 2009).

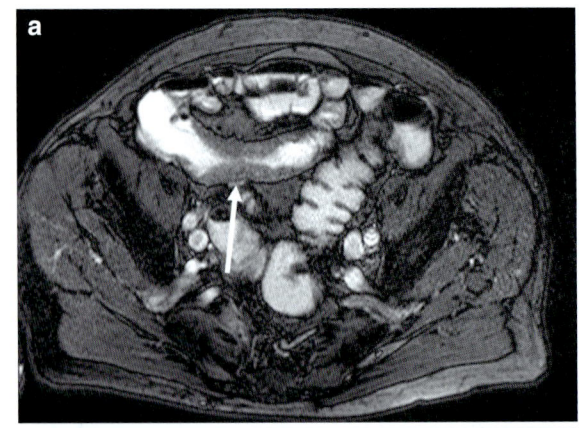

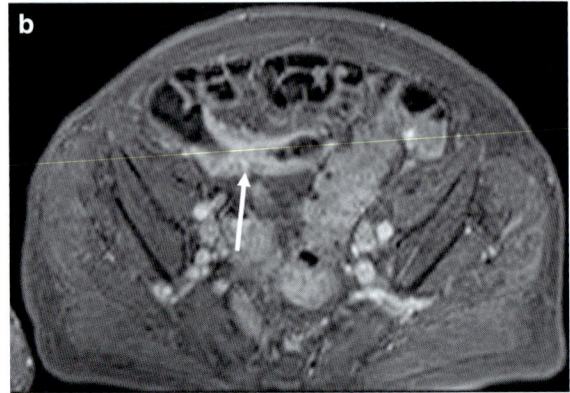

Fig. 8.8. (a) An 80-year-old patient with Crohn's disease. Transverse fat-saturated true-FISP image shows a stenosis of the terminal ileum (*arrow*). (b) Transverse 3D T1w interpolated volume imaging image with fat saturation after intravenous contrast shows enhancement of the stenosis – most prominent at the mucosa – which indicates that the stenosis is caused by inflammation of the ileal wall (*arrow*)

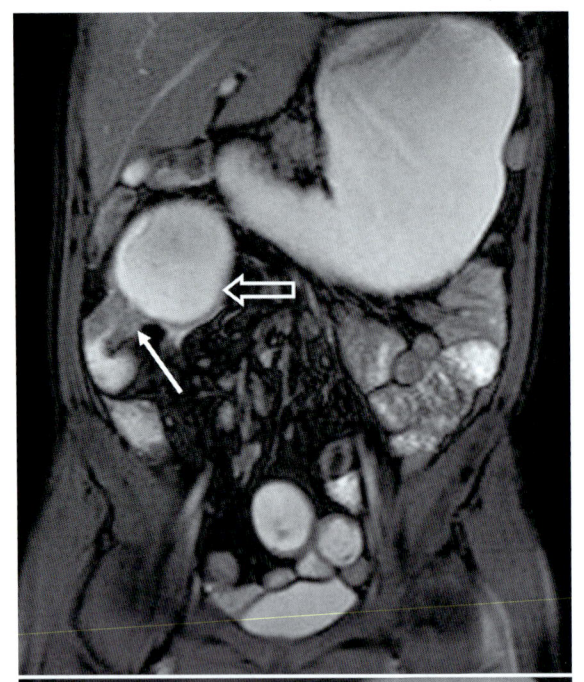

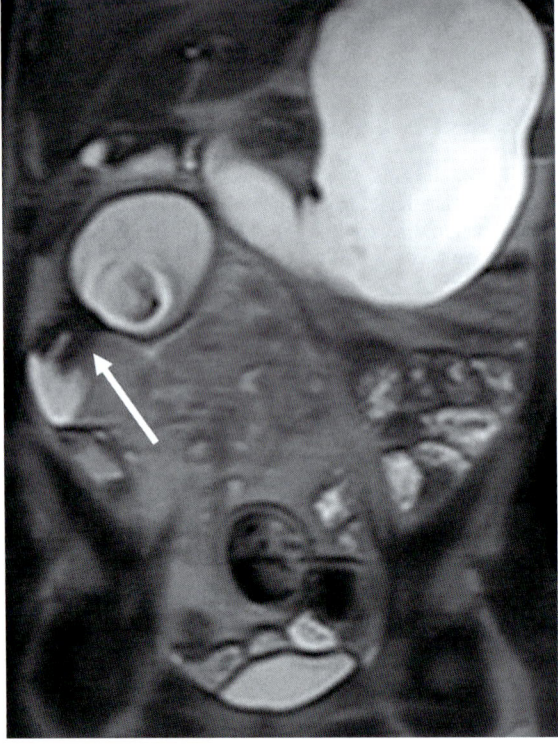

Fig. 8.7. (a) Twenty-three-year-old male patient with Crohn's disease who previously underwent multiple bowel small bowel resections. Coronal fat suppressed true-FISP image shows a stenosis of the proximal jejunum (*arrow*) with an extensive prestenotic dilatation (*open arrow*). Note the distension of the stomach. (b) Coronal HASTE image shows low signal intensity of the stenosis reflecting fibrosis (*arrow*)

For initial assessment of CD activity, one could favor MR enteroclysis as this will give the most extensive evaluation. However, superiority over MR enterography has not been demonstrated. Thereby, subtle abnormalities (erythema, apthous ulcers) will go undetected at MR enteroclysis as well. For these reasons as well as reduced burden and logistical advantages, MR enterography is used as initial examination in many institutions. A strategy with initial MR enterography and subsequent video capsule endoscopy is an alternative approach. MR enterography will demonstrate more extensive disease, including possible stenoses preventing video capsule endoscopy. Video capsule endoscopy is used for detecting subtle changes.

At this moment, there is no established strategy for the initial examination in patients suspected for

CD. The choice whether MR enterography or MR enteroclysis is used will depend on the aforementioned considerations as well as other factors such as disease spectrum.

For clinical follow-up of patients with CD, MR enterography is preferable over MR enteroclysis. The lack of the burden of naso-duodenal intubation, shorter examination time, and no (limited) ionizing radiation exposure are important advantages to the patient and radiologist. This will facilitate more frequent monitoring, which is important given the costs and side effect associated with medical treatment. MR enterography will show the findings demonstrated at an initial MR enterography or MR enteroclysis. Only in the case of subtle findings demonstrated at initial MR enteroclysis, which are not found in small bowel loops collapsed at MR enterography, one could consider to perform an additional MR enteroclysis or alternatively video capsule endoscopy.

Readers are referred to Chap. 10 for more details on the present role of MR enterography in managing CD.

8.4.2
Celiac Disease

Celiac disease is a gluten-sensitive enteropathy of the gastrointestinal tract that affects the small intestine in genetically susceptible individuals. The disease can occur at any age. The diagnosis of celiac disease can be challenging due to a wide range of clinical manifestations and the lack of specificity. Although the diagnosis is confirmed by small-intestine biopsy, patients who are referred for MR enterography with nonspecific gastro-intestinal complaints might have celiac disease as underlying pathology.

Fold pattern abnormalities are most the most specific sign of celiac disease seen on MRI (Paolantonio et al. 2007). These can best be assessed on true-FISP images. A decreased number of jejunal folds (less than threefolds per inch is considered to be decreased) or complete flattening of the folds can be seen in celiac disease. Also, the ileal folds can be increased (more than 5 per inch), this is called "ileal jejunization." Jejunoileal fold pattern reversal is present when both ileal jejunization and a decreased number of jejunal folds are present in the same patient. Less specific for celiac disease is the presence of ileal dilatation (more than 3 cm), intussusception (visible as the "double halo sign" of bowel-within-bowel), and enlarged lymph nodes (>1 cm) (Paolantonio et al. 2007) (see Chap. 10, Fig. 10.13).

Small bowel lymphomas of the T-cell type are associated with the concomitant presence of celiac disease (Chott et al. 1999) and are also called enteropathy-associated T-cell lymphomas. A small study retrospectively analyzed the features of T-cell associated lymphomas in ten patients and found that enteropathy-associated T-cell lymphomas tended to be localized in a single bowel segment and tended to be long (>10 cm) (Lohan et al. 2008) when compared with non-Hodgkin's lymphomas of the B-cell type (see malignant small bowel neoplasms).

8.4.3
Benign Small Bowel Neoplasms

There are syndromes characterized by the occurrence of polyps in the gastrointestinal tract including the Peutz–Jeghers syndrome (PJS), juvenile polyposis, and neurofibromatosis. These syndromes can be subdivided depending on whether the polyps are hamartomas (PJS) or adenomas (familial adenomatous polyposis (FAP)). In patients with PJS, frequent monitoring is necessary because these polyps have a size-related increased risk of malignant degeneration (Spigelman et al. 1989). Lifetime risk for developing small intestinal cancer in PJS patients is 13% (Giardiello et al. 2000). Current guidelines recommend surgical or endoscopic polypectomy for polyps larger than 1.5 cm (Wirtzfeld et al. 2001; Dunlop 2002), although there are no studies performed that provide data on which cut-off point for polypectomy is best.

There is only one study studying MR enterography in patients with PJS. Caspari et al. (2004) included four PJS patients and compared MR enterography with capsule endoscopy for the detection of small bowel polyps. With MRI, polyps larger than 15 mm were all detected, whereas smaller polyps were less well detected with MRI. MRI was not able to detect any polyps smaller than 5 mm (Fig. 8.9).

When all polyps should be identified, MR enterography is not recommended for monitoring because of suboptimal proximal jejunum distension at MR enterography (see Chaps. 9 and 10). MR enteroclysis is then more suited. When the examination is performed at relatively short time intervals and primarily larger polyps are sought for, MR enterography could be used. Also, in patients in whom MR enteroclysis is not possible, MR enterography is an alternative. However, one should be aware that smaller neoplasms may go undetected in reasonable distended loops and larger neoplasms in collapsed loops.

Patients with familial polyposis have adenomatous polyps, mostly located in the colon. Extra-colonic manifestations of FAP are located in the upper gastrointestinal tract, often in the duodenum. Polyps can also occur in the proximal jejunum, but MRI failed to detect these in a series of four patients with small polyps (0–5 mm) (CASPARI et al. 2004). The role of MR enterography for screening of FAP patients has yet to be studied in larger case series. For now, screening guidelines recommend upper endoscopy surveillance in these patients (HIROTA et al. 2006).

8.4.4
Malignant Small Bowel Neoplasms

Primary malignant masses of the small bowel are relatively uncommon. The most common primary neoplasm of the small bowel is carcinoid. These tumors are well-differentiated neuro-endocrine neoplasms that occur mostly in the distal ileum and are almost always malignant. Literature about the MR appearance of carcinoid tumors is scarce. One study reports the MR features of carcinoid tumors in a series of 29 patients (BADER et al. 2001). The tumor had two types of presentations at MRI: it presented as a discrete mass that enhanced on postcontrast T1-weighted images. The appearance on T2-weighted images varied from hyper- to isointense to muscle. The second presentation was as a uniform bowel wall thickening without the presence of a discrete mass. This wall thickening was isointense on T1- and T2-weighted images and enhanced after intravenous contrast administration.

Small bowel lymphomas are mostly of the non-Hodgkin type. They arise from B cells of mucosa-associated lymphoid tissue (B-cell lymphoma). The terminal ileum is the most affected site, as there is a relatively greater amount of lymphoid tissue present. Solitary lesions are most common, but in 10–20% of cases, multiple sites are involved. Most small bowel lymphomas are located within the bowel wall. Obstruction caused by lymphoma is uncommon because the infiltrating tumor weakens the muscularis propria. The formation of cavities is also seen in primary small bowel lymphomas. Initially, these patients have an intramural lymphoma that ulcerates, progresses, and perforates to the mesentery, where it forms a usually sterile abscess (LEVINE et al. 1997). Lymphomas often show enhancement after intravenous contrast administration (Fig. 8.10).

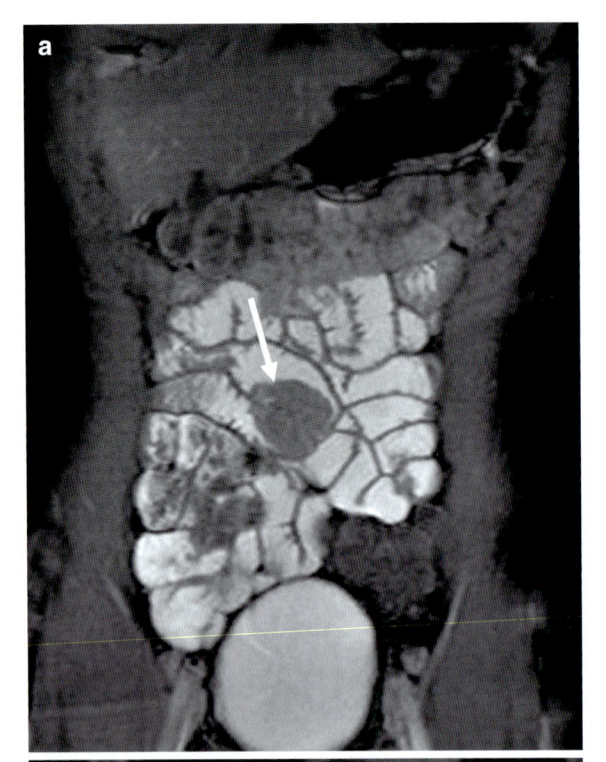

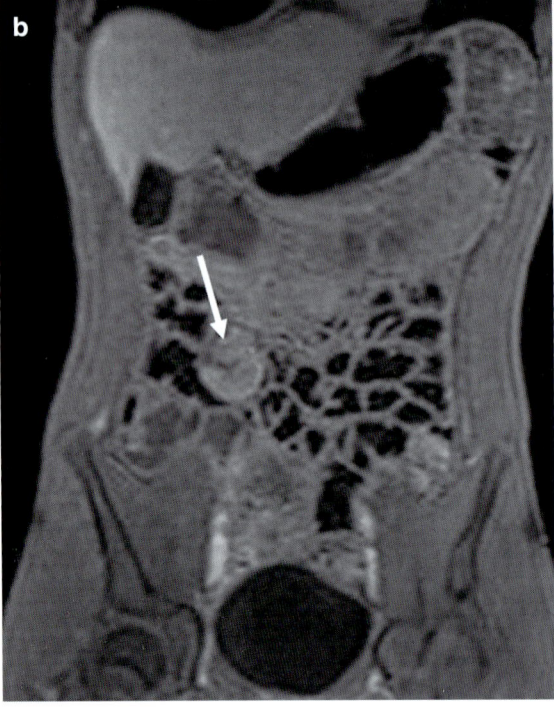

Fig. 8.9. (a) Twenty-year-old male patient clinically suspected for Peutz–Jeghers syndrome. Coronal true-FISP image with fat suppression shows a large polyp (approximately 3/4 cm) in the distal jejunum (*arrow*). Note the good distension in this enterography exam. (b) Coronal 3D T1w interpolated volume imaging image with fat suppression after intravenous contrast shows mild enhancement of the polyp (*arrow*)

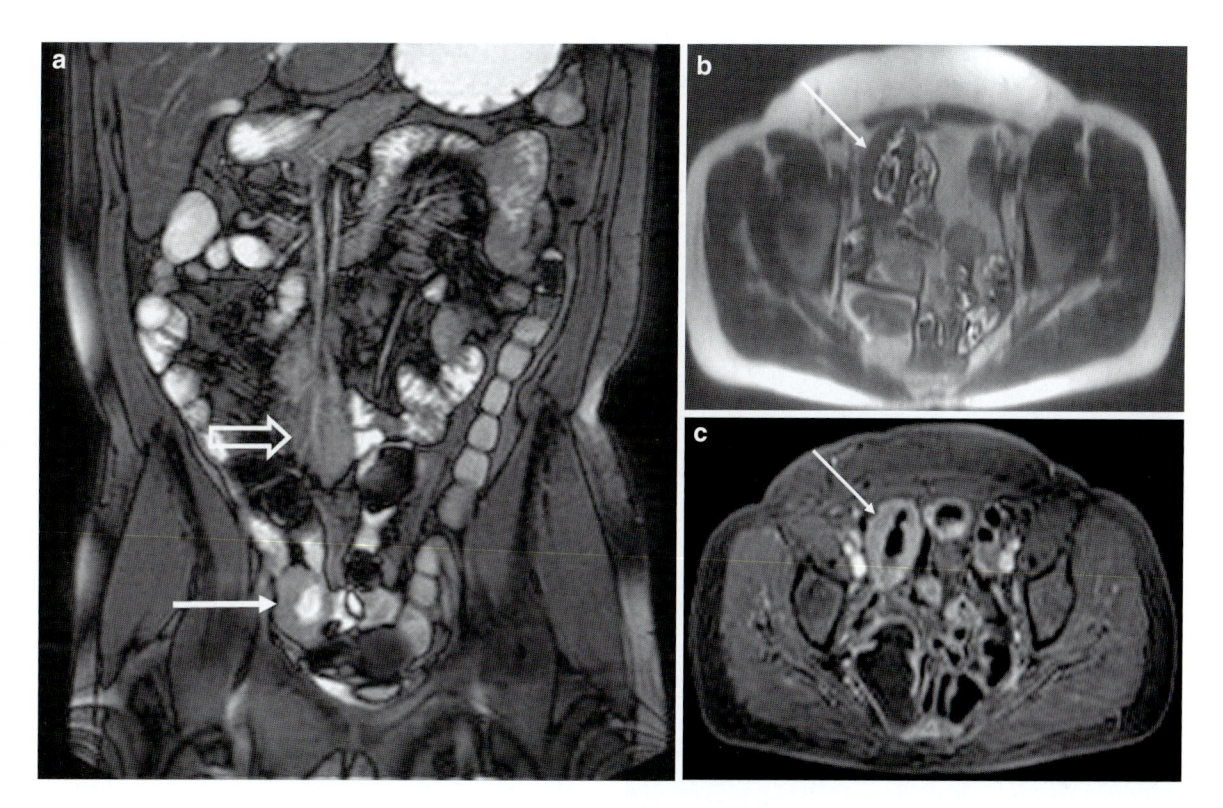

Fig. 8.10. (a) Forty-seven-year-old female patient with a non-Hodgkin lymphoma. Coronal fat suppressed true-FISP image shows a lymphoma, located in the ileal wall (*arrow*). No obstruction. Also seen is a large lymphoma in the mesenteric fat (*open arrow*). (b) Transverse HASTE image shows the lymphoma in the bowel wall as a hypodense structure (*arrow*). (c) Transverse T1-weighted image with fat suppression shows transmural enhancement of the lymphoma after intravenous contrast injection

8.4.5 Miscellaneous

Other small bowel diseases that show changes in bowel wall thickness and enhancement pattern are intestinal infections, ischemic disorders, radiation enteritis (Fig. 8.11), and vasculitis (LAGHI et al. 2009). No studies have been performed that assess the accuracy of MR enterography in these patients. Presently, most experience for assessment of these diseases with imaging is with multidetector CT.

Scleroderma/progressive systemic sclerosis can also be seen on MR enterography in the form of dilatations and pseudodiverticula due to neuropathy and myopathy of the small bowel.

Endometriosis deposits of the small bowel can be seen on MR enterography. Endometriomas have high signal intensity on T1-weighted images with fat saturation. Rare diseases may be encountered as well.

Small bowel obstruction can be assessed with MR enterography, although in patients with an ileus, the administration of oral contrast might be omitted (Fig. 8.7) (see Chap. 16 for more details on bowel obstruction).

Familial Mediterranean fever is a rare autosomal recessive disease that is characterized by attacks of

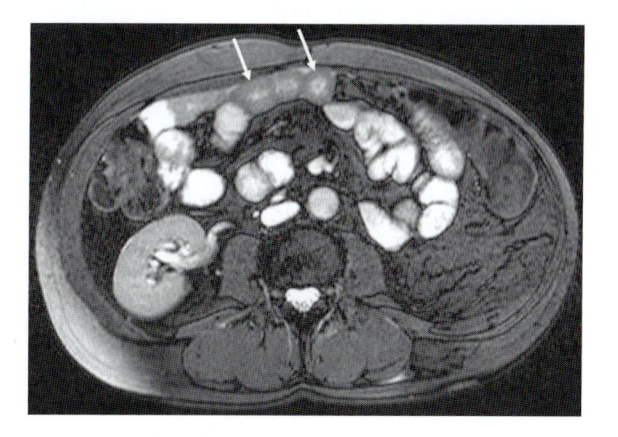

Fig. 8.11. Male patient with previous carcinoma of the pyelum who underwent nefrectomy and radiation. Coronal 3D T1w interpolated volume imaging image after intravenous contrast shows thickened bowel wall of the jejunum (*arrows*), most likely due to radiation enteritis

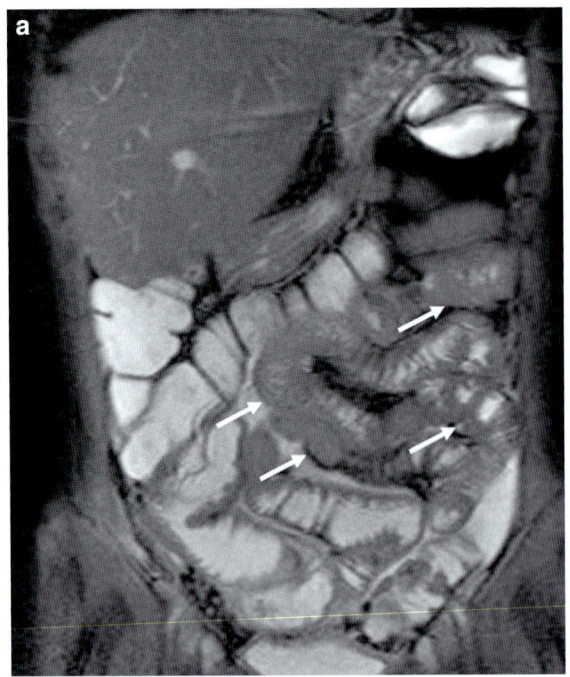

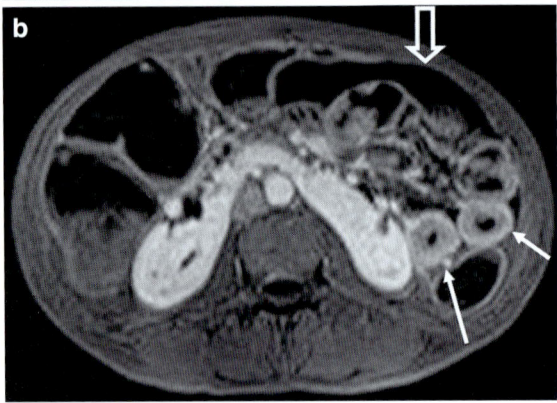

Fig. 8.12. (a) Forty-three-year-old man with familial Mediterranean fever. Coronal fat suppressed true-FISP image shows thickened jejunal bowel loops (*arrows*). (b) Transverse 3D T1w interpolated volume imaging image with fat suppression after intravenous contrast shows enhancing bowel loops, especially serosal enhancement (*arrows*). Also visible is a horse-shoe kidney and free intraperitoneal air (*open arrow*) after previous surgery

tutions. Research now is focused on creating abdominal 3 T protocols (see Chap. 2), studying perfusion and diffusion and obtaining more insight into the role of MRI in determining disease activity in CD. New techniques are being developed to assess bowel wall enhancement in a more objective manner. With the creation of so-called T1-maps, the absolute T1-value can be calculated and therefore the absolute contrast enhancement (HORSTHUIS et al. 2009b). With these data, the enhancement can not only be objectively compared with other MR examinations, but also with other modalities that assess disease severity in CD. Recently, more research is being performed on dynamic contrast-enhanced MRI (DCE-MRI) in CD. Mural hemodynamic parameters derived from DCE-MRI were reported to be correlated with disease chronicity and microvessel density was inversely related to mural blood flow (TAYLOR et al. 2009). This has risen the hypothesis that stenosis-driven hypoxia contributes to angiogenesis in CD. Readers are referred to Chap. 10 for more details on the present role of MR enterography in managing small bowel diseases when compared with other techniques.

In clinical practice, video capsule endoscopy is increasingly used. A recent study recommends video capsule endoscopy as an addition to MRI (TILLACK et al. 2008), but in the future more research will be performed to determine the exact place of these modalities.

The strength and weaknesses of MR enterography in imaging of small bowel diseases when compared with MR enteroclysis and other diagnostic techniques should be determined to full extent.

fever and serosal inflammation. On MR enterography, bowel wall thickening of the jejunum and ileum is seen with serosal enhancement (Fig. 8.12).

8.5
Future Prospects of MR Enterography

MR enterography has become an important diagnostic technique for small bowel diseases in many insti-

References

Bader TR, Semelka RC, Chiu VC, et al (2001) MRI of carcinoid tumors: spectrum of appearances in the gastrointestinal tract and liver. J Magn Reson Imaging 14:261–269

Best WR, Becktel JM, Singleton JW, et al (1976) Development of a Crohn's disease activity index. National Cooperative Crohn's Disease Study. Gastroenterology 70:439–444

Burton SS, Liebig T, Frazier SD, et al (1997) High-density oral barium sulfate in abdominal MRI: efficacy and tolerance in a clinical setting. Magn Reson Imaging 15:147–153

Caspari R, von FM, Krautmacher C, et al (2004) Comparison of capsule endoscopy and magnetic resonance imaging for the detection of polyps of the small intestine in patients with familial adenomatous polyposis or with Peutz-Jeghers' syndrome. Endoscopy 36:1054–1059

Choi D, Jin LS, Ah CY, et al (2003) Bowel wall thickening in patients with Crohn's disease: CT patterns and correlation with inflammatory activity. Clin Radiol 58:68–74

Chott A, Vesely M, Simonitsch I, et al (1999) Classification of intestinal T-cell neoplasms and their differential diagnosis. Am J Clin Pathol 111:S68–S74

Cronin CG, Lohan DG, Mhuircheartaigh JN, et al (2008) MRI small-bowel follow-through: prone versus supine patient positioning for best small-bowel distention and lesion detection. AJR Am J Roentgenol 191:502–506

Del Vescovo R, Sansoni I, Caviglia R, et al (2008) Dynamic contrast enhanced magnetic resonance imaging of the terminal ileum: differentiation of activity of Crohn's disease. Abdom Imaging 33:417–424

Dunlop MG (2002) Guidance on gastrointestinal surveillance for hereditary non-polyposis colorectal cancer, familial adenomatous polypolis, juvenile polyposis, and Peutz-Jeghers syndrome. Gut 51(Suppl 5):V21–V27

Florie J, Horsthuis K, Hommes DW, et al (2005) Magnetic resonance imaging compared with ileocolonoscopy in evaluating disease severity in Crohn's disease. Clin Gastroenterol Hepatol 3:1221–1228

Florie J, Wasser MN, Arts-Cieslik K, et al (2006) Dynamic contrast-enhanced MRI of the bowel wall for assessment of disease activity in Crohn's disease. AJR Am J Roentgenol 186:1384–1392

Froehlich JM, Daenzer M, von WC, et al (2009) Aperistaltic effect of hyoscine N-butylbromide versus glucagon on the small bowel assessed by magnetic resonance imaging. Eur Radiol 19:1387–1393

Giardiello FM, Brensinger JD, Tersmette AC, et al (2000) Very high risk of cancer in familial Peutz-Jeghers syndrome. Gastroenterology 119:1447–1453

Giovagnoni A, Fabbri A, Maccioni F (2002) Oral contrast agents in MRI of the gastrointestinal tract. Abdom Imaging 27:367–375

Girometti R, Zuiani C, Toso F, et al (2008) MRI scoring system including dynamic motility evaluation in assessing the activity of Crohn's disease of the terminal ileum. Acad Radiol 15:153–164

Gourtsoyiannis N, Papanikolaou N, Grammatikakis J, et al (2000) MR imaging of the small bowel with a true-FISP sequence after enteroclysis with water solution. Invest Radiol 35:707–711

Gourtsoyiannis N, Papanikolaou N, Grammatikakis J, et al (2004) Assessment of Crohn's disease activity in the small bowel with MR and conventional enteroclysis: preliminary results. Eur Radiol 14:1017–1024

Hirota WK, Zuckerman MJ, Adler DG, et al (2006) ASGE guideline: the role of endoscopy in the surveillance of premalignant conditions of the upper GI tract. Gastrointest Endosc 63:570–580

Horsthuis K, Bipat S, Stokkers PC, et al (2009a) Magnetic resonance imaging for evaluation of disease activity in Crohn's disease: a systematic review. Eur Radiol 19:1450–1460

Horsthuis K, Nederveen AJ, de Feiter MW, et al (2009b) Mapping of T1-values and Gadolinium-concentrations in MRI as indicator of disease activity in luminal Crohn's disease: a feasibility study. J Magn Reson Imaging 29:488–493

Kaminsky S, Laniado M, Gogoll M, et al (1991) Gadopentetate dimeglumine as a bowel contrast agent: safety and efficacy. Radiology 178:503–508

Kivelitz D, Gehl HB, Heuck A, et al (1999) Ferric ammonium citrate as a positive bowel contrast agent for MR imaging of the upper abdomen. Safety and diagnostic efficacy. Acta Radiol 40:429–435

Koh DM, Miao Y, Chinn RJ, et al (2001) MR imaging evaluation of the activity of Crohn's disease. AJR Am J Roentgenol 177:1325–1332

Laghi A, Carbone I, Catalano C, et al (2001) Polyethylene glycol solution as an oral contrast agent for MR imaging of the small bowel. AJR Am J Roentgenol 177:1333–1334

Laghi A, Paolantonio P, Hassan C (2009) Small bowel imaging. Semin Roentgenol 44:99–110

Lauenstein TC, Ajaj W, Narin B, et al (2005) MR imaging of apparent small-bowel perfusion for diagnosing mesenteric ischemia: feasibility study. Radiology 234:569–575

Lauenstein TC, Schneemann H, Vogt FM, et al (2003) Optimization of oral contrast agents for MR imaging of the small bowel. Radiology 228:279–283

Levine MS, Rubesin SE, Pantongrag-Brown L, et al (1997) Non-Hodgkin's lymphoma of the gastrointestinal tract: radiographic findings. AJR Am J Roentgenol 168:165–172

Lohan DG, Alhajeri AN, Cronin CG, et al (2008) MR enterography of small-bowel lymphoma: potential for suggestion of histologic subtype and the presence of underlying celiac disease. AJR Am J Roentgenol 190:287–293

Lomas DJ, Graves MJ (1999) Small bowel MRI using water as a contrast medium. Br J Radiol 72:994–997

Low RN, Sebrechts CP, Politoske DA, et al (2002) Crohn disease with endoscopic correlation: single-shot fast spin-echo and gadolinium-enhanced fat-suppressed spoiled gradient-echo MR imaging. Radiology 222:652–660

Maccioni F, Bruni A, Viscido A, et al (2006) MR imaging in patients with Crohn disease: value of T2- versus T1-weighted gadolinium-enhanced MR sequences with use of an oral superparamagnetic contrast agent. Radiology 238:517–530

Maccioni F, Viscido A, Broglia L, et al (2000) Evaluation of Crohn disease activity with magnetic resonance imaging. Abdom Imaging 25:219–228

Maglinte DD, Gourtsoyiannis N, Rex D, et al (2003) Classification of small bowel Crohn's subtypes based on multimodality imaging. Radiol Clin North Am 41:285–303

Masselli G, Casciani E, Polettini E, et al (2008) Comparison of MR enteroclysis with MR enterography and conventional enteroclysis in patients with Crohn's disease. Eur Radiol 18:438–447

Miao YM, Koh DM, Amin Z, et al (2002) Ultrasound and magnetic resonance imaging assessment of active bowel segments in Crohn's disease. Clin Radiol 57:913–918

Negaard A, Paulsen V, Sandvik L, et al (2007) A prospective randomized comparison between two MRI studies of the small bowel in Crohn's disease, the oral contrast method and MR enteroclysis. Eur Radiol 17:2294–2301

Negaard A, Sandvik L, Berstad AE, et al (2008) MRI of the small bowel with oral contrast or nasojejunal intubation in Crohn's disease: randomized comparison of patient acceptance. Scand J Gastroenterol 43:44–51

Oto A, Zhu F, Kulkarni K, et al (2009) Evaluation of diffusion-weighted MR imaging for detection of bowel inflammation in patients with Crohn's disease. Acad Radiol 16:597–603

Pallotta N, Baccini F, Corazziari E (1999) Contrast ultrasonography of the normal small bowel. Ultrasound Med Biol 25:1335–1340

Paolantonio P, Tomei E, Rengo M, et al (2007) Adult celiac disease: MRI findings. Abdom Imaging 32:433–440

Prassopoulos P, Papanikolaou N, Grammatikakis J, et al (2001) MR enteroclysis imaging of Crohn disease. Radiographics 21:Spec No S161–S172

Punwani S, Rodriguez-Justo M, Bainbridge A, et al (2009) Mural Inflammation in Crohn Disease: Location-Matched Histologic Validation of MR Imaging Features. Radiology jul 27 Epub ahead of print.

Pupillo VA, Di CE, Frieri G, et al (2007) Assessment of inflammatory activity in Crohn's disease by means of dynamic contrast-enhanced MRI. Radiol Med (Torino) 112: 798–809

Schunk K, Kern A, Oberholzer K, et al (2000) Hydro-MRI in Crohn's disease: appraisal of disease activity. Invest Radiol 35:431–437

Sharman A, Zealley IA, Greenhalgh R, et al (2009) MRI of small bowel Crohn's disease: determining the reproducibility of bowel wall gadolinium enhancement measurements. Eur Radiol 19: 1960–1967

Shoenut JP, Semelka RC, Magro CM, et al (1994) Comparison of magnetic resonance imaging and endoscopy in distinguishing the type and severity of inflammatory bowel disease. J Clin Gastroenterol 19:31–35

Shoenut JP, Semelka RC, Silverman R, et al (1993) Magnetic resonance imaging in inflammatory bowel disease. J Clin Gastroenterol 17:73–78

Spigelman AD, Murday V, Phillips RK (1989) Cancer and the Peutz-Jeghers syndrome. Gut 30:1588–1590

Taylor SA, Punwani S, Rodriguez-Justo M, et al (2009) Mural Crohn disease: correlation of dynamic contrast-enhanced MR imaging findings with angiogenesis and inflammation at histologic examination–Pilot Study. Radiology 251: 369–379

Tillack C, Seiderer J, Brand S, et al (2008) Correlation of magnetic resonance enteroclysis (MRE) and wireless capsule endoscopy (CE) in the diagnosis of small bowel lesions in Crohn's disease. Inflamm Bowel Dis 14:1219–1228

Torkzad MR, Lauenstein TC (2009) Enteroclysis versus enterography: the unsettled issue. Eur Radiol 19:90–91

Wiarda BM, Horsthuis K, de Bruijne-Dobben A, et al (2009) MR imaging of the small bowel with the True FISP sequence: intra- and interobserver agreement of enteroclysis versus imaging without contrast material. Clin. Imaging 33:267–273

Wirtzfeld DA, Petrelli NJ, Rodriguez-Bigas MA (2001) Hamartomatous polyposis syndromes: molecular genetics, neoplastic risk, and surveillance recommendations. Ann Surg Oncol 8:319–327

MRI of the Small Bowel: Enteroclysis

Nickolas Papanikolaou and Sofia Gourtsoyianni

CONTENTS

9.1 Introduction 136

9.2 MR Enteroclysis Technique 136
9.2.1 Duodenal Intubation 136
9.2.2 Intraluminal Contrast Agents 136
9.2.3 Patient's Position 137
9.2.4 Pulse Sequences 137

9.3 Normal Appearances 140

9.4 Interpretation of Imaging Findings 141
9.4.1 Crohn's Disease 141
9.4.2 Small Bowel Neoplasms 145
9.4.3 Intestinal Obstruction 146
9.4.4 Malabsorption Disorders 146

9.5 Limitations and Disadvantages of MR Enteroclysis 147

9.6 Conclusions 147

Abbreviations 147

References 147

Nickolas Papanikolaou, PhD
Department of Radiology, University Hospital of Heraklion, University of Crete, Medical School, Stavrakia 71111, Heraklion, Crete, Greece
Sofia Gourtsoyianni, MD
Department of Radiology, University Hospital of Heraklion, Stavrakia, Heraklion 71111, Crete, Greece

KEY POINTS

MR enteroclysis is an emerging technique for small bowel imaging combining the advantages of conventional enteroclysis with those of cross-sectional imaging. MR enteroclysis is equal to conventional enteroclysis in detecting, localizing, and estimating the length of involved small bowel segments. Early lesions such as thickening and distortion of the valvulae conniventes and superficial-type ulcers are clearly demonstrated on conventional enteroclysis but they are not consistently depicted by MR enteroclysis, due to its inadequate spatial resolution. The valvulae conniventes are shown in their best advantage and distortion of the mucosal folds are easily detected by MR enteroclysis. The characteristic discrete longitudinal or transverse ulcers of Crohn's disease can be demonstrated on MR enteroclysis, guaranteed by satisfactory distention and opacification of the bowel. Cobblestoning is caused by the combination of longitudinal and transverse ulceration, and is easily shown by MR enteroclysis. Bowel wall thickening is clearly shown by all MR enteroclysis sequences. Bowel wall thickness and the length of small bowel involvement can be measured on MR enteroclysis images. Narrowing of the lumen and associated prestenotic dilation are easily recognized on MR enteroclysis images by all sequences. Exoenteric manifestations of the disease are demonstrated in detail on true-FISP images due to the high contrast generated from the bright mesenteric fat. Disease activity can be best appreciated on postgadolinium fat-saturated 2D/3D T1-weighted sequence by the characteristic enhancement patterns of thickened small bowel wall and degree of enhancement of mesenteric lymph nodes compared to adjacent vessel enhancement.

9.1
Introduction

Advances in MRI hardware and software have allowed rapid acquisition of high-resolution images of the gastrointestinal (GI) tract, upgrading the diagnostic role of MRI for the imaging evaluation of patients with intestinal diseases (Gourtsoyiannis et al. 2000, 2001; Umschaden et al. 2000; Prassopoulos et al. 2001). Imaging of the entire small bowel may be challenging and important in view of problematic access of endoscopic methods. Optimal luminal distention is of paramount importance for accurate diagnosis and currently the only technique that can fulfill this requirement is enteroclysis. The combination of ultrafast MRI sequences and duodenal intubation is known as MR enteroclysis (Gourtsoyiannis et al. 2000; Umschaden et al. 2000). Morphologic evaluation of small intestinal diseases, as well as functional information, can be obtained with state-of-the-art MR enteroclysis examinations. The most important advantages of MR enteroclysis include: (a) absence of radiation exposure, (b) rich soft tissue contrast through the utilization of multiple contrast mechanisms, and (c) three-dimensional imaging capabilities. The technical aspects, clinical applications, and limitations of MR enteroclysis are summarized in this chapter.

9.2
MR Enteroclysis Technique

9.2.1
Duodenal Intubation

Duodenal intubation ensures adequate small bowel distention, which is considered a prerequisite for identification of intestinal abnormalities (Gourtsoyiannis et al. 2000; Umschaden et al. 2000). In our institution we currently use the 13 French Maglinte enteroclysis catheter (MEC, Cook, Bloomington, IN). Positioning of the nasojejunal catheter is monitored fluoroscopically. The range of intubation time is 2.5–3.5 min, while radiation dose is kept to a minimum by good collimation, low fluoroscopy current and by using short periods of intermittent fluoroscopy. Although in the beginning MR enteroclysis was performed in association with conventional enteroclysis (CE) (Papanikolaou et al. 2002b), nowadays the standalone MR enteroclysis examination is the mainstream approach (Gourtsoyiannis et al. 2006; Masselli et al. 2009). When MR enteroclysis follows CE, certain adjustments in the selection of the appropriate contrast agent, the amount and route of its administration are important for both examinations to be successful. The patient's tolerance to intubation is related to the examiner's experience and can be considered a drawback of MR enteroclysis. Conscious sedation is advocated in USA (Kohli and Maglinte 2009) to overcome the patient's discomfort during duodenal intubation for performance of CT enteroclysis. Local anesthesia of the pharynx and spending time explaining the procedure in detail to the patient have been proven in our everyday practice equally useful measures to minimize discomfort. Oral contrast administration without intubation is performed to reduce the patient's discomfort (Lomas and Graves 1999) (see Chap. 8). However, small bowel distention is usually not sufficient, primarily at the proximal small bowel. A collapsed or not adequately distended small bowel loop may mask minimal abnormalities or may result in false-positive findings. Without fail, a detailed evaluation of the small intestine requires luminal distention that can be guaranteed by intubation.

9.2.2
Intraluminal Contrast Agents

Intraluminal contrast agents are essential for both lumen opacification and distention. A suitable contrast agent should provide homogeneous opacification throughout the entire small bowel lumen, clear differentiation between the lumen and the bowel wall, and be characterized by minimal mucosal absorption, absence of artifacts formation, no severe adverse effects, and low cost (see also Chap. 3). Various media have been proposed (Table 9.1) as optimal intraluminal contrast agents for small intestinal imaging that can fulfill the previous criteria, but there is no consensus

Table 9.1. The most important intraluminal contrast agents classified according the endoluminal signal intensity changes they induce

Positive	Negative	Biphasic
Gadolinium chelates	SPIO	Methylcellulose
Ferrous ammonium citrates	OMP	Mannitol
Manganese chloride	$BaSO_4$	PEG

Table 9.2. Scan parameters of different sequences utilized in MR enteroclysis protocol

	SSTSE	HASTE	3D FLASH	True-FISP
Scan time (s)	3	1/slice	23	1.5/slice
Slice thickness (mm)	70–100	4–6	2.5	4
Number of slices	1	18	40	12
TR(ms)/TE(ms)/a°	Inf/1200/180	Inf/90/180	4.8/1.8/45	6/3/70
Matrix	240 × 256	256 × 256	256 × 512	512 × 512

on the ideal one, at present. Positive contrast agents render the intestinal lumen with high signal intensity. Negative intraluminal contrast agents result in low intraluminal signal intensity, while biphasic agents are affecting signal intensity depending on the pulse sequence used, usually low on T1- and high on T2-weighted images. These agents are considered more suitable for small bowel imaging, to our experience. Polyethylene glycol water solution with electrolytes is an iso-osmotic, biphasic contrast agent with excellent performance in MR enteroclysis (GOURTSOYIANNIS et al. 2000, 2001).

A controlled infusion is important for a successful MR enteroclysis. Initially a flow rate of 80–120 mL/min is utilized until the contrast reaches the terminal ileum. Subsequently, the flow rate increases up to 200 mL/min to achieve reflex atony that facilitates acquisition of images with minimal motion artifacts. A home-made pump consisting of plastic pneumocolon adapted with plastic tubes can be used to avoid problems with the magnetic field interferences. Alternatively a dedicated enteroclysis pump can be used positioned outside the MRI room.

9.2.3
Patient's Position

Patients can be examined either in prone or supine position. The former is suggested because it exerts mild pressure to the anterior abdominal wall facilitating separation of the small bowel loops, while it decreases the volume of peritoneal cavity to be imaged. As supine position is more comfortable, MR enteroclysis can be performed this way in older and frail patients.

9.2.4
Pulse Sequences

A comprehensive MR enteroclysis examination protocol should include both T1- and T2-weighted images as for example spoiled gradient echo (i.e., FLASH) and single shot turbo spin echo (SSTSE; i.e., HASTE) sequences, respectively (Table 9.2). Incorporating different MR sequences is the most effective way to demonstrate anatomy, identify and characterize abnormalities, and disclose associated extraintestinal manifestations. Sequences should be fast enough to permit comfortable breath-holding; high-performance gradient systems are important for this purpose. Image quality, irrespectively of pulse sequences applied, can significantly be improved when using abdominal phased array RF coils by increasing the signal-to-noise ratio.

Acquisition of SSTSE images (slab thickness 7–10 cm, TR: infinite, TE: 1,200 ms, scan time: 3 s) precedes the main examination to monitor the infusion process. Projectional SSTSE images of the small bowel have been applied for demonstrating small bowel obstruction (UMSCHADEN et al. 2000). Faster versions of SSTSE sequence (MAKKI et al. 2002) may be used for MR fluoroscopy thus providing information about small bowel motility (see also Chap. 14).

True-FISP sequence (TR: 6 ms, TE: 3 ms, flip angle: 70°, slice thickness: 4 mm, scan matrix 256 or 512 and scan time 1.5 s per slice) is a cardinal sequence for MR enteroclysis. It provides motion-free, high-resolution, "T2-like" images of the small intestine, and the mesenteries in a few seconds. The normal bowel wall and valvulae conniventes exhibit moderate signal intensity on true-FISP images, while the intraluminal fluid and the extraluminal fat show high signal intensity favoring the delineation of the bowel wall (Fig. 9.1). Demonstration of the mesenteries is excellent using true-FISP sequence. The high signal intensity of the mesenteric fat provides the ideal background for the depiction of small anatomic structures; small lymph nodes and thin mesenteric vessels including the vasa recta are clearly seen with low signal intensity, especially when a 512 matrix is utilized. The sequence is prone to specific type of artifacts; susceptibility artifacts from trapped air and black boundary artifacts along to the external small bowel wall surface due to chemical shift phenomena may be seen (Fig. 9.2a). However, black boundary artifacts can be clearly differentiated from abnormal bowel wall thickening. The capability to add fat saturation prepulses in the true-FISP sequence may also be used to overcome black boundary artifacts (Fig. 9.2b). The acquisition of multiple images over time at the same slice in a dynamic manner permits the evaluation of local and global small bowel motility patterns. This sequence is termed cine-true-FISP and it has shown to be of help in the differentiation between "soft", inflammatory type of stenosis and fibrostenotic strictures in patients with Crohn's disease.

The most commonly used sequence in small bowel protocols is the HASTE sequence (PRASSOPOULOS et al. 2001; LEE et al. 1998). It can provide heavily T2-weighted images with high contrast resolution in less than 1 s per slice (Fig. 9.3). Imaging parameters may include TE of 90 ms, infinite TR, 4–6 mm slice thickness, 256 × 256–512 scan matrix and scanning time appropriate for breath-hold acquisition of images. HASTE images does not suffer from susceptibility or chemical shift artifacts but are prone to high-order motion usually manifested as intraluminal flow voids (Fig. 9.4a) or blurring of small bowel wall edges (PAPANIKOLAOU et al. 2002a). To overcome this limitation administration of antiperistaltic drugs – as for example 1 mg of glucagon – should precede acquisition of HASTE images. The normal bowel wall is clearly seen on HASTE images with low signal intensity (Fig. 9.3), as opposed to the high signal intensity of the thickened bowel wall that may be observed in patients with active Crohn's disease. This sequence is not appropriate for imaging evaluation of the mesenteries. K-space filtering effects may obscure small anatomic structures and result in decreased definition of larger vessels or lymph nodes (Fig. 9.5a).

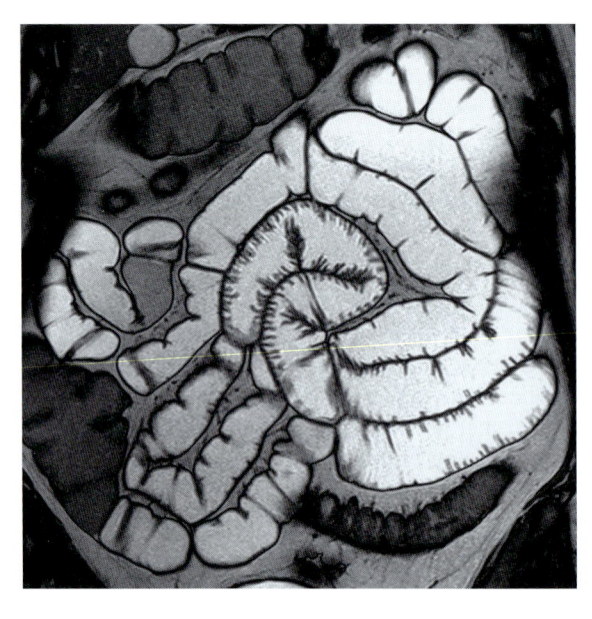

Fig. 9.1. High-quality images of the small intestine can be acquired by combining the true-FISP sequence with PEG as an intraluminal contrast agent

Fig. 9.2. Coronal true-FISP images in a patient with Crohn's disease without (**a**) and with fat-saturation prepulses (**b**). In the native true-FISP image the presence of *black* boundary artifact is evident in voxels were both fat and water protons are coexisting (*arrows*). By adding fat-saturation prepulses (**b**), the black boundary artifacts may be eliminated, permitting accurate wall thickness analysis

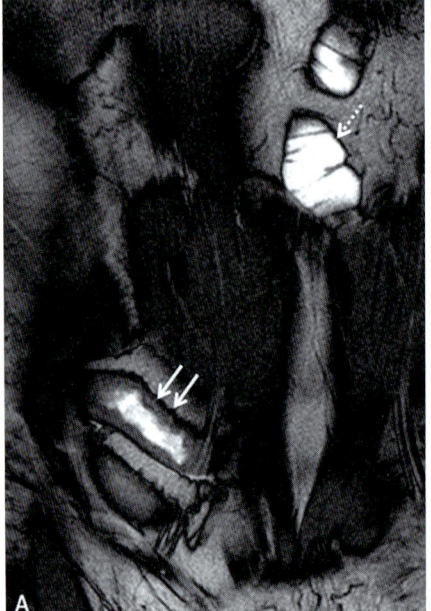

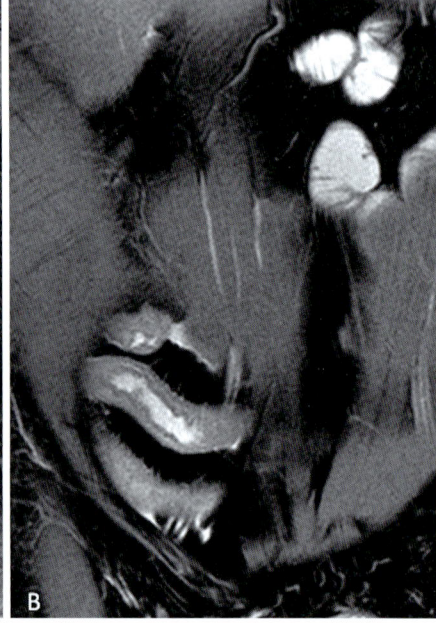

High spatial resolution T1-weighted images of the small bowel can be obtained applying 3D or 2D spoiled gradient echo sequence (GOURTSOYIANNIS et al. 2001; GOURTSOYIANNIS and PAPANIKOLAOU 2008). Fat-saturation prepulses facilitate the demonstration of the bowel wall in combination with a negative intraluminal contrast agent. Thin sections and small pixel size allows for increased definition of the bowel wall. Intravenous administration of gadolinium increases the conspicuity of the normal bowel wall and may permit lesion characterization by evaluating different enhancement patterns. A 3D FLASH sequence with fat saturation may applied with 4.8 ms TR, 1.8 ms TE, 45° flip angle, 2.5 mm slice thickness, 256 × 512 scan matrix and 23 s scan time. Normal bowel wall on contrast-enhanced FLASH images with fat saturation exhibits high signal intensity due to gadolinium uptake and is perfectly delineated between the low signal intensity of the mesenteric fat and the negative intraluminal contrast agent (Fig. 9.6). A scanning delay of 60–80 s post-IV contrast results in maximal contrast between the intestinal

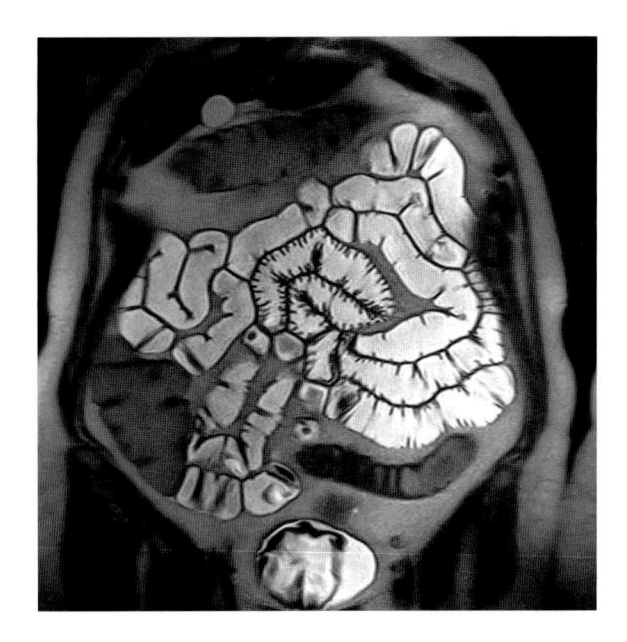

Fig. 9.3. Coronal HASTE image demonstrating T2 contrast and clear depiction of the intestinal wall. Notice the loss of information from the mesenteries due to selective spatial blurring effects

Fig. 9.4. MR enteroclysis: coronal HASTE (**a**) and true-FISP (**b**) images. HASTE is suffering from high-order motion due to peristaltic waves presented as signal voids (*arrows*), while true-FISP sequences are rather insensitive to such artifacts due to flow compensation capabilities in all three axes

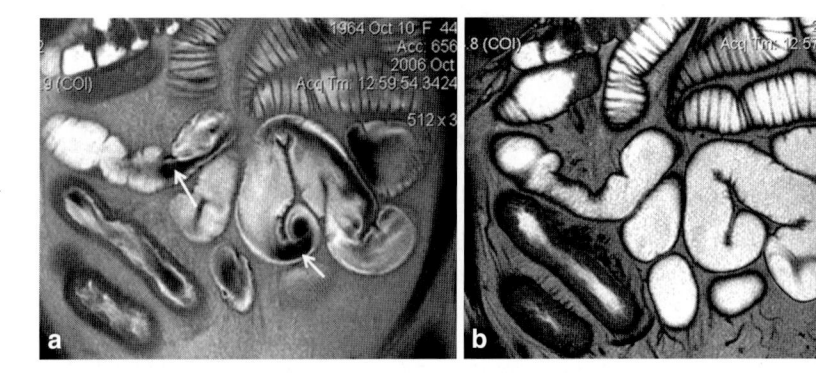

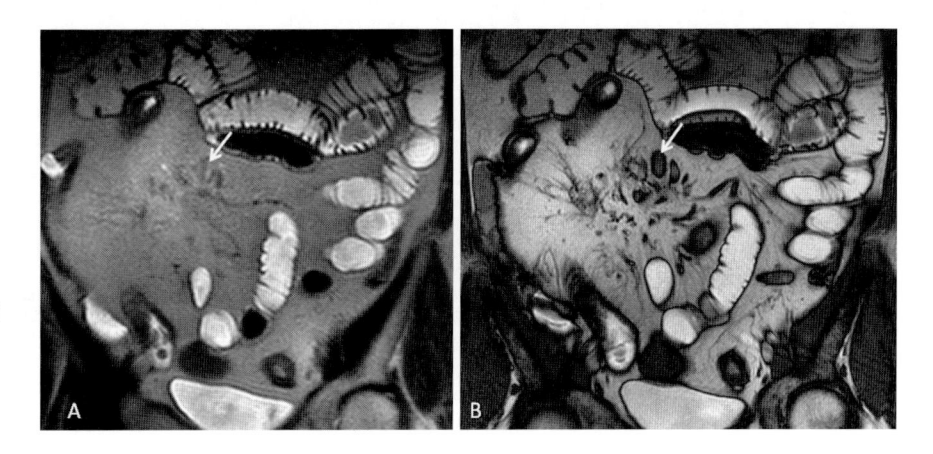

Fig. 9.5. Coronal HASTE (**a**) and true-FISP (**b**) images in a patient with Crohn's disease. Mesenteric lymph nodes (*arrow*) and vessels are poorly depicted with the HASTE sequence due to K-space filtering effects

wall and the lumen (Fig. 9.7). 3D FLASH sequence is sensitive to motion; consequently, antiperistaltic drugs administration should precede the application of the sequence (Fig. 9.8).

Incorporation of different MR sequences – such as SSTSE, true-FISP, HASTE and gadolinium-enhanced FLASH – into a comprehensive MR enteroclysis imaging protocol is important to obtain all the information the method can provide, in a balanced fashion, where disadvantages of one sequence are overcome by the advantages of the other (Table 9.3). For example, susceptibility artifacts on true-FISP images may prevent demonstration of a small portion of small bowel wall that can be evaluated on HASTE or FLASH images, while motion artifacts downgrading image quality on FLASH images do not interfere with true-FISP images. Information from images obtained using different contrast mechanisms increases the confidence in lesion detection and characterization, and provides a completed anatomic demonstration of the intestinal lumen small bowel wall and the mesenteries.

9.3
Normal Appearences

The use of a biphasic intraluminal contrast agent such as PEG results in high signal intensity of the lumen on true-FISP images and low signal intensity on post-gadolinium FLASH images (Figs. 9.1 and 9.6). A very powerful contrast mechanism that MR is offering is the T2 contrast that is based on differences between the T2 relaxation times of tissues. In T2-weighted images, such as HASTE, normal intestinal wall exhibits moderate signal intensity. Normal bowel wall is uniformly thin not exceeding 3 mm in thickness. Normal intestinal folds are visualized as dark linear structures. HASTE provides high contrast between bowel wall and intraluminal fluid. One should be aware that some ultrafast pulse sequences that are routinely utilized for small bowel imaging,

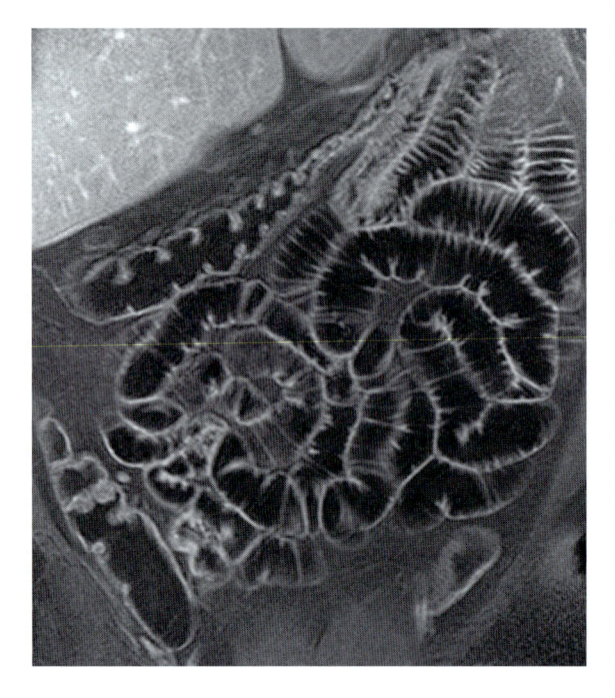

Fig. 9.6. Normal appearance of the small bowel in post-gadolinium coronal FLASH images with fat-saturation pre-pulses. The combination of parallel imaging algorithms and state of the art matrix coils permits the acquisition of 1,024 matrices with sufficient signal-to-noise ratio

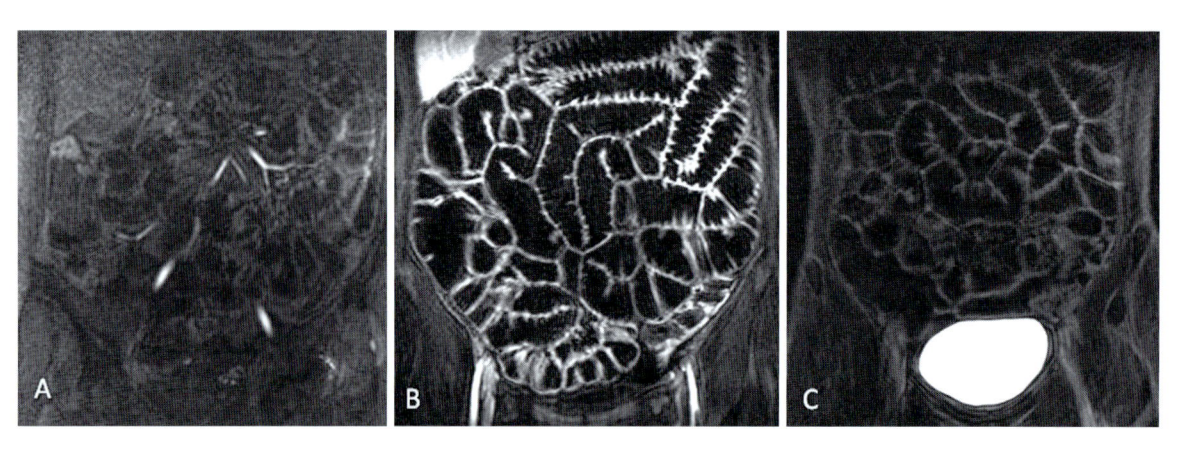

Fig. 9.7. Coronal post-gadolinium FLASH images on different patients acquired at three time points after gadolinium injection at 25 s (**a**), 75 s (**b**) and 180 s (**c**). Optimal contrast between the intestinal wall and surrounding tissues is achieved at 75 s

Fig. 9.8. Coronal post-gadolinium FLASH sequence before (**a**) and after intravenous administration of glucagon (**b**). Peristaltic motion present in (**a**) is resulting in significant blurring

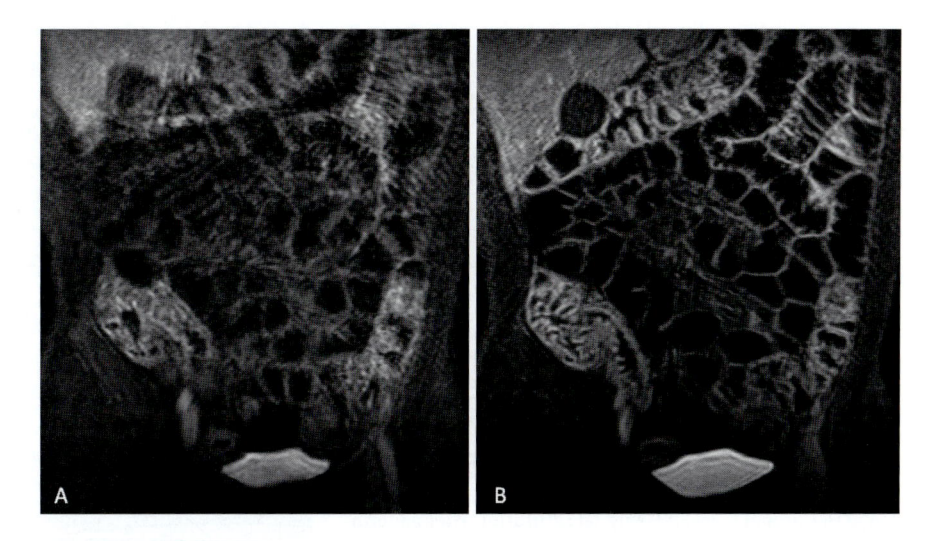

Table 9.3. Comprehensive MR enteroclysis examination protocol

	True-FISP	FLASH	HASTE
Wall depiction	✓	✓	✓
Lumen opacification	✓	✓	
Lesion detection, localization	✓	✓	✓
Lesion characterization		✓	
Detection of mesenteric lesions	✓		
Characterization of mesenteric lesions		✓	
Respiratory artifacts		•	
Black boundary artifacts	•		
Susceptibility artifacts		•	
Intraluminal flow voids			•
K-space filtering			•

Strengths (✓) and weaknesses (•) of each individual sequence

such as true-FISP sequence, deviate in terms of contrast due to T1 interferences. True-FISP is capable of demonstrating normal anatomy and morphology equally well to HASTE; however, the mixed contrast may decrease its potential in tissue characterization. In addition the superb contrast between the bright mesenteric fat and the dark mesenteric vessels or lymph nodes, make it exceptional for the demonstration of extraintestinal anatomy.

In case of postgadolinium FLASH images, normal intestinal wall exhibits moderate homogeneous enhancement while abnormal wall might be expressed by three different enhancement patterns as will be discussed in detail in the next paragraph. Postgadolinium FLASH sequences allow also improved lesion characterization in case of small bowel neoplasms.

9.4
Interpretation of Imaging Findings

9.4.1
Crohn's Disease

Crohn's disease is a preferential field for the application of MR enteroclysis. Different pulse sequences may offer different kind of information that can be intergraded to provide an overall view of mucosal, mural, and extramural abnormalities associated with the disease and complementary information about disease activity and complications. These MR enteroclysis features of Crohn's disease are to a large extent identical to the features of MR enterography.

In a recent study (GOURTSOYIANNIS et al. 2006), a comparison between MR enteroclysis and CE was performed on a sign-by-sign basis in patients with Crohn's disease. A total number of 49 involved segments were disclosed by MR enteroclysis, all of which were confirmed by CE. There was full agreement between MR enteroclysis and CE in determining the length and the site of involvement of the diseased segments.

Early lesions of Crohn's disease, such as thickening and distortion of the valvulae conniventes and superficial types of ulcers that are clearly demonstrated on CE are not consistently depicted by MR

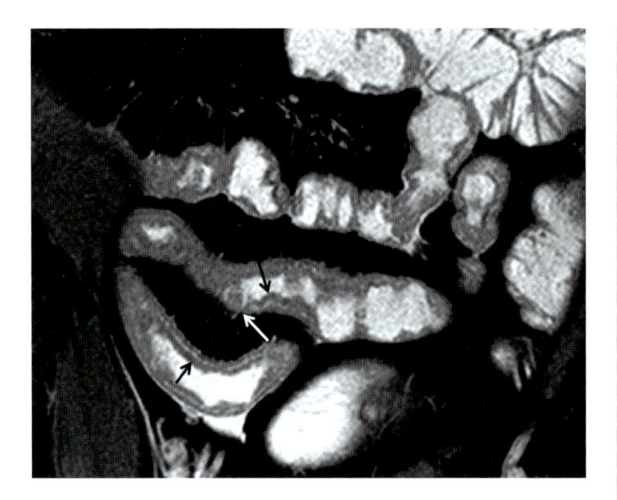

Fig. 9.9. Coronal true-FISP with fat saturation after gadolinium administration. Normal mucosal layer is demonstrated as a black thin line due to T2 shortening effects from increased local concentration of gadolinium (*black arrows*). Discrete ulceration can be discriminated from fold thickening in the basis of preservation of continuity of mucosa. In the area of the discrete ulcer (*white arrow*) the mucosal layer is disrupted

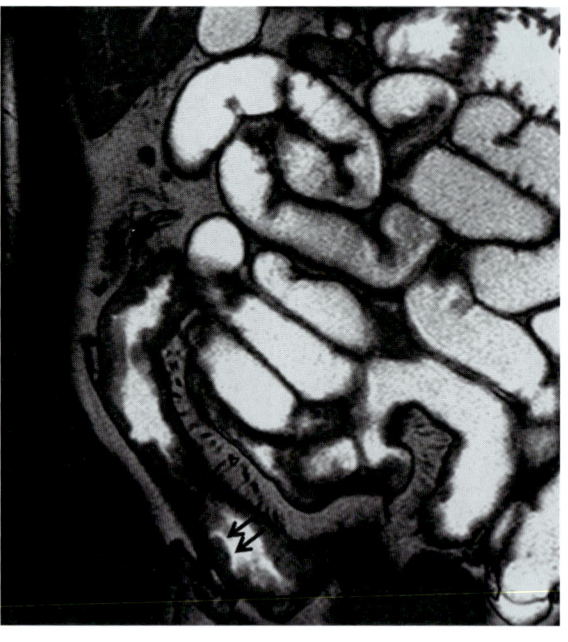

Fig. 9.10. Linear ulcer (*black arrows*) is demonstrated on a patient with active inflammatory subtype of Crohn's disease, on a coronal true-FISP image

enteroclysis (Gourtsoyiannis et al. 2006). This results in an overall sensitivity of less than 50% for MR enteroclysis detecting superficial ulcerations, most probably due to inadequate spatial resolution. Direct imaging techniques such as video capsule endoscopy (VCE) are obviously performing better in detecting such early mucosal abnormalities. It is speculated that dedicated ultrafast, high-resolution sequences and stronger gradients will further improve the detection of such early, but not specific, manifestations of the disease in the near future.

The characteristic discrete, longitudinal, or transverse ulcers of Crohn's disease can be demonstrated on MR enteroclysis, following optimal distention and homogeneous opacification of the bowel lumen (Fig. 9.9). A sensitivity of about 90% in detecting deep ulcers was achieved in a recent study of 52 patients with suspected or established Crohn's disease, and this is probably related to the optimized technique that was utilized (Gourtsoyiannis et al. 2006).

Cobblestoning, a combination of longitudinal and transverse ulceration, can be easily demonstrated by MR enteroclysis. As in the case of discrete ulcers, a tailored MR enteroclysis examination can guarantee a high sensitivity and specificity of 92.3% and 94.4%, respectively, for the demonstration of cobblestoning (Gourtsoyiannis et al. 2006). A true-FISP sequence is known to be superior to HASTE in demonstrating linear ulcers (Fig. 9.10), cobblestoning, and intramural tracts, due to its superb resolution capabilities and its relative insensitivity to motion artifacts, while 3D FLASH sequences are less efficient in depicting such lesions when they are smaller than 3 mm (Prassopoulos et al. 2001). Bowel wall thickening can be clearly detected by all MR enteroclysis sequences. Mural thickening presenting with moderate signal intensity on true-FISP images can be easily differentiated from misregistration due to the black boundary artifacts (Gourtsoyiannis and Papanikolaou 2008). Bowel wall thickness and the length of small bowel involvement can be measured accurately on MR enteroclysis images. Narrowing of the lumen and associated prestenotic dilation (Fig. 9.11), as well as skip or multiple lesions (Fig. 9.12), are routinely recognized on MR enteroclysis images in all sequences. The addition of cine true-FISP sequences that can be used to demonstrate local motility patterns might reduce any potential false-positive results in stenotic lesions due to bowel spasm.

One of the most significant advantages that MR enteroclysis is offering over endoscopic techniques is its capability to demonstrate in the same imaging session exoenteric manifestations of the disease. This can be done in the best of its advantage on true-FISP images

MRI of the Small Bowel: Enteroclysis 143

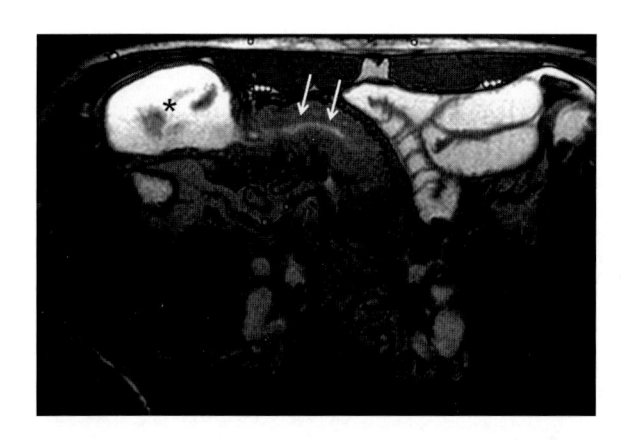

Fig. 9.11. Axial true-FISP image in a patient with fibrostenotic subtype of Crohn's disease. A fibrostenotic lesion is causing significant luminal narrowing (*arrows*) and prestenotic dilation (*asterisk*). The mural signal intensity is moderate reflecting the presence of fibrosis

due to the high contrast generated from the bright mesenteric fat. Complications such as fistulae, phlegmons (Fig. 9.13) or abscesses may be more accurately diagnosed on T1-weighted FLASH images with fat saturation by the characteristic pattern of enhancement after gadolinium administration (Gourtsoyiannis et al. 2006). The latter sequence is additionally useful in active disease because of the marked contrast uptake in the thickened small bowel wall (Lohan et al. 2007; Makki et al. 2002) and mesenteric lymph node enhancement (Fig. 9.14) (Lee et al. 1998). MR enteroclysis imaging signs that are related to active disease have been proposed (Gourtsoyiannis et al. 2004, 2009; Koh et al. 2001; Florie et al. 2006), and this may represent one of the most important indications for the examination in the near future, however there are no universal agreed criteria for such assessment of

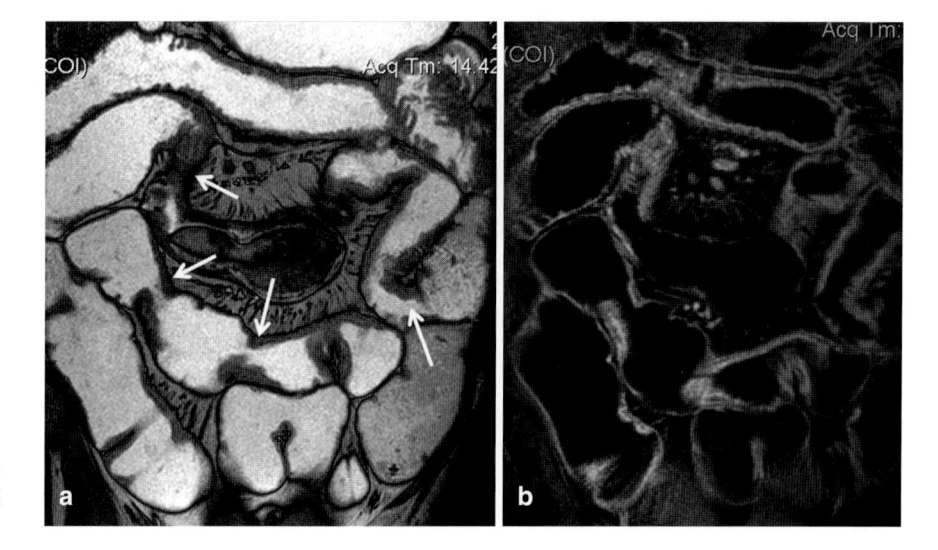

Fig. 9.12. Skip lesions are identified (*arrows*) both on coronal (**a**) true-FISP and (**b**) postgadolinium FLASH with fat-saturation images in a patient with longstanding Crohn's disease

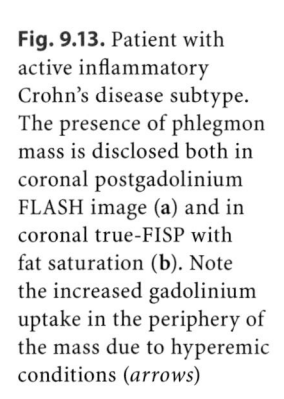

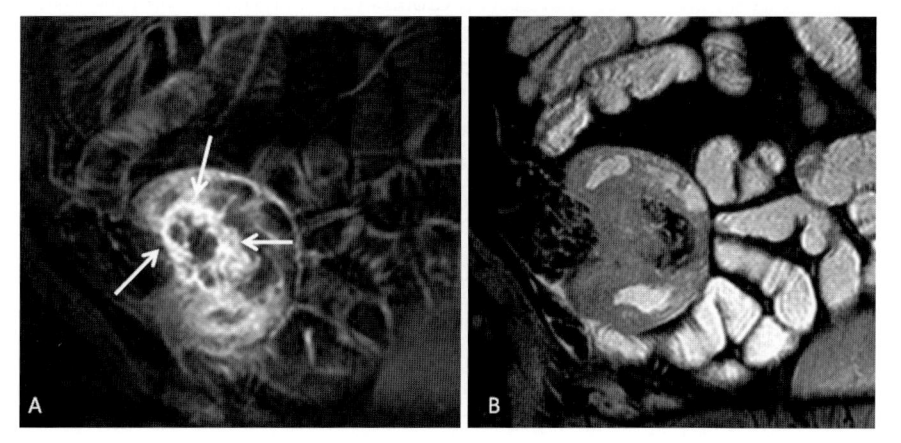

Fig. 9.13. Patient with active inflammatory Crohn's disease subtype. The presence of phlegmon mass is disclosed both in coronal postgadolinium FLASH image (**a**) and in coronal true-FISP with fat saturation (**b**). Note the increased gadolinium uptake in the periphery of the mass due to hyperemic conditions (*arrows*)

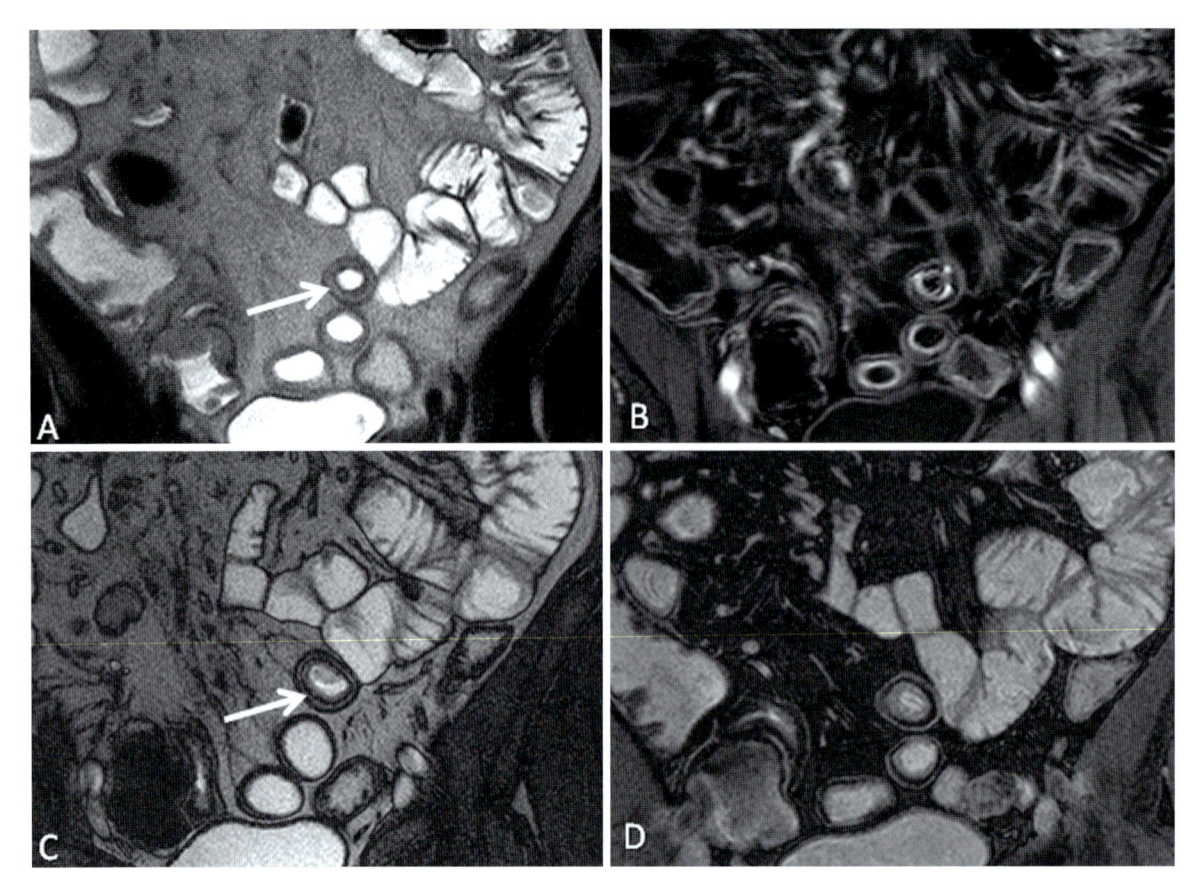

Fig. 9.14. The presence of intramural fat might simulate the appearance of submucosal edema. In HASTE images (**a**) both intramural fat and edema are exhibiting high signal intensity (*arrow*), while on post-gadolinium FLASH images (**b**) with fat saturation fat and edema presents with low signal intensity (*arrows*). True-FISP without or with fat saturation might help to discriminate between fat and edema, since fat is generating the typical black boundary artifact (*arrow* on **c**), or it presents with low signal on fat-saturated true-FISP images (**d**), contrary to edema which on the latter images is bright

disease activity as the protocols of MR enteroclysis or enterography are widely different. According to one study (Gourtsoyiannis et al. 2004), there are criteria, among all possible imaging findings that one encounters on MR enteroclysis in patients with Crohn's disease and in correlation with Crohn's disease activity index (CDAI) that provide a reference to discriminate active from non active disease. These are: (a) more than one transmural ulcer, (b) wall thickness >7 mm, and (c) enhancing mesenteric lymph nodes with a signal intensity enhancement ratio (signal intensity of lymph node/ signal intensity of adjacent vessel) >0.7.

Intramural fat can be accurately identified when combining features from true-FISP and gadolinium-enhanced 3D FLASH images with fat saturation. Discrimination between the deposition of fat and the presence of edema (Fig. 9.15) may be helpful for the disease classification. Collagen is known to result in late gadolinium enhancement (Semelka et al. 2001). In this context, MR has the potential to differentiate fibrostenotic from edematous lesions on the basis of different gadolinium enhancement patterns.

By assessment of Crohn's disease via MR enteroclysis, certain diagnostic tasks can be accomplished including the demonstration of extent of mural and extramural disease, the calculation of disease activity, and the identification of clinical subtypes, a critical point for further patient management. Maglinte et al. (2003) introduced an imaging-based classification of Crohn's disease subtypes constituting of active inflammatory (AI), fibrostenotic (FS), and fistulizing-perforating (FP) subtype. In a recent study (Gourtsoyianni et al. 2009), mesenteric lymph nodes of patients with AI disease presented with the highest enhancement ratio when compared to mesenteric lymph nodes of patients with FP disease, who presented with moderate enhancement ratio and those in patients with FS who presented with the lowest enhancement ratio. The difference in mean values of enhancement ratio between mesenteric lymph nodes of AI and FS subtypes was statistically significant. Thus, according to this study degree of homogeneous uptake is not the same for all different disease subtypes, and therefore quantification of enhancement ratio was proven useful in clinical practice for disease subtype classification.

MR enteroclysis also allows the assessment of Crohn's disease recurrence after ileocolic resection.

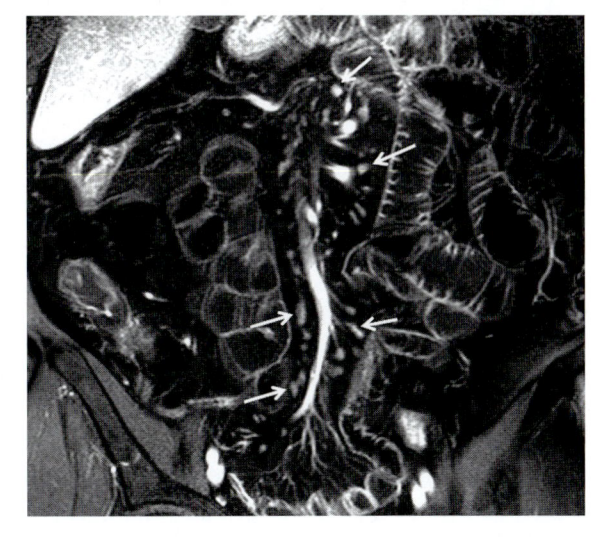

Fig. 9.15. Patient with active inflammatory subtype of Crohn's disease. Multiple, enhancing mesenteric lymph nodes (*arrows*) are easily depicted in a coronal post-gadolinium FLASH image

Sailer et al. (2008) developed a reproducible MR score which showed high agreement with the endoscopic Rutgeerts score, and according to it medical therapy or surgical intervention can be indicated.

MR enteroclysis is an emerging technique for the assessment of small bowel pathology and its clinical applications is so far limited to centers of reference. The method is complementary to CE in detecting superficial or early Crohn's disease, but it is of equal diagnostic accuracy in disclosing transmural disease. In addition, MR enteroclysis can adequately depict mesenteric involvement and extraintestinal complications of Crohn's disease which is an important advantage over CE. Specific MR enteroclysis imaging features may be used to assess disease activity. Furthermore, accurate individual lesion detection, provided by MR enteroclysis, may successfully address clinical questions related to the classification of Crohn's disease subtypes.

9.4.2 Small Bowel Neoplasms

MR enteroclysis may combine the effectiveness of cross-sectional MRI (SEMELKA et al. 1996) with the advantages of CE in the detection and characterization of small bowel neoplasms. Small bowel tumors usually exhibit moderate signal intensity on true-FISP images (Fig. 9.16a) as opposed to the high signal intensity of the distended lumen and the mesenteric fat. Post-gadolinium 3D FLASH sequence with fat

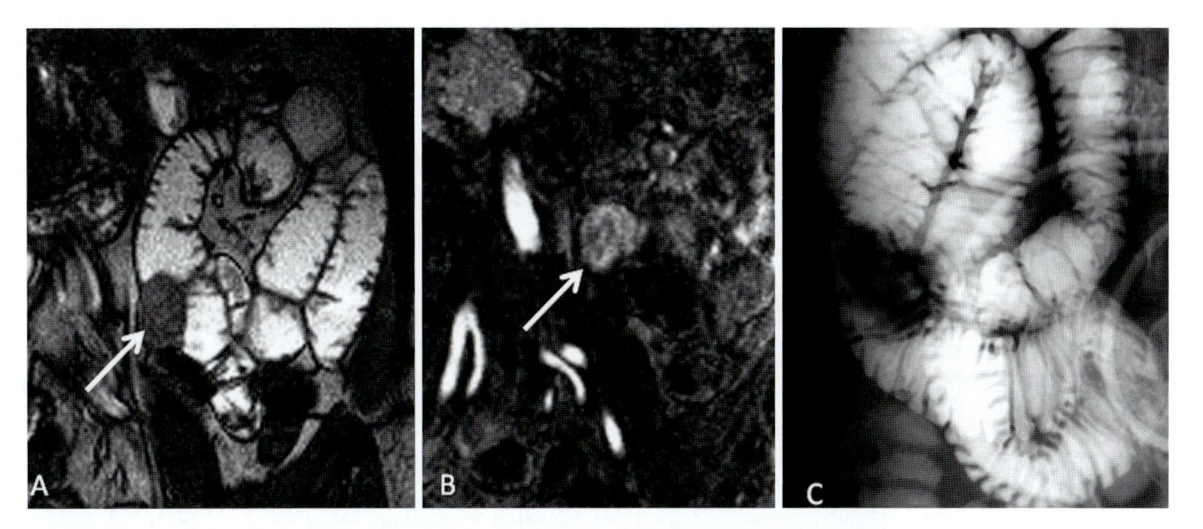

Fig. 9.16. Coronal true-FISP (**a**) and post-gadolinium FLASH (**b**) images are showing a well-defined mass (*arrows*) with moderate signal intensity on true-FISP and increased contrast uptake. The presence of the mass was confirmed on conventional enteroclysis (**c**), and proved to be a benign stromal tumor (with permission from GOURTSOYIANNIS et al. 2001)

saturation may be the most important one (Fig. 9.16b) for the identification and characterization of small bowel tumors. The degree of prestenotic dilation, the peritoneal extension of the neoplasm and the associated lymphadenopathy can be appreciated by all MR enteroclysis sequences. The role of MR enteroclysis in small bowel tumors has not fully established, at present, due to the limited experience on that issue. However the technique is very promising and may be considered as the effective approach for imaging of small bowel neoplasms. Due to the excellent distention and the possibility for repeated imaging with different sequences provided by MR enteroclysis it possible to differentiate with greater certainty between collapsed bowel loops and potential masses. In a more recent study (MASSELI et al. 2009), the accuracy of MR enteroclysis for identification of small bowel neoplasms in symptomatic patients with a size ranging from 8 mm to 7 cm was found to be 97% when compared to histopathological examination. Another study (SCHMID-TANNWALD et al. 2009) concentrated in the ability of MR enteroclysis to identify and localize only primary carcinoid tumors of the small bowel which was found to reach 93% when using contrast enhanced T1-weighted fat-saturated GRE sequences as compared to surgical findings. Primary carcinoid tumors appeared as nodular intraluminal masses in 40% of the cases, as focal wall thickening in 33% and in 20% as both (SCHMID-TANNWALD et al. 2009).

9.4.3
Intestinal Obstruction

MR enteroclysis is very effective in determining the presence and the level (Fig. 9.17) of low-grade small bowel obstruction (LIENEMANN et al. 2000). Initial evaluation of a patient with suspected small bowel obstruction with dynamic SSTSE images is useful for the prompt disclosure of this condition, meanwhile providing information about small bowel motility. In addition, MR enteroclysis may reveal the cause of obstruction. Sequential true-FISP images in a functional cine MRI mode proved highly accurate in small bowel obstruction due to post-surgical adhesions (LIENEMANN et al. 2000), while post-gadolinium 3D FLASH images may demonstrate other than adhesions causes of obstruction. In patients with obvious signs of high-grade obstruction, an MRI examination without enteral contrast administration can be considered.

9.4.4
Malabsorption Disorders

Malabsorption states, and especially celiac disease, are another indication for MR imaging of the small bowel (LAGHI et al. 2003). The role of diagnostic imaging in celiac disease is usually limited, since the final diagnosis is obtained by jejunal biopsy. Decreased number of jejunal folds, reversed jejunal folds, i.e., decreased number of jejunal folds and increased folds in ileum is indicative of celiac sprue due to total villous atrophy, a finding that can be better appreciated by MR enteroclysis than by MR enterography due to excellent distention of the jejunum. MR enteroclysis might be a useful tool both for diagnosis and follow-up, since it can provide, noninvasively, morphologic information such as bowel dilation, ileal jejunization, jejuno-ileal reversal pattern and, at the same time, extraintestinal findings, such as mesenteric vascular congestion,

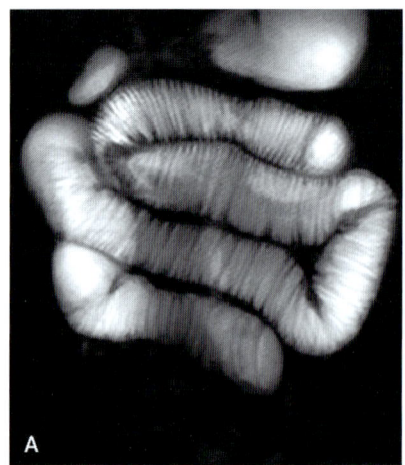

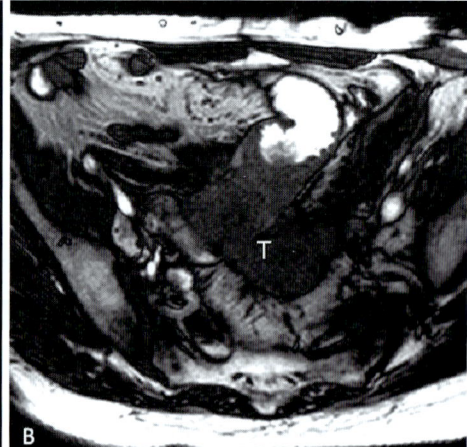

Fig. 9.17. Patient with colonic carcinoma that has invaded a jejunal small bowel loop. (**a**) Coronal projection single shot TSE image demonstrating dilation of jejunal loops and absence of opacification of distal small bowel loops. (**b**) Axial true-FISP image disclosing a large mass (*T*), invading the small bowel, responsible for bowel obstruction

lymphadenopathy, hyposplenism or the presence of intussusception (Laghi et al. 2003). One should aware of lymphomas in patients with celiac disease.

9.5
Limitations and Disadvantages of MR Enteroclysis

MR enteroclysis has not been adequately compared to other techniques for small bowel imaging. Duodenal intubation and inherent very limited radiation exposure are considered drawbacks of MR enteroclysis as compared to MR enterography. Optimal and homogeneous distention throughout the entire small bowel however allow for easier depiction of individual lesions, like discrete ulcerations, avoid misregistration of collapsed or undistended bowel segments, increases confidence in diagnosis for the average practitioner and guarantees better comparison and measurements in follow-up studies after treatment due to consistent optimal image quality. Adequate distention is important to verify the presence of edema in a diseased bowel segment, and therefore aid in patients management in differentiating inflammatory from fibrotic disease. A disadvantage of MR enteroclysis is the limited spatial resolution as compared to CE and multidetector CT. Temporal resolution, even with functional cine MR mode or dynamic SSTSE, is inferior to the real-time imaging provided by CE and ultrasound. The cost-effectiveness of the method has not been evaluated, yet. A technically successful MR enteroclysis examination and correct interpretation of its findings requires familiarity with the technique.

9.6
Conclusions

MR enteroclysis appears very promising for the evaluation of small bowel anatomy, motility, and pathology. Accumulated experience during the past decade shows that MR enteroclysis is well performing in Crohn's disease, tumorous lesions, and small bowel obstruction. MR enteroclysis is a highly specific examination for demonstration of the transmural nature and extent of inflammation. It can depict lesions beyond severe luminal stenosis, can characterize further stenotic lesions (edema vs. fibrosis differentiation), and can identify intraperitoneal extension or extraintestinal manifestations. Various imaging features have been shown to correlate with disease activity, while MR enteroclysis may permit accurate classification in different disease subtypes, affecting directly patient management.

List of Abbreviations

AI	Active inflammatory
CDAI	Crohn's disease activity index
CE	Conventional enteroclysis
FISP	Fast imaging with steady precession
FLASH	Fast low angle shot
FP	Fistulizing-perforating
FS	Fibrostenotic
HASTE	Half Fourier single shot turbo spin echo
GRE	Gradient echo
PEG	Polyethylene glycol
SSTSE	Single shot turbo spin echo
TR	Repetition time
TE	Echo time

References

Florie J, Wasser MN, Arts-Cieslik K, et al (2006) Dynamic contrast-enhanced MRI of the bowel wall for assessment of disease activity in Crohn's disease. AJR Am J Roentgenol 186:1384–1392

Gourtsoyiannis NC, Grammatikakis J, Papamastorakis G, et al (2006) Imaging of small intestinal Crohn's disease: comparison between MR enteroclysis and conventional enteroclysis. Eur Radiol 16:1915–1925

Gourtsoyiannis N, Papanikolaou N (2008) Magnetic resonance enteroclysis of the small bowel. In: Gore RM, Levine MS (eds) Textbook of gastrointestinal radiology. Saunders, Elsevier, Philadelphia, Amsterdam, pp 765–774

Gourtsoyiannis N, Papanikolaou N, Grammatikakis J, et al (2000) Magnetic resonance imaging of the small bowel using a True-FISP sequence after enteroclysis with water solution. Invest Radiol 35:707–711

Gourtsoyiannis N, Papanikolaou N, Grammatikakis J, et al (2001) MR enteroclysis protocol optimization: comparison between 3d FLASH with fat saturation after intravenous gadolinium injection and true-FISP sequences. Eur Radiol 11:908–913

Gourtsoyiannis N, Papanikolaou N, Grammatikakis J, et al (2004) Assessment of Crohn's disease activity in the small bowel with MR and conventional enteroclysis: preliminary results. Eur Radiol 14:1017–1024

Gourtsoyianni S, Papanikolaou N, Amanakis E, et al (2009) Crohn's disease lymphadenopathy: MR findings. Eur J Radiol 69:425–428

Koh DM, Miao Y, Chinn RJ, et al (2001) MR imaging evaluation of the activity in Crohn's disease. AJR Am J Roentgenol 177:1325–1332

Kohli M, Maglinte D (2009) CT enteroclysis in small bowel Crohn's disease. Eur J Radiol 69:398–403

Laghi A, Paolantonio P, Catalano C, et al (2003) MR imaging of the small bowel using polyethylene glycol solution as an oral contrast agent in adults and children with celiac disease: preliminary observations. AJR Am J Roentgenol 180: 191–194

Lauenstein TC, Schneemann H, Vogt FM, et al (2003) Optimization of oral contrast agents for MR imaging of the small bowel. Radiology 228:279–283

Lee JK, Marcos HB, Semelka RC (1998) MR imaging of the small bowel using the HASTE sequence. AJR Am J Roentgenol 170:1457–1463

Lienemann A, Sprenger D, Steitz HO, et al (2000) Detection and mapping of intraabdominal adhesions by using functional cine MR imaging: preliminary results. Radiology 217: 421–425

Lohan D, Cronin C, Meehan C, et al (2007) MR small bowel enterography: optimization of imaging timing. Clin Radiol 62:804–807

Lomas DJ, Graves MJ (1999) Small bowel MRI using water as a contrast medium. BJR 72:994–997

Maglinte D, Gourtsoyiannis N, Rex D, et al (2003) Classification of small bowel Crohn's subtypes based on multimodality imaging. Radiol Clin N Am 41:285–303

Makki M, Graves MJ, Lomas DJ (2002) Interactive body magnetic resonance fluoroscopy using modified single-shot half-Fourier rapid acquisition with relaxation enhancement (RARE) with multiparameter control. J Magn Reson Imaging 16(1):85–93

Masselli G, Polettini E, Casciani E, et al (2009) Small neoplasms: prospective evaluation of MR enteroclysis. Radiology 251:743–750

Papanikolaou N, Prassopoulos P, Grammatikakis I, et al (2002a) Technical challenges and clinical applications of MR enteroclysis. Top Magn Reson Imaging 13:397–408

Papanikolaou N, Prassopoulos P, Grammatikakis J, et al (2002b) Optimization of a contrast medium suitable for conventional enteroclysis, MR enteroclysis, and virtual MR enteroscopy. Abdom Imaging 27:517–522

Patak MA, Froehlich JM, von Weymarn C, et al (2001) Noninvasive distension of the small bowel for magnetic-resonance imaging. Lancet 22:987–988

Prassopoulos P, Papanikolaou N, Grammatikakis J, et al (2001) MR enteroclysis imaging of Crohn disease. Radiographics 21 Spec No:S161–S172

Sailer J, Reinisch W, Vogelsang H, et al (2008) Anastomotic recurrency of Crohn's disease after ileocolic resection: Comparison of MR enteroclysis with endoscopy. Eur Radiol 18:2512–2521

Schmid-Tannwald C, Zech CJ, Panteleon A, et al (2009) Characteristic imaging features of carcinoid tumors of the small bowel in MR enteroclysis. Radiology 49:242–251

Semelka RC, Chung JJ, Hussain SM, et al (2001) Chronic hepatitis: correlation of early patchy and late linear enhancement patterns on gadolinium-enhanced MR images with histopathology initial experience. J Magn Reson Imaging 13:385–391

Semelka RC, John G, Kelekis NL, Burdeny DA, Ascher SM (1996) Small bowel neoplastic disease: demonstration by MRI. J Magn Reson Imaging 6:855–860

Umschaden HW, Szolar D, Gasser J, et al (2000) Small-bowel disease: comparison of MR enteroclysis images with conventional enteroclysis and surgical findings. Radiology 215:717–725

MRI of the Small Bowel: Clinical Role

Damian J.M. Tolan, Stuart A. Taylor, and Steve Halligan

CONTENTS

10.1 Introduction 149
10.2 Small Bowel Imaging: What is the Question? 150
10.3 Choice of Small Bowel Imaging Technique: General Considerations 150
10.3.1 The Radiation Issue 150
10.3.2 Invasive Investigations: Bowel Preparation and Tubes 150
10.3.3 Acute vs. Elective Evaluation 151
10.3.4 Capacity and Hardware 152
10.3.5 Disease Stage 152
10.3.6 Extra Enteric Assessment 152
10.4 Small Bowel Assessment: Head to-Head Comparison-General Considerations 152
10.4.1 MR Enterography or Enteroclysis? 152
10.4.2 Radiology or Endoscopy? 155
10.5 Indications for Small Bowel Imaging 155
10.5.1 Inflammatory Bowel Disease: Crohn's disease 155
10.5.2 Autoimmune Disease: Celiac Disease and Scleroderma/Progressive Systemic Sclerosis 159
10.5.3 Polyposis Syndromes: Familial Adenomatous Polyposis and Peutz-Jeghers Syndrome 160
10.5.4 Malignancy 162
10.5.5 Evaluation of Occult GI Bleeding 163
10.5.6 Other Small Bowel Diseases 165
10.5.6.1 Adhesions 165
10.5.6.2 Radiation Enteritis 165
10.5.6.3 Endometriosis 167
10.6 Conclusion 167
References 168

Damian J. M. Tolan, MD, MBChB, FRCR
Leeds Teaching Hospitals NHS Trust, Jubilee Wing
Leeds General Infirmary, LS1 3EX, Leeds, UK
Stuart A. Taylor, MD, MRCP, FRCR
Steve Halligan, MD, MRCP, FRCR
University College London, 2F Podium, 235 Euston Road, London
NW1 2BU, UK

KEY POINTS

In this chapter, the potential applications for MR examination of the small bowel are assessed along with the strengths and weaknesses of MR enterography vs. enteroclysis and the place of endoscopic evaluation in investigation of small bowel disorders. General considerations when choosing a radiological modality should include radiation dose, the invasiveness of the procedure to the individual, acute vs. elective evaluation of cases, capacity and hardware availability, and requirement for extraenteric assessment. The commonest and most important small bowel diseases are then evaluated, including an appraisal of the roles of different radiological and endoscopic imaging modalities: this includes Crohn's disease, Celiac disease and scleroderma, polyposis syndromes, small bowel malignancy, investigation of unexplained iron deficiency anemia, adhesions, radiation enteropathy, and endometriosis.

10.1
Introduction

Over the last decade, there has been increasing interest in utilizing MRI to investigate small bowel disease. The techniques of enteric MRI, together with clinical results, have been covered elsewhere in this volume (Chaps. 8 and 9). In this chapter, we address the place of MR in the diagnostic armamentarium for small bowel disease with reference to other imaging modalities, elucidating its role and considering its advantages and disadvantages according to clinical indication.

10.2
Small Bowel Imaging: What is the Question?

Diseases of the small bowel include inflammatory diseases, particularly Crohn's disease, Celiac disease and other autoimmune conditions, polyposis syndromes such as Peutz–Jeghers syndrome, primary malignancies including lymphoma and adenocarcinoma, congenital and postoperative adhesions, and infectious diseases. The full range of radiological investigations may be utilized in these conditions, together with endoscopic techniques, notably wireless capsule endoscopy (WCE) and double balloon enteroscopy (DBE).

However, while many of the available tests may be useful, each has its associated strengths and limitations, and it should be remembered that accurate clinical information, including a provisional diagnosis where relevant, is essential when deciding the most appropriate radiological investigation. This can only be achieved via close cooperation with colleagues in gastroenterology and abdominal surgery, together with full consideration of upper and lower gastrointestinal endoscopy findings and histopathology when available. For example, knowledge of postoperative anatomy following prior surgery can be critical when interpreting difficult cases. The formulation of a clear question by the referring clinician is therefore the most important step to allow the radiologist to choose the most appropriate technique to provide the answer to a particular situation. Referring clinicians must also be aware that as the clinical status of an individual patient with a particular condition changes, the appropriateness of an imaging modality may also change, for example where acute complications such as obstruction, acute hemorrhage or hollow viscous perforation are suspected.

The small bowel presents many clinical and radiological diagnostic challenges. Investigations must be both accurate and acceptable to our patients. The following sections examine the main issues to consider when contemplating the use of small bowel MR techniques over other available imaging modalities, with reference to current evidence. It also explores those clinical applications where MR may be more appropriate. The interface between endoscopic imaging and radiology is also examined.

10.3
Choice of Small Bowel Imaging Technique: General Considerations

10.3.1
The Radiation Issue

It is now clear that access to multidetector computed tomography (MDCT) has led to an increase in population radiation exposure (BRENNER and HALL 2007). The benefits of MDCT are well known, including rapid image acquisition, isovoxel reconstruction, and potential for multiphase contrast enhanced acquisition. However, patients with small bowel pathology, particularly those with Crohn's disease, frequently undergo multiple studies over the course of their disease, especially during acute episodes or when complications arise (DESMOND et al. 2008). This can result in significant radiation accumulation; estimated in one study at over 80 mSv in the 9% of patients undergoing five or more CT examinations, rising to over 160 mSv after ten or more CT scans, a dose that has been estimated to impart a lifetime risk of fatal malignancy of 1.6 in 200 (JAFFE et al. 2007; PELOQUIN et al. 2008). Nuclear medicine studies and barium examinations carry a lower but not insignificant radiation burden. Many individuals with small bowel disease are young, so where possible radiation-free imaging is preferable (Fig. 10.1). For this reason, small bowel MRI and ultrasound examinations are advantageous, where clinically appropriate.

10.3.2
Invasive Investigations: Bowel Preparation and Tubes

While a period of fasting is usually required for all small bowel studies, cathartic bowel preparation is unpopular with patients (JENSCH et al. 2008), but may be an important aspect of barium examinations of the small bowel, WCE, and DBE. Purgation is not always necessary prior to CT, nuclear medicine, or MRI studies, depending on the indication and clinician preference, but the bowel distension agent may be a laxative, for example polyethylene glycol (PEG), or have a significant laxative side-effect (e.g., mannitol) (LAUENSTEIN et al. 2003).

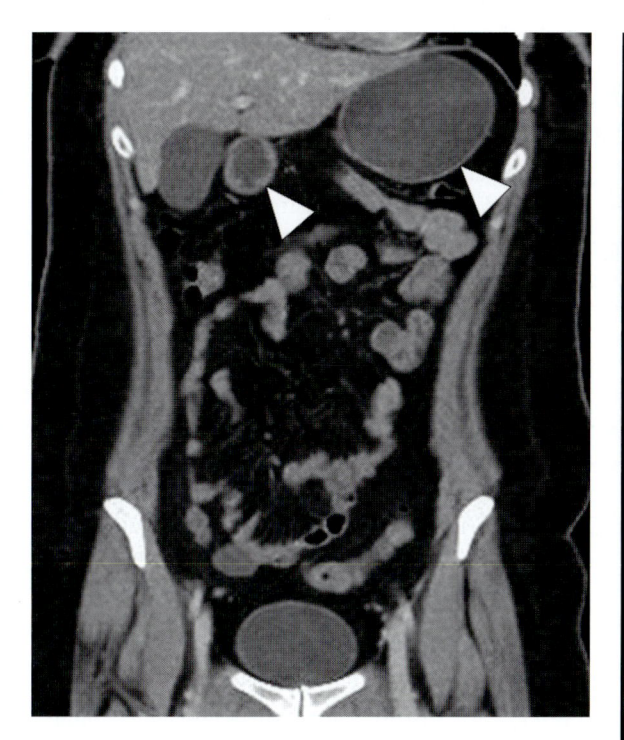

Fig. 10.1. CT enterography for suspected Crohn's disease in a young patient intolerant of nasojejunal tube and MRI. Scan 1h after oral contrast demonstrates gastric stasis (*arrowheads*) and poor small bowel distension

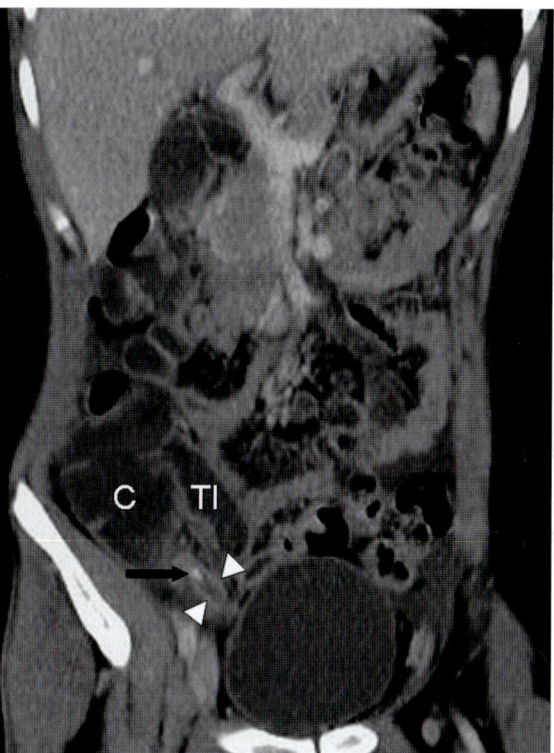

Fig. 10.2. Coronal CT performed acutely in patient with Crohn's disease and bowel obstruction, with suspected acute flare. The appendix lies adjacent to distended cecum (*C*) and terminal ileum (*TI*) and is dilated (*arrowheads*). It contains an appendicolith (*arrow*) – diagnosis appendicitis

In our experience, nasojejunal intubation without sedation for enteroclysis is tolerated but unpopular with both patients and most radiologists, and it also deters some patients from attending for repeat studies. While in expert hands fluoroscopic screening times can be low (Traill and Nolan 1995), tube placement by less experienced operators or in more difficult cases may result in higher screening times, imparting a significant radiation dose and negating the benefit of using MRI to avoid radiation. In a small proportion of patients, jejunal intubation is impossible due to distorted anatomy or patient intolerance. While sedoanesthesia makes the procedure more comfortable for patients, it requires additional monitoring and staff to prevent complications and has implications for the patient following the procedure (e.g., the ability to drive or to go home unaccompanied). In one study comparing two types of sedoanesthesia for CT enteroclysis, while most patients would undergo the procedure again if required, very high mean doses of opiate and benzodiazepines were administered (3.9 mg midazolam and 108 μg fentanyl) and a significant number of patients (25–31%) had oxygen desaturation, indicating potentially dangerous oversedation (Maglinte et al. 2008). MR enteroclysis examinations also result in significantly more discomfort and abdominal pain following the procedure than enterography (Negaard et al. 2008).

10.3.3
Acute vs. Elective Evaluation

Many radiology departments offer 24h access for acute abdominal CT. MDCT is very effective for detection of perforation and abscess, and exclusion of clinically unsuspected pathology outside the bowel (Fig. 10.2) as well as for evaluation of the acute abdomen, particularly when evaluating the site and cause of small bowel obstruction and acute presentations of Crohn's disease (Fig. 10.3) (Vogel et al. 2007).

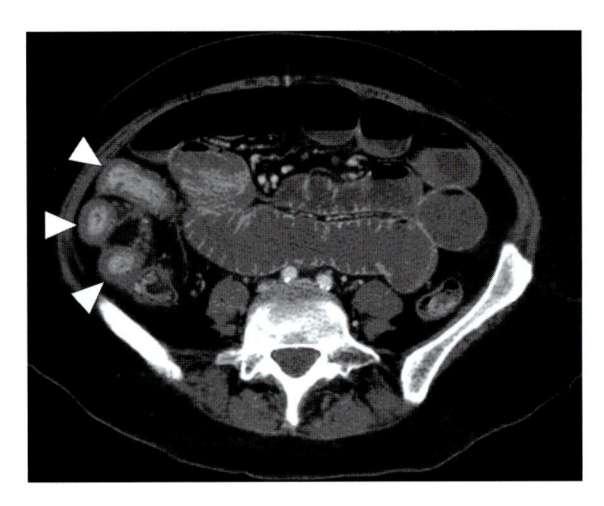

Fig. 10.3. Axial CT in acute flare of Crohn's with small bowel obstruction. Note mural hyperenhancement of diseased distal ileum (*arrowheads*)

While similar out of hours access may be available for ultrasound, the same is not always true for other modalities, particularly MRI. In this setting, considerations of radiation exposure must be tempered by the need for rapid diagnosis. Indeed, MDCT may be more appropriate where hollow viscus perforation is suspected, for example. In acutely unwell patients, a CT scan is quicker and needs fewer breath-holds than MRI, improving patient compliance in what is often a difficult clinical situation. In severely ill patients, the length of examination and limited access for clinical assessment during the scan may render MRI completely inappropriate.

Even in an elective outpatient setting, limited access may restrict the availability to MRI.

10.3.4
Capacity and Hardware

As alluded to above, hardware constraints are a significant factor for many wishing to offer small bowel MRI. The technical requirements for enteric MRI are covered elsewhere in this volume, suffice to say that access to high-quality body surface coils and adequate field strength scanners (1.5 T or higher) are essential. However, negotiating scanning time for these cases is equally important, and developing a new service is a challenge, when balancing ever-increasing MRI service demands for other clinical indications.

10.3.5
Disease Stage

As Crohn's disease is the commonest indication, an ability to detect early disease is important, particularly as interest grows within the gastroenterology community for earlier treatment with potent immunomodulator therapy with the hope of modifying the course of disease. Aphthous ulcers, the earliest manifestation of Crohn's disease, are best demonstrated radiologically with traditional barium studies, and it may be argued that this may protect a role for barium studies in the evaluation of patients with no prior diagnosis of Crohn's disease. However, such early findings are difficult to detect (Liangpunsakul et al. 2003) even in skilled hands and, in the authors' experience, radiologists in training are currently exposed to insufficient cases to achieve competence in interpretation. Furthermore, the majority of newly presenting patients have more advanced findings at diagnosis (such as wall thickening or even fistulation). In reality, the difficulty of diagnosing very early disease using cross-sectional techniques may not have a significant impact in day-to-day clinical practice since the pertinent questions relate more to disease severity, activity, and extent. Indeed, in the authors' practice, barium studies have assumed a secondary role for problem-solving equivocal MRI examinations.

10.3.6
Extra Enteric Assessment

A clear benefit of cross-sectional imaging over barium examinations and ultrasound is the ability to accurately evaluate overlapping or gas-filled bowel loops deep in the pelvis or elsewhere. However, of equal importance, extra enteric abdominal abnormalities may be detected, such as fistulation or abscess (Fig. 10.4), colonic or appendiceal pathology (Fig. 10.5), or staging of metastatic malignancy and these are particular strengths of both MDCT and MRI.

10.4
Small Bowel Assessment: Head-to-Head Comparison – General Considerations

10.4.1
MR Enterography or Enteroclysis?

This section could equally be entitled "zealot or pragmatist?" The techniques of enterography and

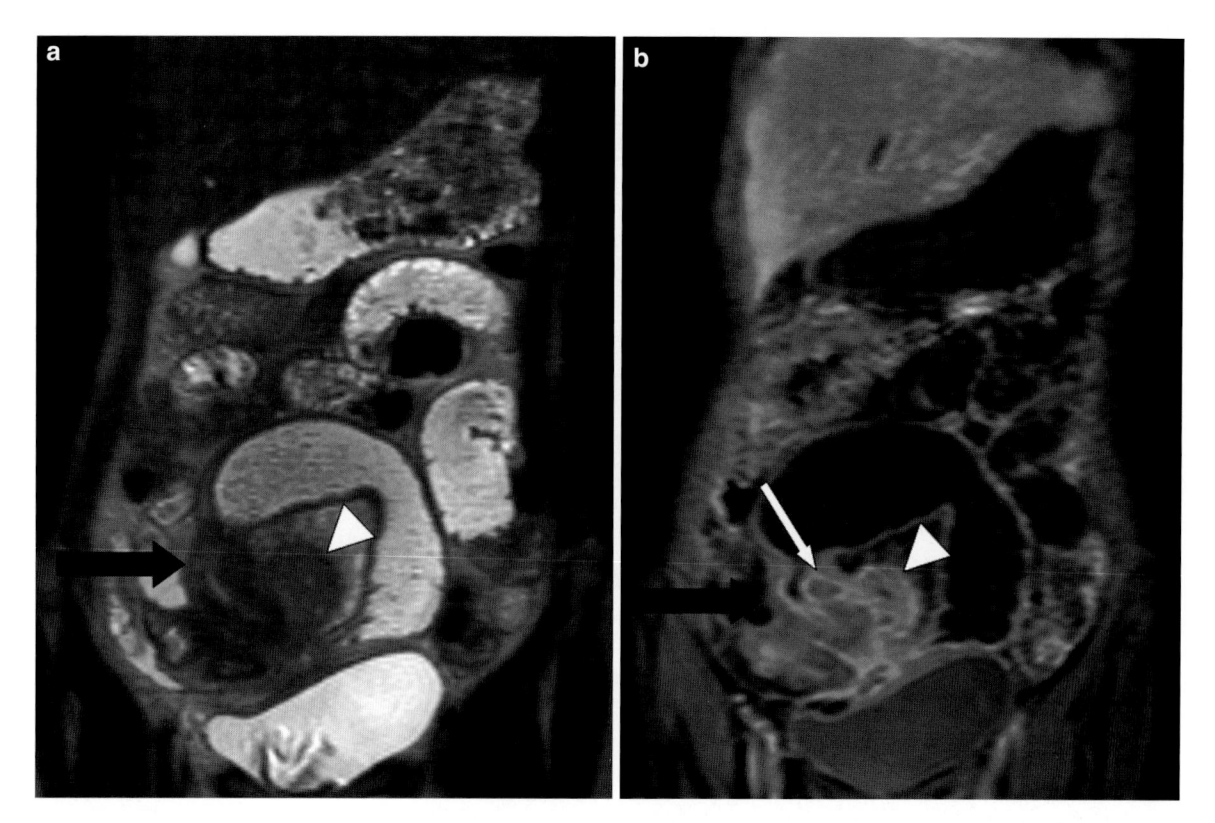

Fig. 10.4. MR enterography with (**a**) coronal HASTE and (**b**) coronal postgadolinium VIBE sequences demonstrate obstruction of a Crohn's terminal ileal segment (*black arrow*) mural hyperenhancement from acute on chronic fibrostenotic disease with a small intramural abscess (*white arrow*) and an inflammatory phlegmon in the mesentery (*arrowhead*)

enteroclysis are comprehensively covered in Chaps. 8 and 9. An ideal technique would maximize bowel distension to facilitate detection of small bowel pathology, while optimizing patient tolerance and minimizing cost and resource use. Unfortunately, there is very little comparative data in the literature to guide radiologists as to the optimum technique according to the differing indications. In reality, as will be discussed, the choice of one technique over another is largely governed by personal opinion and preference, and available expertise and infrastructure.

Neither MR enteroclysis nor enterography have a clear advantage over each other for all indications. While enteroclysis is inherently invasive, usually unpopular with patients (Negaard et al. 2008) and incurs additional financial cost and radiation exposure, distension is undoubtedly superior, particularly in the jejunum (Masselli et al. 2008; Negaard et al. 2007). Bowel distension is a prerequisite for successful small bowel MRI examination. This superiority may make enteroclysis more suitable for patients with celiac disease or intestinal polyposis, for example, where jejunal disease is more common. Enterography conversely may be more suited to patients with disease affecting the distal small bowel as the advantages conveyed by enteroclysis are less obvious (Masselli et al. 2008), notably ileal Crohn's disease. There is, therefore, a reasonable argument that the superior quality of MR enteroclysis justifies its invasiveness in the first diagnosis of polyposis syndromes, with enterography more suited to follow-up of patients with established disease. Enterography is, however, highly advantageous in a paediatric population (Laghi et al. 2003) and in other patients where nasojejunal intubation is unsuitable or not tolerated. It is also less time-consuming for radiologists and there is no doubt that the vast majority of radiologists are unprepared to perform intubation when faced with the easier alternative of enterography; the historical overwhelming preponderance of barium follow-through over barium enteroclysis is proof of this. Inclusion of dynamic gradient echo acquisitions may in part compensate for suboptimal distension, improving sensitivity for jejunal pathology by demonstrating normal peristalizing collapsed loops (Torkzad et al. 2007), compared to aperistaltic diseased segments (Kitazume et al. 2007).

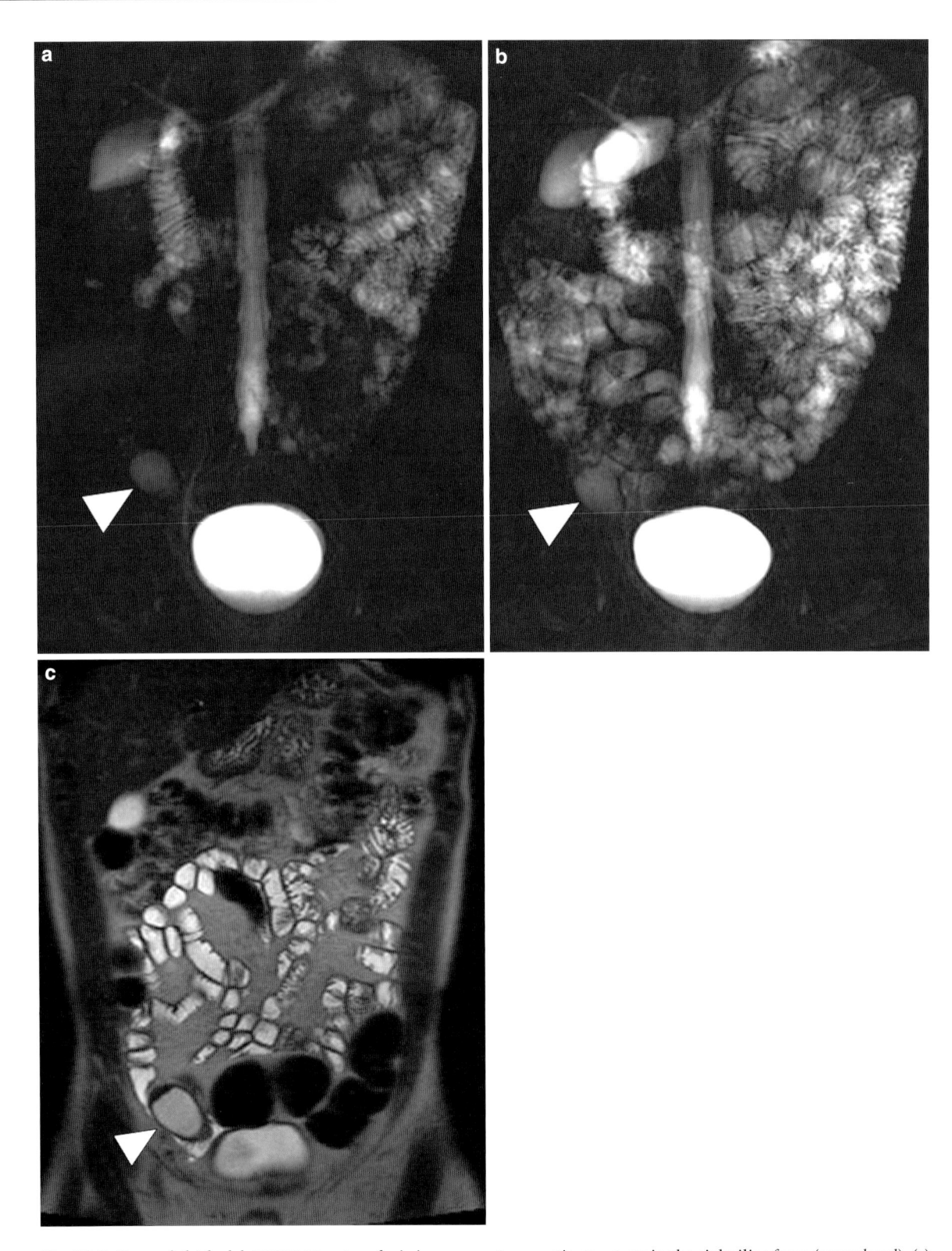

Fig. 10.5. Coronal thick slab T2W MR enteroclysis images, (**a**) early and (**b**) late after infusion of methylcellulose, show a 4 cm cystic structure in the right iliac fossa (*arrowhead*). (**c**) Coronal HASTE sequence confirms an appendix mucocele

Until the literature demonstrates significant and clear advantages of one examination over the other, a pragmatic and tailored approach to technique may be required according to indication, personal experience and patient preference. With respect to demonstrating an advantage, it is worth noting that very few randomized studies of barium studies have been performed, and those that were found follow-through superior (BERNSTEIN et al. 1997). In reality, the vast majority of the literature constitutes personal case-series from highly competent gastrointestinal radiologists, with the result that the reported test characteristics can be accused of clear spectrum bias.

10.4.2
Radiology or Endoscopy?

Endoscopic evaluations of the small bowel (WCE and DBE) are largely complementary to radiological investigations, as each has different strengths and weaknesses. An obvious advantage of endoscopic techniques is direct visualization of the enteric mucosa and the ability to detect subtle lesions beyond the resolution of radiological investigations, including telangectasias, mucosal hyperaemia (the earliest visible sign of Crohn's disease), and aphthous ulcers (FUKUMOTO et al. 2009b). With the advent of DBE, pan-endoscopy of the small bowel is potentially achievable in a high proportion of individuals (over 70%), albeit requiring considerable expertise and both per oral and per anal intubation for a complete examination (ARAKI et al. 2009). Other endoscopic possibilities include biopsy, polypectomy, ablation of vascular malformations, and tattooing to aid identification of pathology for laparoscopic resection. However, examinations are often long, due to the complexity of navigating the small bowel with the endoscope and overshoot, and require considerable patient sedation or anesthesia. As with any new interventional (or radiological) technique, there is a significant learning curve for new practitioners (GROSS and STARK 2008), and the range of interventional tools is more limited than colonoscopy, where extensive endoscopic mucosal resection of early tumors is possible. Access to DBE is also currently limited in many hospitals, services often being concentrated in major referral centres. The same is true regarding WCE, with expensive equipment and consumables, and limited expertise (POSTGATE et al. 2009). WCE is a less invasive examination, but reading time for studies is long (often over 1 h), a significant drawback (WESTERHOF et al. 2009a). Computer-aided detection technology may reduce reading times and improve accuracy in the future, but remains within the research domain at present (LI and MENG 2009).

DBE requires sedoanaesthesia and WCE carries a risk of retention/obstruction in stricturing small bowel disease (see below), and both usually require bowel purgation. Although WCE offers high-resolution images, there are limitations: localization signals within the abdomen from the capsule are not easily anatomically co-located to a specific bowel segment, so radiologic imaging may be required to determine the precise site of disease (HARA et al. 2005). Proximal lesions, such as those in the duodenum, may be missed due to rapid transit through the segment (CLARKE et al. 2008; POSTGATE et al. 2008), and as battery life is limited, prolonged gut transit may result in the capsule shutting down before the colon is reached (WESTERHOF et al. 2009b). Of course, unlike cross-sectional radiological techniques such as MRI, both WCE and DBE fail to provide any information beyond the bowel lumen and as such are insensitive to mural disease deep to the bowel mucosa, and extraenteric complications. In practical terms, less invasive WCE and radiological techniques can offer targets for DBE to biopsy or to ablate focal lesions.

Extraluminal complications are best assessed by cross-sectional imaging, and although visualization of mucosal disease is superior with endoscopy, inaccessible lesions and poorly visualized bowel segments are not uncommon (FUKUMOTO et al. 2009a). Overall, multimodality assessment is the rule rather than the exception, particularly for difficult cases: radiology and endoscopy are frequently interdependent in such cases (MAGLINTE et al. 2007).

10.5
Indications for Small Bowel Imaging

We will now assess the role of MRI with reference to the main indications for small bowel imaging.

10.5.1
Inflammatory Bowel Disease: Crohn's disease

Direct comparisons between the various imaging modalities in Crohn's disease are conspicuously lacking within the current literature, especially randomized studies. Most studies are small and compare one or two imaging techniques at a single center, usually very experienced in one of the techniques under examination.

One of the greatest drawbacks of any study of inflammatory bowel disease is the lack of a reliable reference standard, as there is discrepancy between clinical disease activity scores, radiological, endoscopic, and biopsy activity even in the same individual at the same timepoint. A recent meta-analysis compared the accuracy of MRI in the assessment of Crohn's disease with other radiological modalities (Horsthuis et al. 2008). Bearing these biases in mind and allowing for the marked variability in standard of reference for the primary component studies, a meta-analysis performed by Horsthuis and colleagues assessed 33 studies with prospective recruitment and over 15 subjects, utilizing CT, MRI, ultrasound, or scintigraphy. While per-patient analysis yielded uniformly high sensitivity across modalities (around 90%) with similar specificity, per-segment sensitivity revealed lower results ranging from 77% for scintigraphy to 67% for CT, while maintaining high specificity (over 90%). CT was least sensitive and specific when compared with MRI and scintigraphy (Horsthuis et al. 2008), an important observation given the high radiation burden of CT. There was no attempt to assess the relative performance of barium studies. As we are aiming to use nonionizing examinations wherever possible, these data suggest MRI and ultrasound are attractive methods of assessing nonacute patients (Figs. 10.6 and 10.7). With no compelling evidence supporting the superiority of either ultrasound or MRI over the other, implementation is currently dependent on local facilities and available expertise. The dependence of ultrasound on the expertise of the practitioner is well described (Sheridan et al. 1993), together with the known difficulties when evaluating deep pelvic loops and the more proximal small bowel.

The superior distension afforded by enteroclysis compared with enterography results in the former probably having a greater accuracy in depicting diseased segments (Masselli et al. 2008). However as noted above, the disadvantages of enteroclysis are significant enough to render it impractical to offer enteroclysis as the sole small bowel MRI technique within most institutions. Enterography is intuitively a more acceptable modality both for patients and radiologists and clearly more generalizable. Pragmatically, enteroclysis could be reserved for first disease staging/diagnosis, particularly in patients with suspicion of jejunal disease or patients who cannot manage to drink oral contrast due to nausea. Such an approach is advocated by leading proponents of the enteroclysis technique. Others, including the authors, use MR enterography as the first technique for all small bowel

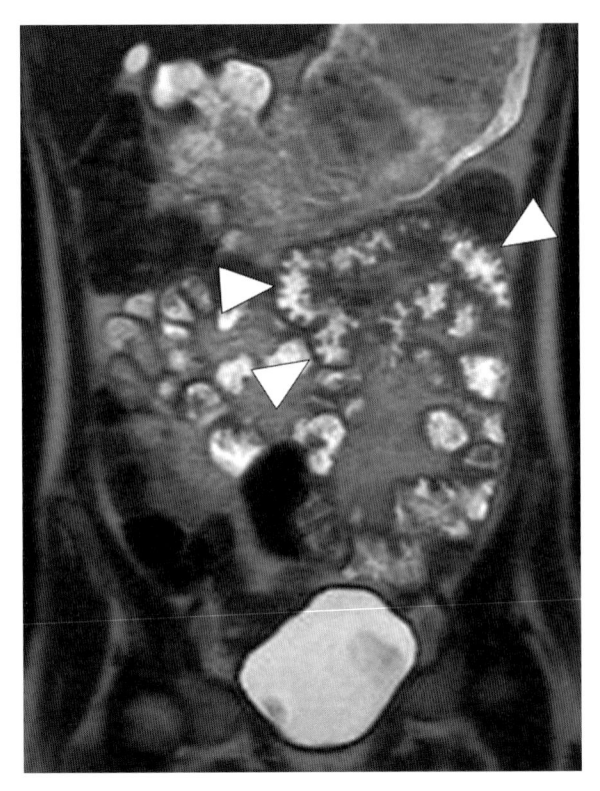

Fig. 10.6. Clinical suspicion of Crohn's in a patient with normal small bowel meal, upper and lower GI endoscopy. Coronal HASTE from MR enterography in a well-distended jejunum shows nodular thickening of folds (*arrowheads*) (and enlarged enhancing mesenteric nodes – not shown). Enteroscopy confirmed diffuse Crohn's disease

MRI referrals in Crohn's disease, for the reasons described in Sect. 11.1.4. One additional significant benefit of MRI over other examinations is the ability to accurately define fistulizing perianal disease as an addition to the small bowel examination.

The ability of cross-sectional techniques to assess Crohn's disease activity is also worthy of consideration. In a further meta-analysis, Horsthuis et al. analysed the ability of MRI to determine disease activity. Pooling 140 patients from seven studies, MRI correctly graded disease activity in 91% of cases with frank disease, but only 62% or patients in remission or with mild disease and, when incorrect, tended to over-stage disease in 38% of patients in remission and 21% with mild disease (Horsthuis et al. 2009a). Actively inflamed bowel segments exhibit higher mural T2 signal and may have higher gadolinium concentrations after contrast administration (Horsthuis et al. 2009b), both of which can be subjectively assessed during interpretation of disease activity. Generally, hyperenhancement, particularly when layered/stratified, indicates active

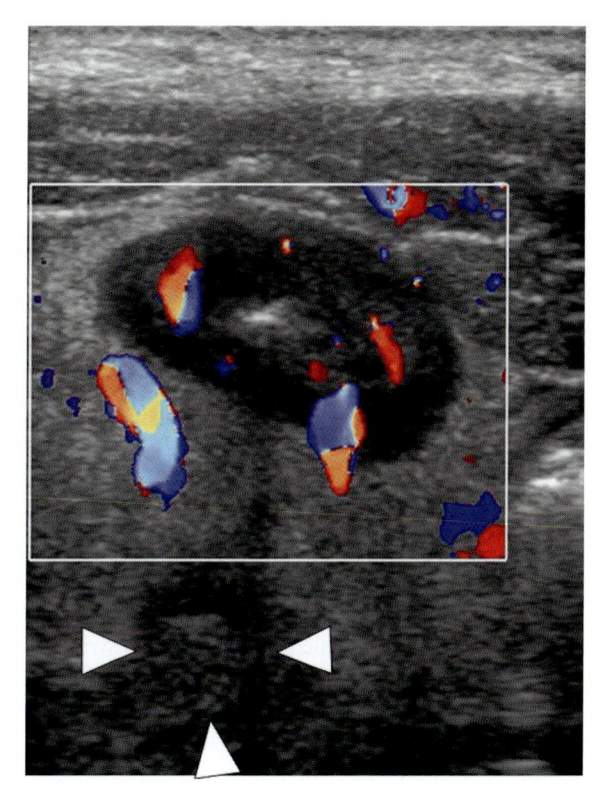

Fig. 10.7. Axial high-frequency ultrasound, in a male with acute right iliac fossa pain. The terminal ileum is thickened, with increased Doppler color flow. Echogenic fibrofatty mesentery and small abscess (*arrowheads*) from short segment Crohn's disease

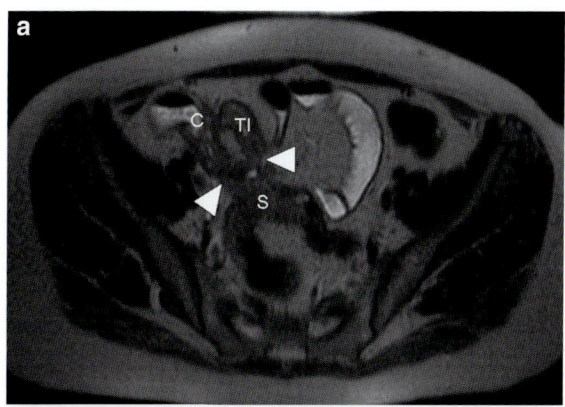

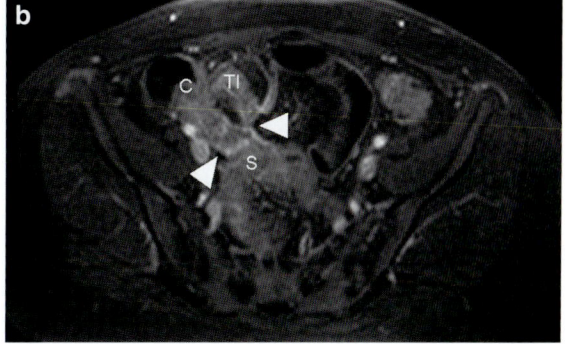

Fig. 10.8. New presentation with obstructing Crohn's sigmoid stricture at colonoscopy. MR enterography (**a**) axial HASTE and (**b**) postcontrast VIBE shows complex cecosigmoidileal fistula (*arrowheads*) with hyperenhancement from active disease

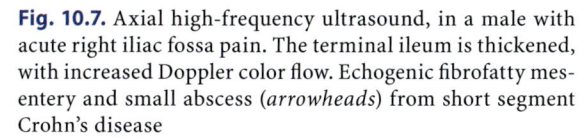

disease on MR or CT evaluations (Fig. 10.8) (Sempere et al. 2005). Low-level heterogeneous enhancement often indicates inactive or fibrostenotic disease (Fig. 10.9). It should be noted that layered enhancement may persist when inflammation has resolved (Sempere et al. 2009). Ultrasound allows demonstration of increased vascularity by increased power or color Doppler signal (Fig. 10.6) (Fraquelli et al. 2008), and isotope studies can also depict increased focal uptake.

Rimola and colleagues have proposed that MR enterography is sufficiently accurate for it to be a viable alternative to endoscopy in patients with established Crohn's disease (Rimola et al. 2009).

While there is reasonable evidence supporting MR small bowel techniques for the assessment of established Crohn's disease, the role in the first diagnosis of those with suspected disease is less clear-cut. Small comparative studies between MRI and fluoroscopic enteroclysis suggest that the latter has greater sensitivity for early mucosal disease (Gourtsoyiannis et al. 2004). This raises the possibility that MR may miss the diagnosis of Crohn's disease in those presenting with subtle mucosal disease only. However, there is also growing evidence of the failings of small bowel barium examinations (Maglinte 2005). This is perhaps multifactorial and an intrinsic limitation of the technique, resulting from overlapping pelvic loops hiding disease, inadequate distension of jejunal loops, and subtle early disease also being missed. A recent study comparing sequential barium follow through with CT and MR enterography and ileocolonoscopy showed similar accuracy in the detection of Crohn's disease, but cross-sectional imaging demonstrated more extraenteric complications (Lee et al. 2009). While this latter finding is perhaps intuitive, it is a clear weakness of barium examinations and may relegate them in the future to a problem-solving modality, assuming the competence to interpret them exists. The study also confirmed that, in the main, patients with symptoms suggestive of Crohn's disease usually have demonstrable disease on cross-sectional imaging techniques.

Nuclear medicine examinations can play a role for assessment of disease activity in Crohn's disease, with

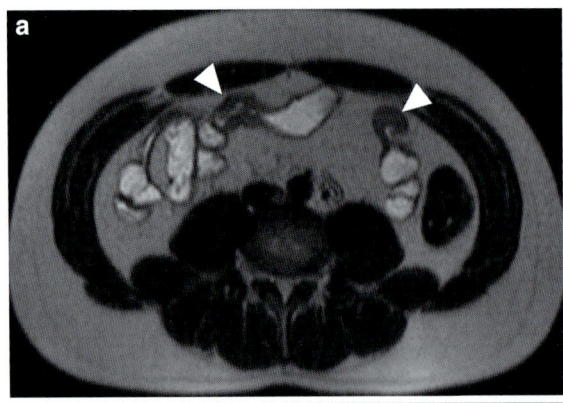

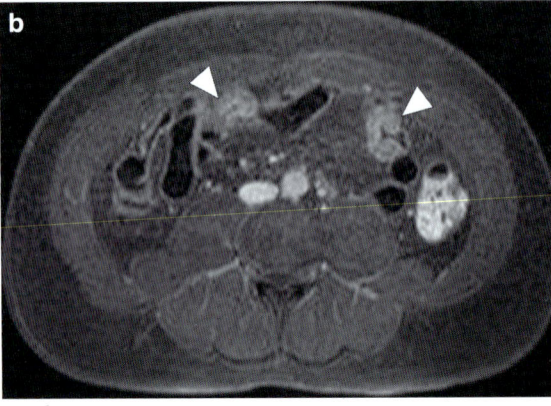

Fig. 10.9. Known Crohn's disease with new symptoms. MR enterography demonstrates two short strictures (*arrowheads*) on (**a**) axial HASTE and (**b**) postcontrast VIBE but no enhancement – fibrostenotic disease

either Technitium-99m-HMPAO (Giaffer et al. 1996) or Indium-111 (Nelson et al. 1990) or Technitium-99m-DMSA used to detect inflamed bowel segments (Koutroubakis et al. 2003). While the diagnostic accuracy for inflammatory bowel disease is similar to other modalities, the techniques are limited by an inability to reliably detect complications such as abscess, obstruction or fistula. Hybrid single photon emission computerized tomography with CT fusion (SPECT/CT) may overcome this limitation and improves discrimination of bowel from bone marrow uptake in the pelvis (Biancone et al. 2005) and detection of complications (Filippi et al. 2006). While some authors have investigated more complex fusion techniques to improve diagnostic accuracy of nuclear medicine studies, such as CT PET enteroclysis (Das et al. 2007), the long examination time, radiation requirement, and invasive nature probably preclude practical application of this technique. For this reason, and the consequent radiation burden, the role of isotope studies is likely to be extremely limited.

WCE has also been proposed as a first-line investigation for suspected Crohn's disease. Meta-analysis data suggests that WCE has superior sensitivity for the diagnosis of Crohn's disease over both radiological and conventional endoscopic techniques (Triester et al. 2006). Furthermore, preliminary health economic data suggest that WCE may be a cost-effective first-line test in the work-up of those with suspected Crohn's disease (Goldfarb et al. 2004). However, the required infrastructure and expertise needed to perform high volumes of WCE are currently lacking in most healthcare systems, limiting widespread adoption for this indication. WCE is therefore often reserved for cases when high clinical suspicion remains but conventional endoscopy and imaging have been negative or inconclusive. In patients without obstructive symptoms, capsule retention rates are low. While the use of WCE as a first-line test for the diagnosis of Crohn's disease may increase, capsule retention due to stricture formation is a problem (Cave et al. 2005), with the greatest risk around 8% in those with a prior history of surgery (Westerhof et al. 2009b). In these cases, it may be sensible to perform enteroclysis to exclude stricture before proceeding with a capsule study (Fig. 10.10), as normal barium follow through does not adequately exclude stricture, although MR enterography may be an effective alternative to exclude significant Crohn's strictures prior to WCE. An even simpler approach is to use a patency capsule.

Ileocolonoscopy allows high ileal intubation rates (~95%) in expert hands (Terheggen et al. 2008), but examination of the ileum is necessarily limited to the terminal ileum. Conventional colonoscopy is thus usually supplemented by a small bowel imaging test, either because it has not been possible to intubate the ileum or because the proximal extent of terminal ileal disease cannot be seen. Small bowel imaging is also necessary where the terminal ileum is normal on ileoscopy but where there is a clinical possibility of proximal disease, e.g., in the jejunum in younger patients. DBE offers examination of the more proximal ileum but is more invasive, and is likely to be reserved for cases where differentiation of inflammatory from malignant strictures is necessary, based on inconclusive radiological imaging characterization.

A flowchart is provided for a suggested patient pathway to investigate known or suspected Crohn's disease (Fig. 10.11).

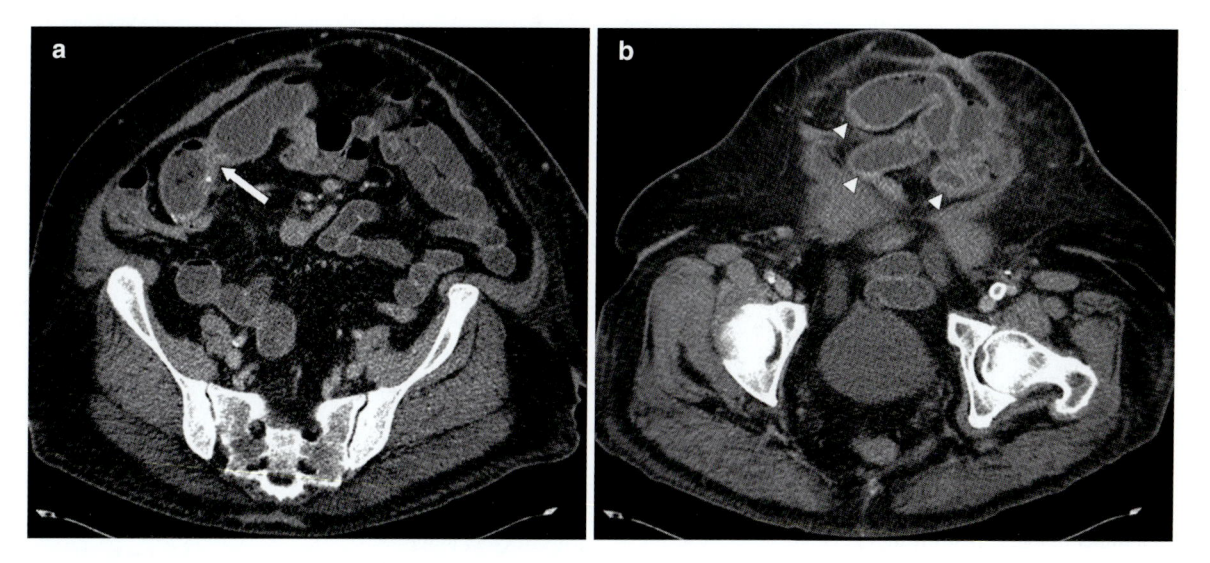

Fig. 10.10. Limited ileal resection for Crohn's disease 30 years prior, with new refractory anaemia. (a) CT enteroclysis (requested prior to WCE) demonstrates tight stricture at anastomosis (arrow), increasing risk of capsule retention/obstruction, and (b) long segment thickening and enhancement (arrowheads) from recurrent Crohn's disease

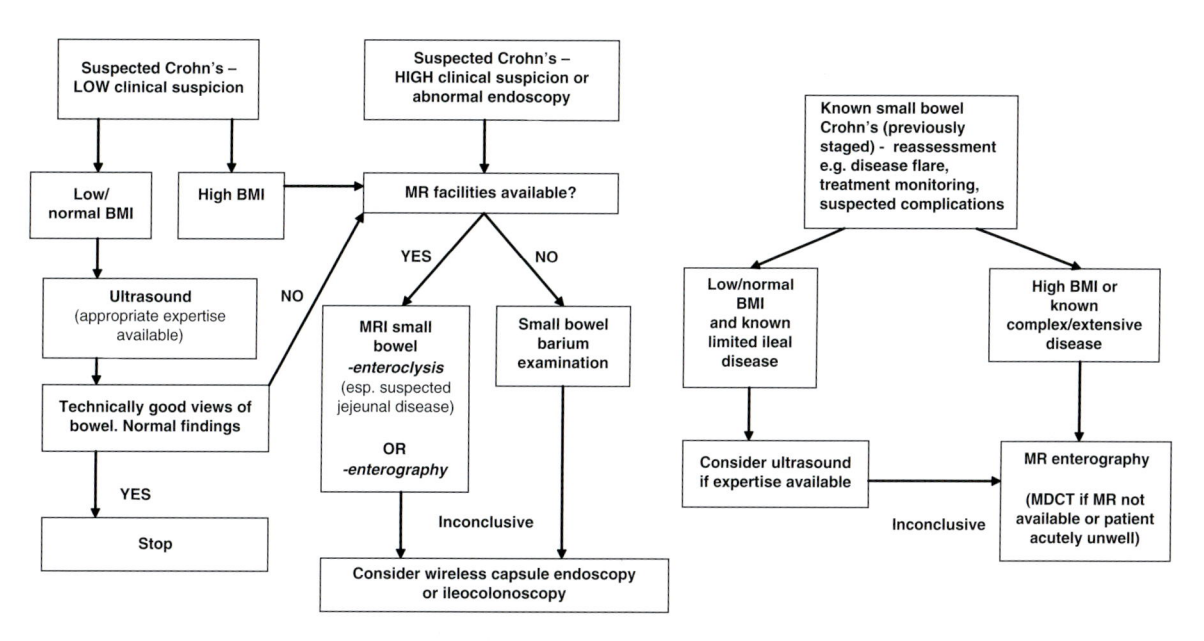

Fig. 10.11. Suggested flowchart for investigation of small bowel Crohn's disease

10.5.2
Autoimmune Disease: Celiac Disease and Scleroderma/Progressive Systemic Sclerosis

Celiac disease is caused by gluten insensitivity, and produces a range of abnormalities in the GI tract, centred on the proximal small bowel. The mainstay of diagnosis relies upon positive serology for endomysial antibody or elevated tissue transglutaminase, with duodenal biopsy confirmation (Di and Corazza 2009; Jones and Sleet 2009). As for Crohn's disease, endoscopic and WCE examinations have the ability to depict more subtle disease (sensitivity 87.5%, specificity 90.9%) (Rondonotti et al. 2007). The role of radiology is thus to detect complications, particularly in those patients who become refractory to dietary control or where there is specific concern for underlying malignancy, notably gastrointestinal lymphoma,

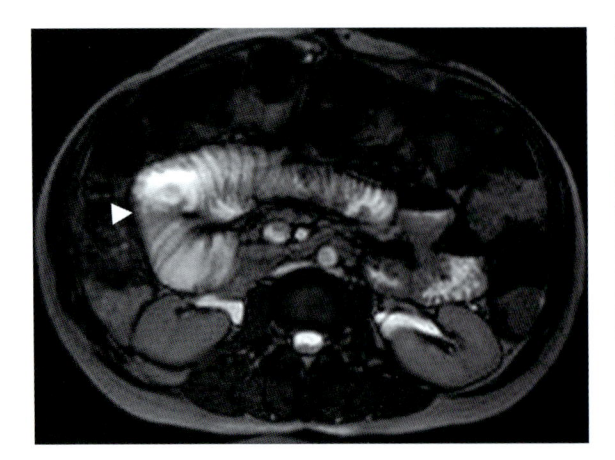

Fig. 10.12. MR enterography in refractory Celiac disease. Axial FISP shows dilated proximal jejunum and reduction in number of folds (*arrowhead*)

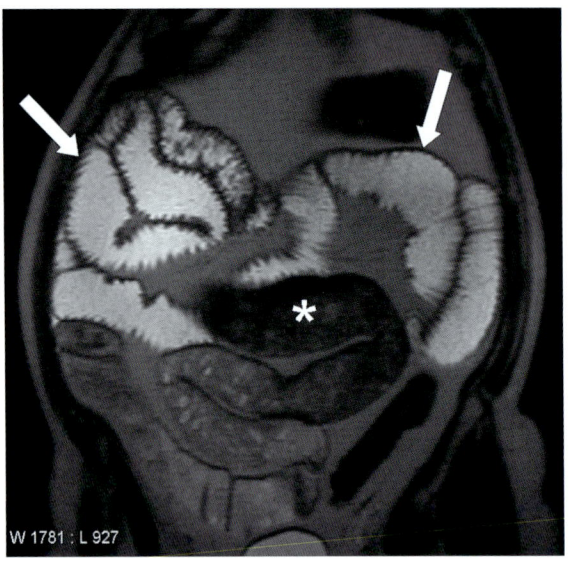

Fig. 10.13. Diffuse dilatation of small bowel in Scleroderma (*arrowheads*) shown at coronal HASTE. There is no wall thickening and folds are preserved. Note stasis of bowel content (*asterisk*) due to reduced peristalsis

or adeno/squamous cell carcinomas. The imaging findings associated with celiac disease are well described and include focal dilatation, jejunalization of the ileum, flattening of jejunal folds, intussusception, lymphadenopathy, hyposplenism, and focal wall thickening (Fig. 10.12) (Paolantonio et al. 2007). Given that diagnosis or exclusion of malignancy is the key role for radiology, rather than diagnosis, an ability to detect other extraenteric complications (such as cavitating lymph node syndrome) is an advantage (Boudiaf et al. 2004) – barium studies are once again displaced by newer technologies.

While there are no large studies of radiology for investigation of possible malignancy in Celiac disease, Masselli et al. have shown MR enteroclysis to be highly accurate for diagnosis of small bowel neoplasia (Masselli et al. 2009). It would therefore seem prudent to use enteroclysis rather than enterography for this indication, while awaiting more data on MR enterography (Lohan et al. 2008). CT enteroclysis and standard MDCT also both have a role (Boudiaf et al. 2004; Mallant et al. 2007; Soyer et al. 2008), and are likely to be at least as sensitive as MRI. Again the choice is largely pragmatic, although ionizing radiation should be avoided whenever possible in a young patient cohort at higher risk of malignant transformation.

Scleroderma/Progressive Systemic Sclerosis is another multisystem autoimmune disease, which affects the gastrointestinal tract in up to 80% cases (Domsic et al. 2008). Antinuclear and anti-scl70 antibodies are usually positive, with the disease process resulting in enteric neuropathy and myopathy, the latter causing replacement of the muscular layer by fibrotic tissue (Young et al. 1996). This results in bowel hypocontractility and dilatation, which in turn promotes bacterial overgrowth and malabsorption (Fig. 10.13) (Ebert 2008). Although evidence on the diagnostic performance of imaging modalities is limited and warrants further research, the expected findings of dilatation, reduced peristalsis, and pseudodiverticula formation are probably equally well seen with both barium (Pickhardt 1999) and MR examinations, the latter with the addition of cine MR sequences to allow a functional assessment.

10.5.3
Polyposis Syndromes: Familial Adenomatous Polyposis and Peutz–Jeghers Syndrome

Polyposis syndromes present interesting challenges for radiology. *Familial adenomatous polyposis coli (FAP)* is typically diagnosed in young adults following screening colonoscopy, although some sporadic cases are detected in individuals presenting without a family history, due to spontaneous mutations in the APC (adenomatous polyposis coli) gene. While radiology has little role in monitoring colonic disease (except where frank malignancy has developed), it has significant input beyond the colon, given the wide ranging manifestations and complications of the condition.

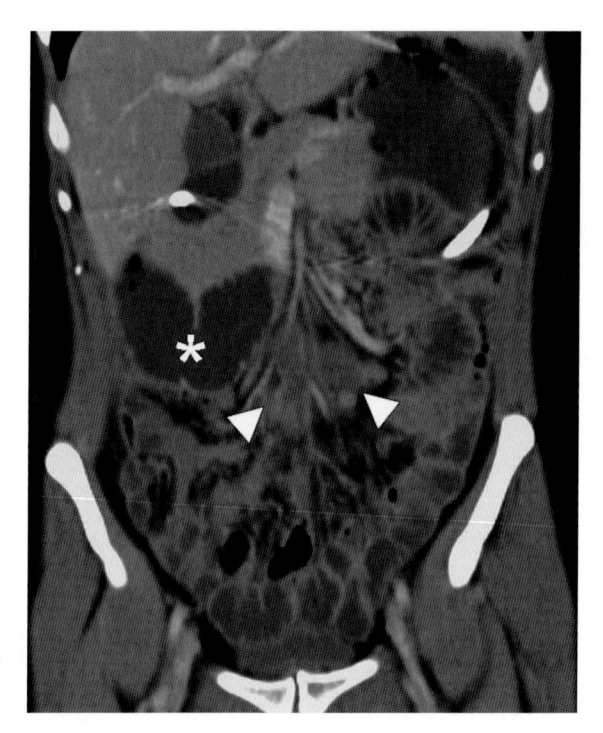

Fig. 10.14. Obstructive symptoms in a postcolectomy patient with FAP and duodenal polyposis. CT enteroclysis shows no jejunal polyps, but a desmoid tumor lies in the small bowel mesentery (*arrowheads*), obstructing the jejunum, resulting in duodenal dilatation (*asterisk*)

the Spiegelman classification for each individual patient. Polyposis may extend to involve the jejunum and ileum, which necessitates a more extensive enteric evaluation than that offered by standard upper GI endoscopy alone (IAQUINTO et al. 2008a). WCE allows such an evaluation and is safe, although it does not assess the duodenum adequately, the commonest site of disease (IAQUINTO et al. 2008b). Furthermore, routine WCE risks obstruction in postcolectomy patients who have desmoid tumors or adhesions (PENNAZIO et al. 2008).

Enteroclysis has advantages over enterography in that jejunal (and by implication duodenal) distension is superior and the cross-sectional imaging capability of CT and MR allows simultaneous assessment of desmoid tumors. There is the some data that MRI is more accurate than CT for the assessment of desmoid disease (LEE et al. 2006) and therefore MR enteroclysis is very likely to be the superior radiological method to assess this subgroup of patients, particularly in those with obstructive symptoms. Barium enteroclysis does not have adequate sensitivity or specificity for even large polyps over 10 mm, and so cannot be recommended for this indication (PLUM et al. 2009). However, the superior spatial resolution of MDCT suggests the CT enteroclysis may have a role, and both MDCT and MRI will also allow detection of the pancreatic and adrenal tumors that may also complicate this syndrome.

Peutz–Jeghers Syndrome (PJS) results in hamartomatous polyposis of the GI tract, particularly affecting the small bowel and colon, due to mutation of the STK11 (serine/threonine kinase) gene. Important complications are obstruction, intussusception, and hemorrhage from large polyps, and patients often present with small bowel obstruction in childhood. (VIDAL et al. 2009). There is therefore a role for imaging to evaluate the presence, size, and distribution of polyps to determine whether elective DBE polypectomy is appropriate, and for planning whether an antegrade or retrograde route will be required to achieve this (PLUM et al. 2007). Enteroclysis most accurately depicts polyposis, by optimizing jejunal distension, and although CT offers better spatial resolution than MR, both techniques are satisfactory. WCE outperforms radiological investigation for confirming polyposis, and particularly for detection of smaller polyps (<5 mm) (CASPARI et al. 2004), but these are rarely symptomatic. Larger polyps may be missed with capsule examinations (POSTGATE et al. 2008) and imaging may demonstrate complications, such as intussussception. MRI also more accurately defines the true size and location of larger polyps (CASPARI et al. 2004). As with Crohn's

Desmoid tumors are benign fibrous tumors but are locally aggressive, and are a major and life-threatening complication in patients with FAP. There is a tendency to develop following surgical trauma, notably panproctocolectomy, and in approximately 10% of cases overall, desmoids result in significant comorbidity and mortality due to pressure effects on adjacent organs and insidious infiltration resulting in obstruction of small bowel, blood vessels, or renal tract (ARVANITIS et al. 1990). Both CT and MRI can demonstrate desmoids and their precursor lesions accurately (Fig. 10.14) (AZIZI et al. 2005; KAWASHIMA et al. 1994), which is important to allow planning for surgical resection (LATCHFORD et al. 2006b). A further concern in patients with FAP is the strong association with duodenal polyposis and carcinoma, a common cause of noncolorectal cancer death, and patients usually need screening of upper GI endoscopy at regular intervals (BULOW et al. 2004). Radiology has a subsequent role in the assessment of established duodenal malignancy.

Endoscopic evaluation is more sensitive than radiology for the assessment of duodenal polyposis in FAP, with the distinct advantage that biopsy to detect dysplasia and field change is necessary to establish

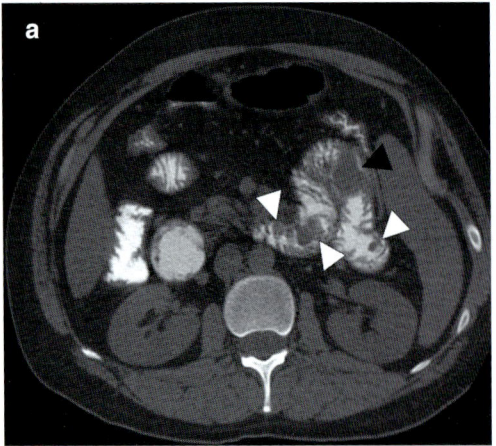

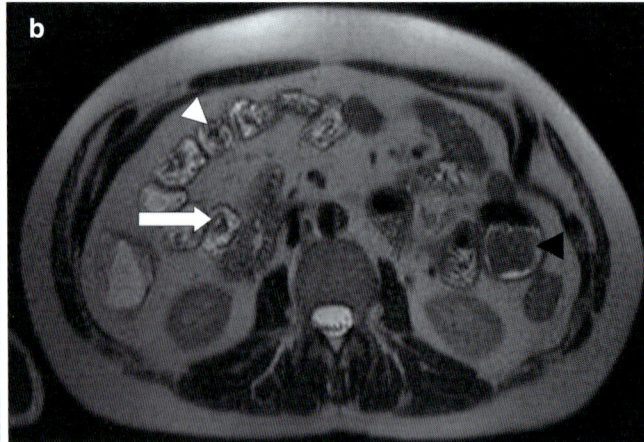

Fig. 10.15. Peutz–Jegher syndrome small bowel assessment. (a) Baseline CT enteroclysis demonstrates multiple polyps (*white arrowheads*) with the largest lesion indicated (*black arrowhead*). (b) There is interval growth to 3 cm at 2-year follow-up MR enterography examination. Note small pedunculated polyp (*arrowhead*). DBE polypectomy was performed for relief of obstructive symptoms

disease, after a baseline enteroclysis examination, follow-up enterography may be appropriate to monitor the diameter of known polyps in patients scheduled for surveillance rather than polypectomy (e.g., polyps <2 cm diameter) (Fig. 10.15), but hard evidence supporting this approach is limited.

One of the greatest concerns for PJS patients is the development of malignancy. GI tract cancers are common (57% of PJS cases by age 70) with colorectal cancer occurring most frequently (39% by age 70). However, other abdominal sites are also at risk, including the stomach and small bowel, pancreas and gynecological organs, as well as breast tumors occurring in 50% of females reaching 60 years (HEARLE et al. 2006). Cross-sectional imaging therefore presents a possible opportunity to search for these complications. While there is no current evidence to support a particular screening programme in terms of modality or screening interval, MRI may have a role, allowing assessment of both small bowel and solid organ sites. Further research and analysis of cost-effectiveness is required to evaluate such a strategy (LATCHFORD et al. 2006a). In a young patient cohort, avoidance of high-dose ionizing radiation by avoiding MDCT is quite likely to be a key concern in the screening setting.

10.5.4
Malignancy

Data are emerging to define the role of imaging in the assessment of small bowel malignancy. This is an important area because, although uncommon, the

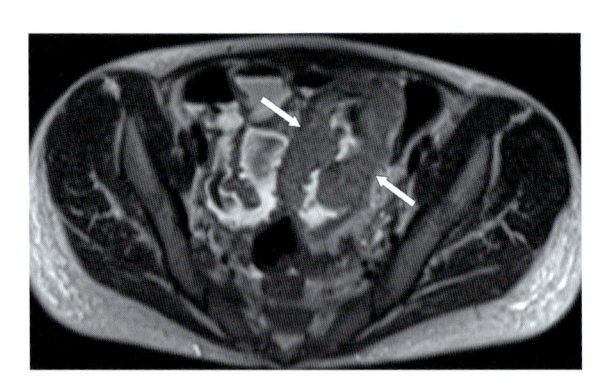

Fig. 10.16. MR enterography axial HASTE with focal shouldered ileal stricture (*arrows*) and preserved lumen with no obstruction, typical of lymphoma

incidence of small bowel malignancy is currently increasing while survival rates remain unchanged (GUSTAFSSON et al. 2008). Primary (adenocarcinoma, lymphoma, stromal, and carcinoid tumors) and secondary tumors may involve the small bowel. All primary tumors are uncommon, and no large direct comparative studies have been performed with respect to MR and MDCT in their evaluation. While standard MDCT and MR enterography can localize and stage tumors (Fig. 10.16) (LOHAN et al. 2008; MINORDI et al. 2007), the largest series utilize enteroclysis to optimize their detection and any data confirming superiority over enterography is limited (RYAN and HEASLIP 2008).

Masselli and colleagues recently published their experience of MR enteroclysis in 150 patients with a

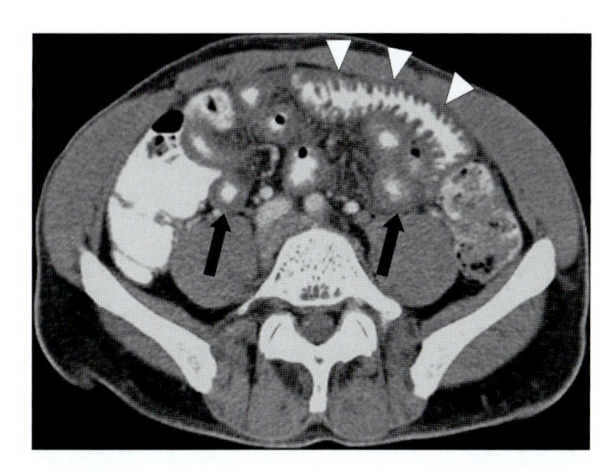

Fig. 10.17. CT enteroclysis (positive enteric contrast) with diffuse ileal wall (*arrows*) and fold thickening (*arrowheads*) from lymphomatous infiltration

clinical suspicion small bowel neoplasia. All patients had prior negative upper and lower GI endoscopy, and follow-up WCE, surgery, clinical follow-up, or endoscopic biopsy. MR enteroclysis detected 19 of 22 tumors (prevalence 15%), with false-positive diagnosis in two cases, giving 86% sensitivity, 98% specificity, and 97% accuracy for MRI (Masselli et al. 2009). Pilleul and colleagues evaluated CT enteroclysis in 219 patients, with a higher tumor prevalence (27%) and found comparable results, with lesions detected in 50 of 59 cases and false-positive diagnosis in five, giving 85% sensitivity, 97% specificity, and 93% accuracy (Fig. 10.17) (Boudiaf et al. 2004; Masselli et al. 2009; Pilleul et al. 2006).

It is important to consider WCE in the context of possible small bowel tumors.

While capsule retention is a risk, occurring in up to 25% of cases in one series, the risk of obstruction is low (Pennazio et al. 2008). Both DBE and WCE have similar diagnostic yields, but WCE is less invasive (Pasha et al. 2008). Like CT and MRI, WCE is also hindered by false-positive and negative diagnoses. In one analysis, WCE was normal in 1.5% of cases with a proven tumor, and failed to detect an abnormality in 10% of instances where one was present (Lewis et al. 2005) and other false-negative studies have been reported by other authors (Postgate et al. 2008). WCE visualizes tumors either as polyps/masses, ulcers or strictures. Accurate anatomic localization and sizing can be difficult, and imaging is usually required for staging and surgical planning, or to guide DBE or push enteroscopy for biopsy confirmation. While WCE is undoubtedly the highest yield single investigation, in any patient with unexplained ongoing symptoms and a negative WCE, where concern persists for small bowel malignancy, further radiological investigation is appropriate.

10.5.5
Evaluation of Occult GI Bleeding

Occult bleeding must be differentiated from active overt bleeding, for which IV contrast enhanced MDCT, labelled red cell scanning and mesenteric angiography, are the primary investigative tools where endoscopy has been negative (Laing et al. 2007).

Occult bleeding is most commonly caused by angiodysplasia, with tumors, ulceration, Meckel's diverticulum, and Crohn's disease less common causes. In patients with negative prior upper and lower GI endoscopy, the typical yield of radiological investigations of all types is low; only 5% for standard barium examinations rising to 10–20% with barium and CT enteroclysis (Moch et al. 1994; Rex et al. 1989; Voderholzer et al. 2003). These data are in stark contrast to WCE where diagnostic yield is as high as 45–76% (Costamagna et al. 2002; Hartmann et al. 2003).

This is in part explained by detection of vascular lesions too small or subtle to detect radiologically, such as angiodysplasia and Dieulafoy lesions (Blecker et al. 2001; Foutch 1993), but the additional yield of WCE over all other investigations (40% vs. push enteroscopy, 37% vs. barium small bowel studies, 31% vs. CT enterography) makes a compelling case for using it as the first-line investigation for this indication (Triester et al. 2005). Rajesh and colleagues, with particular expertise in small bowel imaging, obtained similar yield to WCE for both barium-air enteroclysis and CT enteroclysis (Rajesh et al. 2009), but these data have not been replicated by other workers.

The available literature on occult GI bleeding does not yet include MR examinations of the small bowel in significant numbers, although there is clearly overlap in the setting of possible small bowel neoplasia (Masselli et al. 2009). It is therefore appropriate that WCE is the first-line investigation for occult GI bleeding, unless there are other symptoms that indicate MRI. For example, where there is specific suspicion of Crohn's disease or small bowel neoplasia, MDCT or MR enteroclysis are appropriate first-line investigations. MDCT or MR enteroclysis may also be used for cases of occult bleeding where WCE has been negative (Maglinte et al. 2007). In the authors' experience, MDCT may have theoretical advantages over MR for detection of small, more subtle, hypervascular

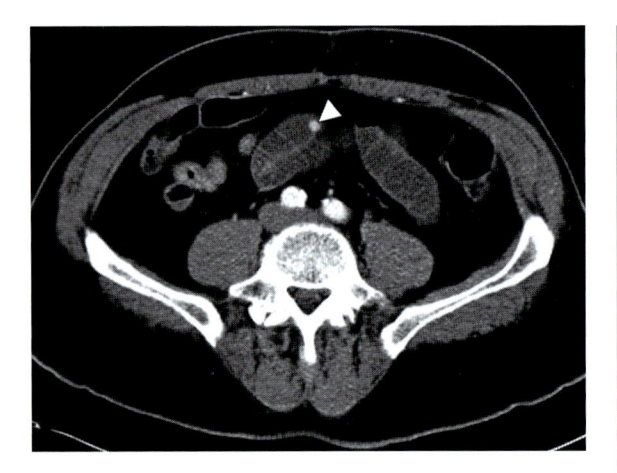

Fig. 10.18. Patient with transfusion-dependent anemia, referred for CT enteroclysis due to lack of local capacity for WCE. A 6 mm hyperenhancing vascular malformation is identified in mid small bowel (*arrowhead*), subsequently ablated with DBE. Distension is critical to identify these lesions (normal prior CT)

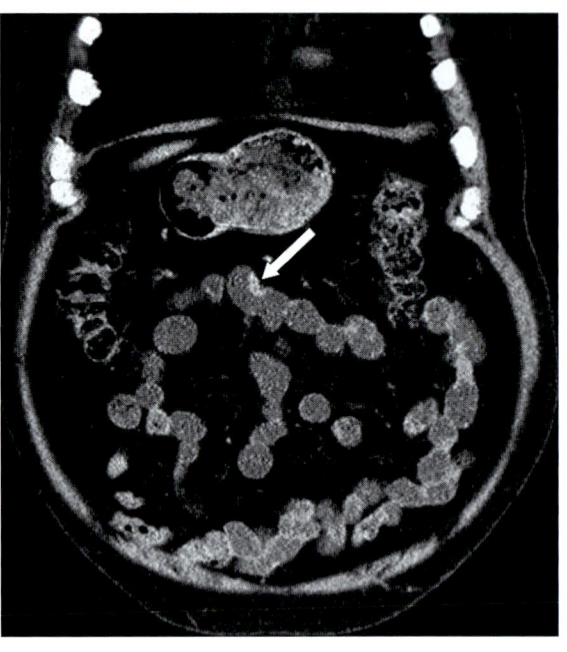

Fig. 10.19. CT enteroclysis localizes a hyperenhancing venous malformation in the mid-jejunum after abnormal WCE, to plan an antegrade DBE for combined DBE/laparoscopic resection

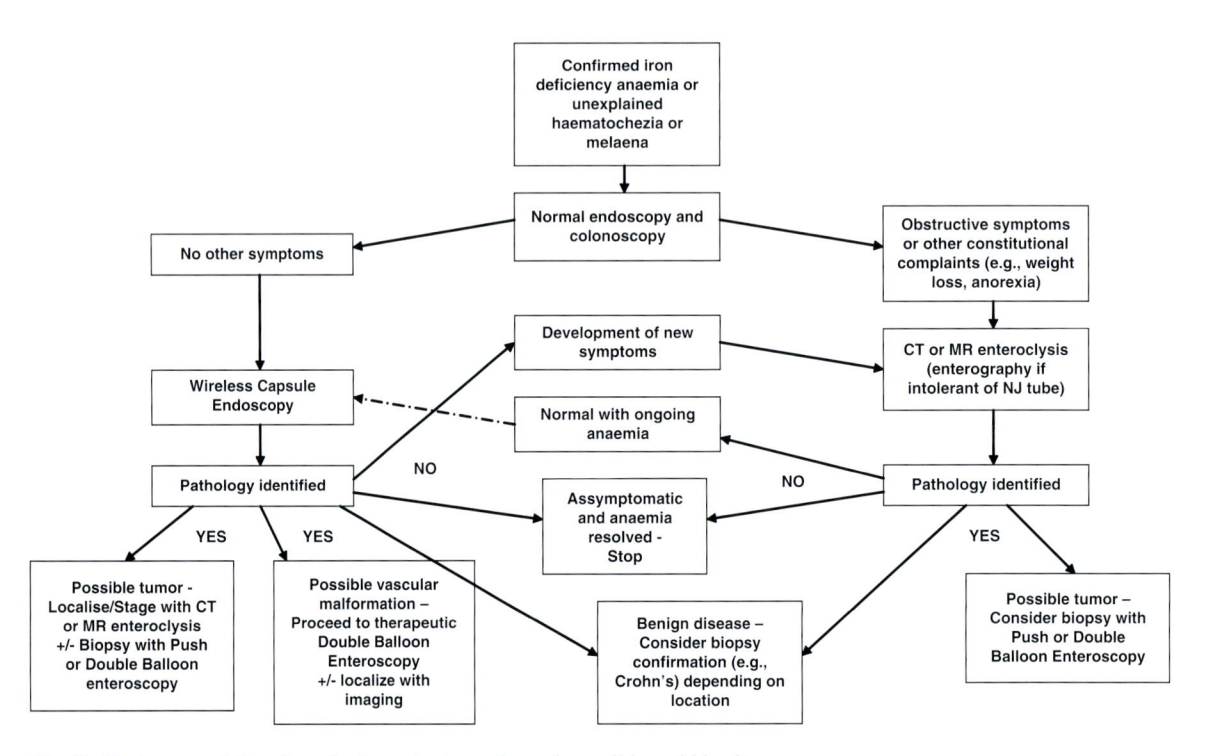

Fig. 10.20. Suggested flowchart for investigation of occult small bowel bleeding

tumors due to superior spatial resolution and less susceptibility to motion artifact following contrast enhancement (Figs. 18 and 19).

An algorithm is provided as a guide to investigate patients using these modalities (Fig. 10.20).

10.5.6
Other Small Bowel Diseases

10.5.6.1
Adhesions

The MR imaging of adhesions will be dealt with in detail in Chap. 16. WCE is not indicated, due to retention risk, but DBE can offer balloon dilatation of focal strictures, for example those related to surgical anastomoses. Imaging has the preeminent role in obstruction. In acute high-grade obstruction, MDCT can define the site, underlying cause, and detect complications (Maglinte et al. 1993; Fukuya et al. 1992; Megibow et al. 1991). Some authors recommend CT enteroclysis in this setting, with overnight drainage to decompress dilated proximal loops and infusion of positive contrast to determine whether conservative management is likely to succeed (predicted by passage of contrast beyond the stricture at 3 h) (Maglinte et al. 2007). For most workers, this is a labour-intensive approach and clinical benefit over standard MDCT is unclear in high-grade obstruction. Acute MRI examination of the small bowel, to detect obstruction, has a role, particularly in patients where ionizing radiation exposure is undesirable (e.g., pregnancy) (Witherspoon et al. 2009; Mckenna et al. 2007).

Low-grade obstruction can be missed with standard MDCT, and the distension offered by enteroclysis can reveal adhesions in this context (Rajesh and Maglinte 2006et al. 1998). However, functional cine MR as part of an MR enterography examination depicts physiological peristalsis and normal bowel motion within the abdomen, including "visceral slide," which is the normal movement of bowel loops relative to each other (Lienemann et al. 2000). Fixity and lack of peristalsis in a bowel loop indicates adhesion (Fig. 10.21). However, it is not possible to differentiate symptomatic from asymptomatic adhesions with this technique (Buhmann-Kirchoff et al. 2008), and MR enteroclysis may add value in this setting (Gourtsoyiannis et al. 2002). Again, research is lacking with respect to direct comparison of these imaging techniques for low-grade obstruction.

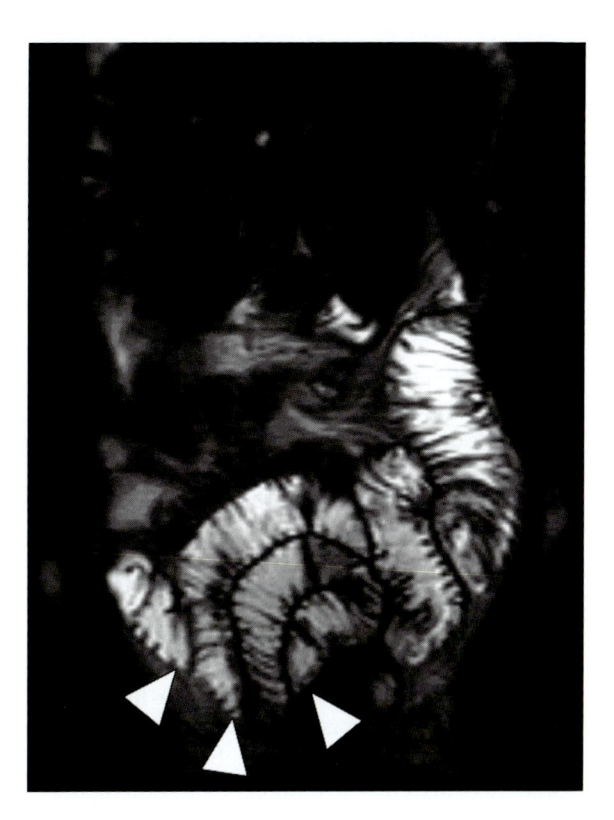

Fig. 10.21. MR enterography coronal HASTE in patient with obstructive symptoms and prior subtotal colectomy for Crohn's disease. Sharply angulated small bowel loops, with dilatation due to adhesions (*arrowheads*), but no thickening to indicate Crohn's disease

10.5.6.2
Radiation Enteritis

Increasing utilization of high-dose fractionated radiotherapy in the curative treatment of pelvic malignancies, such as cervical, prostate, and rectal cancers, comes at the expense of toxicity. At doses over 5,000 mGy, the risk of bowel complications increases significantly, with other risk factors for bowel injury, including older age and anal excision (Miller et al. 1999), presence of adhesions from previous surgery, and increasing irradiated small bowel volume (Gunnlaugsson et al. 2007).

Radiation enteritis typically affects the distal ileum and is often associated with rectosigmoid involvement (Palmer and Bush 1976). The rectum is affected more frequently than the small bowel in pelvic radiotherapy, where proctitis is estimated to occur in 19% of cases (Miller et al. 1999). While acute symptoms occur soon after treatment and often resolve, chronic enteritis manifests 9–24 months, or even longer, after treatment, secondary to an obliterative endarteritis.

Acute symptoms only progress to chronic enteritis in a minority of cases (MILLER et al. 1999) with severe complications (e.g., fistula or obstruction) presenting at a mean interval of 18 months (LIBOTTE et al. 1995). Radiotherapy produces mucosal inflammation, reduced secretion, and hypomotility of affected segments (MACNAUGHTON 2000). Severe complications requiring surgical therapy are uncommon, but these data may be biased by an understandable reluctance to not operate in this context, where surgery is known to be very difficult. A review of 14,791 patients receiving radiotherapy found that 25 patients required surgical referral after failure of conservative management. Complications included radiation enteritis (60%), strictures (53%), fistulae (17%), nonhealing wounds (15%), and de novo cancers in irradiated fields (10%) (TURINA et al. 2008).

The role of imaging is to diagnose the presence and extent of small bowel involvement and complications, since the rectosigmoid is easily accessible to endoscopy. The choice of modality will be influenced by patient presentation. In cases with clear clinical evidence of high-grade obstruction or sepsis/abscess, MDCT will allow confirmation of site of pathology and exclusion of recurrent or metastatic malignancy, which is the main concern in this patient cohort. In some cases, pelvic MRI or CT/PET may be required where there is a lack of fat to provide the intrinsic contrast to allow CT characterization.

Once more, clear evidence of superiority of one cross-sectional modality or method of bowel distension is lacking. In the elective outpatient setting, a wider range of imaging options is available. While the distal ileum is the usual disease site due to proximity to the radiation field, multifocal disease does occur and jejunal loops may lie in the pelvis. If surgical treatment is planned for obstructive symptoms, an accurate roadmap of strictures is highly desirable. For this reason, enteroclysis may be appropriate, particularly where very short segments are involved or where long segments of disease necessitate accurate assessment of normal bowel length to predict "short bowel" after surgical resection. MRI offers better tissue contrast than MDCT, which is an advantage in patients suffering malabsorption and anorexia due to small bowel disease with lack of fat and soft tissue edema (Figs. 10.22 and 10.23). Not all patients may find enteroclysis acceptable, and so pragmatism is necessary. Enterography may offer similar accuracy, but hard research data to support this assumption is lacking.

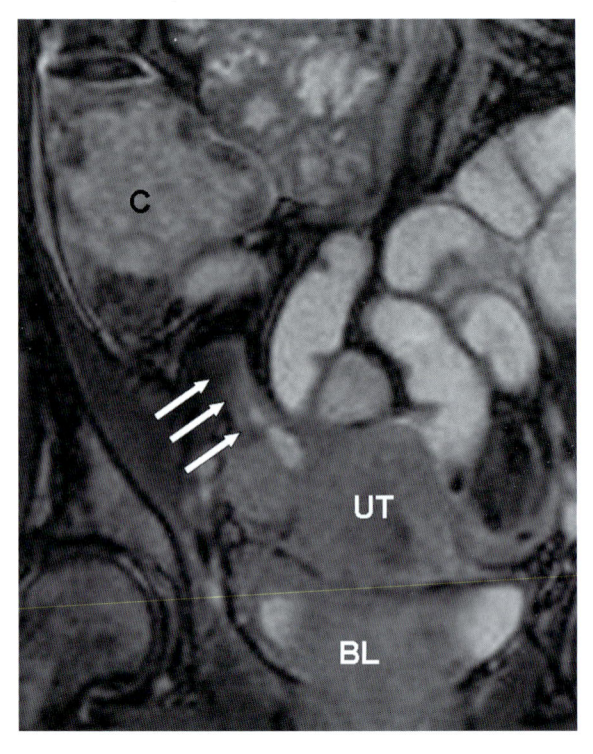

Fig. 10.22. Female patient with intermittent obstructive symptoms, 18 months postradical chemoradiotherapy forcervical carcinoma. Coronal FISP from MR enteroclysisdemonstrates a single 3 cm non distending stricture of the distal ileum (*arrows*), adjacent to uterus (UT), bladder (BL) and caecum (C). Proximal dilatation is consistent with subacute obstruction from radiation enteritis

The main imaging findings are wall thickening and edema, stricture and obstruction, deep ulceration and fistulation to adjacent organs (HORTON et al. 1999). The main indicator for the diagnosis is a prior history of radiotherapy and abnormality conforming to radiation field. Care is required to exclude malignancy, suggested by mass-like thickening, infiltration of adjacent tissues, and nodal enlargement.

It is clear that WCE should be used with caution in this patient group. Capsule retention resulting in bowel obstruction is well recognized, due to radiation-induced stricture (ROGERS et al. 2008; LEE et al. 2004; LIN et al. 2007), and so the role of WCE is probably restricted to the assessment for small bowel telangectasia (from radiotherapy) in patients with occult GI bleeding and a normal cross-sectional enteroclysis examination. DBE can access the terminal ileum for both diagnosis and intervention (PASHA et al. 2007), without risk of obstruction, but requires bowel cleansing that is unnecessary with radiological evaluation.

cological symptoms. The gynecological organs are most often affected, followed by dependent abdominopelvic structures, including bowel. While the rectosigmoid is the commonest intestinal location (85%), the small bowel (7%) cecum and appendix (3% each) are recognized sites (MACAFEE et al. 1960). The terminal ileum is the most likely small bowel location (MELODY 1956) and obstruction may occur from adhesions, due to recurrent bleeding, or due to infiltration or annular involvement by endometrioma.

A specific imaging diagnosis can be difficult without a suggestive history. A bowel mass with stricture may suggest malignancy if blood products are not looked for specifically. MR evaluation with fat-saturated T1W sequences display characteristic high signal in endometriomas due to degrading blood products (DEL FRATE et al. 2006), with additional supporting evidence for the diagnosis when associated with gynecological findings such as uterine adenomyosis, endometriotic ovarian cysts, or hydrosalpinges (GHATTAMANENI et al. 2009). While the bowel serosa and muscularis are involved, the mucosa is usually intact, producing a characteristic crennulated appearance on barium studies, that cannot be appreciated with other imaging modalities. One group has evaluated MDCT, supplemented with colonic water enema, showing 98.7% sensitivity with 100% specificity for bowel involvement (BISCALDI et al. 2007). This suggests that bowel distension may aid diagnosis, and would be worthy of further research.

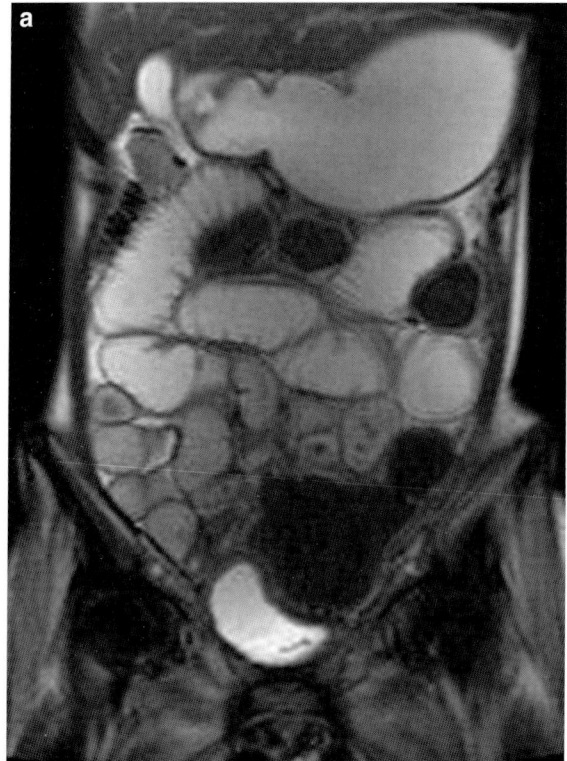

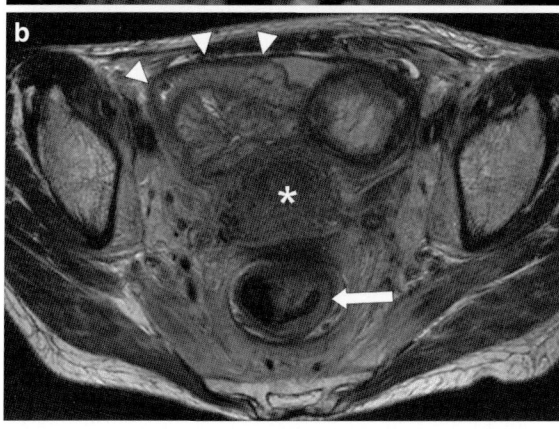

Fig. 10.23. Post-radical chemoradiotherapy for cervical carcinoma with increasing diarrhoea. (**a**) Coronal HASTE indicates subacute obstruction. (**b**) Axial T2W TSE sequence shows thickening and wall oedema of the distal ileum (*arrowheads*) and rectosigmoid (*arrow*) lying within the radiation field (uterus – *asterisk*) consistent with radiation enterocolitis

10.5.6.3
Endometriosis

In women of reproductive age, endometriosis is a significant cause of pelvic symptoms, including cyclical pain, bowel obstruction (WICKRAMASEKERA et al. 1999) and altered bowel habit, as well as gyne-

10.6
Conclusion

MR of the small bowel offers sensitive and radiation-free imaging for a wide range of disorders. While its role for some indications remains unclear, and the evidence limited, Crohn's disease, Celiac disease, and exclusion of malignancy are well-established indications, and evidence supporting its use continues to accumulate. Integration of radiological and endoscopic evaluation of the small intestine and a balanced approach, including a thorough understanding of the strengths and weaknesses of different tests in a particular clinical scenario, are essential to optimize patient management and their clinical outcomes. While the arguments pitching MR enterography against MR enteroclysis await definitive resolution, we can be confident that MR imaging of the small bowel will assume the primary role in the diagnosis and follow-up of small bowel diseases in the very near future.

References

Araki A, Tsuchiya K, Okada E, Suzuki S, Oshima S, Yoshioka S, Yoshioka A, Kanai T, Watanabe M (2009) Single-operator double-balloon endoscopy (DBE) is as effective as dual-operator DBE. J.Gastroenterol.Hepatol.

Arvanitis ML, Jagelman DG, Fazio VW, Lavery IC, McGannon E (1990) Mortality in patients with familial adenomatous polyposis. Dis.Colon Rectum 33:639–642

Azizi L, Balu M, Belkacem A, Lewin M, Tubiana JM, Arrive L (2005) MRI features of mesenteric desmoid tumors in familial adenomatous polyposis. AJR Am.J.Roentgenol. 184:1128–1135

Bernstein CN, Boult IF, Greenberg HM, van der PW, Duffy G, Grahame GR (1997) A prospective randomized comparison between small bowel enteroclysis and small bowel follow-through in Crohn's disease. Gastroenterology 113: 390–398

Biancone L, Schillaci O, Capoccetti F, Bozzi RM, Fina D, Petruzziello C, Geremia A, Simonetti G, Pallone F (2005) Technetium-99m-HMPAO labeled leukocyte single photon emission computerized tomography (SPECT) for assessing Crohn's disease extent and intestinal infiltration. Am.J.Gastroenterol. 100:344–354

Biscaldi E, Ferrero S, Fulcheri E, Ragni N, Remorgida V, Rollandi GA (2007) Multislice CT enteroclysis in the diagnosis of bowel endometriosis. Eur.Radiol. 17:211–219

Blecker D, Bansal M, Zimmerman RL, Fogt F, Lewis J, Stein R, Kochman ML (2001) Dieulafoy's lesion of the small bowel causing massive gastrointestinal bleeding: two case reports and literature review. Am.J.Gastroenterol. 96:902–905

Boudiaf M, Jaff A, Soyer P, Bouhnik Y, Hamzi L, Rymer R (2004) Small-bowel diseases: prospective evaluation of multi-detector row helical CT enteroclysis in 107 consecutive patients. Radiology 233:338–344

Brenner DJ, Hall EJ (2007) Computed tomography--an increasing source of radiation exposure. N.Engl.J.Med. 357: 2277–2284

Buhmann-Kirchhoff S, Lang R, Kirchhoff C, Steitz HO, Jauch KW, Reiser M, Lienemann A (2008) Functional cine MR imaging for the detection and mapping of intraabdominal adhesions: method and surgical correlation. Eur. Radiol. 18:1215–1223

Bulow S, Bjork J, Christensen IJ, Fausa O, Jarvinen H, Moesgaard F, Vasen HF (2004) Duodenal adenomatosis in familial adenomatous polyposis. Gut 53:381–386

Caspari R, von FM, Krautmacher C, Schild H, Heller J, Sauerbruch T (2004) Comparison of capsule endoscopy and magnetic resonance imaging for the detection of polyps of the small intestine in patients with familial adenomatous polyposis or with Peutz-Jeghers' syndrome. Endoscopy 36:1054–1059

Cave D, Legnani P, de FR, Lewis BS (2005) ICCE consensus for capsule retention. Endoscopy 37:1065–1067

Clarke JO, Giday SA, Magno P, Shin EJ, Buscaglia JM, Jagannath SB, Mullin GE (2008) How good is capsule endoscopy for detection of periampullary lesions? Results of a tertiary-referral center. Gastrointest.Endosc. 68: 267–272

Costamagna G, Shah SK, Riccioni ME, Foschia F, Mutignani M, Perri V, Vecchioli A, Brizi MG, Picciocchi A, Marano P (2002) A prospective trial comparing small bowel radiographs and video capsule endoscopy for suspected small bowel disease. Gastroenterology 123:999–1005

Das CJ, Makharia G, Kumar R, Chawla M, Goswami P, Sharma R, Malhotra A (2007) PET-CT enteroclysis: a new technique for evaluation of inflammatory diseases of the intestine. Eur.J.Nucl.Med.Mol.Imaging 34:2106–2114

Del Frate C, Girometti R, Pittino M, Del FG, Bazzocchi M, Zuiani C (2006) Deep retroperitoneal pelvic endometriosis: MR imaging appearance with laparoscopic correlation. Radiographics 26:1705–1718

Desmond AN, O'Regan K, Curran C, McWilliams S, Fitzgerald T, Maher MM, Shanahan F (2008) Crohn's disease: factors associated with exposure to high levels of diagnostic radiation. Gut 57:1524–1529

Di SA, Corazza GR (2009) Coeliac disease. Lancet 373: 1480–1493

Domsic R, Fasanella K, Bielefeldt K (2008) Gastrointestinal manifestations of systemic sclerosis. Dig.Dis.Sci. 53:1163–1174

Ebert EC (2008) Gastric and enteric involvement in progressive systemic sclerosis. J.Clin.Gastroenterol. 42:5–12

Filippi L, Biancone L, Petruzziello C, Schillaci O (2006) Tc-99m HMPAO-labeled leukocyte scintigraphy with hybrid SPECT/CT detects perianal fistulas in Crohn disease. Clin. Nucl.Med. 31:541–542

Foutch PG (1993) Angiodysplasia of the gastrointestinal tract. Am.J.Gastroenterol. 88:807–818

Fraquelli M, Sarno A, Girelli C, Laudi C, Buscarini E, Villa C, Robotti D, Porta P, Cammarota T, Ercole E, Rigazio C, Senore C, Pera A, Malacrida V, Gallo C, Maconi G (2008) Reproducibility of bowel ultrasonography in the evaluation of Crohn's disease. Dig.Liver Dis. 40:860–866

Fukumoto A, Tanaka S, Shishido T, Takemura Y, Oka S, Chayama K (2009a) Comparison of detectability of small-bowel lesions between capsule endoscopy and double-balloon endoscopy for patients with suspected small-bowel disease. Gastrointest.Endosc. 69:857–865

Fukumoto A, Tanaka S, Shishido T, Takemura Y, Oka S, Chayama K (2009b) Comparison of detectability of small-bowel lesions between capsule endoscopy and double-balloon endoscopy for patients with suspected small-bowel disease. Gastrointest.Endosc. 69:857–865

Fukuya T, Hawes DR, Lu CC, Chang PJ, Barloon TJ (1992) CT diagnosis of small-bowel obstruction: efficacy in 60 patients. AJR Am.J.Roentgenol. 158:765–769

Ghattamaneni S, Bhuskute NM, Weston MJ, Spencer JA (2009) Discriminative MRI features of fallopian tube masses. Clin. Radiol. 64:815–831

Giaffer MH, Tindale WB, Holdsworth D (1996) Value of technetium-99m HMPAO-labelled leucocyte scintigraphy as an initial screening test in patients suspected of having inflammatory bowel disease. Eur.J.Gastroenterol.Hepatol. 8:1195–1200

Goldfarb NI, Pizzi LT, Fuhr JP, Jr., Salvador C, Sikirica V, Kornbluth A, Lewis B (2004) Diagnosing Crohn's disease: an economic analysis comparing wireless capsule endoscopy with traditional diagnostic procedures. Dis.Manag. 7:292–304

Gourtsoyiannis N, Papanikolaou N, Grammatikakis J, Prassopoulos P (2002) MR enteroclysis: technical considerations and clinical applications. Eur.Radiol. 12:2651–2658

Gourtsoyiannis N, Papanikolaou N, Grammatikakis J, Papamastorakis G, Prassopoulos P, Roussomoustakaki M (2004) Assessment of Crohn's disease activity in the small bowel with MR and conventional enteroclysis: preliminary results. Eur.Radiol. 14:1017–1024

Gross SA, Stark ME (2008) Initial experience with double-balloon enteroscopy at a U.S. center. Gastrointest.Endosc. 67:890–897

Gunnlaugsson A, Kjellen E, Nilsson P, Bendahl PO, Willner J, Johnsson A (2007) Dose-volume relationships between enteritis and irradiated bowel volumes during 5-fluorouracil and oxaliplatin based chemoradiotherapy in locally advanced rectal cancer. Acta Oncol. 46:937–944

Gustafsson BI, Siddique L, Chan A, Dong M, Drozdov I, Kidd M, Modlin IM (2008) Uncommon cancers of the small intestine, appendix and colon: an analysis of SEER 1973-2004, and current diagnosis and therapy. Int.J.Oncol. 33:1121–1131

Hara AK, Leighton JA, Sharma VK, Heigh RI, Fleischer DE (2005) Imaging of small bowel disease: comparison of capsule endoscopy, standard endoscopy, barium examination, and CT. Radiographics 25:697–711

Hartmann D, Schilling D, Bolz G, Hahne M, Jakobs R, Siegel E, Weickert U, Adamek HE, Riemann JF (2003) Capsule endoscopy versus push enteroscopy in patients with occult gastrointestinal bleeding. Z.Gastroenterol. 41:377–382

Hearle N, Schumacher V, Menko FH, Olschwang S, Boardman LA, Gille JJ, Keller JJ, Westerman AM, Scott RJ, Lim W, Trimbath JD, Giardiello FM, Gruber SB, Offerhaus GJ, de Rooij FW, Wilson JH, Hansmann A, Moslein G, Royer-Pokora B, Vogel T, Phillips RK, Spigelman AD, Houlston RS (2006) Frequency and spectrum of cancers in the Peutz-Jeghers syndrome. Clin.Cancer Res. 12:3209–3215

Horsthuis K, Bipat S, Bennink RJ, Stoker J (2008) Inflammatory bowel disease diagnosed with US, MR, scintigraphy, and CT: meta-analysis of prospective studies. Radiology 247:64–79

Horsthuis K, Bipat S, Stokkers PC, Stoker J (2009a) Magnetic resonance imaging for evaluation of disease activity in Crohn's disease: a systematic review. Eur.Radiol.

Horsthuis K, Nederveen AJ, de Feiter MW, Lavini C, Stokkers PC, Stoker J (2009b) Mapping of T1-values and Gadolinium-concentrations in MRI as indicator of disease activity in luminal Crohn's disease: a feasibility study. J.Magn Reson. Imaging 29:488–493

Horton KM, Corl FM, Fishman EK (1999) CT of nonneoplastic diseases of the small bowel: spectrum of disease. J.Comput. Assist.Tomogr. 23:417–428

Iaquinto G, Fornasarig M, Quaia M, Giardullo N, D'Onofrio V, Iaquinto S, Di BS, Cannizzaro R (2008a) Capsule endoscopy is useful and safe for small-bowel surveillance in familial adenomatous polyposis. Gastrointest.Endosc. 67:61–67

Iaquinto G, Fornasarig M, Quaia M, Giardullo N, D'Onofrio V, Iaquinto S, Di BS, Cannizzaro R (2008b) Capsule endoscopy is useful and safe for small-bowel surveillance in familial adenomatous polyposis. Gastrointest.Endosc. 67:61–67

Jaffe TA, Gaca AM, Delaney S, Yoshizumi TT, Toncheva G, Nguyen G, Frush DP (2007) Radiation doses from small-bowel follow-through and abdominopelvic MDCT in Crohn's disease. AJR Am.J.Roentgenol. 189:1015–1022

Jensch S, de Vries AH, Pot D, Peringa J, Bipat S, Florie J, van Gelder RE, Stoker J (2008) Image quality and patient acceptance of four regimens with different amounts of mild laxatives for CT colonography. AJR Am.J.Roentgenol. 191:158–167

Jones R, Sleet S (2009) Coeliac disease. BMJ 338:a3058

Kawashima A, Goldman SM, Fishman EK, Kuhlman JE, Onitsuka H, Fukuya T, Masuda K (1994) CT of intraabdominal desmoid tumors: is the tumor different in patients with Gardner's disease? AJR Am.J.Roentgenol. 162:339–342

Kitazume Y, Satoh S, Hosoi H, Noguchi O, Shibuya H (2007) Cine magnetic resonance imaging evaluation of peristalsis of small bowel with longitudinal ulcer in Crohn disease: preliminary results. J.Comput.Assist.Tomogr. 31:876–883

Koutroubakis IE, Koukouraki SI, Dimoulios PD, Velidaki AA, Karkavitsas NS, Kouroumalis EA (2003) Active inflammatory bowel disease: evaluation with 99mTc (V) DMSA scintigraphy. Radiology 229:70–74

Laghi A, Borrelli O, Paolantonio P, Dito L, Buena de MM, Falconieri P, Passariello R, Cucchiara S (2003) Contrast enhanced magnetic resonance imaging of the terminal ileum in children with Crohn's disease. Gut 52:393–397

Laing CJ, Tobias T, Rosenblum DI, Banker WL, Tseng L, Tamarkin SW (2007) Acute gastrointestinal bleeding: emerging role of multidetector CT angiography and review of current imaging techniques. Radiographics 27:1055–1070

Latchford A, Greenhalf W, Vitone LJ, Neoptolemos JP, Lancaster GA, Phillips RK (2006a) Peutz-Jeghers syndrome and screening for pancreatic cancer. Br.J.Surg. 93:1446–1455

Latchford AR, Sturt NJ, Neale K, Rogers PA, Phillips RK (2006b) A 10-year review of surgery for desmoid disease associated with familial adenomatous polyposis. Br.J.Surg. 93:1258–1264

Lauenstein TC, Schneemann H, Vogt FM, Herborn CU, Ruhm SG, Debatin JF (2003) Optimization of oral contrast agents for MR imaging of the small bowel. Radiology 228:279–283

Lee DW, Poon AO, Chan AC (2004) Diagnosis of small bowel radiation enteritis by capsule endoscopy. Hong.Kong. Med.J. 10:419–421

Lee JC, Thomas JM, Phillips S, Fisher C, Moskovic E (2006) Aggressive fibromatosis: MRI features with pathologic correlation. AJR Am.J.Roentgenol. 186:247–254

Lee SS, Kim AY, Yang SK, Chung JW, Kim SY, Park SH, Ha HK (2009) Crohn Disease of the Small Bowel: Comparison of CT Enterography, MR Enterography, and Small-Bowel Follow-Through as Diagnostic Techniques. Radiology

Lewis BS, Eisen GM, Friedman S (2005) A pooled analysis to evaluate results of capsule endoscopy trials. Endoscopy 37:960–965

Li B, Meng M (2009) Computer Aided Detection of Bleeding Regions for Capsule Endoscopy Images. IEEE Trans. Biomed.Eng

Liangpunsakul S, Chadalawada V, Rex DK, Maglinte D, Lappas J (2003) Wireless capsule endoscopy detects small bowel ulcers in patients with normal results from state of the art enteroclysis. Am.J.Gastroenterol. 98:1295–1298

Libotte F, Autier P, Delmelle M, Gozy M, Pector JC, Van HP, Gerard A (1995) Survival of patients with radiation enteritis of the small and the large intestine. Acta Chir Belg. 95:190–194

Lienemann A, Sprenger D, Steitz HO, Korell M, Reiser M (2000) Detection and mapping of intraabdominal adhesions by using functional cine MR imaging: preliminary results. Radiology 217:421–425

Lin OS, Brandabur JJ, Schembre DB, Soon MS, Kozarek RA (2007) Acute symptomatic small bowel obstruction due to capsule impaction. Gastrointest.Endosc. 65:725–728

Lohan DG, Alhajeri AN, Cronin CG, Roche CJ, Murphy JM (2008) MR enterography of small-bowel lymphoma: potential for suggestion of histologic subtype and the presence of underlying celiac disease. AJR Am.J.Roentgenol. 190:287–293

Macafee CH, Greer HL (1960) Intestinal endometriosis. A report of 29 cases and a survey of the literature. J.Obstet. Gynaecol.Br.Emp. 67:539–555

MacNaughton WK (2000) Review article: new insights into the pathogenesis of radiation-induced intestinal dysfunction. Aliment.Pharmacol.Ther. 14:523–528

Maglinte DD, Applegate KE, Rajesh A, Jennings SG, Ford JM, Savabi MS, Lappas JC (2008) Conscious sedation for patients undergoing enteroclysis: Comparing the safety and patient-reported effectiveness of two protocols. Eur.J.Radiol.

Maglinte DD, Gage SN, Harmon BH, Kelvin FM, Hage JP, Chua GT, Ng AC, Graffis RF, Chernish SM (1993) Obstruction of the small intestine: accuracy and role of CT in diagnosis. Radiology 188:61–64

Maglinte DD, Sandrasegaran K, Chiorean M, Dewitt J, McHenry L, Lappas JC (2007) Radiologic investigations complement and add diagnostic information to capsule endoscopy of small-bowel diseases. AJR Am.J.Roentgenol. 189:306–312

Maglinte DDT (2005) Invited Commentary. Radiographics 25:711–718

Mallant M, Hadithi M, Al-Toma AB, Kater M, Jacobs M, Manoliu R, Mulder C, van Waesberghe JH (2007) Abdominal computed tomography in refractory coeliac disease and enteropathy associated T-cell lymphoma. World J. Gastroenterol. 13:1696–1700

Masselli G, Casciani E, Polettini E, Gualdi G (2008) Comparison of MR enteroclysis with MR enterography and conventional enteroclysis in patients with Crohn's disease. Eur. Radiol. 18:438–447

Masselli G, Polettini E, Casciani E, Bertini L, Vecchioli A, Gualdi G (2009) Small-Bowel Neoplasms: Prospective Evaluation of MR Enteroclysis. Radiology

McKenna DA, Meehan CP, Alhajeri AN, Regan MC, O'Keeffe DP (2007) The use of MRI to demonstrate small bowel obstruction during pregnancy. Br.J.Radiol. 80:e11–e14

Megibow AJ, Balthazar EJ, Cho KC, Medwid SW, Birnbaum BA, Noz ME (1991) Bowel obstruction: evaluation with CT. Radiology 180:313–318

Melody GF (1956) Endometriosis causing obstruction of the ileum. Obstet.Gynecol. 8:468–472

Miller AR, Martenson JA, Nelson H, Schleck CD, Ilstrup DM, Gunderson LL, Donohue JH (1999) The incidence and clinical consequences of treatment-related bowel injury. Int.J.Radiat.Oncol.Biol.Phys. 43:817–825

Minordi LM, Vecchioli A, Mirk P, Filigrana E, Poloni G, Bonomo L (2007) Multidetector CT in small-bowel neoplasms. Radiol.Med. 112:1013–1025

Moch A, Herlinger H, Kochman ML, Levine MS, Rubesin SE, Laufer I (1994) Enteroclysis in the evaluation of obscure gastrointestinal bleeding. AJR Am.J.Roentgenol. 163:1381-1384

Negaard A, Paulsen V, Sandvik L, Berstad AE, Borthne A, Try K, Lygren I, Storaas T, Klow NE (2007) A prospective randomized comparison between two MRI studies of the small bowel in Crohn's disease, the oral contrast method and MR enteroclysis. Eur.Radiol. 17:2294–2301

Negaard A, Sandvik L, Berstad AE, Paulsen V, Lygren I, Borthne A, Klow NE (2008) MRI of the small bowel with oral contrast or nasojejunal intubation in Crohn's disease: Randomized comparison of patient acceptance. Scand.J.Gastroenterol. 43:44–51

Nelson RL, Subramanian K, Gasparaitis A, Abcarian H, Pavel DG (1990) Indium 111-labeled granulocyte scan in the diagnosis and management of acute inflammatory bowel disease. Dis.Colon Rectum 33:451–457

Palmer JA, Bush RS (1976) Radiation injuries to the bowel associated with the treatment of carcinoma of the cervix. Surgery 80:458–464

Paolantonio P, Tomei E, Rengo M, Ferrari R, Lucchesi P, Laghi A (2007) Adult celiac disease: MRI findings. Abdom.Imaging 32:433–440

Pasha SF, Harrison ME, Leighton JA (2007) Obscure GI bleeding secondary to radiation enteritis diagnosed and successfully treated with retrograde double-balloon enteroscopy. Gastrointest.Endosc. 65:552–554

Pasha SF, Leighton JA, Das A, Harrison ME, Decker GA, Fleischer DE, Sharma VK (2008) Double-balloon enteroscopy and capsule endoscopy have comparable diagnostic yield in small-bowel disease: a meta-analysis. Clin. Gastroenterol.Hepatol. 6:671–676

Peloquin JM, Pardi DS, Sandborn WJ, Fletcher JG, McCollough CH, Schueler BA, Kofler JA, Enders FT, Achenbach SJ, Loftus EV, Jr. (2008) Diagnostic ionizing radiation exposure in a population-based cohort of patients with inflammatory bowel disease. Am.J.Gastroenterol. 103:2015–2022

Pennazio M, Rondonotti E, de FR (2008) Capsule endoscopy in neoplastic diseases. World J.Gastroenterol. 14:5245–5253

Pickhardt PJ (1999) The "hide-bound" bowel sign. Radiology 213:837–838

Pilleul F, Penigaud M, Milot L, Saurin JC, Chayvialle JA, Valette PJ (2006) Possible small-bowel neoplasms: contrast-enhanced and water-enhanced multidetector CT enteroclysis. Radiology 241:796–801

Plum N, May AD, Manner H, Ell C (2007) [Peutz-Jeghers syndrome: endoscopic detection and treatment of small bowel polyps by double-balloon enteroscopy]. Z.Gastroenterol. 45:1049–1055

Plum N, May A, Manner H, Ell C (2009) Small-bowel diagnosis in patients with familial adenomatous polyposis: comparison of push enteroscopy, capsule endoscopy, ileoscopy, and enteroclysis. Z.Gastroenterol. 47:339–346

Postgate A, Despott E, Burling D, Gupta A, Phillips R, O'Beirne J, Patch D, Fraser C (2008) Significant small-bowel lesions detected by alternative diagnostic modalities after negative capsule endoscopy. Gastrointest.Endosc. 68:1209–1214

Postgate A, Haycock A, Thomas-Gibson S, Fitzpatrick A, Bassett P, Preston S, Saunders BP, Fraser C (2009) Computer-aided learning in capsule endoscopy leads to improvement in lesion recognition ability. Gastrointest.Endosc. 70:310–316

Rajesh A, Maglinte DD (2006) Multislice CT enteroclysis: technique and clinical applications. Clin.Radiol. 61:31–39

Rajesh A, Sandrasegaran K, Jennings SG, Maglinte DD, McHenry L, Lappas JC, Rex D (2009) Comparison of capsule endoscopy with enteroclysis in the investigation of small bowel disease. Abdom.Imaging 34:459–466

Rex DK, Lappas JC, Maglinte DD, Malczewski MC, Kopecky KA, Cockerill EM (1989) Enteroclysis in the evaluation of suspected small intestinal bleeding. Gastroenterology 97:58–60

Rimola J, Rodriguez S, Garcia BO, Ordas I, Ayala E, Aceituno M, Pellise M, Ayuso C, Ricart E, Donoso L, Panes J (2009) Magnetic resonance for assessment of disease activity and severity in Crohn disease. Gut

Rogers AM, Kuperman E, Puleo FJ, Shope TR (2008) Intestinal obstruction by capsule endoscopy in a patient with radiation enteritis. JSLS. 12:85–87

Rondonotti E, Spada C, Cave D, Pennazio M, Riccioni ME, De V, I, Schneider D, Sprujevnik T, Villa F, Langelier J, Arrigoni A, Costamagna G, de FR (2007) Video capsule enteroscopy in the diagnosis of celiac disease: a multicenter study. Am.J.Gastroenterol. 102:1624–1631

Ryan ER, Heaslip IS (2008) Magnetic resonance enteroclysis compared with conventional enteroclysis and computed tomography enteroclysis: a critically appraised topic. Abdom.Imaging 33:34–37

Sempere GA, Martinez S, V, Medina CE, Benages A, Tome TA, Canelles P, Bulto A, Quiles F, Puchades I, Cuquerella J, Celma J, Orti E (2005) MRI evaluation of inflammatory activity in Crohn's disease. AJR Am.J.Roentgenol. 184:1829–1835

Sheridan MB, Nicholson DA, Martin DF (1993) Transabdominal ultrasonography as the primary investigation in patients with suspected Crohn's disease or recurrence: a prospective study. Clin.Radiol. 48:402–404

Soyer P, Boudiaf M, Fargeaudou Y, Dray X, Hamzi L, Vahedi K, Lavergne-Slove A, Rymer R (2008) Celiac disease in adults: evaluation with MDCT enteroclysis. AJR Am.J.Roentgenol. 191:1483–1492

Terheggen G, Lanyi B, Schanz S, Hoffmann RM, Bohm SK, Leifeld L, Pohl C, Kruis W (2008) Safety, feasibility, and tolerability of ileocolonoscopy in inflammatory bowel disease. Endoscopy 40:656–663

Torkzad MR, Vargas R, Tanaka C, Blomqvist L (2007) Value of cine MRI for better visualization of the proximal small bowel in normal individuals. Eur.Radiol. 17:2964–2968

Traill ZC, Nolan DJ (1995) Technical report: intubation fluoroscopy times using a new enteroclysis tube. Clin.Radiol. 50:339–340

Triester SL, Leighton JA, Leontiadis GI, Fleischer DE, Hara AK, Heigh RI, Shiff AD, Sharma VK (2005) A meta-analysis of the yield of capsule endoscopy compared to other diagnostic modalities in patients with obscure gastrointestinal bleeding. Am.J.Gastroenterol. 100:2407–2418

Triester SL, Leighton JA, Leontiadis GI, Gurudu SR, Fleischer DE, Hara AK, Heigh RI, Shiff AD, Sharma VK (2006) A meta-analysis of the yield of capsule endoscopy compared to other diagnostic modalities in patients with non-stricturing small bowel Crohn's disease. Am.J.Gastroenterol. 101:954–964

Turina M, Mulhall AM, Mahid SS, Yashar C, Galandiuk S (2008) Frequency and surgical management of chronic complications related to pelvic radiation. Arch.Surg. 143:46–52

Vidal I, Podevin G, Piloquet H, Le RM, Fremond B, Aubert D, Leclair MD, Heloury Y (2009) Follow-up and surgical management of Peutz-Jeghers syndrome in children. J.Pediatr. Gastroenterol.Nutr. 48:419–425

Voderholzer WA, Ortner M, Rogalla P, Beinholzl J, Lochs H (2003) Diagnostic yield of wireless capsule enteroscopy in comparison with computed tomography enteroclysis. Endoscopy 35:1009–1014

Vogel J, da Luz MA, Baker M, Hammel J, Einstein D, Stocchi L, Fazio V (2007) CT enterography for Crohn's disease: accurate preoperative diagnostic imaging. Dis.Colon Rectum 50:1761–1769

Westerhof J, Koornstra JJ, Weersma RK (2009a) Can we reduce capsule endoscopy reading times? Gastrointest.Endosc. 69:497–502

Westerhof J, Weersma RK, Koornstra JJ (2009b) Risk factors for incomplete small-bowel capsule endoscopy. Gastrointest.Endosc. 69:74–80

Wickramasekera D, Hay DJ, Fayz M (1999) Acute small bowel obstruction due to ileal endometriosis: a case report and literature review. J.R.Coll.Surg.Edinb. 44:59–60

Witherspoon P, Chalmers AG, Sagar PM (2009) Successful pregnancy after laparoscopic ileal pouch-anal anastomosis complicated by small bowel obstruction secondary to a single band adhesion. Colorectal Dis.

Young MA, Rose S, Reynolds JC (1996) Gastrointestinal manifestations of scleroderma. Rheum.Dis.Clin.North Am. 22:797–823

MRI of the Colon (MR Colonography): Technique

11

Sonja Kinner and Thomas C. Lauenstein

CONTENTS

11.1 Introduction 173

11.2 Basics for the Scan: Hardware 174
11.2.1 Main Magnet 174
11.2.2 Gradient System 174
11.2.3 HF-System 174

11.3 Patient Preparation and Prerequisites 175
11.3.1 Bowel Preparation 175
11.3.1.1 Bowel Cleansing 175
11.3.1.2 Fecal Tagging 176
11.3.2 Bowel Distention 177
11.3.2.1 Water-Based Distension 177
11.3.2.2 Other Distension Media 177
11.3.2.3 Impact of Spasmolytic Agents 178
11.3.3 Image Contrast 179
11.3.3.1 Bright Lumen MRC 179
11.3.3.2 Dark Lumen MRC 179

11.4 The Scan: Performance of MRC 180

11.5 After the Scan: Postprocessing and Image Analysis 181

11.6 Particularities of MR of the Colon at 3 T 182

References 183

KEY POINTS

MR of the colon with bowel preparation and distension (MR colonography) has gained access into clinical routine as a diagnostic tool for the evaluation of the large bowel. MR colonography can be used as an alternative for optical colonoscopy and computed tomography colonography, particularly in patients with incomplete optical colonoscopy. In addition, MR colonography is studied as a screening tool combining noninvasiveness and no ionizing radiation. The lack of ionizing radiation exposition makes MR colonography attractive to be used in young patients with IBD as well. This chapter focuses on technical aspects of MRI of the colon, including MR colonography, and the following aspects will be discussed: hardware requirements, patient preparation, examination proceedings as well as image analysis and interpretation.

Sonja Kinner, MD
Department of Diagnostic and Interventional Radiology and Neuroradiology, University Hospital Essen, Hufelandstrasse 55, 45122 Essen, Germany
Thomas C. Lauenstein, MD
Privatdozent, Department of Radiology, University Hospital Essen, Hufelandstrasse 55, 45122 Essen, Germany

11.1 Introduction

Optical colonoscopy is regarded as the reference standard for the assessment of colorectal pathology (colorectal neoplasia; bowel wall inflammation) and subsequent biopsies. Virtual colonography (virtual colonoscopy) has advantages over optical colonoscopy as it is less invasive and less burdensome. Furthermore, analysis is not limited to the bowel itself. Rather, all surrounding abdominal structures can be assessed as well. Because of economical rationale and higher clinical availability, most strategies of colonography have focused on CT colonography in the past. Several studies in screening populations have demonstrated the potential of CT colonography, but ionizing radiation exposure remains a drawback of CT colonography. Thus, MR colonography (MRC) has gained increasing interest. In addition to the lack of ionizing radiation, MRI allows a high soft tissue contrast (T1w/T2w imaging). Perfusion information can be obtained after the intravenous administration of gadolinium. This chapter focuses on technical aspects of MRI of the colon, including MRC, and the following aspects will be discussed: hardware requirements, patient preparation, examination proceedings, image analysis and interpretation as well as an overview of typical indications of MRC. Current available evidence on results of MRI of the colon, including MRC, will be reviewed in Chap 12.

11.2
Basics for the Scan: Hardware

To visualize the entire colon, a large field of view (FOV) in z-direction is needed. Usually, an FOV of 45 cm is sufficient to display the entire cranio-caudal length of the large bowel. In particularly large patients, an FOV of 45 cm may not be sufficient. In these cases, the examination should be split into two blocks, namely (a) the upper part of the abdomen, which normally includes the distal part of the ascending colon, transverse colon, and the proximal part of the descending colon and (b) the lower abdomen/pelvis, which in case of a normal anatomical setting, comprises the cecal area, the proximal part of the ascending colon, distal part of the descending colon, sigmoid, and rectum. The following system components have to fulfill special requirements for MRI of the colon:

1. The main magnet with its homogeneity of the magnetic field for the complete imaging volume
2. The gradient system with its linearity for the imaging volume
3. The high frequency (HF) system with its HF-signal homogeneity and signal susceptibility for the imaging volume

11.2.1
Main Magnet

The magnet of a magnetic resonance scanner used for MRI of the colon should feature a high magnetic field strength to allocate adequate magnetization and guarantee a high signal-to-noise-ratio (SNR) for good image quality. Magnets with field strengths from 1 T – preferably 1.5 T – are currently the clinical standard and may be complemented in clinical practice by 3 T magnets, as outlined in Sect. 11.6. The advantage of 1.5 T systems is related to combination of two facts: First, short acquisition times of single-shot or gradient echo sequences can be achieved, which should not exceed 15–20 s as data collection is performed under breath-hold conditions. This prerequisite can often not be met by a 1 T scanner. Second, image robustness is high and prevalence of artifacts is low when 1.5 T systems are used, compared with 3 T systems.

The basic magnetic field should show a high homogeneity for the whole examined volume to ensure minor imaging distortion and high signal homogeneity. The FOV should be at least 45 cm in z-direction to cover the whole imaging region abdomen/pelvis. A cylindrical configuration of the main magnet is conducive for these requirements and is currently the most encountered magnet configuration.

11.2.2
Gradient System

Special needs have to be fulfilled to ensure a high spatial resolution during one single breath-hold for MRI of the colon

A rapid slew rate (mT/m/ms) in combination with a high gradient amplitude (mT/m) are prerequisites for short repetition and echo times (TR and TE). Thus, short acquisition times can be coupled with the coverage of a large imaging volume during one single breath-hold. In addition, the use of short TR is needed to obtain highly T1-weighted images to guaranty for a high contrast display of the contrast-enhanced bowel wall after intravenous gadolinium administration. Furthermore, short TR and TE times are a prerequisite to perform fast imaging with balanced steady-state precession sequences (TrueFISP, Balanced Fast Field Echo, or FIESTA), which are part of the standard MRC protocol. Furthermore, the gradient system should deliver a high gradient linearity for a high volume to minimize image distortion at the border of the imaging range. These prerequisites can be best realized using a cylindrical configuration of the gradient coil.

11.2.3
HF-System

A homogeneous HF signal reception is important. For signal reception, the whole body HF coil integrated in

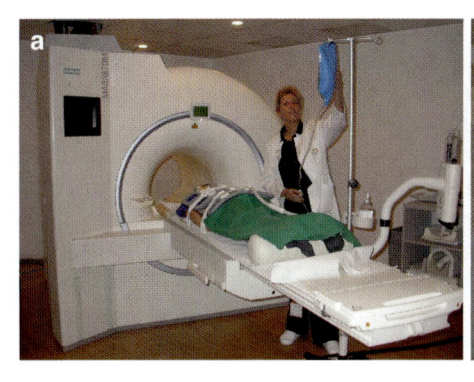

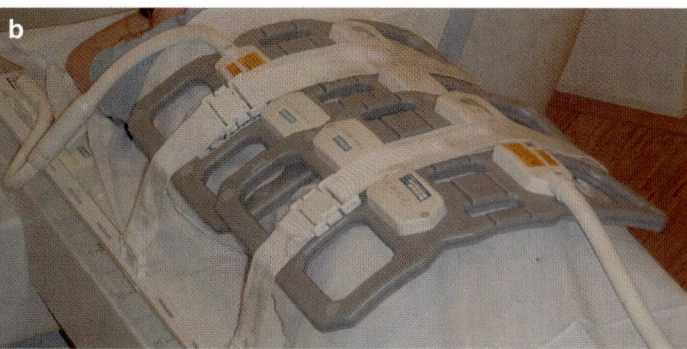

Fig. 11.1. For MR colonography (MRC), patients are usually scanned in prone position (**a**). The rectal enema consisting of warm tap water is administered via an enema bag using hydrostatic pressure. A combination of two flex surface array coils (**b**) is placed on the patient's back to cover the whole abdomen and pelvis

the magnet is limited concerning signal-to-noise ratio (SNR). Therefore, a combination of different HF surface coils should be used. These surface coils receive signal from surrounding tissue while detecting only noise from a limited area, which leads to a relatively high SNR. To cover larger anatomical areas, coil elements have to be combined to phased array coils (Fig. 11.1). These phased array coils are the basis for the application of parallel imaging techniques (Griswold et al. 2002). With parallel imaging techniques, larger anatomical areas can be captured per time unit. Alternatively, the spatial resolution can be increased for the same acquisition time or a combination of both can be applied. Thus, a combination of two prerequisites can be accomplished. MR images from the entire abdomen and pelvis can be collected during one single breath. Furthermore, a high spatial resolution of MR images can be achieved and even relatively small lesions of the bowel wall (<5 mm) can be visualized.

11.3
Patient Preparation and Prerequisites

In a first step, general contraindications for MR imaging like presence of pacemakers, heart defibrillators, or other electrical implants have to be excluded. Claustrophobia, existence of hip prosthesis, or other metal implants are relative contraindications and a decision to examine these patients has to be discussed in clinical context (Lauenstein 2006). To achieve good image quality and to ensure diagnostic assessment of the colon, several conditions have to be considered, which are described below.

11.3.1
Bowel Preparation

Depending on the clinical indication, patients can be subjected to bowel preparation schemes. In case of performing MRC, several methods can be applied. Each approach has its strengths and weaknesses regarding image quality and patient acceptance.

11.3.1.1
Bowel Cleansing

For evaluation of MRC, a large contrast between bowel wall and bowel contents is mandatory. Most obvious approach is that patients have to undergo bowel purgation similar to the procedure as applied prior to colonoscopy. This process should begin on the afternoon before the MR scan. Several different substances for bowel cleansing are commercially available (Tan and Tjandra 2006). Those can be mainly subdivided into polyethylene–glycol–elyte (PEG) solutions and sodium phosphate based solutions. Both solutions show equal results for bowel cleansing and can be used alternatively except for pediatric and elderly patients, patients with bowel obstruction, and other structural intestinal disorders, gut dysmotility, renal failure, congestive heart failure, or liver failure as sodium phosphate based solutions are hyperosmolar and can lead to electrolyte disturbances.

When a bowel purgation protocol is used, MRC should be performed in the morning to avoid unnecessary patient discomfort. Insufficient bowel cleansing and presence of residual fecal material may result in diagnostic difficulties. Residual stool can impede the assessment of the bowel wall and lead to false-negative (if stool masks pathologies) or false-positive (if stool mimics pathologies like polyps/masses) findings. In general, this type of bowel preparation is widely used in CT colonography and double contrast barium enema and has good results with regard to cleansing. However, patient acceptance is comparable with standard colonoscopy cleansing, the most burdensome part of a colonoscopy procedure.

11.3.1.2
Fecal Tagging

Up to 75% of patients undergoing bowel cleansing complain about various symptoms related to the cleansing procedure (Thomeer et al. 2002). These side-effects include symptoms such as "feeling unwell" and "the inability to sleep." Therefore, patient acceptance is negatively impacted. Elimination of bowel cleansing therefore would theoretically result in a higher patient acceptance of MRC. "Fecal tagging" is such a concept avoiding bowel purgation (Bielen et al. 2003; Papanikolaou et al. 2003). Based on the ingestion of contrast compounds to regular meals prior to the examination, signal intensity of fecal material is modified and adapted to the signal properties of the rectal enema. Hence, fecal material becomes "virtually invisible." First approaches were based on the ingestion of gadolinium-labeled foodstuff in conjunction with a gadolinium-based rectal enema (bright lumen MRC). However, this strategy was costly and was given up as bright lumen MRC is less utilized nowadays.

Highly concentrated barium sulfate has been proposed for fecal tagging in several volunteers and patient studies providing diagnostic image quality for dark lumen MRC (Lauenstein et al. 2001, 2002). Patients were asked to ingest 200 ml of barium sulfate (Micropaque, Guerbet) with each main meal within 48 h prior to the MR scan. On T1w images, the fecal material has a low signal intensity and facilitate evaluation of the bowel wall, with good differentiation between the homogeneously "dark" colonic lumen and the contrast-enhanced bowel wall. However, it has been demonstrated that ingestion of (100 vol%) barium-based substances can result in limited patient acceptance as well (Goehde et al. 2005). Thus, other tagging substances were to be evaluated. Several requirements need to be fulfilled: tagging substances must mix well with foodstuff and stool, they must not be reabsorbed in the GI tract, must alter signal characteristics of fecal material adequately, and must be easy for the patients to be ingested.

Another tagging strategy uses a solution containing 5% gastrografin, 1% barium, and 0.2% locust bean gum. This fecal tagging approach has been tested with regard to patient acceptance (Kinner et al. 2007). A total of 284 asymptomatic patients have been evaluated with this approach. The tagging solution (250 cc) was ingested with every main meal starting 2 days before the MR examination. MRC was performed on a 1.5-T MR system in conjunction with a rectal enema of tap water. Ingestion of the tagging solution led to a low signal of fecal material on T1w images (Fig. 11.2) and thus allowed a good differentiation between the dark lumen (filled with tagged stool and water) and the bright bowel wall (after i.v. gadolinium administration). Optical colonoscopy (in conjunction with bowel purgation) was performed within 1 month after MRC. Each 24 h following both examinations, patient acceptance was assessed based on a standardized questionnaire. Patients rated the bowel cleansing prior to optical colonoscopy significantly more unpleasant when compared with the ingestion of the tagging agent for MRC.

The question still remains whether fecal tagging should always be used for MRC bowel preparation.

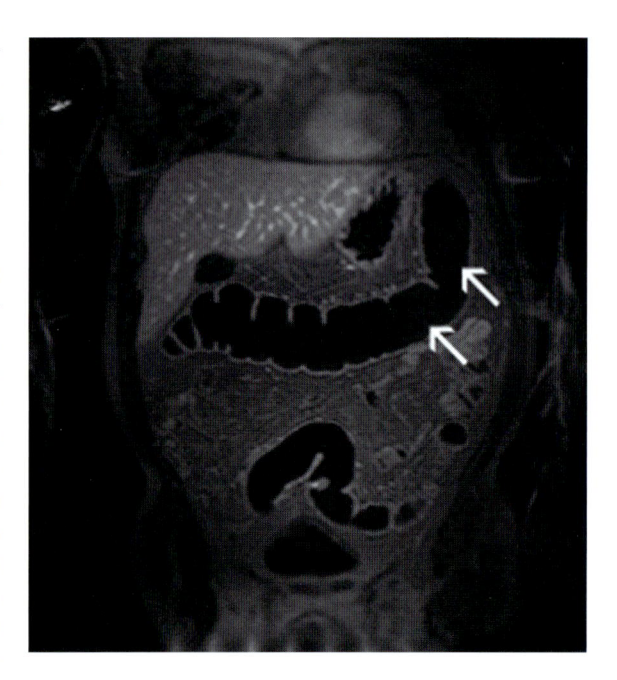

Fig. 11.2. Fifty-four-year-old male patient undergoing MRC for colorectal cancer screening. A fecal tagging approach was used for bowel preparation. On the gadolinium enhanced T1w images, signal of stool (e.g., in the distal transverse colon; *arrows*) is almost as low as the signal of the rectal water enema. Thus, the colonic lumen appears homogeneously dark and can be easily differentiated from the bright colonic wall

We believe that both methods (fecal tagging and bowel purgation) have their value. If applied in detecting colorectal polyps and colorectal cancer, fecal tagging should be preferably applied in screening patients (with a low expected prevalence of colorectal lesions). However, bowel purgation should be applied for patients with a high-risk profile (e.g., in the context of clinical symptoms or patient history). Whenever a colorectal mass is seen on MRC, the patient can directly undergo colonoscopy for polypectomy or tissue sampling without the need of an additional bowel preparation.

11.3.2
Bowel Distention

Most colonic loops are collapsed under physiological conditions. Hence, bowel loops have to be distended to differentiate the bowel wall (and pathologic findings arising from it) from the bowel lumen (DACHMAN et al. 2007). Insufficient bowel distension may result in both false-positive and/or false-negative findings: unfolded bowel segments may mimic bowel thickening leading to a misinterpretation of colonic inflammation or tumor (KINNER and LAUENSTEIN 2007; ROTTGEN et al. 2003). Even larger masses can be missed in nondistended bowel segments. In a study by Kay et al. (2000), 2 out of 24 colorectal lesions were missed by MRC due to collapsed bowel segments. Some centers propose the colon to be imaged without rectal contrast, for example in conjunction with MR enterography or enteroclysis. However, a poor distension may harbor the risk of reduced diagnostic accuracy.

The application of different liquid contrast agents (water, barium solutions) via a rectal tube or the insufflation of air/CO_2 has been proposed to ensure adequate bowel distension (LOMAS et al. 2001; AJAJ et al. 2004).

11.3.2.1
Water-Based Distension

Tap Water

Most departments use tap water at a comfortable temperature for bowel distension, because a consistently high distension can be achieved, while CO_2 is easily reabsorbed in the colon. A further advantage of water as a distension medium is related to its biphasic signal character. Because of the high T2 signal of water, the colonic lumen can be easily differentiated from the low-signal bowel wall on T2w images. CO_2, however, is dark on T2w MRI, thereby limiting the value of T2w MRC. Usually 1,500 mL of water is administered to ensure sufficiently high bowel distension.

Water-Based Barium Solutions

Initial strategies of MRC (LAUENSTEIN et al. 2001) used barium-based rectal enemas (1% barium sulfate). However, this strategy is not used anymore as water-based rectal enemas result in the same signal properties and water is less expensive.

Water/Gadolinium Mixture

Applying this technique, the colon is filled in prone position via a rectal catheter with 1,500–2,000 mL of a water-based enema. The water is to be labeled 1:100 with a gadolinium-containing contrast agent (LUBOLDT et al. 2000). On the T1w data sets, only the colonic lumen containing the enema is bright, whereas all other tissues remain low in signal intensity. This "bright lumen" technique relies on the visualization of filling defects. Bowel wall and enhancement characteristics cannot be assessed by using this technique. Another negative aspect is the higher cost of gadolinium.

11.3.2.2
Other Distension Media

CO_2

CO_2 can be alternatively used for colonic distension. This approach was introduced by Lomas et al. (2001). They examined seven patients with known colonic tumors using a CO_2 enema. MRC was evaluated for depiction of tumor and adjacent structures using surgical findings as the reference standard. In all seven patients, the tumor was demonstrated, and in four patients breach of the muscularis propria was correctly predicted. Although a promising tool, this technology is only rarely used. The underlying reason is the relatively complex technical procedure of CO_2 insufflation as MRI compatible insufflators have to be used. When adjusted for use near an MRI suite, a constant intracolonic pressure is obtained with such an insufflator compensating for colonic absorption, ileocecal reflux, and incontinence for gas.

Air

The group of Morrin et al. described first the implementation of MRC with air insufflation. They could prove that MRC using room air was a feasible virtual colonoscopy technique. Air distention was well tolerated by patients and resultant images provided adequate luminal distention and wall conspicuity (Morrin et al. 2001).

Ajaj et al. (2004) compared MRC in conjunction room air insufflations to water-based MRC in terms of image quality and patient acceptance. No significant differences were seen between the two techniques with regard to discomfort levels and image quality. The presence of air in the colonic lumen did not result in the presence of susceptibility artifacts. Interestingly, contrast to noise ratio (CNR) of the contrast-enhanced colonic wall as well as bowel distension were superior on air-distended 3D data sets. This can be explained by the low T1 signal of air, while water (especially when mixed with residual fecal material) may show an intermediate T1 signal. The better distension of MRC with room air can be attributed to the low colonic reabsorption of air (in contrast to CO_2). Authors concluded that MRC can be performed using either water or air for colonic distension. Both techniques permit assessment of the colonic wall and identification of colorectal masses.

Other

Zhang et al. evaluated in 2007 the feasibility of detection of colorectal pathologies with fat enema in MRC using T1-weighted fast spoiled gradient-echo with inversion recovery sequence (Zhang et al. 2007). Following the placement of a rectal enema tube (Shuangling Medical Device, China), fat contrast medium (Kangque; Atai medical system, Inner Mongolia, China) was gently administered into the colon at up to 1 m of hydrostatic pressure with the patient lying in the prone position. The fat contrast medium mainly contained salad oil, acacia, menthol, and distilled water. Neoplasms >10 mm could be detected correctly while patients tolerated this technique well.

11.3.2.3
Impact of Spasmolytic Agents

Spasmolytic agents (e.g., 20 mg scopolamine or 1 mg glucagon) should be administered intravenously (Rogalla et al. 2005). They provide greater bowel distention, obviate bowel spasms, and minimize artifacts caused by bowel motion. In addition, patient acceptance of a rectal enema will increase after spasmolysis. The administration should be started prior to the rectal filling process. As half-life of some spasmolytic agents is low, a second injection can be performed prior to the data acquisition of the T1w gradient echo sequences.

Glucagon

Glucagon (GlucaGen, Novo Nordisk Pharma) is a polypeptide hormone, which – apart from the effect of rising blood glucose levels – can relax smooth muscles. However, the colon has been found to be least sensitive to the effects of glucagon compared with other parts of the gastrointestinal tract (Chernish and Maglinte 1990; Morrin et al. 2002). Adverse reactions rarely occur and present mainly with nausea, vomiting, and headache. Usage of Glucagon is contraindicated in patients with pheochromocytoma, insulinoma, poorly controlled diabetes, or a former adverse reaction to glucagon. Usually, a dosage of 1 mg is intravenously administered. The half-life is short ranging from 8 to 18 min (http://www.glucagenhypokit.com/Hypokit_Pi.pdf).

Butylscopolamine

Butylscopolamine is also known as scopolamine butylbromide and hyoscine butylbromide. It is a quaternary ammonium compound and a semisynthetic derivative of scopolamine with an antimuscarinic, anticholinergic effect. The blockade of parasympathetic ganglia causes relaxation of smooth muscle. While it is not FDA approved and therefore not used in the US, Butylscopolamine is widely utilized in Europe and Asia. In different studies, butylscopolamine has proven to be more effective than glucagon in distending the colon (Goei et al. 1995; Rogalla et al. 2005). Butylscopolamine is contraindicated for patients with glaucoma, obstructive uropathy, gastrointestinal tract obstruction or ileus, as well as myasthenia gravis and unstable cardiac disease. A frequent side effect is blurred vision. Furthermore, tachycardia, dry mouth, and acute urinary retention can occur. Usually, a dosage of 20 mg is given intravenously. Some authors have proposed the intramuscular injection of the substance (Wagner et al. 2008). The intravenous administration of the substance results in a rapid distribution in the whole body. In blood, the half-life time for the substance is only 4 min (http://ch.oddb.org/de/gcc/resolve/pointer/!fachinfo). Hence, a second injection prior to the acquisition of the contrast-enhanced T1w images should be considered.

11.3.3
Image Contrast

A high contrast between bowel lumen and wall is crucial to visualize pathologies arising from the bowel wall. This can be achieved in two different ways either using a dark colonic lumen and bright colonic wall or vice versa. The contrast mechanisms depend on the sequence types and the applied rectal and intravenous contrast media.

11.3.3.1
Bright Lumen MRC

First MRC approaches were implemented using a bright lumen technique. The colon is filled with 2,000 cc of an enema consisting of water labeled 1:100 with a gadolinium-containing contrast agent. After finishing the bowel filling process, a T1w data set of the abdomen encompassing the entire colon is collected. To compensate for the presence of residual air exhibiting no signal within the colon, the data acquisition needs to be performed in both the prone and supine position. On the T1w data sets, only the colonic lumen containing the enema is bright whereas all other tissues remain low in signal intensity. Differential diagnostic considerations for luminal filling defects within the bright colonic lumen include residual air, residual fecal material, or a polypoid colonic mass. Differentiating aspects for residual air and residual stool include the gravity-dependent position, i.e., the motion from prone to the supine data set. On the other hand, polyps remain largely unchanged in position in both prone and supine data sets.

Another "bright lumen" MRC technique is based on the acquisition of TrueFISP or HASTE sequences. Using a rectal water-enema, the contrast mechanism is comparable with that of the approach in conjunction with a paramagnetic contrast enema and the acquisition of T1w GRE sequences. Again, data acquisition must be performed in both prone and supine position. Main drawback of the bright lumen technology remains the limited sensitivity and specificity for the detection of colorectal masses: both false-positive or false-negative results can be frequently seen: polyps with a long stalk may move sufficiently to be disregarded as residual stool, while stool adherent to the colonic wall may not move at all and thus falsely impress as a polyp (LAUENSTEIN et al. 2005).

11.3.3.2
Dark Lumen MRC

The detection of colorectal lesions with "bright lumen" MRC relies on the visualization of filling defects. "Dark lumen" MRC, however, is based on a contrast mechanism generated between a brightly enhancing colonic wall and a homogeneously dark colonic lumen. Instead of using a gadolinium enema, only water or air is rectally applied rendering low-signal on T1-weighted 3D GRE acquisitions. To obtain a bright colonic wall, a paramagnetic contrast compound is applied intravenously. After a first precontrast T1-weighted 3D gradient echo data set, paramagnetic contrast should be administered i.v. at a dosage of 0.1–0.2 mmol/kg. The 3D acquisition should be repeated in the coronal plane after a delay of 70 and 120 s. We additionally recommend taking advantage of the contrast injection and the relatively long delay before the first contrast-enhanced coronal 3D data set. Thus, the liver can be imaged in an arterial phase (e.g., after a contrast delay of 20 s) using the same sequence. This sequence should be additionally collected after 180 s to provide information of an equilibrium contrast phase. This is especially important for fibrotic changes of the bowel wall (e.g., in patients with CED), which show some form of late enhancement. Since residual air exhibits no signal in the colonic lumen, the examination has to be performed in either prone or supine position. Furthermore, the "dark lumen" technique copes with the problem of residual stool in an easy way: if the lesion enhances it is a polyp or carcinoma, if it does not enhance it represents stool. Potential colorectal lesions have to be analyzed by comparing signal intensities on the pre- and postcontrast images. If analysis were limited to the postcontrast data set, bright stool could be misinterpreted as a polyp. Comparison with the precontrast images documents the lack of contrast enhancement, which assures the correct diagnosis. The use of intravenously administered contrast material significantly improves reader confidence in the assessment of bowel wall conspicuity and the ability to depict medium-sized polyps in suboptimally prepared colons. Besides, "dark lumen" MRC permits a direct analysis of the bowel wall. This facilitates the evaluation of inflammatory changes in patients with

IBD. Increased contrast uptake and bowel wall thickening is an indicator for the degree of inflammation. Furthermore, the intravenous application of paramagnetic contrast permits a more reliable assessment of parenchymal abdominal organs contained within the FOV. Particularly, the liver can be accurately evaluated regarding the presence and type of concomitant pathology such as metastatic disease.

11.4
The Scan: Performance of MRC

Patients have to be informed about the procedure and the risks and adverse effects of intravenous contrast administration. An intravenous access should be placed in an arm vein prior to the scan. The patient has to be placed in lateral position on the scanner table. Drapery for potentially leaking distension media has to be on the table if tap water or watery solutions are used. The radiologist now carefully performs a rectal examination and subsequently places a rectal tube or a Foley catheter in the rectum. The patient turns hereafter in prone position. Supine position can also be used, as it may be perceived more comfortably by the patient and breath-hold instructions can be easily met. However, prone position harbors some advantages as the distension may be increased (Cronin et al. 2008).

Two body surface coils for signal reception should be used to ensure the coverage of the entire abdomen and pelvis. Subsequently, the patient is moved into the scanner. The image center should be on the level of the kidneys. A localizer sequence is applied to ensure full coverage of the colon in craniocaudal direction. The application of the rectal enema should only be started after i.v. spasmolysis. We propose the use of a tap water enema of approximately 1,500–2,000 mL. Instillation of the enema should be carried out in stages over a 1-min period to reduce discomfort and bowel cramping. However, the filling process should be stopped if the patient complains about pain or abdominal cramps. By means of fast T2-weighted sequences (e.g., RARE or FISP sequences), the degree of filling can be controlled.

MRC sequences should be collected during one breath-hold. Thus, mainly three sequences are appropriate (Fig. 11.3), which constitute our standard protocol: A T2-weighted single-shot-fast-spin-echo (SSFSE) sequence with fat saturation in coronal and/or axial plane are acquired. These sequences are important to depict edema in or adjacent to the bowel wall, to detect active inflammation of the bowel wall. Afterwards, the acquisition of 2D and/or 3D fast imaging with balanced steady-state precession sequences in the coronal plane should be performed. This sequence should be performed without fat saturation as the technique allows good visualization not only of the colon but also of the mesentery, including mesenteric lymph nodes, which can be a helpful indicator of pericolonic inflammation. Different vendor names are used for this sequences type: TrueFISP (Siemens Medical Solution, Erlangen, Germany), Balanced Fast Field Echo (Philips

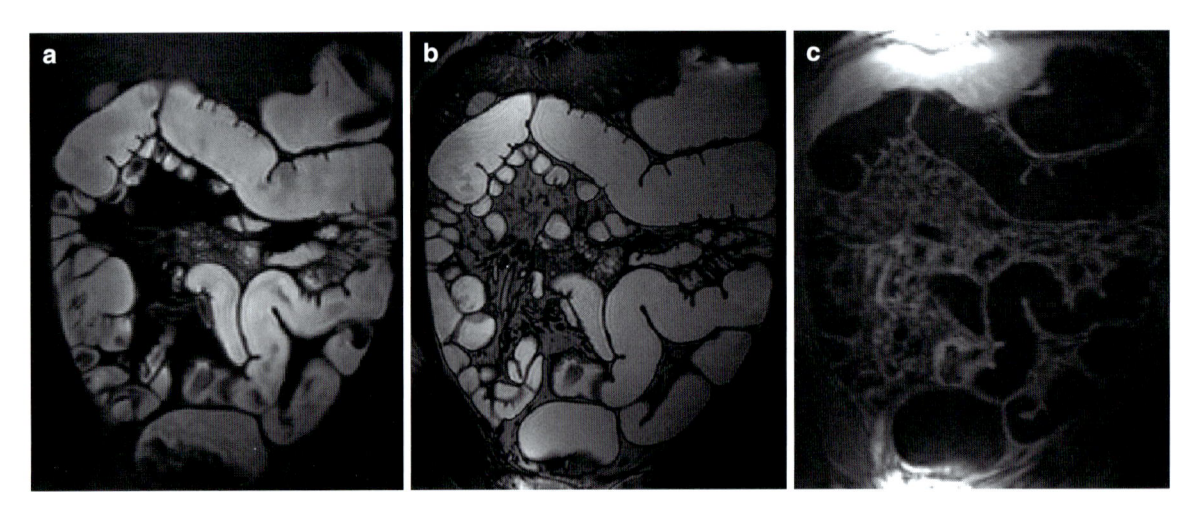

Fig. 11.3. Sixty-year-old male screening patient. Typical sequences used for MRC: (**a**) T2-weighted single-shot-fast-spin-echo (SSFSE) sequence with fat saturation (bright-lumen MRC); (**b**) fast imaging with steady-state precession (FISP) sequence (bright-lumen MRC); (**c**) T1-weighted sequences (3D gradient echo sequence) before and – as shown here – after i.v. gadolinium contrast injection (dark-lumen MRC)

Fig. 11.4. Seventy-two-year-old male screening patient. Motion artifacts can hamper image analysis in GRE-T1-w sequences due to motion/breathing artifacts (**a**: dark-lumen MRC). FISP sequences (**b**: bright-lumen MRC) is less sensitive to motion is exhibits a more robust image quality in this patient

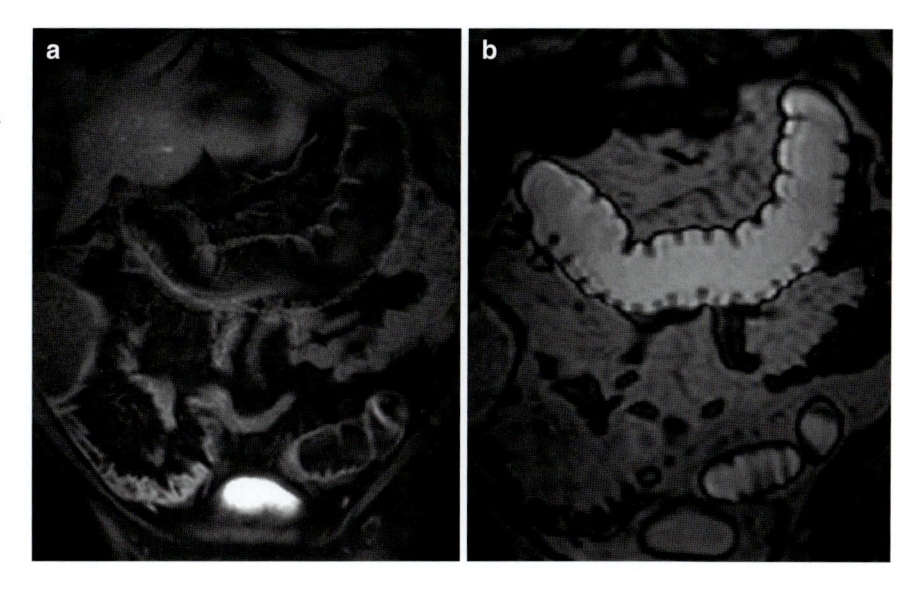

Medical Systems, Best, the Netherlands), or FIESTA (GE Medical Systems, Milwaukee, Wisconsin). Images are characterized by a mixture of both T1 and T2 contrast, creating a homogeneous bright signal of the colonic water-filled lumen. One main advantage of True-FISP is its robustness as it is insensitive to motion and thus particularly helpful in patients unable to hold their breath (Fig. 11.4).

Finally, dynamic T1-weighted sequences (3D gradient echo sequence) should be collected in coronal plane. After a first nonenhanced scan, gadolinium should be administered intravenously and the 3D acquisition should be repeated at several time points (see "Butylscopolamine"). After the last coronal scan, an additional axial scan for the whole FOV can be performed. Sequence parameters are shown in Table 11.1. Once data collection is finished, the enema is drawn back into the enema bag. The rectal tube or catheter is removed and the patient can leave the scanner. Mean examination time of an MRC amounts to 20–25 min.

11.5
After the Scan: Postprocessing and Image Analysis

All data sets should be analyzed on a postprocessing or a good PACS workstation. 3D T1-weighted MR data sets before and after contrast administration can be viewed in a multiplanar reformation mode. Image interpretation should be initially based on contrast-enhanced T1-weighted data sets. If a suspicious

Table 11.1. Sequence parameters for MR Colonography

	2D T2w SSFSE with fat saturation	2D FISP without fat saturation	3D T1w GRE with fat saturation
TR (ms)	1,200	4.5	3.1
TE (ms)	60	2.3	1.3
Flip (degree)	90	60	10
Slice thickness (mm)	6	3	1.8
FOV (mm)	500	500	400
Matrix	256	256	256

SSFSE steady-state fast spin echo; *True-FISP* fast imaging with steady-state precession; *GRE* gradient recalled echo; *TE* echo time; *TR* repetition time; *FOV* field of view; *2D* two-dimensional; *3D* three-dimensional

colorectal lesion is detected, a comparison with the unenhanced scan should be performed to prove contrast uptake of the lesion. Carcinoma and polyps always show contrast uptake while stool residuals appear with high signal intensities on unenhanced and enhanced scans. Thus, false-positive results can be prevented (Figs. 11.5 and 11.6). Fat-saturated T2-weighted sequences will help to differentiate between active and inactive inflammatory processes, as active inflammation shows high signal intensity due to edema in or next to the bowel wall (Fig. 11.7). If the patient is incompliant, the FISP sequence can be of help because of its robustness and

Fig. 11.5. Fifty-seven-year-old female screening patient. Residual stool (*arrows*) may mimic colonic lesions on T1-weighted images after i.v. contrast injection (**a**: dark-lumen MRC). A comparison with the precontrast scan (**b**: dark-lumen MRC) reveals lack of enhancement and high signal even in the noncontrast scan. Thus, fecal material can be accurately differentiated from polyps

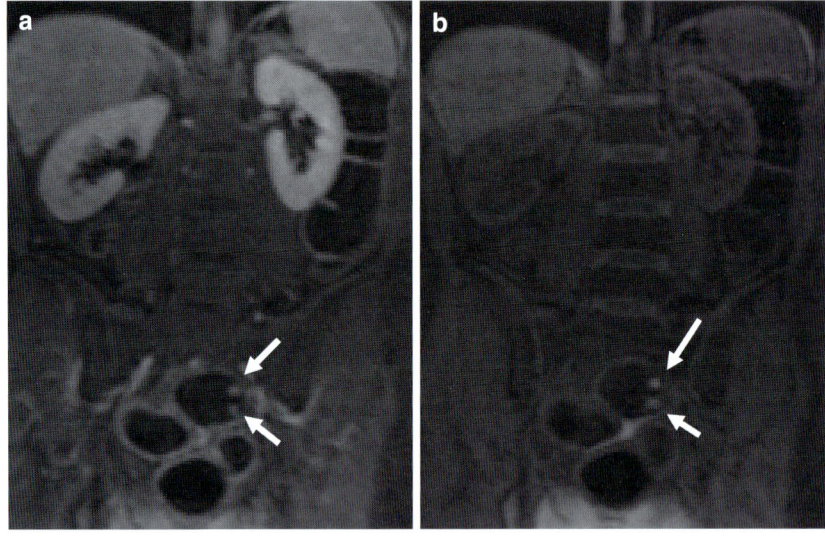

Fig. 11.6. Imaging examples show a rectal polyp in a 58-year-old male patient undergoing MRC for colorectal cancer screening. Note the contrast enhancement after i.v. contrast injection (**b**: dark-lumen MRC) compared with the unenhanced scan (**a**: dark-lumen MRC). Thus, a polyp (*arrows*) can be accurately differentiated from stool residuals

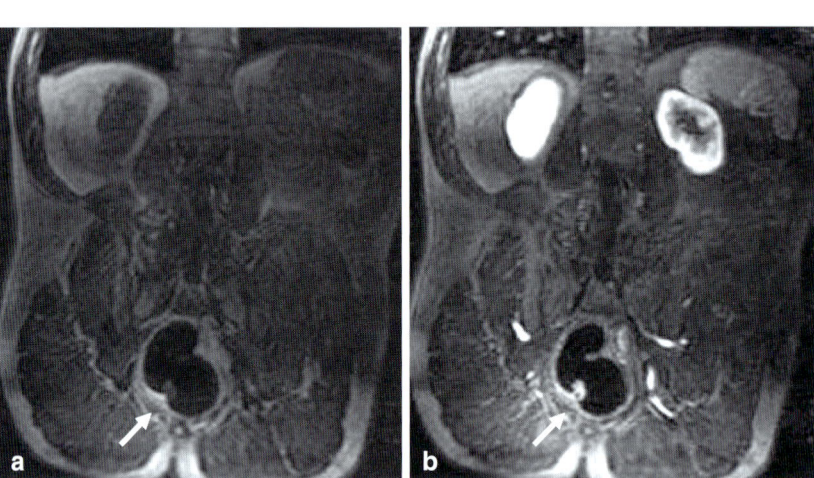

minor sensitivity for motion artifacts (LAUENSTEIN et al. 2005). Also, chronic inflammatory processes as well as fistulas can be detected with FISP sequences (GOURTSOYIANNIS and PAPANIKOLAOU 2005) (Fig. 11.8). Additionally, software tools allow for processing 3D data sets to virtually endoscopic interior views. While these virtual endoscopic flights are routinely used for CT colonoscopy, image analysis of MR data should primarily be based on source data. This as signal intensity fluctuations hamper 3D fly through.

11.6
Particularities of MR of the Colon at 3 T

Sequence protocols for MR of the colon have to be modified for the application at 3 T and cannot be fully adopted from 1.5 T (see also Chap. 2) (MERKLE et al.

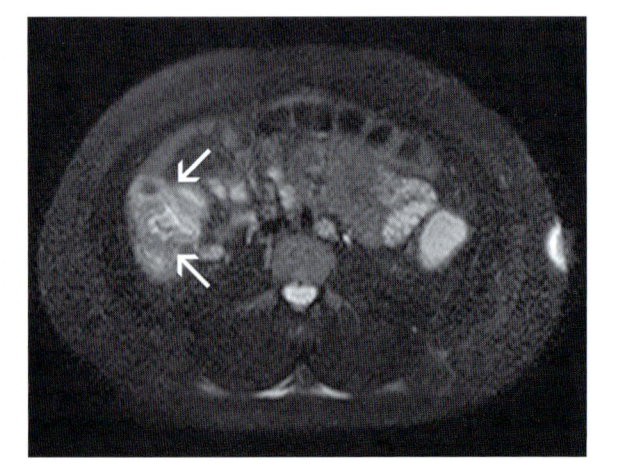

Fig. 11.7. Twenty-eight-year-old female patient with abdominal pain and diarrhea. Edema can be depicted in and adjacent to the bowel wall on fat-suppressed T2-weighted images (bright-lumen MRC; *arrows*). This is a sensitive indicator of active inflammatory disease

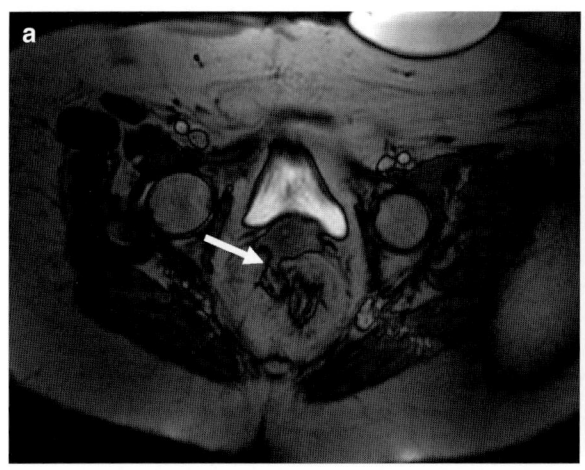

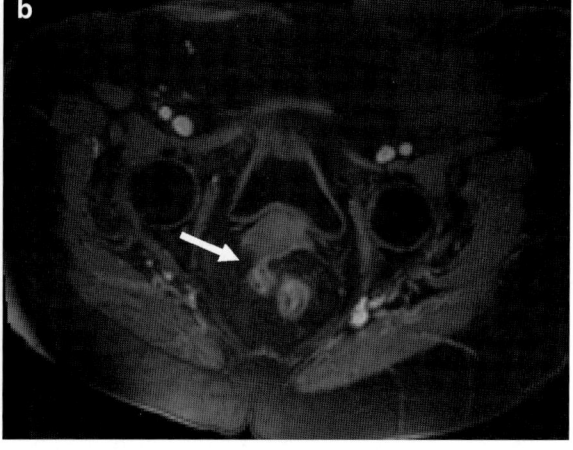

Fig. 11.8. Thirty-five-year-old female patient with Crohn's disease. FISP images (**a**: bright-lumen MRC) show fistula between the rectum and the uterus (*arrow*), which can also be detected by T1-weighted GRE sequence after i.v. gadolinium injection (**b**, **a**: dark-lumen MRC)

2006). Especially, problems with image artifacts, specific absorption rates (SAR) as well as hardware requirements have to be considered. At 3 T, the imaging signal is theoretically fourfold higher compared with that at 1.5 T. However, the signal-to-noise ratio (SNR) only doubles as the imaging noise also increases by factor of 2. The increased SNR can be used to increase spatial resolution or to decrease acquisition times.

MRC at 3 T is more prone to susceptibility artifacts than at 1.5 T. This is particularly true for the border of air and soft tissue. Although in most cases, water is used as rectal distension medium, appearance of residual air bubbles in the colon cannot be fully avoided. Thus, this can result in inferior visualization of colonic segments.

The specific sequence types have to be adapted to the conditions at 3 T. For the T2-weighted SSFSE sequences, times of repetition (TR) at 1.5 T range between 700 and 1,000 ms. Thus, short acquisition times can be associated with a satisfactory T2 signal. SAR limits the minimal TR at 3 T (approximately 1,500 ms). Therefore, an image is acquired only every 1.5 s, which makes it impossible to acquire the whole colon in one single breath-hold. Additionally, due to an intensified $T2^*$ effect, more imaging blurring can occur. Parallel imaging techniques can present a solution for this problem. With the help of parallel imaging techniques, the echo train length can be shortened, effective echo time (TE) can be decreased and allowed for sharper imaging resolution.

Other problems occur with the application of FISP sequences. Banding artifacts occur frequently at the edge of the FOV as these sequences are very susceptible to field inhomogeneities. These artifacts are pronounced at 3 T imaging. A solution for this problem is to subdivide the acquisition into multiple blocks along the z-axis. Hereby repeated centering can be performed, which enhances field homogeneity. Furthermore, differences of imaging contrast at FISP sequences have to be considered. In general, imaging contrast increases with lower TR and TE and higher flip angles. Lower flip angles have to be chosen at 3 T due to SAR limits. However, banding patterns also change at lower flip angles. Therefore, a low RF pulse should be applied and lower TR and TE can be chosen. To compensate for contrast loss, higher slice thicknesses for the FISP sequence at 3 T should be used.

Image quality can be considerably affected by alterations of TE for 3D T1-weighted gradient echo sequences at 3 T. Therefore, a high bandwidth should be chosen to ensure the use of a low TE. The advantage of robust image quality overbalances the reduction of SNR. In summary, application of 3D T1-weighted GRE sequences at 3 T are advantageous as a higher SNR can be achieved.

References

Ajaj WLT, Pelster G, Goehde SC, et al (2004) MR colonography: how does air compare to water for colonic distention? J Magn Reson Imaging 19(2):216–221

Bielen D, Thomeer M, Vanbeckevoort D, et al (2003) Dry preparation for virtual CT colonography with fecal tagging using water-soluble contrast medium: initial results. Eur Radiol 13(3):453–458

Chernish SM, Maglinte DD (1990) Glucagon: common untoward reactions–review and recommendations. Radiology 177(1):145–146

Cronin CG, Lohan DG, Mhuircheartaigh JN, et al (2008) MRI small-bowel follow-through: prone versus supine patient positioning for best small-bowel distention and lesion detection. AJR Am J Roentgenol 191(2):502–506

Dachman AH, Dawson DO, Lefere P, et al (2007) Comparison of routine and unprepped CT colonography augmented by low fiber diet and stool tagging: a pilot study. Abdom Imaging 32(1):96–104

Goehde SC, Descher E, Boekstegers A, et al (2005) Dark lumen MR colonography based on fecal tagging for detection of colorectal masses: accuracy and patient acceptance. Abdom Imaging 30(5):576–583

Goei R, Nix M, Kessels AH, et al (1995) Use of antispasmodic drugs in double contrast barium enema examination: glucagon or buscopan? Clin Radiol 50(8):553–557

Gourtsoyiannis NC, Papanikolaou N (2005) Magnetic resonance enteroclysis. Semin Ultrasound CT MR 26(4):237–246

Griswold MA, Jakob PM, Heidemann RM, et al (2002) Generalized autocalibrating partially parallel acquisitions (GRAPPA). Magn Reson Med 47(6):1202–1210

http//ch.oddb.org/de/gcc/resolve/pointer/!fachinfo.

http://www.glucagenhypokit.com/Hypokit_Pi.pdf.

Kay CL, Kulling D, Hawes RH, et al (2000) Virtual endoscopy– comparison with colonoscopy in the detection of space-occupying lesions of the colon. Endoscopy 32(3):226–232

Kinner S, Lauenstein TC (2007) MR colonography. Radiol Clin North Am 45(2):377–387

Kinner S, Kuehle CA, Langhorst J, et al (2007) MR colonography vs. optical colonoscopy: comparison of patients' acceptance in a screening population. Eur Radiol 17(9):2286–2293

Lauenstein T, Holtmann G, Schoenfelder D, et al (2001) MR colonography without colonic cleansing: a new strategy to improve patient acceptance. Am J Roentgenol 177(4):823–827

Lauenstein TC (2006) MR colonography: current status. Eur Radiol 16(7):1519–1526

Lauenstein TC, Goehde SC, Ruehm SG, et al (2002) MR colonography with barium-based fecal tagging: initial clinical experience. Radiology 223(1):248–254

Lauenstein TC, Ajaj W, Kuehle CA, et al (2005) Magnetic resonance colonography: comparison of contrast-enhanced three-dimensional vibe with two-dimensional FISP sequences: preliminary experience. Invest Radiol 40(2):89–96

Lomas DJ, Sood RR, Graves MJ, et al (2001) Colon carcinoma: MR imaging with CO_2 enema – Pilot Study. Radiology 219(2):558–562

Luboldt W, Bauerfeind P, Wildermuth S, et al (2000) Colonic masses: detection with MR colonography. Radiology 216(2):383–388

Merkle EM, Dale BM, Paulson EK (2006) Abdominal MR imaging at 3 T. Magn Reson Imaging Clin N Am 14(1):17–26

Morrin MM, Hochman MG, Farrell RJ, et al (2001) MR colonography using colonic distention with air as the contrast material: work in progress. AJR Am J Roentgenol 176(1):144–146

Morrin MM, Farrell RJ, Keogan MT, et al (2002) CT colonography: colonic distention improved by dual positioning but not intravenous glucagon. Eur Radiol 12(3):525–530

Papanikolaou N, Grammatikakis J, Maris T, et al (2003) MR colonography with fecal tagging: comparison between 2D turbo FLASH and 3D FLASH sequences. Eur Radiol. 13(3):448

Rogalla P, Lembcke A, Ruckert JC, et al (2005) Spasmolysis at CT colonography: butyl scopolamine versus glucagon. Radiology 236(1):184–188

Rottgen R, Schroder RJ, Lorenz M, et al (2003) [CT-colonography with the 16-slice CT for the diagnostic evaluation of colorectal neoplasms and inflammatory colon diseases]. Rofo 175(10):1384–1391

Tan JJ, Tjandra JJ (2006) Which is the optimal bowel preparation for colonoscopy – a meta-analysis. Colorectal Dis 8(4):247–258

Thomeer M, Bielen D, Vanbeckevoort D, et al (2002) Patient acceptance for CT colonography: what is the real issue? Eur Radiol 12(6):1410

Wagner M, Klessen C, Rief M, et al (2008) High-resolution T2-weighted abdominal magnetic resonance imaging using respiratory triggering: impact of butylscopolamine on image quality. Acta Radiol 49(4):376–382

Zhang S, Peng JW, Shi QY, et al (2007) Colorectal neoplasm: magnetic resonance colonography with fat enema-initial clinical experience. World J Gastroenterol 13(40):5371–5375

MRI of the Colon (Colonography): Results

Frank M. Zijta and Jaap Stoker

CONTENTS

12.1 Introduction 186

12.2 When to Perform MR of the Large Bowel 186

12.3 Detection of Precursors of Colorectal Cancer 186
12.3.1 Intermediate and Large Polyps 187
12.3.2 Image Interpretation 187
12.3.3 High Prevalence Population 188
12.3.3.1 Bright Lumen Strategy 188
12.3.3.2 Dark Lumen Strategy 190
12.3.3.3 Fecal Tagging 192
12.3.4 Low Prevalence Population 194
12.3.4.1 Screening MR Colonography 194

12.4 Colorectal Cancer (CRC) 194
12.4.1 Clinical Staging 194

12.5 Inflammatory Bowel Disease (IBD) 194
12.5.1 MRI of the Colon in Inflammatory Bowel Disease (IBD) 194
12.5.2 MR Colonography in IBD 195

12.6 Diverticular Disease (DD) and Acute Colonic Diverticulitis 198

12.7 Incomplete Colonoscopy 199

12.8 Patient Acceptance in MR Colonography 200
12.8.1 Bowel Preparation 200
12.8.2 Colonic Distension 201

12.9 Conclusion 201

References 202

KEY POINTS

Magnetic resonance imaging (MRI) has been increasingly studied as a diagnostic tool for the evaluation of the colon. Without the use of intraluminal colonic distension methods or following colonic distension with the use of either positive or negative luminal contrast medium (MR colonography), cross-sectional images can be acquired of the entire abdomen. Subsequent evaluation of the complete colonic wall can be executed using multiplanar reformations of the source data set with optional three dimensional (3D) rendering, in the case of a MR colonography data set. Although most investigators primarily focused on the ability of detecting colorectal polyps and masses using MR colonography, a wide spectrum of colorectal disorders can be evaluated by utilizing MRI to examine the colon.

Until now, no consensus has been reached regarding the technique and optimal bowel preparation of MR colonography. Current evidence suggests that MR colonography has sufficient accuracy for detecting colorectal cancer and clinical significant polyps. Efforts are made to replace rectal enemas by gaseous distension as in CT colonography, which may improve acceptance of MR colonography. The wide ranges of fecal tagging schemes give the possibility of limited bowel preparation in MR colonography. In addition, MR has a potential role in determining disease activity in inflammatory bowel disease of the colon and in incomplete colonoscopy.

Frank M. Zijta, MD
Jaap Stoker, MD, PhD
Department of Radiology, Academic Medical Center, Meibergdreef 9, Amsterdam, the Netherlands

12.1
Introduction

Radiological evaluation of the colon using MR imaging, has been increasingly applied over the last decade. Advances in MR technology, particularly the advent of faster T1 pulse sequences, resulted in reduced physiological artifacts and consequently facilitate bowel imaging and assessment. Although the examination can be performed without or with the rectal administration of a luminal contrast medium (MR colonography), most of the available literature reports on MR colonography. Yet it should be remembered that this selection primarily depends on the type of clinical indication, together with available expertise in this field.

When applying colonic distension, MRI offers a method for colon imaging comparable to computed tomography (CT) colonography. This method is considered to optimize MRI evaluation and results in – when compared to colonoscopy – a minimally invasive tool for evaluating the entire colon, permitting multiplanar imaging, and potentially enables three-dimensional (3D) rendering during postprocessing. Additionally, it provides information of the extra colonic organs which are not visible during colonoscopy. Advantage of MR colonography over CT colonography is the lack of the use of ionizing radiation and the high inherent soft tissue contrast, which allows the use of a wide range of "fecal tagging" regimes for bowel preparation. Whereas colonic distension in CT colonography typically entails the rectal administration of carbon dioxide or air, in MR colonography colonic distension is often acquired with the administration of a water-based enema and only few studies have reported on the usage of gaseous agents for colonic distension.

Since the introduction of MR colonography (Luboldt et al. 1997), research in this field is mainly focused at outlining its role in the detection of colorectal masses and subsequently describe the future potentials of this modality in screening for colorectal carcinoma (CRC) as it has proved to be accurate in detecting clinical relevant precursors of CRC (Zijta et al. 2009). However, the clinical indications for performing MR colonography reach beyond this and cover indications that are applied for both colonoscopy and CT colonography.

As outlined in Chap. 11, a variety of acquisition methods are described to perform MR colonography, but to date none of the different approaches have been shown to be superior. Regardless of the applied technique, prerequisite is a well distended colon, which is either cleansed or homogenously tagged, to permit an adequate assessment in an MR colonography setting.

This chapter presents an overview of the results of MR imaging of the large bowel on the basis of current evidence from literature at the moment of writing (June 2009). In the first part of this chapter, the diagnostic value of the techniques will be discussed for various clinical indications. The second part of the chapter will concern the patient's acceptance of the various techniques, as applied in MR colonography. Finally, future potentials and recommendations will be outlined.

12.2
When to Perform MR of the Large Bowel

The indications for performing MRI of the colon merely cover the indications that are applied for colonoscopy and/or CT colonography and can therefore include the diagnostic assessment of the colorectum of symptomatic patients for CRC, the colorectal assessment of asymptomatic individuals who are at average or increased risk for CRC, clinical staging evaluation in patients with CRC, assessment of colorectal involvement in patients with recognized or suspected inflammatory bowel disease (IBD), the evaluation of patients with incomplete or failed colonoscopy, and the evaluation of patients with suspected diverticular disease (DD) and acute colonic diverticulitis.

12.3
Detection of Precursors of Colorectal Cancer

In many western countries, colorectal cancer (CRC) is presently one of the leading causes of death from cancer in both men and women. If the disease is diagnosed in a localized stage, the 5-year survival is high. However, the 5-year survival rate drops to less than 10% if distant metastases are present (O'Connell et al. 2004).

Primary goals of CRC screening are to reduce both morbidity and mortality through a reduction in the incidence of the advanced staged disease and prevention of CRC by removal of benign precursors (adenomas). In screening for colonic cancer different techniques exists, of which fecal occult blood test (FOBT), double-contrast barium enema (DCBE), sigmoidoscopy, and colonoscopy are practicable techniques and more recently CT colonography was added to the list of CRC screening techniques of the American Cancer Society (Levin et al. 2008). Prospective randomized trials have demonstrated significant mortality reduction with FOBT screening. This as FOBT screening leads to earlier detection of invasive disease and removal of adenomatous polyps (Mandel et al. 2000).

12.3.1
Intermediate and Large Polyps

Histologically, colorectal polyps can be divided into adenomatous and hyperplastic in which adenomatous polyps comprise nearly two-third of all colorectal polyps. According to the adenoma-carcinoma sequence, adenomatous polyps have the potential to progress to CRC.

The potential risk for developing CRC from colorectal adenomas is related to both size and histology. Colonography enables the detection and size estimation of colorectal polyps and can therefore trigger future polypectomy at colonoscopy. Importantly, no histological distinction can be applied using colonography and size remains the most important criterion to estimate the potential to evolve into malignancy. Therefore, it is essential to define the potential CRC risk associated with each polyp size category, before data on MR colonography polyp detection rates (see Sects. 12.4.1 and 12.4.2) can be interpreted in their clinical context.

Irrespective of histology, colorectal polyps can be stratified into three generally accepted size thresholds, reflecting the potential risk to contain or progress into cancer. Large polyps are defined as polyps with a size of 10 mm or larger (≥10 mm) and a recent study demonstrated carcinoma in 2.6% and advanced histology in 30.6% of all polyps ≥10 mm. Of the 13 992 asymptomatic patients who underwent colonoscopy, malignancy was demonstrated in 0.2% of the intermediate polyps (6–9 mm), and the likelihood that polyps smaller than 5 mm ("diminutive" lesions) harbored malignancy was less than 0.1% (Lieberman et al. 2008).

A recently published simulation, which has inherent limitations, estimated the associated risk for a large colorectal adenomatous polyp (≥10 mm) to evolve into CRC, as approximately 16% in 10 years. The estimated risk potential for intermediate (6–9 mm) and diminutive lesions is substantially smaller (0.7 and 0.08%, respectively) (Pickhardt et al. 2008). Histological features that have been associated with a higher risk for CRC include high-grade of dysplasia (HGD) and villous element (Winawer and Zauber 2002). Neoplasia can, therefore, be classified into "advanced" (i.e., adenocarcinoma and advanced adenomas: all adenomas ≥10 mm, adenomas with HGD or containing villous element (>25%)) and therefore clinically significant, or "not advanced."

General guidelines regarding relevance of lesion size for colonography are presented by the recently published consensus proposal for CT colonography. These recommendations propose that patients with polyps ≥10 mm as found with colonography, should be referred for polypectomy at colonoscopy. In addition, patients with intermediate polyps (6–9 mm) should either be referred for colonoscopy or undergo CT colonography on a custom bases (Zalis et al. 2005). Though, in daily practice frequently a more stringent approach is applied, resulting in the removal of any polyp >6 mm during colonoscopy. Small polyps (≤5 mm) are considered clinically not important, because of their very low risk for development of CRC. Recommendations have been proposed concerning data reporting in colonography, which encompasses the presentation of outcomes regarding different polyp size categories and additional data for histological subset analyses (Halligan et al. 2005).

Finally, an overall subdivision can be applied into (1) symptomatic patients for CRC (e.g., abdominal pain, changing bowel habits, rectal bleeding, and anemia) with recognized symptoms for CRC, (2) asymptomatic subjects at increased risk for CRC (e.g., family history of familial adenomatous polyposis (FAP), first degree relative with CRC, personal and/or family history of CRC, or polyps, IBD), and (3) asymptomatic subject at average risk for CRC (age >50 years). The latter is considered a screening population with a relatively low prevalence of disease.

12.3.2
Image Interpretation

Proper colonic distension is the key element for adequate visualization of colorectal polyps and cancers. Inferior distension or segmental collapse will ultimately lead to false-positive and false-negative findings. This as the observer is not optimal able to detect lesions that may intrude into the colonic lumen, and otherwise a segment that is collapsed may simulate pathological bowel wall thickening.

Similar to CT colonography, in MR colonography the postprocedural display techniques for detecting colorectal polyps and masses recognize two principles and is performed on a postprocessing workstation with dedicated software. Firstly, two-dimensional (2D) data sets will be evaluated using a 2D method, which facilitates the evaluation of both the colon and extracolonic organs. 3D data sets can be evaluated two-dimensionally in each orthogonal anatomical plane (i.e., transverse, sagittal, and coronal), using multiplanar reformation (MPR). When a colorectal lesion is detected, the reviewer is able to score the localization and morphological features of the abnormality. Subsequently, colorectal lesions can be measured and classified into three predefined polyp categories (Zalis et al. 2005). Again, polyps <6 mm can be ignored in this setting, as the likelihood for the presence of advanced neoplasia is extremely low (Pickhardt et al. 2008). Most MR colonography studies report the solitary use of MPR data set interpretation.

An additional principle of data evaluation entails the application of virtual colonoscopy in which the MR colonography dataset is used to construct a 3D rendering. However, technical limitations hamper the application of this method in MR colonography, which is widely applied in CT colonography, whereas in CT colonography this endoluminal view is typically based on data thresholding, high variation in signal value precludes such a straightforward approach for MRI data. These fluctuations in MRI signal might originate both from global (e.g., distance to the antenna) as well as from local effects (inhomogeneities in bowel content), and are difficult to overcome. Nonetheless, several authors report on the use of a 3D surface rendering during review and can be used for problem solving (Lauenstein et al. 2002, 2005; Kuehle et al. 2007).

12.3.3
High-Prevalence Population

12.3.3.1
Bright Lumen Strategy

In the late 1990s and early 2000s, several investigators identified MR colonography as a potential diagnostic method for the detection of colorectal polyps and cancer in symptomatic patients and patients at increased risk for CRC (Luboldt et al. 1998, Lauenstein et al. 2001). Initial research was performed with the use of bright lumen MR colonography in which the colonic lumen appears hyperintense on T1-weighted sequences by the rectal administration of a gadolinium based enema, as outlined in Chap. 11 (Fig. 12.1).

Among the first prospective studies using bright lumen MR colonography was a paper by Luboldt et al., who reported a high sensitivity (93%) and a high specificity (99%) for detecting patients with large colorectal lesions (≥10 mm). 1.5 T MR colonography was compared with colonoscopy in 117 symptomatic patients referred for colonoscopy, using a rectal enema that contained 3 L of water and 60 mL of 0.5 mol/L Magnevist (gadopentetate dimeglumine). However, a moderate sensitivity was demonstrated (75%) when a cut-off value of 7 mm was applied (Luboldt et al. 2000). Pappalardo and colleagues studied 70 patients at increased risk for CRC, who underwent 1.0 T MR colonography using a comparable bright lumen approach. High diagnostic outcomes were found (sensitivity 96% and specificity 93%) for detecting patients with polyps of all sizes (Pappalardo et al. 2000). In this study, 125 endoluminal lesions were found in 54 patients of which 94 lesions were >10 mm in size.

These results demonstrated the ability of MR colonography to detect colorectal lesions exceeding the size of 10 mm with acceptable diagnostic accuracy. This encouraged study groups to investigate MR colonography as alternative diagnostic tool in this field, particularly the value of this modality in detecting intermediate polyps (6–9 mm).

While earlier studies typically used the bright lumen variant with promising outcomes, currently the dark lumen method is mostly applied (see Sect. 12.3.3.2). This change in acquisition method, however, was initially more based on practical reasons (costs of contrast agent) than on extensive series. Some research was performed on different type of MR colonography regimes by Florie et al., who demonstrated diagnostic yield for the bright lumen strategy (Florie et al. 2007c). In this study, three different MR colonography strategies, which consisted of two dark lumen (water-based and air-based colonic distension) and one bright lumen strategy with fecal tagging as bowel preparation (see Sect. 12.3.3.2), were compared. Forty-five subjects at increased risk for CRC were subjected to both MR colonography and colonoscopy. While the diagnostic confidence of both the bright lumen and dark lumen strategy using air for colonic distension was rated best by two independent observers, patient acceptance in the bright

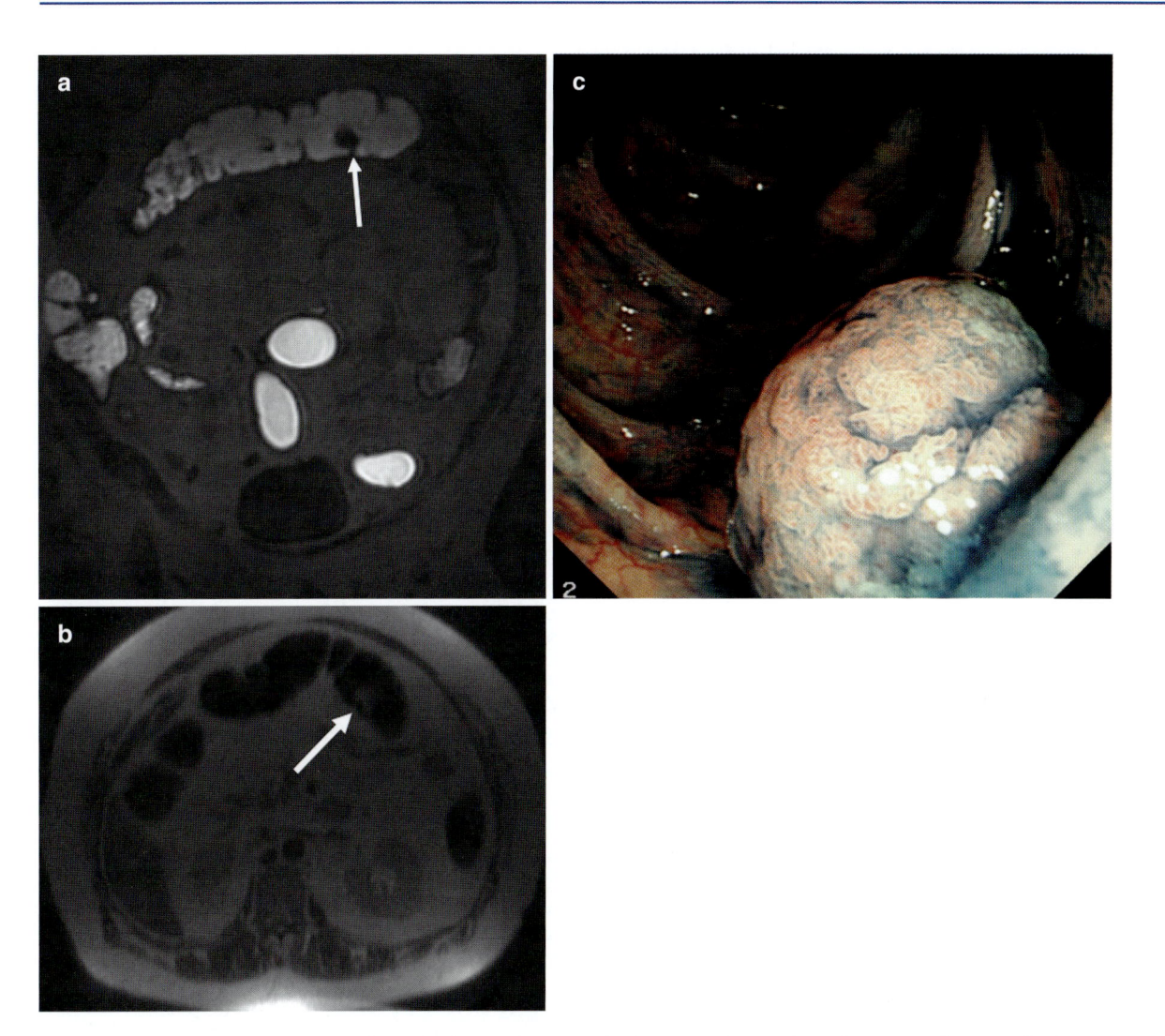

Fig. 12.1. (**a**) T1-weighted 3D coronal fast field echo (FFE) image of a 56-year-old patient with suspicion of a hyperplastic polyposis syndrome. MR colonography visualized a hypo-intense lesion which protrudes into the "bright" colonic lumen (*arrow*), in the distal part of the transverse colon. Suspicious of a pedunculated polyp. (**b**) The presence of a lesion is also confirmed at an axial T2-weighted two-dimensional (2D) fast spin echo (FSE) image, with relative high signal intensity on this sequence (*arrow*). (**c**) The presence of a 15-mm pedunculated polyp was confirmed at colonoscopy. Histology analysis confirmed the diagnosis of a hyperplastic polyp

lumen method proved less burdensome as compared to the other two dark lumen strategies. The latter was mainly due to the better tolerance of the bowel preparation method, which is outlined in Sect. 12.7.1.

In a further prospective study in 200 patients at increased risk for CRC, bright lumen MR colonography using gadolinium/water mixture for colonic distension, was compared to findings with colonoscopy (FLORIE et al. 2007b). Results in this study showed only moderate sensitivity in detecting patients with polyps ≥10 mm (75%). Specificity for these clinical significant polyps was 93%; however, a high number of false-positive findings reduced specificity for polyps ≥6 mm to 67%. The latter was mostly related to both air pockets and motion artifacts. This study was performed in primarily high-risk patients for CRC who took part in a surveillance program. Interestingly, the prevalence of patients with polyps >10 mm in this cohort who underwent colonoscopy surveillance was only 6%, which might have influenced test outcome.

Another prospective study, conducted in 120 symptomatic patients and patients at increased risk, using the "bright lumen" approach with standard bowel preparation, showed adequate detection rates for patients with present polyps or lesions with any size. Forty-seven of 56 patients with colonoscopically confirmed colorectal lesions, were correctly identified to have lesions using bright lumen MR colonography, and 94% of lesions ≥10 mm were depicted (SAAR et al. 2007). Additionally, MR colonography was able to detect all seven CRCs.

Limitations in these studies concern the technical ability of the used technique to correctly identify flat polyps/adenomas and small polyps, which is also frequently reported in CT colonography in surveillance populations (VAN GELDER et al. 2004, JENSCH et al. 2008). But more importantly, small air pockets and nontagged fecal residue are reported as a constant source of false positive findings in recent bright lumen MR colonography studies (Fig. 12.2).

12.3.3.2
Dark Lumen Strategy

The first published article on the use of dark lumen MR colonography appeared in 2001 and suggested promising results regarding diagnostic accuracy, acquisition time, and review time. Initially following a standard preparation for bowel cleansing, a water enema was used which consisted of the rectal administration of 3,000 mL of warm tap water followed by a pre- and post-(IV)contrast T1-weighted 3D gradient echo data acquisition (LAUENSTEIN et al. 2001a). The use of water results in a homogenously low signal throughout the colonic lumen at T1-weighted sequences and allows depiction of enhancing abnormalities originating from the colonic wall after

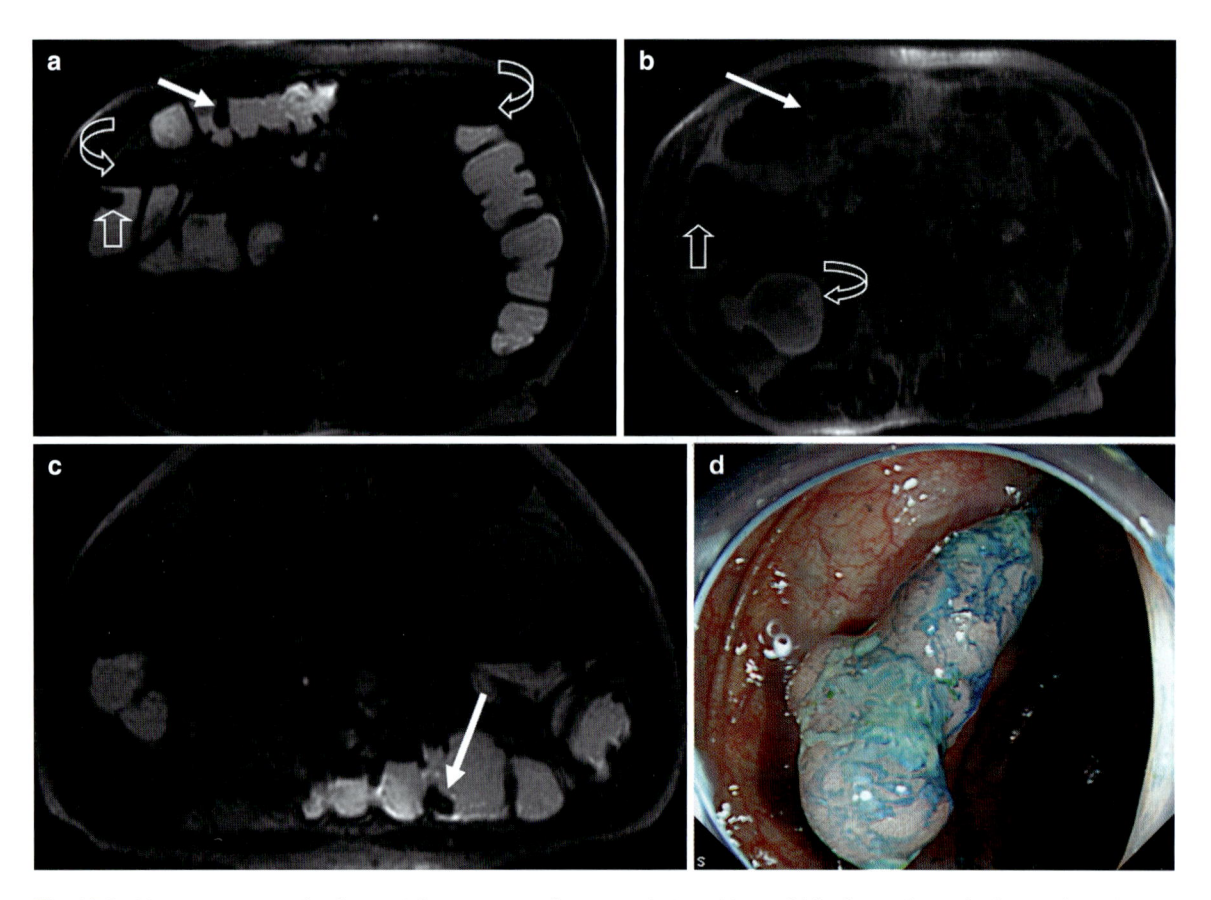

Fig. 12.2. (a) Supine T1-weighted 3D axial FFE image of an 84-year-old male with multiple polyps in the right colon. "Bright lumen" MR colonography visualized a lesion in the proximal aspect of the transverse colon (*arrow*) and a lesion in the ascending colon (*open arrow*). Several air filled areas are present which might lead to false negative findings in this position (*curved arrows*). (b) The polyps are also visualized on the corresponding axial T2w 2D FSE image in supine position, which show relative high signal on this sequence (*arrows*). Hydronefrosis of the right kidney (*curved open arrow*). (c) Corresponding prone T1w 3D axial FFE image shows the somewhat elongated polyp on the anterior aspect of the transverse colon (*arrow*) (d) Colonoscopy confirmed the presence of a pedunculated 10 mm polyp in the proximal aspect of the transverse colon. Also the polyp in the ascending colon was confirmed at colonoscopy (not shown)

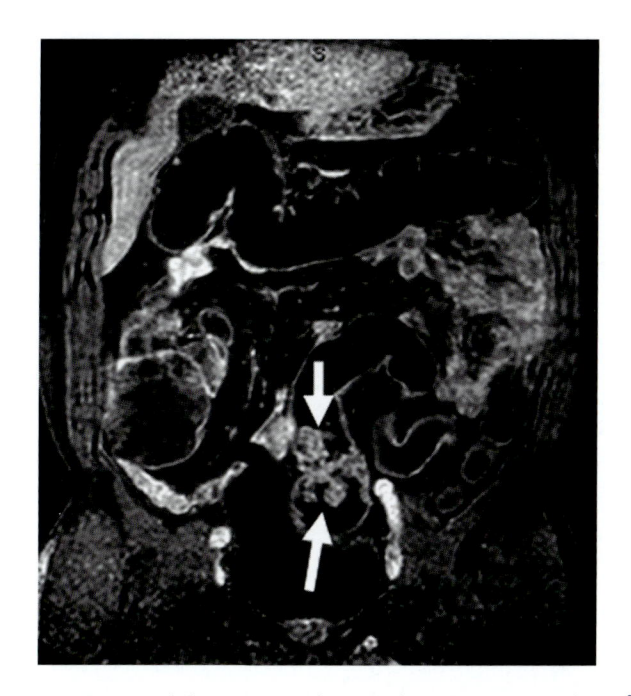

Fig. 12.3. Dark lumen MR colonography using 3DT1 turbo field echo (TFE) sequence with additional fat saturation. Sequential parameters: TR/TE = 4.6/2.2 ms; FOV = 420 mm; FA = 10; slice thickness = 3 mm. (a) Sixty-year-old male patient who presented with weight loss and rectal bleeding. MR colonography visualized the presence of a 5–6-cm large intraluminal, enhancing tumor just above the recto-sigmoid junction (*arrows*) (images by Dr. Achiam, Herlev, Denmark)

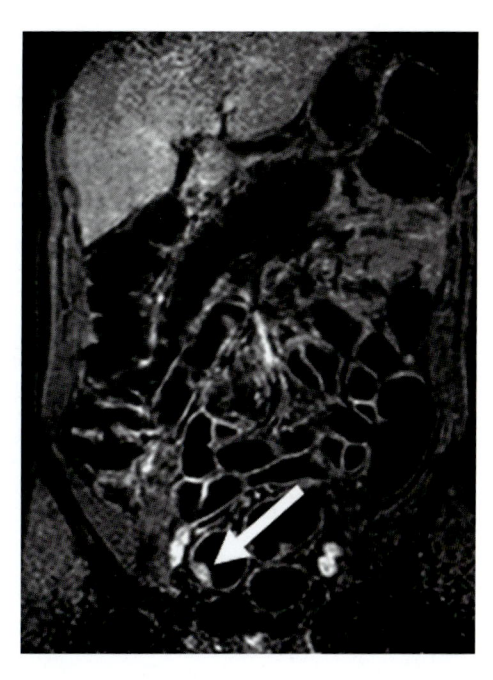

Fig. 12.4. A fifty-eight-year-old male who presented with fatigue and changed bowel habits. Dark lumen MR colonography visualized an enhancing lesion in the sigmoid colon (*arrow*). The presence of a 12-mm polyp was confirmed at colonoscopy (images by Dr. Achiam, Herlev, Denmark)

the intravenous administration of contrast agent (Figs. 12.3–12.5).

As the increase in signal-to-noise ratio (SNR) is significant between pre- and postcontrast series, this technique will in theory leads to better diagnostic accuracy. Interestingly, three of twelve patients included in this study underwent additional bright lumen MR colonography in a further session, which in turn resulted in two false-positive findings in one patient. On the contrary in dark lumen MR imaging no false-negative findings were reported.

Studies specifically evaluating the value of dark lumen MR colonography, using standardized bowel cleansing and water-based enema for colonic bowel distension, have been conducted. In one study, 122 subjects underwent MR colonography prior to colonoscopy. Adequate colonic distension and the absence of significant disturbing artifacts resulted in a high diagnostic confidence in practically all acquired examinations. All nine carcinomas and 89% (16/18) of all intermediate polyps (5–10 mm) and 100% (2/2) of polyps ≥10 mm at colonoscopy were detected with MR colonography performed in prone position (Ajaj et al. 2003).

A more recent prospective study by Hartmann et al. found comparable results for the detection of intermediate, large adenomatous polyps and CRCs (84, 100 and 100%, respectively). Ninety-two patients underwent both dark lumen colonography and colonoscopy, using standard bowel preparation and colonic distension method (Hartmann et al. 2006). Yet, these studies have reported on populations that are characterized with a relatively high prevalence of colorectal polyps and malignancy and the results, therefore, apply to these populations only. Feasibility of this technique is far from established and prospective studies with predefined endpoints are necessary to validate its use.

So far only few studies focused on the use of gaseous agents for colonic distension, which subsequently results in a dark appearing colonic lumen at both T1-weighted and T2-weighted sequences. For this purpose, both room air and carbon dioxide (CO_2) are applicable agents (Fig. 12.6).

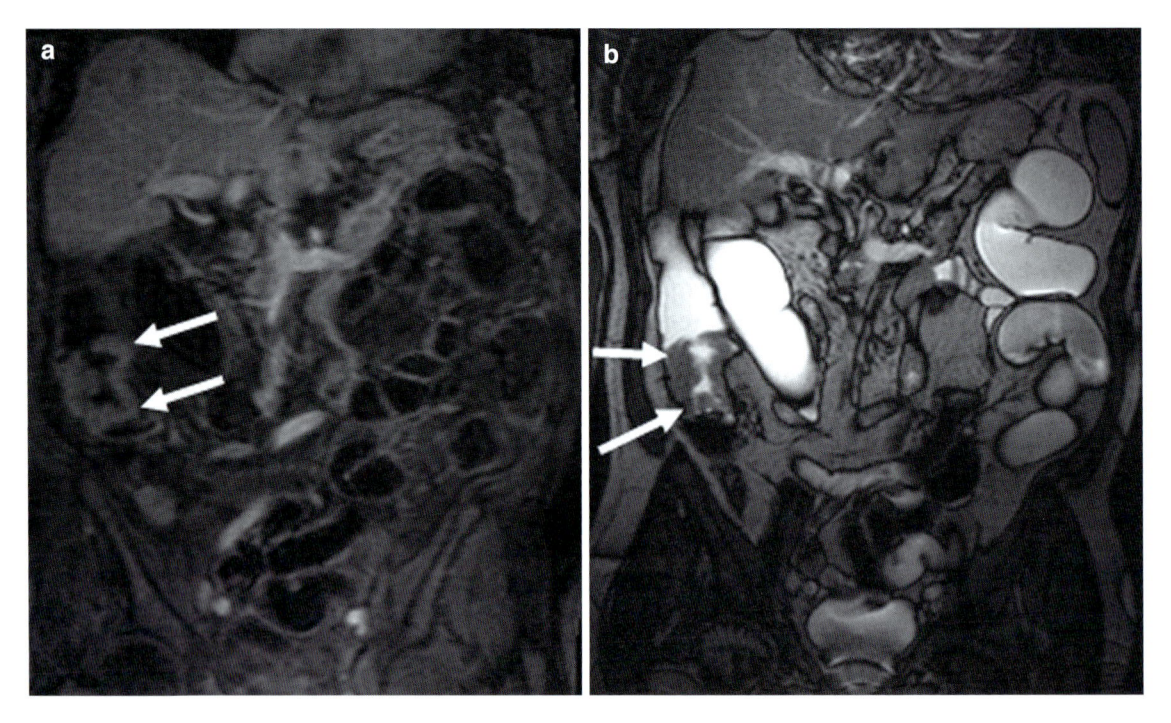

Fig. 12.5. MR colonography in a patient with incomplete endoscopy due to an elongated colon. (**a**) Coronal 3DT1-weighted sequence with additional fat saturation after administration of intravenous contrast agent. A circumferential enhancing tumor was found in the proximal part of the ascending colon (*arrows*). (**b**) True FISP sequence of the same patient, showing a bright lumen appearance with evident filling defect at the level of the tumor (*arrows*) (images by Dr. Kinner, Essen, Germany)

If comparing these two entities, diffusion through the bowel wall favors the application of CO_2 as this ultimately leads to better patient acceptance (Sumanac et al. 2002). Overall, the gas insufflation is considered less burdensome for patients if compared to a water-enema (see Sect. 12.8.2). Additionally, gas distension is thought to allow better colonic distension, yet this assumption has not been established in MR colonography (Rodriguez Gomez et al. 2008).

In a study of 156 patients at average and increased risk of CRC, MR colonography correctly depicted only four out of 31 colorectal polyps of any size, which resulted in poor overall diagnostic outcomes. In this study room, air was manually inflated for luminal distension and was compared with colonoscopy findings. Factors that negatively affected MR colonography performance included physiological artifacts, moderate colonic distension, and the presence of fecal residue (Leung et al. 2004), whereas CO_2 for colonic distension is now standard in CT colonography (Taylor et al. 2007), in MR colonography it has been reported once in a series of six patients with known CRC (Lomas et al. 2001). Although the included population in this study was small, the results are encouraging.

12.3.3.3
Fecal Tagging

As previously outlined, one of the key elements for performing MR colonography is an optimal differentiation between bowel wall and lumen. To correctly identify colonic wall-related pathology, adequate cleansing, or homogenous tagging of residual feces of the bowel is essential. In most earlier studies, a standardized polyethylene glycol electrolyte lavage solution was orally administrated for proper cleansing, which goes together with abdominal discomfort and nausea, and eventually leads to limited patient acceptance and compliance.

Fecal tagging refers to the labeling of the fecal residue and is similar to the method as applied in CT colonography. The administration of an oral-tagging agent results in either low or high signal intensity of the bowel in MR colonography, with a better differentiation between bowel wall and bowel content, and ultimately less false-positive findings as result. Importantly, this enables the use of a limited bowel preparation regime and thus obviates cathartic preparation (Weishaupt et al. 1999, Lauenstein et al. 2002). Fecal tagging can be implemented in bright

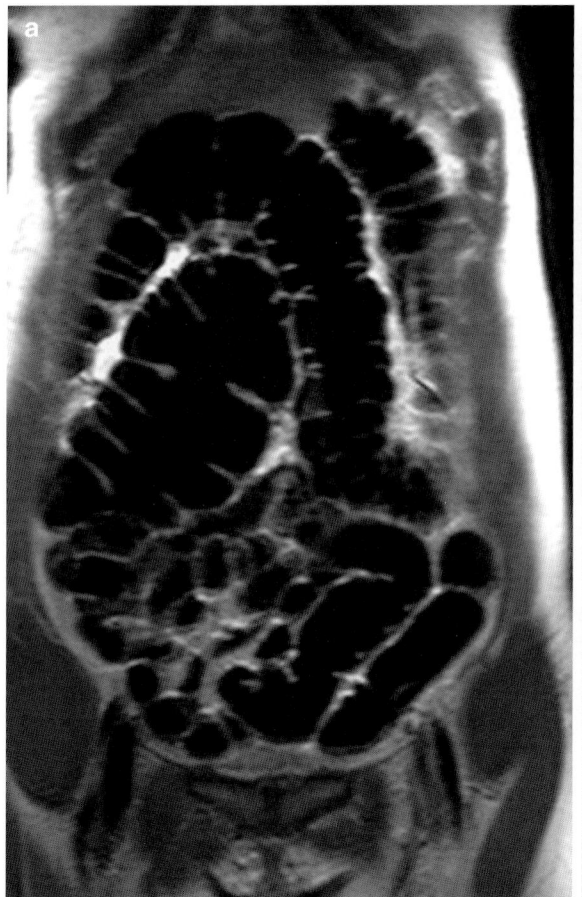

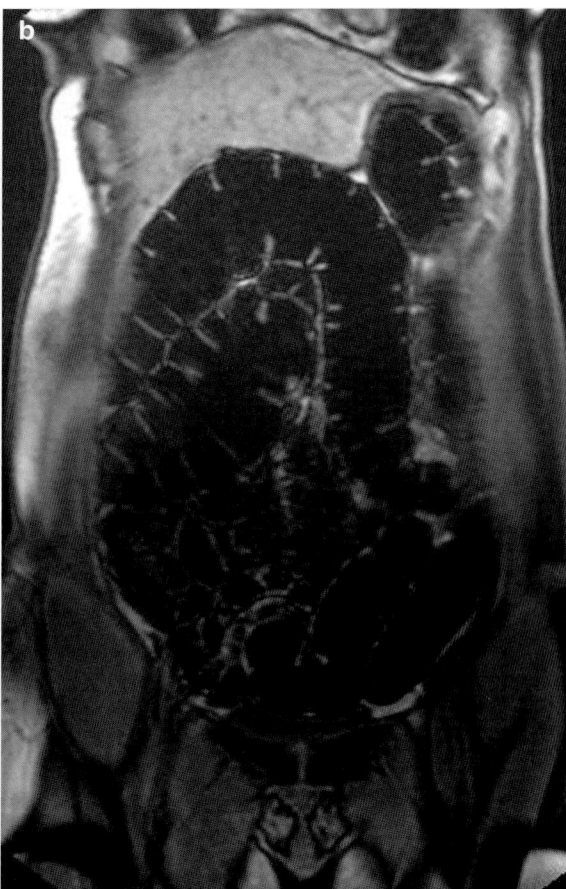

Fig. 12.6. MR colonography after the automatic insufflation of carbon-dioxide (CO_2) in a normal volunteer, results in an optimal distension in all colonic segments. The lumen shows a low signal on both 2D T2-weighted (**a**) and 3D T1-weighted (**b**) sequences, without the presence of disturbing artifacts. Both shown images allow an adequate differentiation between the colonic lumen and colonic wall, even without the administration of an intravenous paramagnetic contrast agent

lumen and dark lumen techniques and was evaluated both on diagnostic outcomes and patient acceptance. The latter is outlined in Sect. 12.8.

Lauenstein et al. proposed a concentrated barium sulfate contrast agent for fecal tagging, which resulted in a homogenously low signal intensity of the colonic lumen, and additionally high contrast-to-noise ratios were measured following to the intravenous administration of T1-shortening paramagnetic contrast agent. Twenty-four symptomatic patients were included in this prospective study, presenting with only mild symptoms. MR colonography demonstrated a high sensitivity (91%) for detecting patients with any sized colorectal lesions and the absence of false-positive findings resulted in an excellent specificity. Though these study results were substantially biased by the high prevalence of large abnormalities as >90% of the colorectal lesions consisted of polyps >8 mm and carcinomas (LAUENSTEIN et al. 2002).

Initial optimism regarding the barium-based fecal tagging approach was tempered by a study reported by Goehde et al, who stopped inclusion of patients in a study owing to inferior MR performance. The diagnostic performance was mainly affected by the high signal intensity of fecal residue throughout the colon on the T1-weighted sequences, which hampered reliable polyp detection in one out of every five included patients. This is reflected in the low sensitivity of lesions >10 mm (50%) (GOEHDE et al. 2005).

Adjusting the barium-based fecal tagging protocol thereby reducing the amount of barium sulfate and add ferumoxsil (GastroMark®, Lumirem®) has been reported to improve patient acceptance (see Sect. 12.8.1). This preparation technique was compared with colonoscopy in 56 patients. For intermediate and large polyps,

MR colonography had a sensitivity of 86% and 81%, respectively. The results improved if these were calculated on a per patient bases, resulting in a high sensitivity (100%) and specificity (91.4%) for depicting patients with polyps ≥10 mm (Achiam et al. 2008a).

In summary, diagnostic outcomes in studies using barium sulfate-based fecal tagging method vary considerably and are therefore difficult to interpret. This emphasizes the necessity to further investigate and optimize this approach.

12.3.4
Low Prevalence Population

12.3.4.1
Screening MR Colonography

Even though most investigators evaluated MR colonography in relatively high prevalence populations, to date one study solely has evaluated MR colonography in a screening population. In this single center prospective study, dark lumen MR colonography without bowel cleansing was compared to colonoscopy in an asymptomatic average risk population of 315 subjects (Kuehle et al. 2007). The overall prevalence of patients with polyps ≥10 mm within this population was 6.3% (20/315). In this study, fecal tagging was applied using a modified barium-based solution (5% Gastrografin/1% barium/0.2% locust bean gum). Sensitivity for the detection of patients with polyps ≥10 mm and patients with intermediate polyps (5–10 mm) was 70% and 60%, respectively. The sensitivity of MR colonography for the detection of patients with adenomatous polyps at least 10 mm in diameter was 87% and 81% for patients with intermediate polyps. Specificity for polyps ≥10 mm and polyps 5–10 mm was 100 and 98% respectively. Recently published data of a multicenter CT colonography screening study (Johnson et al. 2008), reported a comparable sensitivity in identifying asymptomatic patients with adenomas with a size of 10 mm or more and 6 mm in size or more (90% and 78%, respectively).

Evidence on MR colonography in screening is very limited, and only concerns the aforementioned single center study. Current limited evidence, the lack of an established technique, the costs and rather limited access make MR colonography at the moment of writing less suited for screening. Still the use of nonionizing radiation and the wide range of possible limited bowel preparation schemes make MR colonography a potential diagnostic alternative to CT colonography.

12.4
Colorectal Cancer (CRC)

12.4.1
Clinical Staging

In a clinical setting abdominal MR imaging is often used in the pretreatment staging of patients with identified CRC, as it is able to accurately predict the degree of tumor infiltration (T-stage) together with a potential superior visualization of hepatic metastases (Cantwell et al. 2008). However the vast majority of the available literature focus on the most distal colonic segment, since about 40–50% of CRCs are located in the rectum. This subject will be covered in detail in Chap. 13 on MRI of the rectum.

With regard to peritumoral nodal metastasis in the context of CRC, it is important to consider the potential difficulties to depict malignancy within normal sized lymph-nodes. This seems particularly applicable for colon cancer, probably due to the more complex distribution of pericolonic lymph nodes as compared to the relatively fixed perirectal lymph nodes (Low et al. 2003).

Yet new MR techniques are emerging to improve evaluation of preoperative TNM staging and the postoperative follow-up of CRC. The application of ultrasmall superparamagnetic iron oxide particles (USPIO), which is a nanoparticle contrast medium, is increasingly evaluated as potential MR lymphographic agent for the assessment of nodal involvement (Koh et al. 2009). Furthermore, the usefulness of diffusion-weighted imaging (DWI) for preoperative clinical staging for CRC is currently investigated with promising results (Shinya et al. 2009). Consequently, evidence of recent developments is at the time of writing rather limited and future research will demonstrate whether these approaches will gain benefit in clinical staging for CRC.

12.5
Inflammatory Bowel Disease (IBD)

12.5.1
MRI of the Colon in Inflammatory Bowel Disease (IBD)

Gastrointestinal endoscopy (gastroscopy, ileocolonoscopy, and double balloon enteroscopy) with biopsy is

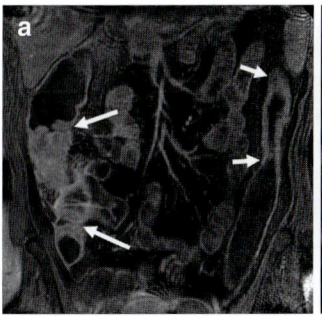

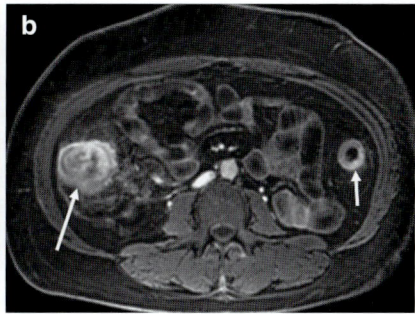

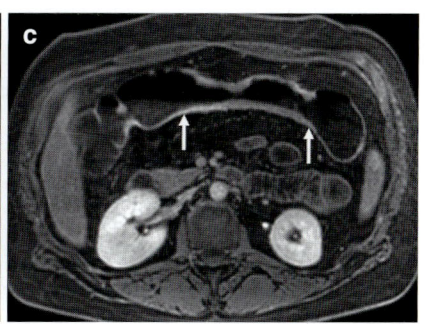

Fig. 12.7. A forty-two-year-old female patient with CD of the terminal ileum and colon underwent routine MR enterography, without the use of a rectal enema. (**a**) Coronal postcontrast T1-weighted MRI showed wall thickening, stenosis, and increased enhancement at the terminal ileum and more distally in the cecum and proximal part of the ascending colon (*arrows*). Additional bowel wall thickening and increased bowel wall enhancement is seen at the proximal descending colon over a length of 5 cm (*small arrows*). (**b**) Circumferential bowel wall thickening with increased enhancement at the ileocecal area, with evident infiltration of the right pericolic area (*long arrow*). No pericolic infiltration is present at the left pericolic area (*small arrow*). (**c**) In the transverse colon, stenosis over a length of 4 cm is observed within an area of circumferential bowel wall thickening and pathological bowel wall enhancement (*small arrows*). Colonoscopy revealed ulcerative stenotic lesions in the descending colon, which prevented a complete examination of the colon

the primary tool, used to make the diagnosis of IBD in patients with clinical suspicion for the disease. Importantly, to date there is no radiological surrogate for this combined initial endoscopic evaluation and histological diagnosis. Nonetheless, some findings of IBD cannot be evaluated using endoscopy.

MRI has the potential to display both the gastrointestinal tract and the extra-luminal structures with substantial anatomical detail. Therefore, it can provide valuable information which is not appreciated using endoscopy, i.e. intramural changes and extraluminal abnormalities including abscesses. Therefore, MRI studies are currently considered to be an adjunct to gastrointestinal endoscopy. As previously outlined in Chaps. 8, 9, and 10, MRI has emerged as diagnostic technique to assess the small bowel for disease activity in patients with suspected IBD.

This section elucidates the role of MRI for the assessment of IBD in the large bowel. Both data on MR imaging of the colon in IBD patients with and without the use of a rectal enema are available. In this section, we will concentrate on reports in which no colonic luminal distension method was applied, frequently this will comprise studies diagnosing IBD or studies evaluating disease activity of the terminal ileum and colon during MR enteroclysis or MR enterography. Criteria used for subjective and objective disease assessment in IBD patients using MRI of the bowel in different approaches, entails bowel wall enhancement, bowel wall thickness, presence of stenosis, ulceration, cobblestoning, target sign, extra enteric findings, lymphadenopathy, and increased vascularization.

In early studies, high sensitivities were reported for differentiating type and severity of IBD. Without reported use of bowel preparation methods and the solely use of intravenous contrast medium, the authors concluded a comparable diagnostic accuracy of MRI as compared to endoscopy (SHOENUT et al. 1994). More recent studies, evaluating the colon without rectal administrated distension, tend to support (FLORIE et al. 2005) or decline these findings (DURNO et al. 2000). In a recent meta-analysis, Horsthuis et al. determined the accuracy of MRI in evaluating disease activity. Six of the seven studies examined both the small and large bowel, and in only two included studies a water-based enema was applied. MRI correctly graded 91% of frank disease and 62% of patients with mild disease or in remission (HORSTHUIS et al. 2009). These data suggest MRI is an potential effective method even without the administration of intraluminal colonic contrast agent (Fig. 12.7).

12.5.2
MR Colonography in IBD

Bowel distension has proved to be a key element for MR imaging in small bowel diseases although the required level of distension is debated (see Chaps. 7, 8, and 9). Most likely this will apply to the diagnostic value of MRI of the large bowel as well (KOH et al. 2001). Effectively, the additional administration of a rectal enema in MR enterography has proved advantageous, leading to better colonic distension and higher diagnostic accuracy in both the colon and ileocecal area (AJAJ et al. 2005a) (Fig. 12.8).

To date, only limited scientific data is reported on the diagnostic role of MR colonography in the assessment of colonic involvement in IBD, primarily ulcerative colitis (UC) and Crohn's disease (CD). Conclusions and recommendations brought up by the different investigators diverge. Important advantage of MR colonography to CT colonography or routine barium enema is the lack of use of nonionizing radiation. This is especially important in young patients in their reproductive age requiring repeated evaluations over time for evaluation of their disease activity, which in IBD is often the case (JAFFE et al. 2007). Similar to MR colonography, only a few studies report on the performance of CT colonography in IBD.

Two research groups from Germany independently investigated whether the extent of inflammatory activity could be assessed with MR colonography using colonoscopy as the reference standard. Schreyer et al. used a bright lumen MR colonography approach with full bowel preparation, enrolling 22 consecutive patients with highly suspected or known IBD (SCHREYER et al. 2005b). In this study, patients had bowel preparation with a gadolinium/water enema for luminal distension and additional intravenous administration of gadolinium. Bowel wall contrast enhancement and bowel wall thickening were used as MRI features of inflammation. Based on these features a three-point scale was used to assess inflammation, with 0 = no inflammation and 2 = inflammation for each colonic segment and terminal ileum. A poor sensitivity in detecting segmental inflammation in CD patients (31.6%) and only moderate (58.8%) sensitivity for identifying segmental inflammation in UC patients were found in the 154 totally evaluated bowel segments.

One of the limitations is the usage of a bright lumen approach which reduces differentiation between hyperintense colonic lumen and enhanced colonic bowel wall. Though this alone will not explain the considerable difference in reported results and associated conclusions, as the same group applied dark lumen MR colonography in another study with only slight improvement in overall segmental inflammation detection (SCHREYER et al. 2005c). Other factors such as that active inflammation is characterized by superficial

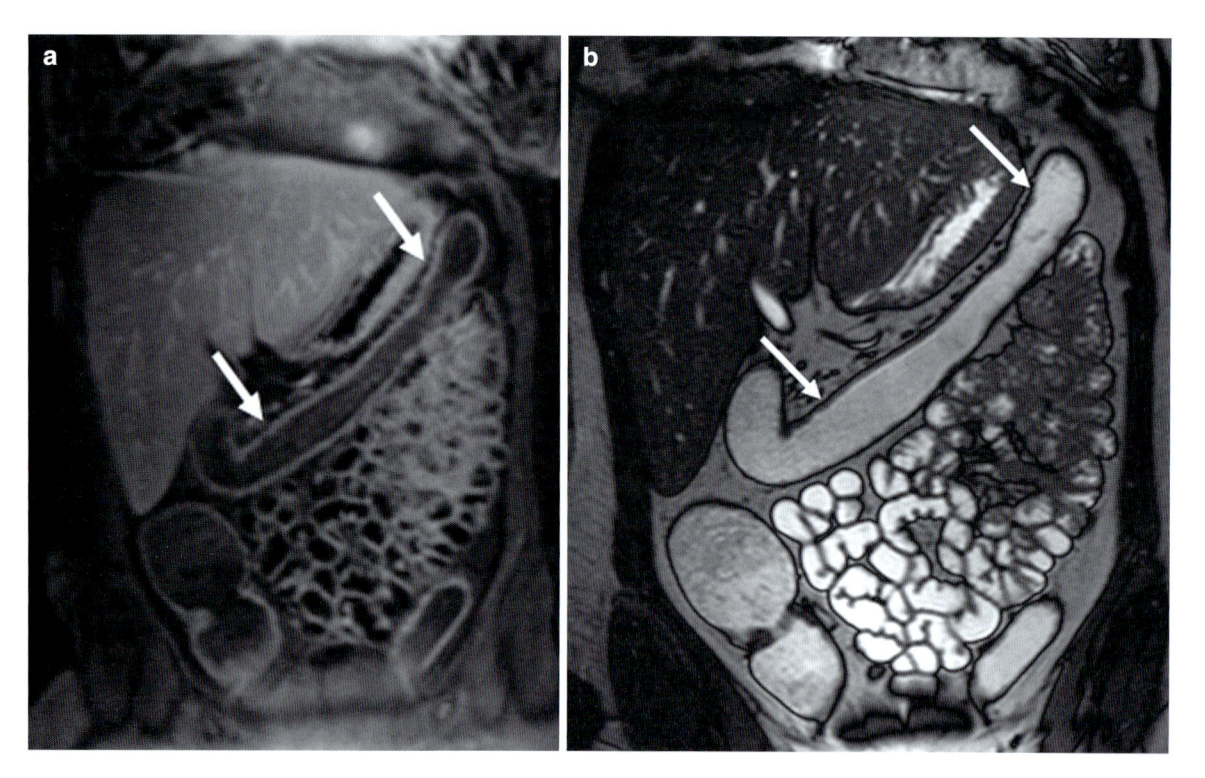

Fig. 12.8. Patient with known ulcerative colitis. (**a**) 3DT1w image after intravenous contrast injection, with hypo intense colonic lumen and uniform slight enhancement of the colonic wall. Altered anatomical appearance of the transverse colon, however no signs of active inflammation. (**b**) Balanced steady-state free precession (true FISP) sequence after the rectal administration of a water based enema, resulting in a hyper-intense appearance of the colonic lumen. Evident loss of the normal anatomical folding in the transverse colon (*arrows*) (images by Dr. Kinner, Essen, Germany)

inflammation rather than by bowel wall thickening, might contribute to this relatively low correlation.

These findings were in sharp contrast with a study in which 15 healthy volunteers and 23 patients with known IBD affecting the colon were subjected to dark lumen MR colonography and colonoscopy (AJAJ et al. 2005c). A comparable study design and determinants of inflammation were used. The authors in this study concluded that MR colonography can be regarded as a possible alternative to endoscopy, with a high sensitivity (87%) in identifying segmental IBD changes. However, some remarks should be placed relating to the methodological set-up, as only the colonic segments that endoscopically appeared inflamed were biopsied, potentially leading to bias (GASCHE et al. 2005). Based on these results, the diagnostic value of MRI for non-affected intestinal segments cannot be determined. Therefore, the results do not define a clear picture of the possibilities and limitations of MRI in detecting disease activity in IBD (Fig. 12.9).

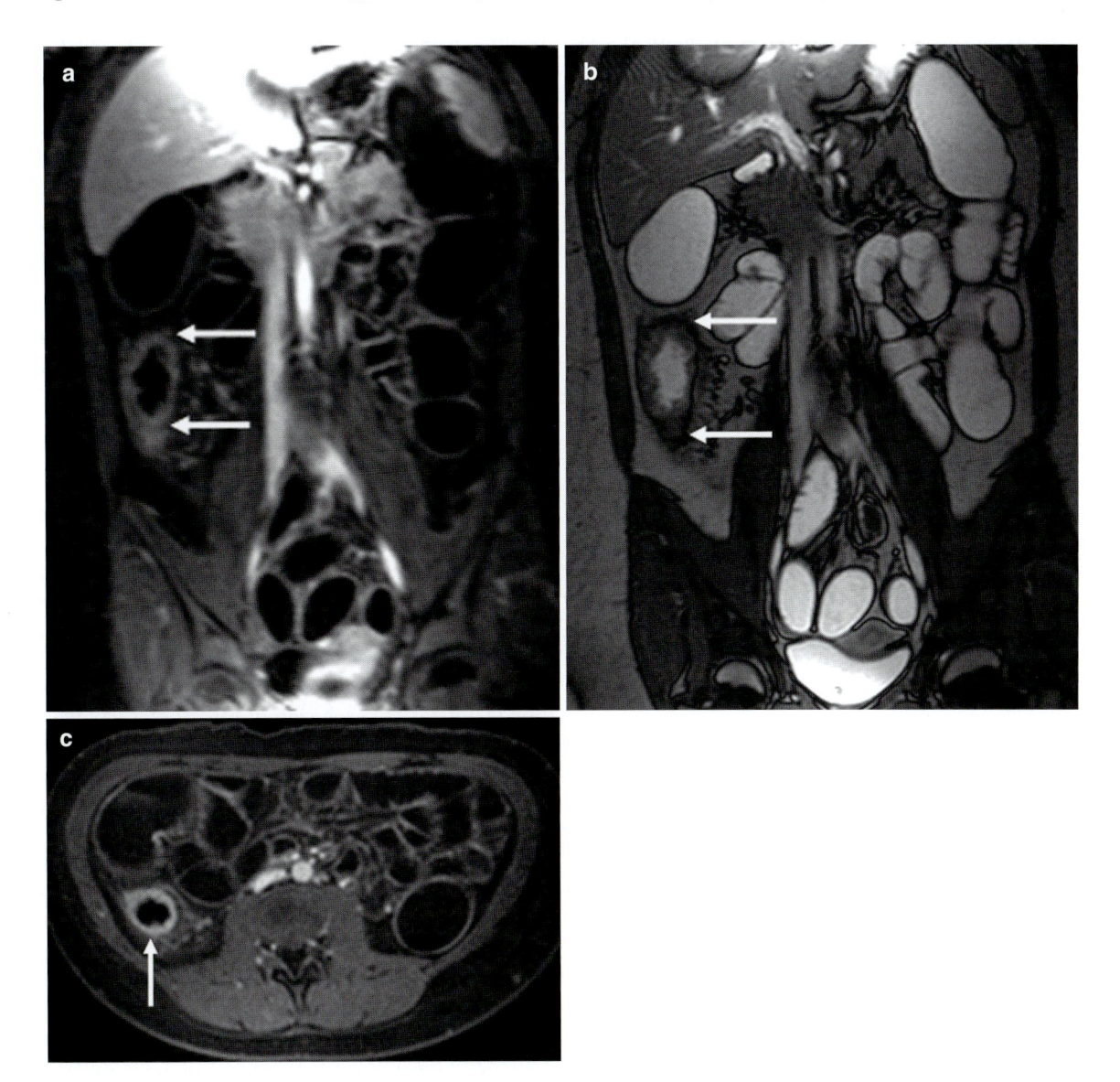

Fig. 12.9. Young patient with CD presented with acute abdominal pain. (**a**) Coronal 3DT1w sequence showed pathological bowel wall thickening and increased bowel wall enhancement after the administration of intravenous contrast, which is suspected of active inflammation (*arrows*). Fat infiltration is seen around the right hemicolon. (**b**) Balanced steady-state free precession (true FISP) sequence demonstrates the high signal intensity colonic lumen and thickened wall of the ascending colon (images by Dr. Kinner, Essen, Germany) (*arrow*). (**c**) In the axial plane, the pathological changes results in a circumferential bowel wall thickening with increased enhancement

More recently, investigators studied MR colonography for quantification of IBD. Langhorst et al. have prospectively compared the performance of MR colonography with colonoscopy, using increased bowel wall contrast enhancement, bowel wall thickening, presence of mesenterial lymph nodes and the absence of the normal haustral pattern as MRI features of active inflammation. (LANGHORST et al. 2007). Twenty-nine patients with IBD were included and bowel preparation for MR colonography entailed barium-based fecal tagging. MR colonography demonstrated an overall sensitivity and specificity of 32% and 88%, respectively. This was combined with a poor patient acceptance for the applied fecal-tagging method (see Sect. 12.7.1).

For predicting disease activity in IBD by the evaluation of bowel wall enhancement, other authors chose to measure bowel wall contrast enhancement on the T1-weighted 3D SPGR and compare pre- and post-contrast sequences (ROTGGEN et al. 2006). Significant statistical correlation was shown with the colonoscopic findings. For the evaluation of quantitative determinants of colonic inflammation, other authors retrospectively used a similar method to quantify signal intensity index and used a bowel wall thickness index (BWTI) to measure bowel wall thickness. BWTI was defined as mean wall thickness to luminal diameter in correspondent colonic segment, to compensate for insufficient distension (ERGEN et al. 2008). Unfortunately, these quantitative parameters demonstrated moderate sensitivity (63%) and adequate specificity (80%) in this cohort of 37 patients with suspected or known IBD. In both studies, bowel wall attenuation was subjectively assessed, in the absence of predefined criteria.

Recently, Rimola and colleagues demonstrated that MR enterography in combination with a water-based enema is adequately able to assess disease activity in patients with established CD (RIMOLA et al. 2009). It should be noted that a potential contribution to the reported high diagnostic accuracy might be the use of a 3.0-T MR unit which allows improvement of spatial resolution if compared to lower magnetic field strength units (i.e., 1.5 T)

Although current evidence suggest adequate accuracy in evaluating disease activity in established IBD patients, so far the role of MRI in the initial diagnosis of those with suspected IBD and the additional differentiation between UC and CD has not been defined yet. Given the present role of MR in small bowel CD, there might be a similar role for MR colonography in colonic IBD. Though available research studying MR imaging of the large bowel with colonoscopy, and in particular MR colonography, is limited and therefore warrants further research to define its position.

12.6
Diverticular Disease and Acute Colonic Diverticulitis

The algorithm for the diagnosis of acute colonic diverticulitis, primarily includes patient history and the physical examination. However, to exclude potential other causes of an acute abdomen and/or to confirm the diagnosis of acute diverticulitis, radiologic evaluation of the abdomen is generally accepted. This radiologic evaluation mostly includes routine abdominal and chest radiographs, although this has very limited value (LAMÉRIS et al. 2009). Both ultrasound (US) and CT with administration of i.v. contrast medium are valuable in these patients (RAO et al. 1998; AMBROSETTI et al. 2002; LAMERIS et al. 2008). CT, however, gives significant more information on alternative diagnoses. New evidence has indicated that a strategy with initial ultrasound and CT in negative or inconclusive US cases, is the best approach (LAMÉRIS et al. 2009).

Major impetus to evaluate the role of MRI in the diagnosis of acute colonic diverticulitis is the lack of ionizing radiation as compared to CT. Furthermore, the superior soft tissue resolution permits adequate visualization of the region of interest, and is able to detect complications of diverticulitis (e.g. free abdominal fluid, abscess formation, and fistulas) (BUCKLEY et al. 2007). Moreover, optimal differentiation facilitates the exclusion of other potential diagnoses of an acute abdomen (see Chap. 17). To compete, MRI should therefore prove to have comparable diagnostic accuracy as found with CT in the detection of patients with acute colonic diverticulitis.

In a recent prospective evaluation, authors have proposed that MRI should primarily be implemented in all patients with suspected acute diverticulitis (HEVERHAGEN et al. 2008). In this study, 55 patients with clinical suspected diverticulitis underwent routine abdominal MRI without the use of a luminal distension method, with high sensitivity (94%) and specificity (88%) for the diagnosis of acute diverticulitis.

Only a few studies have evaluated the potential role of MR colonography in this acute clinical entity. Schreyer et al. reported a similar depiction of diverticulosis and inflammatory bowel changes, if compared to contrast

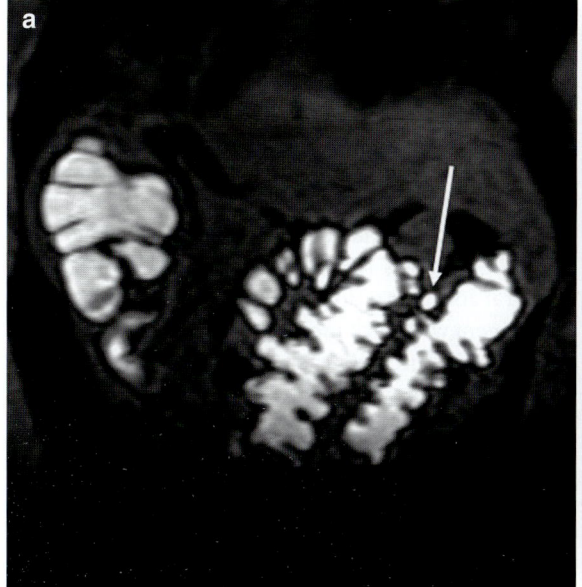

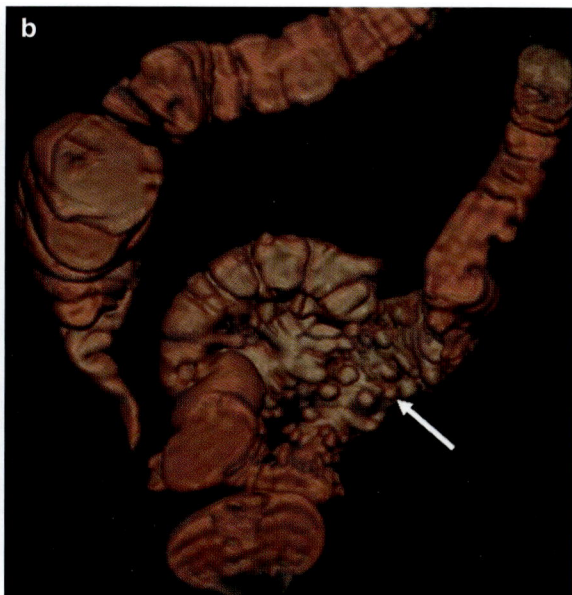

Fig. 12.10. (a) Coronal 3D Flash sequence showing multiple diverticula of the sigmoid colon (*arrow*). (b) Posterior view of a 3D rendering in the same patient, nicely illustrating diverticular disease of the sigmoid colon and descending colon (*arrows*). This 3D postprocessing facilitates presurgical planning (images by Prof. Schreyer, Regensburg, Germany)

enhanced CT. Conventional CT was considered as the reference standard in this prospective study and was performed prior to MR colonography. To prevent complications during the rectal enema, patients were excluded from the study if a perforation was suspected on CT. 3D rendering allowed surgical planning and therefore substituted the necessitate for an additional barium enema (SCHREYER et al. 2004) (Fig. 12.10).

In 40 patients with suspected, known and/or a history of sigmoid diverticulitis and without clinical suspicion of perforation, Ajaj et al. reported high sensitivity and specificity (86% respectively 92%) for detecting diverticular disease and active inflammatory changes. In this study, water-based dark lumen MR colonography was compared to colonoscopy as the reference standard. The authors concluded that MR colonography can be regarded as accurate in the detection of colonic diverticulitis, although MR colonography was not accurate in distinguishing diverticulitis from invasive colorectal malignancy (AJAJ et al. 2005d).

In these two MR studies, the presence of colonic diverticula and secondary signs of inflammation (i.e., enlarged lymph nodes, mesenteric infiltration, bowel wall contrast enhancement, and bowel wall thickening) were assessed. These are similar determinants as used in CT for the evaluation of acute diverticulitis (GOH et al. 2007). Nonetheless, CT enables therapeutical options, allowing direct drainage of abscesses in severe diverticulitis, which can be regarded as important advantages of this modality. As seen in the diagnostic assessment of IBD, MRI can be used as diagnostic tool in identifying patients with active inflammatory changes. The role of MRI in the acute abdomen is increasing, but not clearly defined except for appendicitis (STOKER 2008). The value of an additional water-based enema is questionable as this will hamper patient acceptance and increases examination time as compared to standard radiologic techniques. Readers are referred to Chap. 17 for more detail on MRI in acute gastrointestinal diseases.

12.7
Incomplete Colonoscopy

Colonoscopy is reported to be inadequate or incomplete in up to 19% of patients (DAFNIS et al. 2005), the reasons for initial colonoscopy failure include patient discomfort, colonic elongation, abdominal adhesions, and inadequate bowel preparation. Although incomplete colonoscopy can occur in any patient group, reported series in MR colonography concern patients with symptoms of CRC. Presently, CT-colonography has replaced double contrast barium enema (DCBE) to evaluate the proximal colon in patients with symptoms of CRC (Martinez et al. 2005; Macari et al. 1999; Neri et al. 2002). Hartmann et al. proposed dark lumen water-based MR colonography in 32 patients with symptoms for CRC and an incomplete colonoscopy. In this study, MR colonography correctly identified and located all high-grade stenosis and demonstrated two metastases, peritoneal dissemination and nine polyps (≥7 mm), which were located in the proximal colon (Hartmann et al. 2005).

In 37 patients with incomplete colonoscopy, including 21 patients with high grade stenosis and 16 patients due to patient discomfort and colonic elongation, Ajaj et al. found two lesions suspected for carcinoma, five polyps and four segments suspected of being affected by colitis (Ajaj et al. 2005b). However, the latter was not confirmed with a follow-up colonoscopy or peroperative findings, which concerns a substantial limitation to this study.

Similarly to CT colonography, MR colonography permits a complete evaluation of the colon and enables additional extra colonic evaluation. If the diagnostic accuracy in detecting colorectal pathology of both modalities proves to be comparable, then there will be preference for the modality without the use of ionizing radiation. In particular, in young patients with IBD who have failed colonoscopy.

12.8
Patient Acceptance in MR Colonography

Several investigators have focused on the degree of comfort, acceptance, and future preferences of MR colonography, if compared to conventional colonoscopy. Here we focus on two aspects of the examination, namely patient acceptance regarding bowel preparation and colonic distension.

12.8.1
Bowel Preparation

As previously outlined, one prerequisite for a high-quality MR colonography is a clean or homogenously tagged colon. This as residual feces can both conceal and simulate bowel wall pathology, which potentially leads to false-negative and false-positive findings. In the earlier studies, patient preparation for MR colonography was similar to the bowel preparation as applied for conventional colonoscopy. This ultimately could influence future preferences for this modality, since bowel purgation is rated as one of the most unpleasant parts during conventional colonoscopy. With the introduction of fecal tagging in MR colonography, a method was described that obviated the application of a complete bowel cleansing approach.

Since 1999, several fecal tagging strategies have been evaluated, for both bright lumen and dark lumen approaches (Weishaupt et al. 1999; Lauenstein et al. 2001b). Initial approach in dark lumen MR colonography, as reported by Lauenstein et al, was the oral administration of 200 mL barium-based contrast agent with each meal, starting 36 h for the examination and proved feasible. In this study, patient acceptance was thought to improve; however, this was not thoroughly investigated (Lauenstein et al. 2001b). From the same research group, Goehde et al. used a comparable bowel preparation strategy, which consisted of the administration of 150 mL barium-sulfate in six consecutive oral intakes. Opposite conclusions were drawn from this study as this technical approach resulted in only moderate diagnostic accuracy, poor image quality in approximately 20% of the MR examinations, moreover the total MR colonography examination was graded more uncomfortable as conventional colonoscopy. The barium intake was graded as most disturbing factor (Goehde et al. 2005). The taste of barium sulfate is generally considered unpleasant, and especially the viscous texture might lead to some degree of discomfort. Adjustments in this barium-sulfate regime have been reported. Adding ferumoxsil (GastroMark®, Lumirem®) and reducing the amount of barium sulfate results in improved patient acceptance of the bowel preparation (Achiam et al. 2008b).

A modified barium-based fecal-tagging protocol – consisting of 5% Gastrografine, 1% barium and 0.2% locust bean gum – has been described by a research group in two different studies. In 29 patients with IBD, this fecal tagging preparation was rated significantly less bothersome than bowel purgation (Langhorst et al. 2007). However, overall patient acceptance, based on preparation protocol and examination procedures, was in favor of colonoscopy. Patient acceptance of MR colonography in a screening population was reported for a series of 248 patients using the modified barium fecal tagging regime with colonoscopy as the reference standard (Kinner et al. 2007). Important conclusions in this study entailed the comparable patient acceptance of MR colonography and colonoscopy and the comparable future patient preferences for MR colonography and colonoscopy. A better patient acceptance than colonoscopy would be a major factor favoring MR colonography for screening. Given the wide range of possible limited bowel strategies for MR colonography, efforts should be made to study regimes with a lower burden to be applied for screening.

A prospective study was performed comparing three different fecal tagging strategies with respect to image quality and patient acceptance in a series of 45 patients at increased risk (surveillance) (FLORIE et al. 2007c). The study was executed using two dark lumen approaches with barium-based (3 × 200 mL) fecal tagging strategy and one bright lumen approach with gadolinium (3 × 10 mL) as oral tagging agent, in combination with a low-fiber diet. The bright lumen strategy resulted in better outcomes regarding the diagnostic confidence and acceptance of bowel preparation and, therefore, this protocol was used in the following trial in which MR colonography was preferred above conventional colonoscopy (FLORIE et al. 2007d). Experience from 209 patients regarding bowel preparation and the overall procedure were rated better directly after finishing the examinations, and 5 weeks after both examinations.

12.8.2
Colonic Distension

Another important aspect which influence patient acceptance is colonic distension method. A frequently used method for colonic distension is the administration of a water-based enema, which mostly consists of warm tap water (dark lumen) or gadolinium/water mixture (bright lumen). However, enemas are relative uncomfortable. Insufflation of gas for colonic distension most likely leads to less patient burden, as is common practice in CT-colonography. However, initial studies did not use gas because of substantial susceptibility artifacts at gas soft tissue interfaces and movement artifacts. Improved techniques with data acquisition with short echo times has enabled the performance of MR colonography without important susceptibility artifacts and/ or movement artifacts. Considering these factors, gas-based distension methods are evaluated to improve image quality and patient acceptance in MR colonography.

In a single prospective experience in 165 individuals at both high risk and average risk for CRC, no significant differences in discomfort was found between MR colonography using air for colonic distension and colonoscopy with identical bowel preparation (LEUNG et al. 2003). However interestingly a significant proportion of the individuals preferred colonoscopy to MR colonography. The authors suggest that this finding might be related to the fact that all individuals received sedation during colonoscopy and the examination time was shorter for colonoscopy.

Other authors used air-based MR colonography to compare feasibility and patients acceptance with both water-based colonic distension and colonoscopy in a randomized study, studying five volunteers and 50 patients at high risk for CRC with similar bowel preparation technique (AJAJ et al. 2004). Water-based and air-based colonic distensions were rated comparable, regarding the degree of discomfort. This is in contrast with studies evaluating patient acceptance in CT colonography and DCBE (GLUECKER et al. 2003). These results indicate a better tolerance of air-based colonic distension.

Another feasible way to improve patient acceptance might be a combined fecal tagging strategy and air-based colonic distension. However, comparable patient acceptance with the water-based alternative and significant better examination tolerance compared to colonoscopy, was combined with inferior image quality of air-based MR colonography (GOMEZ et al. 2008).

Considering patient acceptance, the potential better tolerance of using air for colonic distension instead of a water-based enema has not been evidently demonstrated in MR colonography literature. Moreover, so far there is no available evidence on the patient acceptance of CO_2 in MR colonography, the colonic distension method frequently applied in CT colonography.

12.9
Conclusion

MR imaging of the colon can be applied for a wide spectrum of indications. The current available evidence, however, is rather limited, and therefore its role for detecting different types of colonic disorders is far from established. Whereas additional administration of a rectal enema seems legitimated for improving detection of colorectal polyps, the beneficial effect for other indications, i.e., acute diverticulitis and in particular IBD, remains unclear.

To date most of the MR colonography research is aimed at the detection of (precursors of) CRC. Although no consensus has been reached regarding important elements of the exam, current evidence suggests sufficient accuracy in detecting clinical significant polyps. Yet at this point we are far from the implementation of an established diagnostic tool, such as presently observed in CT colonography for screening.

Nonetheless, the increasing availability of higher magnetic field-strength MR units allows better image quality and ultimately leads to improving accuracy in the assessment of the colon. The wide range of limited bowel preparation regimes gives ample opportunity to find a bowel preparation with very limited discomfort. Together with novice developments, i.e., the implementation of DWI, MR lymphography and molecular imaging, MRI of the colon may gain a prominent role in the radiological evaluation of IBD and patients at risk for CRC.

References

Achiam MP, Løgager VB, Chabanova E, et al (2008a) Diagnostic accuracy of MR colonography with fecal tagging. Abdom Imaging PMID:18452023

Achiam MP, Løgager V, Chabanova E, et al (2008b) Patient acceptance of MR colonography with improved fecal tagging versus conventional colonoscopy. Eur J Radiol PMID: 19041207

Ajaj W, Lauenstein TC, Langhorst J, et al (2005a) Small bowel hydro-MR imaging for optimized ileocecal distension in Crohn's disease: should an additional rectal enema filling be performed? J Magn Reson Imaging 22(1):92–100

Ajaj W, Lauenstein TC, Pelster G, et al (2005b) MR colonography in patients with incomplete conventional colonoscopy. Radiology 234(2):452–459

Ajaj WM, Lauenstein TC, Pelster G, et al (2005c) Magnetic resonance colonography for the detection of inflammatory diseases of the large bowel: quantifying the inflammatory activity. Gut 54(2):257–263

Ajaj W, Pelster G, Treichel U, et al (2003) Dark lumen magnetic resonance colonography: comparison with conventional colonoscopy for the detection of colorectal pathology. Gut 52(12):1738–1743

Ajaj W, Ruehm SG, Lauenstein T, et al (2005d) Dark-lumen magnetic resonance colonography in patients with suspected sigmoid diverticulitis: a feasibility study. Eur Radiol 15(11):2316–2322

Ambrosetti P, Becker C, Terrier F (2002) Colonic diverticulitis: impact of imaging on surgical management – a prospective study of 542 patients. Eur Radiol 12:1145–1149

Buckley O, Geoghegan T, McAuley G, et al (2007) Pictorial review: magnetic resonance imaging of colonic diverticulitis Eur Radiol 17:221–227

Cantwell CP, Setty BN, Holalkere N, et al (2008) Liver lesion detection and characterization in patients with colorectal cancer: a comparison of low radiation dose non-enhanced PET/CT, contrast-enhanced PET/CT, and liver MRI. J Comput Assist Tomogr 32(5):738–744

Dafnis G, Granath F, Påhlman L, et al (2005) Patient factors influencing the completion rate in colonoscopy. Dig Liver Dis 37(2):113–118

Durno CA, Sherman P, Williams T, et al (2000) Magnetic resonance imaging to distinguish the type and severity of pediatric inflammatory bowel diseases. J Pediatr Gastroenterol Nutr 30(2):170–174

Ergen FB, Akata D, Hayran M, et al (2008) Magnetic resonance colonography for the evaluation of colonic inflammatory bowel disease: correlation with conventional colonoscopy. J Comput Assist Tomogr 32(6):848–854

Florie J, Birnie E, van Gelder RE, et al (2007a) MR colonography with limited bowel preparation: patient acceptance compared with that of full-preparation colonoscopy. Radiology 245(1):150–159

Florie J, Horsthuis K, Hommes DW, et al (2005) Magnetic resonance imaging compared with ileocolonoscopy in evaluating disease severity in Crohn's disease. Clin Gastroenterol Hepatol 3(12):1221–1228

Florie J, Jensch S, Nievelstein RA, et al (2007b) MR colonography with limited bowel preparation compared with optical colonoscopy in patients at increased risk for colorectal cancer. Radiology 243(1):122–131

Florie J, van Gelder RE, Haberkorn B, et al (2007c) Magnetic resonance colonography with limited bowel preparation: a comparison of three strategies. J Magn Reson Imaging 25(4): 766–774

Gasche C, Turetschek K (2005) Value of MR colonography for assessment of inflammatory bowel disease? Believe what you see-see what you believe. Gut 54(2):181–182

Gluecker TM, Johnson CD, Harmsen WS, et al (2003) Colorectal cancer screening with CT colonography, colonoscopy, and double-contrast barium enema examination: prospective assessment of patient perceptions and preferences. Radiology 227(2):378–384

Goehde SC, Descher E, Boekstegers A, et al (2005) Dark lumen MR colonography based on fecal tagging for detection of colorectal masses: accuracy and patient acceptance. Abdom Imaging 30(5):576–583

Goh V, Halligan S, Taylor SA, et al (2007) Differentiation between diverticulitis and colorectal cancer: quantitative CT perfusion measurements versus morphologic criteria–initial experience. Radiology 242(2):456–462

Halligan S, Altman DG, Taylor SA, et al (2005) CT colonography in the detection of colorectal polyps and cancer: systematic review, meta-analysis, and proposed minimum data set for study level reporting. Radiology 237(3): 893–904

Hartmann D, Bassler B, Schilling D, et al (2005) Incomplete conventional colonoscopy: magnetic resonance colonography in the evaluation of the proximal colon. Endoscopy 37(9):816–820

Hartmann D, Bassler B, Schilling D, et al (2006) Colorectal polyps: detection with dark-lumen MR colonography versus conventional colonoscopy. Radiology 238(1):143–149

Heverhagen JT, Sitter H, Zielke A, et al (2008) Prospective evaluation of the value of magnetic resonance imaging in suspected acute sigmoid diverticulitis. Dis Colon Rectum 51(12):1810–1815

Horsthuis K, Bipat S, Stokkers PC, et al (2009) Magnetic resonance imaging for evaluation of disease activity in Crohn's disease: a systematic review. Eur Radiol 19(6):1450–1460

Jaffe TA, Gaca AM, Delaney S, et al (2007) Radiation doses from small-bowel follow-through and abdominopelvic MDCT in Crohn's disease. AJR Am J Roentgenol 189(5): 1015–1022

Jensch S, de Vries AH, Peringa J, et al (2008) CT colonography with limited bowel preparation: performance characteristics in an increased-risk population. Radiology 247(1): 122–132

Johnson CD, Chen MH, Toledano AY, et al (2008) Accuracy of CT colonography for detection of large adenomas and cancers. N Engl J Med 359(12):1207–1217

Kinner S, Kuehle CA, Langhorst J, et al (2007) MR colonography vs. optical colonoscopy: comparison of patients' acceptance in a screening population. Eur Radiol 17(9):2286–2293

Koh DM, Brown G, Collins DJ (2009) Nanoparticles in rectal cancer imaging. Cancer Biomark 5(2):89–98

Koh DM, Miao Y, Chinn RJS, et al (2001) MR imaging evaluation of the activity of Crohn's disease. AJR Am J Roentgenol 177: 1325–1332

Kuehle CA, Langhorst J, Ladd SC, et al (2007) Magnetic resonance colonography without bowel cleansing: a prospective cross sectional study in a screening population. Gut 56(8):1079–1085

Laméris W, van Randen A, Bipat S, et al (2008) Graded compression ultrasonography and computed tomography in acute colonic diverticulitis: meta-analysis of test accuracy. Eur Radiol 18(11):2498–2511

Laméris W, van Randen A, van Es HW, et al (2009) Imaging strategies for the detection of urgent conditions in patients with acute abdominal pain. BMJ 339:b2431

Langhorst J, Kühle CA, Ajaj W, et al (2007) MR colonography without bowel purgation for the assessment of inflammatory bowel diseases: diagnostic accuracy and patient acceptance. Inflamm Bowel Dis 13(8):1001–1008

Lauenstein TC, Goehde SC, Ruehm SG, et al (2002) MR colonography with barium-based fecal tagging: initial clinical experience. Radiology 223(1):248–254

Lauenstein TC, Herborn CU, Vogt FM, et al (2001a) Dark lumen MR colonography: initial experience. Rofo 173(9): 785–789

Lauenstein TC, Holtmann G, Schoenfelder D, et al (2001b) MR Colonography without colonic cleansing: a new strategy to improve patient acceptance. AJR Am. J Roentgenol 177: 823–827

Levin B, Lieberman DA, McFarland B, et al (2008) Screening and surveillance for the early detection of colorectal cancer and adenomatous polyps, 2008: a joint guideline from the American Cancer Society, the US Multi-Society Task Force on Colorectal Cancer, and the American College of Radiology. CA Cancer J Clin 58(3):130–160

Lieberman D, Moravec M, Holub J, et al (2008) Polyp size and advanced histology in patients undergoing colonoscopy screening: implications for CT colonography. Gastroenterology 135(4):1100–1105

Lomas DJ, Sood RR, Graves MJ, et al (2001) Colon carcinoma: MR imaging with CO_2 enema–pilot study. Radiology 219 (2):558–562

Low RN, McCue M, Barone R, et al (2003) MR staging of primary colorectal carcinoma: comparison with surgical and histopathologic findings. Abdom Imaging 28(6):784–793

Luboldt W, Bauerfeind P, Steiner P, et al (1997) Preliminary assessment of three-dimensional magnetic resonance imaging for various colonic disorders. Lancet 349(9061): 1288–1291

Luboldt W, Bauerfeind P, Wildermuth S, et al (2000) Colonic masses: detection with MR colonography. Radiology 216(2): 383–388

Luboldt W, Steiner P, Bauerfeind P, et al (1998) Detection of mass lesions with MR colonography: preliminary report. Radiology 207(1):59–65

Macari M, Berman P, Dicker M, et al (1999) Usefulness of CT colonography in patients with incomplete colonoscopy. AJR Am J Roentgenol 173(3):561–564

Mandel JS, Church TR, Bond JH, et al (2000) The effect of fecal occult-blood screening on the incidence of colorectal cancer. N Engl J Med 343(22):1603–1607

Martinez F, Kondylis P, Reilly J (2005) Limitations of barium enema performed as an adjunct to incomplete colonoscopy. Dis Colon Rectum 48(10):1951–1954

Neri E, Giusti P, Battolla L, et al (2002) Colorectal cancer: role of CT colonography in preoperative evaluation after incomplete colonoscopy. Radiology 223(3):615–619

O'Connell JB, Maggard MA, Ko CY, et al (2004) Colon cancer survival rates with the new American Joint Committee on Cancer sixth edition staging. J Natl Cancer Inst 96(19): 1420–1425

Pappalardo G, Polettini E, Frattaroli FM, et al (2000) Magnetic resonance colonography versus conventional colonoscopy for the detection of colonic endoluminal lesions. Gastroenterology 119(2):300–304

Pickhardt PJ, Hassan C, Laghi A, et al (2008) Small and diminutive polyps detected at screening CT colonography: a decision analysis for referral to colonoscopy. AJR Am J Roentgenol 190:136–144

Rao PM, Rhea JT, Novelline RA, et al (1998) Helical CT with only colonic contrast material for diagnosing diverticulitis: prospective evaluation of 150 patients. AJR Am J Roentgenol 170(6):1445–1449

Rimola J, Rodríguez S, García Bosch O, et al (2009) Magnetic resonance for assessment of disease activity and severity in Crohn disease. Gut PMID 19136510

Rodriguez Gomez S, Pagés Llinas M, Castells Garangou A, et al (2008) Ark-lumen MR colonography with fecal tagging: a comparison of water enema and air methods of colonic distension for detecting colonic neoplasms. Eur Radiol 18(7): 1396–1405

Saar B, Meining A, Beer A, et al (2007) Prospective study on bright lumen magnetic resonance colonography in comparison with conventional colonoscopy. Br J Radiol 80(952): 235–241

Schreyer AG, Fürst A, Agha A, et al (2004) Magnetic resonance imaging based colonography for diagnosis and assessment of diverticulosis and diverticulitis. Int J Colorectal Dis 19(5):474–480

Schreyer AG, Gölder S, Scheibl K, et al (2005a) Dark lumen magnetic resonance enteroclysis in combination with MRI colonography for whole bowel assessment in patients with Crohn's disease: first clinical experience. Inflamm Bowel Dis 11(4):388–394

Schreyer AG, Rath HC, Kikinis R, et al (2005b) Comparison of magnetic resonance imaging colonography with conventional colonoscopy for the assessment of intestinal inflammation in patients with inflammatory bowel disease: a feasibility study. Gut 54(2):250–256

Shinya S, Sasaki T, Nakagawa Y, et al (2009) The efficacy of diffusion-weighted imaging for the detection of colorectal cancer. Hepatogastroenterology 56(89):128–132

Shoenut JP, Semelka RC, Magro CM, et al (1994) Comparison of magnetic resonance imaging and endoscopy in distinguishing the type and severity of inflammatory bowel disease. J Clin Gastroenterol 19(1):31–35

Stoker J. (2008) Magnetic resonance imaging and the acute abdomen. Br J Surg 95(10):1193–1194

Sumanac K, Zealley I, Fox BM, et al (2002) Minimizing post-colonoscopy abdominal pain by using CO(2) insufflation: a prospective, randomized, double blind, controlled trial evaluating a new commercially available CO(2) delivery system. Gastrointest Endosc 56(2):190–194

Taylor SA, Laghi A, Lefere P, et al (2007) European Society of Gastrointestinal and Abdominal Radiology (ESGAR): consensus statement on CT colonography. Eur Radiol 17(2): 575–579

Van Gelder RE, Nio CY, Florie J, et al (2004) Computed tomographic colonography compared with colonoscopy in patients at increased risk for colorectal cancer. Gastroenterology 127(1):41–48

Weishaupt D, Patak MA, Froehlich J, et al (1999) Faecal tagging to avoid colonic cleansing before MRI colonography. Lancet 354(9181):835–836

Winawer SJ, Zauber AG (2002) The advanced adenoma as the primary target of screening. Gastrointest Endosc Clin N Am 12(1):1–9

Zalis ME, Barish MA, Choi JR, et al (2005) CT colonography reporting and data system: a consensus proposal. Radiology 236(1):3–9

Zijta FM, Bipat S, Stoker J (2009) Magnetic resonance (MR) colonography in the detection of colorectal lesions: a systematic review of prospective studies. Eur Rad (in press)

MRI of the Rectum

Doenja M.J. Lambregts, Monique Maas and Regina G.H. Beets-Tan

CONTENTS

13.1 Introduction/Clinical Background 205
13.2 Standard MR Protocol for Rectal Cancer Staging 208
13.3 MR Anatomy of the Rectum and Mesorectum 209
13.3.1 Rectum 209
13.3.2 Mesorectum 210
13.3.3 Peritoneum 211
13.3.4 Blood Supply 211
13.4 Risk Assessment with MR Imaging 211
13.4.1 T-Stage 212
13.4.2 CRM 212
13.4.3 Lymph Nodes 214
13.4.3.1 Extramesorectal Lymph Nodes 215
13.5 Restaging Rectal Cancer 216
13.5.1 The yT-Stage 217
13.5.2 Tumor Regression from the Mesorectal Fascia 218
13.5.3 The yN Stage 220
13.6 Other Imaging Modalities 220
13.6.1 Endorectal Ultrasound (EUS) 220
13.6.2 CT 220
13.6.3 PET-CT 221
13.7 Future Perspectives 221
13.8 Conclusions and Recommendations for Rectal Cancer Management 222
13.9 Anorectal Fistulas 222
13.10 Endometriosis 224
13.10.1 MRI of "Deep Endometriosis" 225

List of Abbreviations 226

References 226

Doenja M.J. Lambregts, MD
Monique Maas, MD
Regina G.H. Beets-Tan, MD
Department of Radiology, Maastricht University Medical Center, Maastricht, The Netherlands

KEY POINTS

MRI of the rectum primarily concerns MRI in rectal cancer. The primary goal of accurate imaging staging of rectal cancer is to identify the risk factors for local recurrence in order to offer patients a tailored treatment, based on their individual risk profile. The role of the radiologist has thus emerged from a report only to a full consulting role as sparring partner of the treating clinicians in the multidisciplinary team, where he can influence the treatment choice based on his imaging findings. Patients with small, low-risk tumors are most accurately selected with endorectal ultrasound. For evaluation of the larger tumors and the circumferential resection margins, MRI is the optimal imaging technique. At present, no imaging technique is reliable for determining the nodal status. Restaging of rectal cancer after neoadjuvant treatment is becoming a more relevant issue, since further tailoring of treatment is increasingly being considered after neoadjuvant treatment. The main problem after chemoradiation is the discrimination of residual tumor in areas of fibrotic scar tissue. New imaging techniques combining anatomical and functional data require further investigation to solve these issues.

13.1

Introduction/Clinical Background

Colorectal cancer is the third most common cancer in men (after prostate and lung cancer) and the second most common cancer in women (after breast cancer). Rectal cancer comprises approximately 20% of all colorectal cancers. In the United Kingdom (UK), the incidence of rectal cancer in 2005 was 8,361 in males and 5,657 in females. The age-adjusted death rate was

23.7 per 100,000 males and 12.8 per 100,000 females (UK cancer research, website accessed 14 April 09). In the United States, an incidence of 148,810 in 2008 was estimated and the age-adjusted death rate from 2001 to 2005 was 50.6 per 100,000 (National Cancer Institute United States, website accessed 14 June 09).

The etiology of rectal cancer is still unclear, but is probably multifactorial. Environmental factors such as diet, smoking, obesity, but also age, inflammatory bowel disease, and genetic factors are believed to be associated with the development of rectal cancer. Patients usually present with rectal bleeding or changed bowel habits. At colonoscopy, a rectal tumor is found and biopsies are taken. If the diagnosis of rectal cancer is confirmed, the patient's risk profile is evaluated in a multidisciplinary team (MDT) meeting and the most optimal treatment strategy is chosen in consensus by the MDT members. An MDT for colorectal cancer generally consists of a surgeon, a radiation oncologist, a medical oncologist, a pathologist and a radiologist. The role of the radiologist has changed from a report only role to a full consulting one. The radiologist has become a full sparring partner in the disease management team. The primary goal of accurate imaging staging of rectal cancer is to identify risk factors for local recurrence (and/or distant metastases). So, the role of the radiologist with the introduction of neoadjuvant treatment in rectal cancer patients has become an important one: he can influence the treatment choice based on his imaging findings.

The main concern after rectal cancer surgery is the high local recurrence rate reported to vary between <10 and 41%. Local recurrences are mainly caused by incomplete surgical resection (QUIRKE et al. 1986). With the introduction of the "total mesorectal excision" (TME), local recurrence rates have dropped to less than 10% in some specialized centers (HEALD and RYALL 1986). With this TME technique, the whole mesorectal compartment that is the rectum with the surrounding fat and lymph nodes is resected along the mesorectal fascia (MRF) (Fig. 13.1).

The Swedish Rectal Cancer Trial (1997) found that preoperative 5 × 5 Gy in clinically resectable tumors resulted in a decrease of 58% of the local recurrence rate in the irradiated group when compared with the surgery only arm, with minimal 5 years of follow-up. SAUER et al. (2004) conducted a randomized controlled trial comparing preoperative chemoradiation with postoperative chemoradiation for locally advanced rectal cancer. Patients who underwent preoperative chemoradiation had a significantly lower risk for local recurrence than patients who underwent

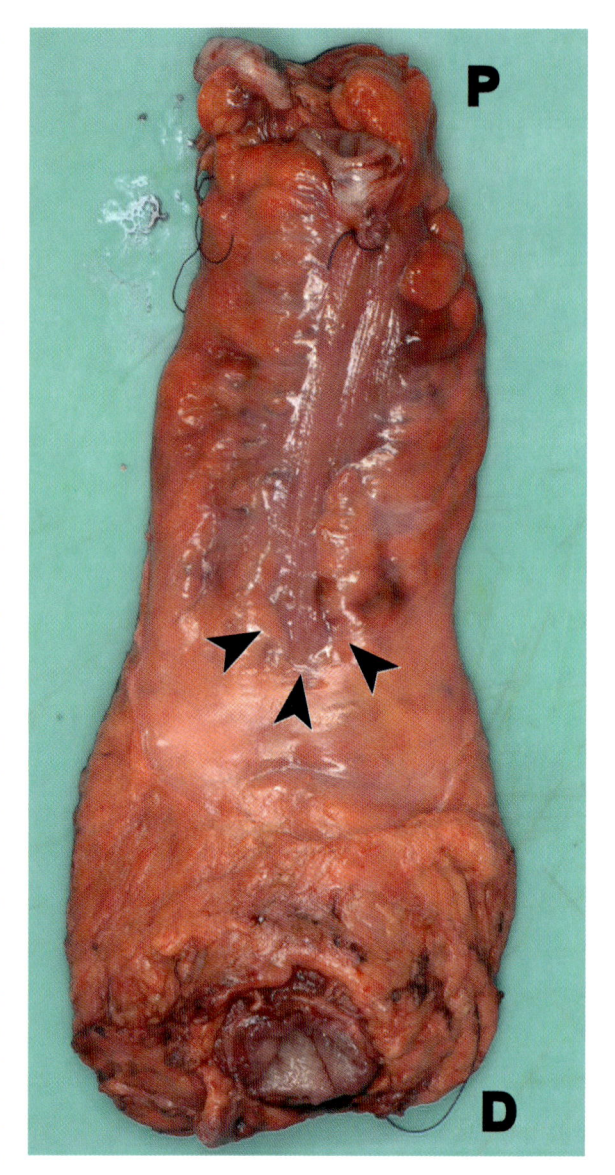

Fig. 13.1. Anterior view of a TME specimen. The entire mesorectal compartment is removed with sharp dissection along the mesorectal fascia. D indicates the distal and P the proximal resection margin. The peritoneal reflection is visualized on the anterior side (*arrowheads*)

postoperative treatment (6% vs. 13%) at a median follow-up of 45.8 months. A randomized controlled trial that evaluated preoperative radiotherapy for clinically resectable rectal cancer versus postoperative chemoradiation for patients with involved circumferential resection margins at pathologic examination has recently reported 5 year local recurrence rates of 11.5% for the postoperative chemoradiation group when compared with 4.7% for the preoperative radiotherapy group ($p < 0.0001$) (SEBAG-MONTEFIORE et al. 2009). From these studies, we learned that preoperative radiotherapy is more effective than a postoperative regimen for reducing the overall local recurrence rate, although survival benefit was only seen with the Scandinavian trial.

A Dutch TME trial compared TME only with preoperative 5 × 5 Gy + TME and found a significant reduction of the risk for local recurrence from 26 to 9% in the preoperative 5 × 5 Gy arm when compared with the surgery only arm. Therefore, even with improved surgery such as TME, preoperative radiotherapy is still beneficial for overall reduction of local recurrence rates. However, from the results we also learned that there were subgroups with different risks for local recurrences. Patients with stage I disease (T1–2N0) did not benefit from radiotherapy, because they were already at low risk for local recurrences, whereas patients with malignant nodes (TxN+, stage III) benefited most from radiotherapy, although these stage III patients still had a relatively high recurrence rate despite the preoperative 5 × 5 Gy (11.2%). More intensive neoadjuvant treatment such as long course preoperative radiotherapy with concurrent chemotherapy could be considered for improvement of local control in these high-risk stage III rectal cancer patients (Kapiteijn et al. 2001; Sauer et al. 2004).

Thus, different risk groups for local recurrences exist. Present day modern imaging techniques are known to accurately select these groups: (1) the low-risk group (T1–2N0) with small tumors that are confined to the bowel wall (Fig. 13.2), (2) the intermediate-risk group (T3N0) with larger tumors and free circumferential resection margins (CRM) (Fig. 13.3), and (3) the high-risk group (T3–4Nx) with locally advanced tumors, that threaten or involve the CRM (Fig. 13.4), or TxN2 tumors with involved nodes (Fig. 13.5). Staging is generally performed with EUS and/or MRI for local staging and with ultrasound of the liver plus chest X-ray or CT of the liver and chest for distant staging.

In this chapter, the emphasis will be on local staging of rectal cancer with MRI. A baseline state-of-the-art MR rectal protocol is given (Table 13.1). The MRI-anatomy of the rectum, MR image evaluation of T-stage, N-stage, and CRM involvement will be addressed. A separate section will address the issue of restaging of locally advanced rectal tumors after neoadjuvant treatment. Finally, the role of CT, EUS, and PET-CT and future perspectives for imaging of rectal cancer will be discussed. In addition, other diseases of the rectum, for which MRI has proven to be beneficial–fistulas and endometriosis–will briefly be addressed.

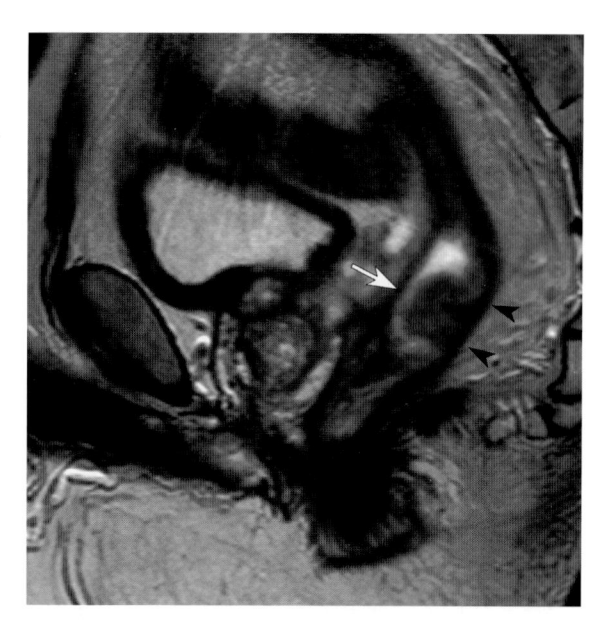

Fig. 13.2. Sagittal T2-weighted FSE image of a male patient with a low-risk rectal tumor stratified for immediate TME. There is a polypoid tumor mass in the mid rectum (*white arrow*) arising from the dorsal rectal wall. The tumor is surrounded by a hypointense line, suggesting a tumor limited to the bowel wall (*black arrowheads*), which was confirmed at histologic evaluation

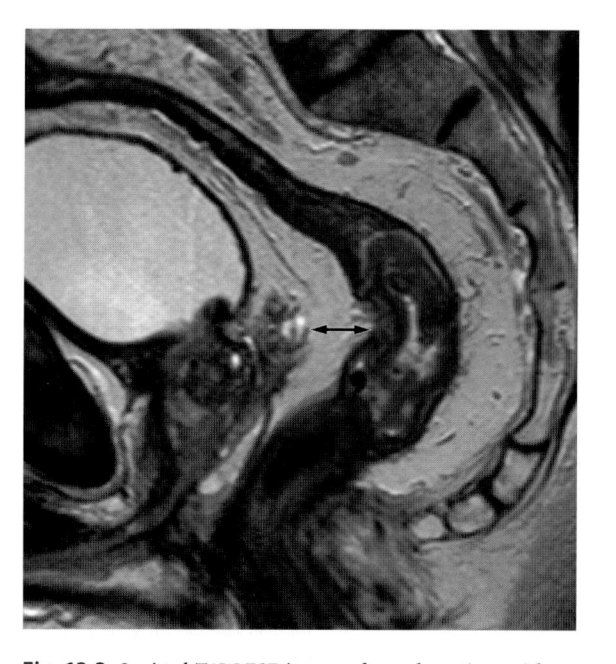

Fig. 13.3. Sagittal T2W FSE image of a male patient with an intermediate risk rectal tumor stratified for a short course of 5 × 5 Gy + TME. There is a tumor in the mid-rectum. On the anterior side the rectal wall is not sharply delineated, suggesting a T3 tumor with ingrowth in the mesorectal fat. A wide margin is observed between the tumor and the mesorectal fascia (*double arrow*). Histologic evaluation confirmed a T3 tumor with wide margins

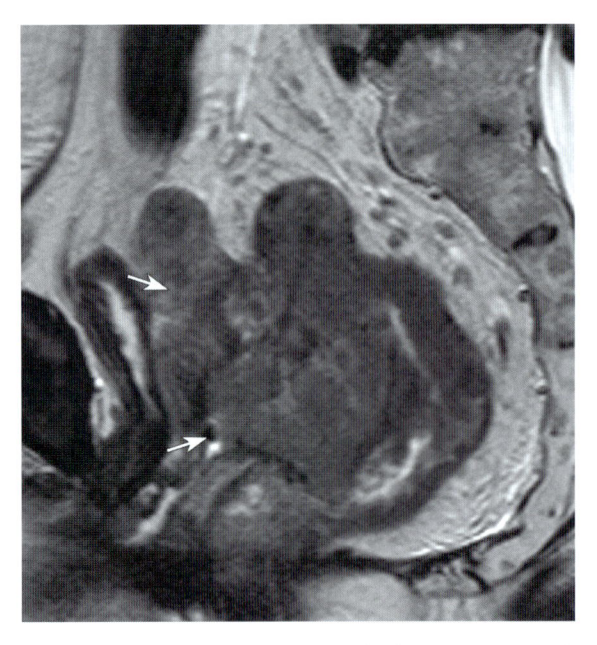

Fig. 13.4. Sagittal T2W FSE image of a female patient with a high-risk rectal tumor stratified for long course chemoradiation. There is a bulky rectal tumor located in the mid-rectum that grows through the mesorectal fascia anteriorly and invades the uterus (*arrows*) and vagina

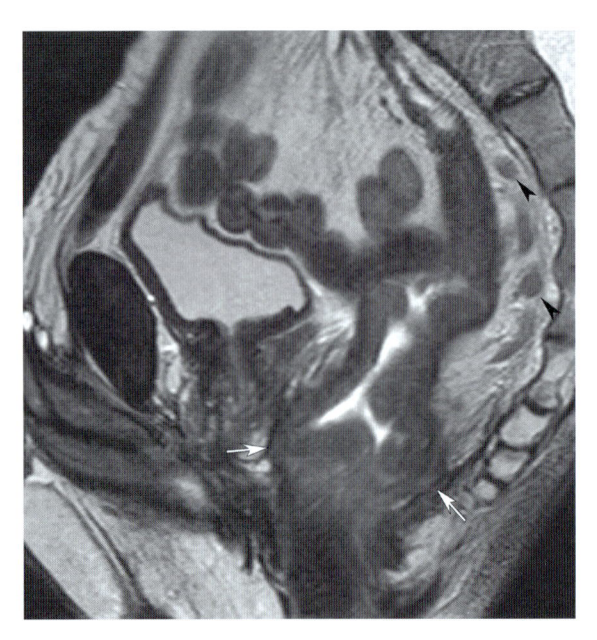

Fig. 13.5. Sagittal T2W FSE image of a male patient with a high-risk rectal tumor stratified for long course chemoradiation. There is a bulky T3 tumor in the distal and mid-rectum. At the distal tumor margin, there is a close or involved resection margin, both at the anterior and posterior site (*white arrows*). Note the suspicious lymph nodes in the presacral region (*black arrowheads*)

13.2
Standard MR Protocol for Rectal Cancer Staging

MRI using new generation external phased array coils has improved signal-to-noise ratio and generates high spatial and contrast resolution images. Phased array MRI has become the standard MR technique for state-of-the-art staging of rectal cancer, except in the selection of the very superficial T1N0 tumors, where EUS still plays the main role. MRI using an endorectal coil, although as accurate as EUS for assessment of tumor ingrowth in the bowel wall, has not really gained worldwide acceptance because of several reasons. First of all, an endorectal staging technique is mainly performed for selection of superficial tumors for local excision instead of TME. This selection in many centers is performed during the first visit of the patient at the MDT clinics and EUS-guided biopsies are often taken at the same time. The endorectal MRI would therefore be a cost-inefficient surplus exam to the standard EUS for selection of superficial cancers and is furthermore cumbersome in application and less patient friendly than an EUS technique. With an endorectal technique, accurate positioning of the coil is often difficult and in high and/or stenosing tumors sometimes not even possible.

For phased array MRI, no bowel preparation is required nor are spasmolytics routinely given. However, occasionally spasmolytics may be helpful in patients presenting with high anteriorly located tumors to reduce the motion artefacts that are caused by adjacent small bowel loops. Although the use of endorectal contrast such as iron oxide enema has been described to be very useful, the rationale for doing so is mainly to provide radiologists a more confident assessment of the exact location of the tumor, especially in small tumors (WALLENGREN et al. 2000). However, the tumor location is most often known to clinicians by their endoscopic exam. The main reason why MRI is requested is to identify the high-risk tumors; those tumors that are threatening or involving the CRM and those that extent far into the perirectal fat. Stretching of the rectal wall by endorectal contrast would cause overstaging of the CRM involvement (SLATER et al. 2006). Furthermore, distension of the rectal wall would compress the mesorectal fat, hampering an accurate evaluation of the mesorectal nodes. A standard rectal MR protocol thus comprises T2-weighted Fast Spin Echo (T2W

Table 13.1. Scan parameters for a standard 2D T2-weighted fast spin echo sequence of the pelvic region.

2D T2W FSE	
Repetition time/echo time (ms)	3427/150
Number of slices	22
Slice thickness	5
Slice gap	2
Flip angle (degrees)	90
Matrix	175 × 256
FOV (mm)	200
Echotrain length	25
Number of signal averages (NSA)	6
Acquisition time (s)	308

FSE) sequences in three planes (Table 13.1). T2W FSE images allow for a good contrast between tumor, surrounding high signal of mesorectal fat and the very thin mesorectal fascia. In this respect, fat suppression sequences are not recommended, as on fat suppression images the anatomy of the mesorectal fascia is not as well respected (Fig. 13.6). A sagittal T2W FSE sequence should first be obtained in order to locate the tumor. Based on the sagittal sequence, axial and coronal T2W FSE sequences are planned and it is especially crucial to angle the axial and coronal plane exactly perpendicular and parallel to the tumor axis. High-resolution images with a slice thickness of 4 mm or less and a field of view (FOV) that covers the promontory and L5 cranially, the anal canal caudally, the symphysis anteriorly and the sacral bone posteriorly are preferred. At the time of writing, diffusion weighted imaging (DWI) sequences are obtained mainly in research protocol settings and their value for rectal cancer staging has not yet been established. Gadolinium contrast administration has not proven to be beneficial for T-stage and CRM evaluation (VLIEGEN et al. 2005). Total acquisition time of a standard rectal MRI does not need to exceed 25 min.

13.3
MR Anatomy of the Rectum and Mesorectum

13.3.1
Rectum

The rectum extends from the anorectal junction to the rectosigmoid junction (usually arbitrarily defined as 15 cm from the anal verge, corresponding to the level of the third sacral vertebra). On T2W images, two layers can be identified within the normal rectal wall: (1) the inner mucosal layer, that can be seen as a line of intermediate signal and (2) the outer muscularis propria layer that can be seen as a hypointense line surrounding the rectum (Fig. 13.7). In case of submucosal edema (due to inflammation), a third layer (the submucosa) can be visualized as an area of high signal between the inner and outer layer (Fig. 13.8).

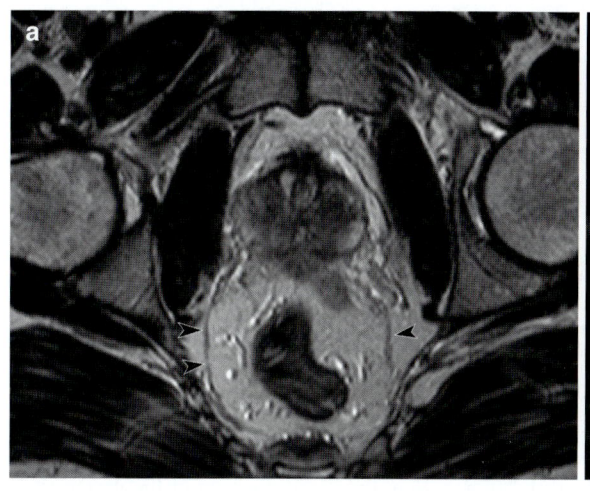

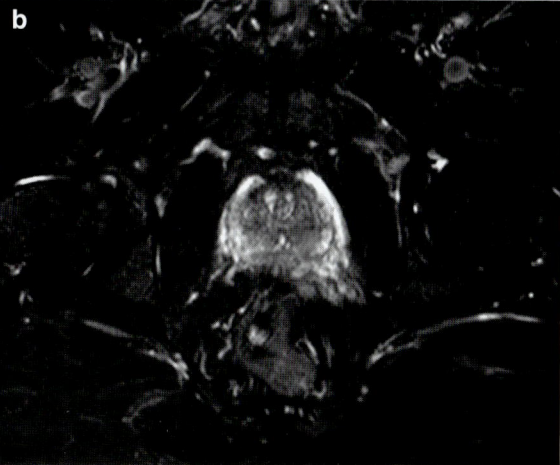

Fig. 13.6. Axial MR images without (**a**) and with fat suppression (**b**). Note how the mesorectal fascia can be clearly identified as a hypointense line on the image without fat suppression (*black arrowheads*). On the fat suppression image, it is hardly visualized

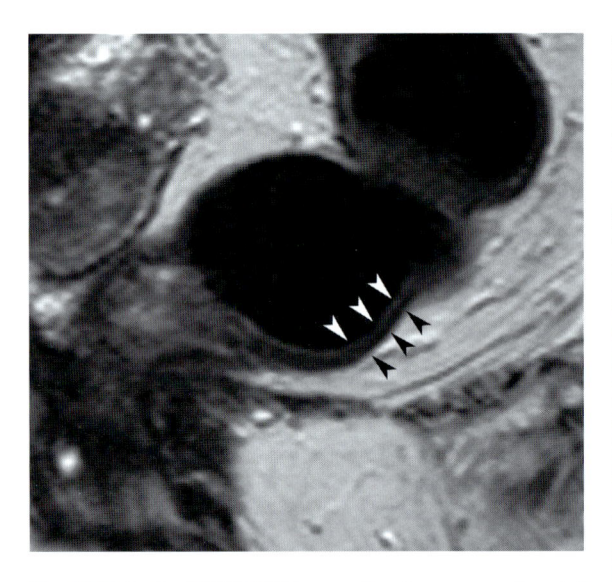

Fig. 13.7. Sagittal T2W FSE image showing a normal rectal wall in a male patient. The inner mucosal layer of the rectal wall is visualized as a line of intermediate signal intensity (*white arrowheads*). The outer layer, the muscularis propria recti, can be seen as a hypointense line surrounding the rectum (*black arrowheads*)

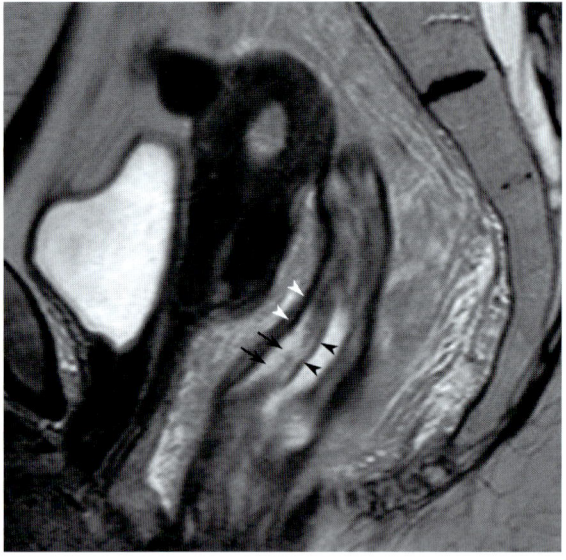

Fig. 13.8. Sagittal T2W FSE MR image of a female patient, showing a layer of high signal intensity (*black arrows*) corresponding to an edematous submucosal layer between the inner mucosal layer (*black arrowheads*) and the muscularis propria (*white arrowheads*)

13.3.2
Mesorectum

The mesorectum entails the rectum, mesorectal fat, lymph nodes, and blood and lymphatic vessels. The mesorectal compartment is bounded by the mesorectal fascia. The mesorectal fascia (MRF) is a thin fibrous structure that on T2W FSE MR images can be seen as a very thin line of hypointense signal intensity when compared with the surrounding high signal fat tissue (Fig. 13.6a). The mesorectal fascia constitutes the surgical resection plane along which a total mesorectal excision is performed. On the anterior side, the mesorectal fat is thinner than on the lateral and posterior side. Therefore, a close relation exists between the anterior rectal wall and the prostate and seminal vesicles in men and the vagina and cervix in women. Distally, the thickness of the mesorectal fat surrounding the rectal wall decreases, due to the tapering of the mesorectum. Thus, near the pelvic floor and anorectal junction, there is a close relation between the rectal wall and mesorectal fascia as well as the pelvic floor muscles (Fig. 13.9). Tumors that are located in the low and anterior rectum consequently are at higher risk for tumor involvement of the MRF.

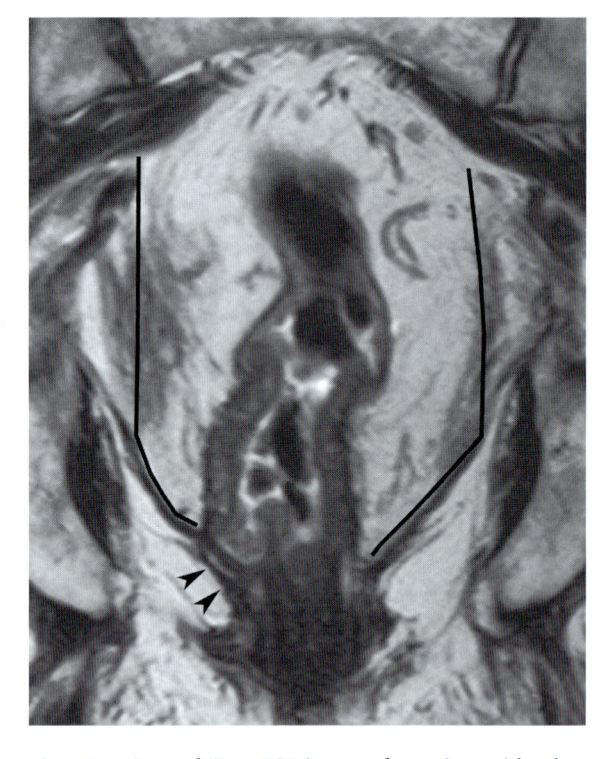

Fig. 13.9. Coronal T2W FSE image of a patient with a low rectal tumor. Note the distal tapering of the mesorectum (*black lines*), causing a close topographical relation of the distal rectal wall and tumor to the pelvic floor muscles (*black arrowheads*)

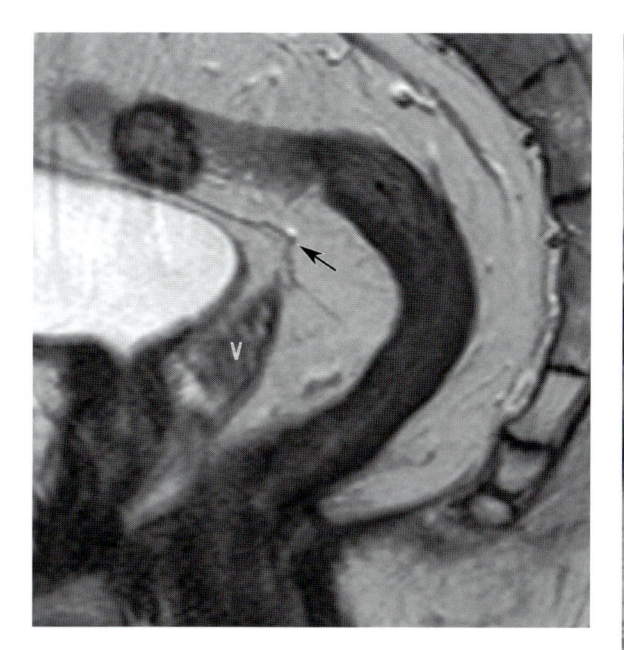

Fig. 13.10. Sagittal T2W FSE image of a male patient. The peritoneal reflection appears as a line of low signal intensity (*black arrow*) proximal to the level of the seminal vesicles (*V*)

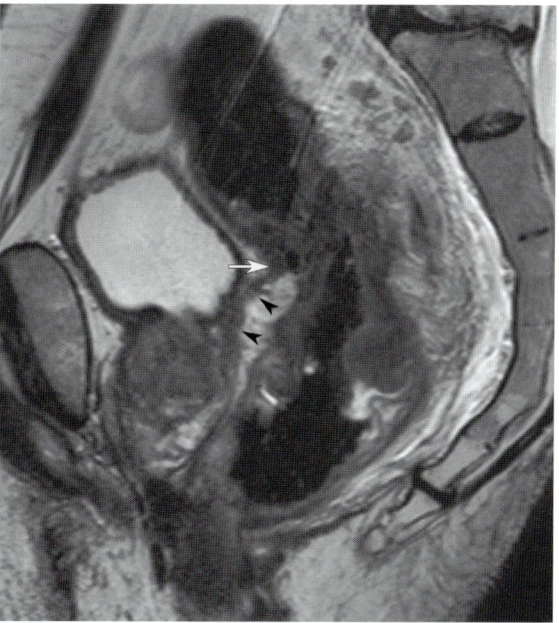

Fig. 13.11. Sagittal T2W FSE image of a male patient with a bulky rectal tumor in the mid-rectum. The tumor grows into the mesorectal fat and invades the mesorectal fascia at the level of the peritoneal fold (*white arrow*). Note the thickened mesorectal fascia (*black arrowheads*)

13.3.3
Peritoneum

In the upper two-thirds of the rectum, the mesorectum is embedded by the parietal and visceral peritoneum. The peritoneum folds anteriorly at the level of the seminal vesicles in men and the posterior vaginal wall in women to form the rectovesical pouch in men or recto-uterine pouch (of Douglas) in women (Fig. 13.10). When the tumor is located anteriorly, its relation to the peritoneal fold is important for surgical planning (Fig. 13.11). Tumors located anteriorly and below the level of the peritoneal fold have a likelihood of invasion of the MRF for which the surgeon will perform a wider excision. Tumors that are located anteriorly but above the visceral peritoneum are above this level and thus hardly ever alter the standard surgical procedure (TME).

13.3.4
Blood Supply

The blood supply of the rectum originates embryologically from the inferior mesenteric artery. The superior rectal artery – a branch of the inferior mesenteric artery – is the main feeding artery of the rectum. On T2W FSE images, the superior rectal artery and its branches are visualized as hypointense tubular structures located in the presacral region. The superior rectal vein runs on the dorsal and left lateral side of the artery (Fig. 13.12). The distal part of the rectum receives additional blood supply from the middle rectal artery, an inconsistent branch from the internal iliac artery.

13.4
Risk Assessment with MR Imaging

The main goal of staging by imaging is to provide the surgeon, radiotherapist, and other members of the multidisciplinary team accurate information about the risk factors for local recurrence, in order to choose the most optimal (curative) treatment strategy for the patient.

The risk factors for local recurrence that can be assessed by imaging methods are (a) the local extent of the tumor (T-stage), (b) circumferential resection margin involvement, and (c) nodal involvement (N-stage). Thus, imaging reports should always provide the answers to the following relevant clinical questions: What is the T-stage? Is the circumferential

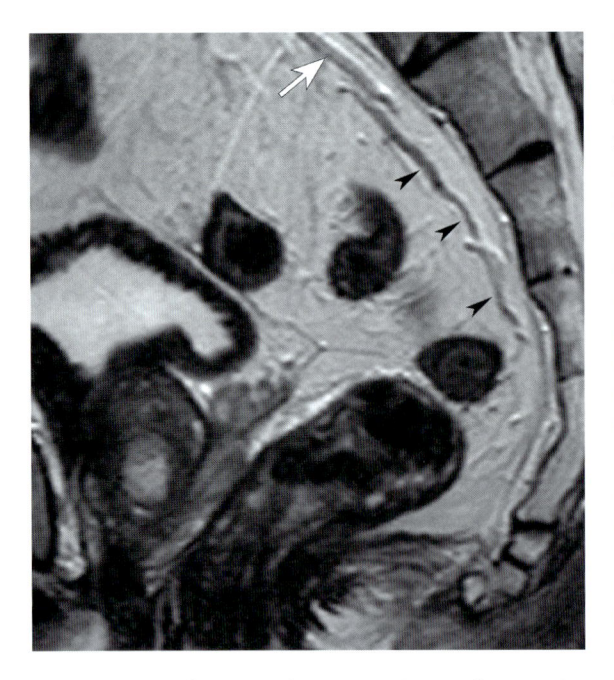

Fig. 13.12. On this sagittal T2W FSE image the superior rectal artery and its branches can be identified as tubular structures with hypointense signal located in the presacral region (*black arrowheads*). The superior rectal vein (*white arrow*) runs on the left and dorsal site of the artery

resection margin involved? Are there nodes inside and outside the mesorectum and if so are they involved? This subsection deals with the role of MRI in the evaluation of these main risk factors for local recurrence: the tumor stage, the circumferential resection margin, and the nodal stage.

13.4.1
T-Stage

The local extent of the tumor (the T-stage) is subdivided into four categories:

T1 tumors limited to the submucosa, T2 tumors invading the muscularis propria, T3 tumors penetrating the muscular rectal wall and extending into the perirectal fat, and T4 tumors invading adjacent organs. Overall accuracy for T-stage prediction with phased array MRI varies between 67 and 83% (BEETS-TAN et al. 2001). There are several reasons for this wide range in accuracies. Staging difficulties are known to occur in the MR distinction between T1 vs. T2 and T2 vs. borderline T3 tumors. The main explanation is the two-layered MR appearance of the rectal wall (Fig. 13.7). Because the submucosal layer of the rectal wall is not visualized on phased-array MRI (except when there is edema), the distinction between a T1 tumor that is limited to the submucosa and a T2-tumor that is outgrowing the submucosa and invading the muscular bowel wall can be very difficult. Thus, the role of imaging for selection of superficial T1 tumors that can be considered for local excision has never been given to MRI but rather remains with EUS. Indeed endorectal MRI can better discriminate between T1 and T2 tumors, with sensitivities and specificities comparable with endorectal ultrasound, (BLOMQVIST et al. 2000); however, the technique has never gained wide popularity because it is more cumbersome than EUS (HÜNERBEIN et al. 2000). Overstaging errors of borderline tumors with desmoplastic reactions are the major cause of difficulties in differentiation between T2 and borderline T3 tumors. Desmoplastic reactions in front of a tumor that are free from tumor nests (pT2) cannot be discriminated from desmoplastic reactions that do contain tumor nests (pT3). To be on the safe side, it is often better to overstage a desmoplastic pT2 tumor as T3 than to understage (Fig. 13.13). A recent study, however, has shown that MRI can select tumors limited to the bowel wall (pT1–2) with high sensitivity. When the bowel wall on T2-weighted MR images can be seen as an intact hypointense line around the tumor, this is a predictive criterion for tumors confined to the bowel wall with a positive predictive value (PPV) of 86–91% (DRESEN et al. 2009) (Fig. 13.14). Large T3 (Fig. 13.15) and T4 tumors (Fig. 13.16) can accurately be identified with MRI, with sensitivities of 74 and 82% and specificities of 76 and 96% for T3 and T4, respectively (BIPAT et al. 2004).

13.4.2
CRM

Preoperative knowledge of tumor involvement of the MRF is crucial to obtain a complete resection (R0 resection) of the tumor. When a tumor extends within 2 mm of the MRF, the circumferential resection margin is close or threatened. When the tumor invades the MRF, the CRM is definitely involved (Fig. 13.17a). The CRM is considered wide when the closest distance from the tumor to the MRF is larger than 2 mm (Fig. 13.17b). When the tumor is surrounded by an intact bowel wall, as described in the previous section (Fig. 13.14), the tumor is limited to the bowel wall and the CRM will always be free (BEETS-TAN et al. 2001). Many single-center studies including our own have shown that MRI is very accurate in predicting

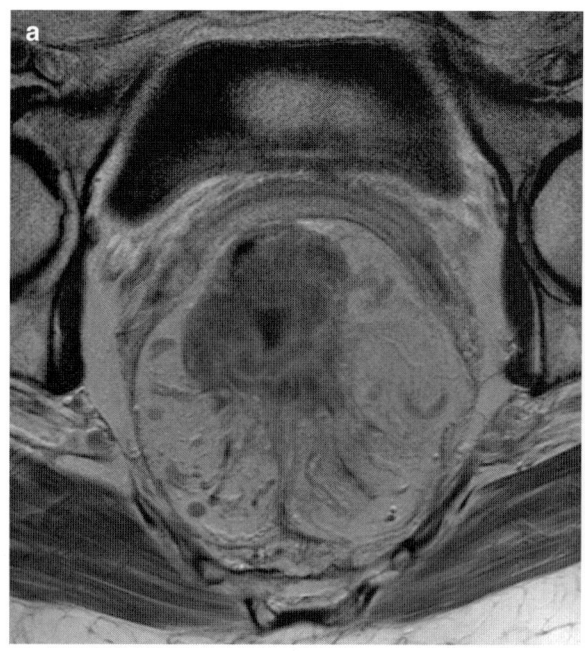

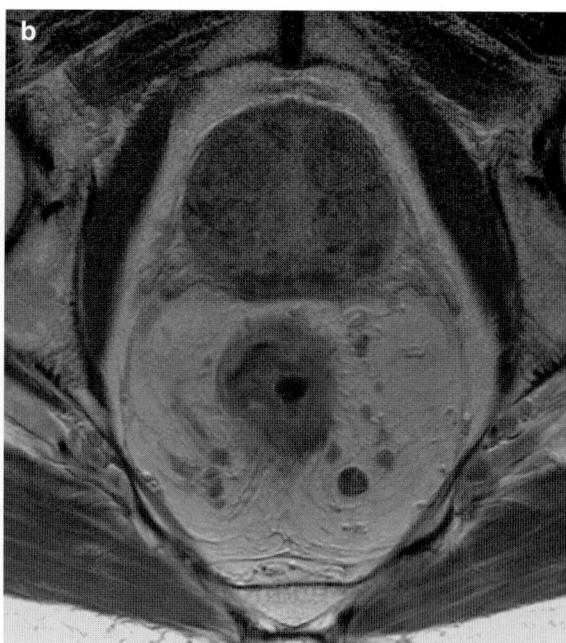

Fig. 13.13. Axial MR images of two patients with rectal tumors that show desmoplastic strands growing into the perirectal fat. (**a**) Shows a pT2 tumor while (**b**) is a pT3 tumor. Note that it is not possible to distinguish between a T2 and T3 tumor on these images. When a tumor shows desmoplasia, MRI cannot differentiate between desmoplasia without (**a**) and with (**b**) tumor (published with permission from BEETS-TAN et al. 2001)

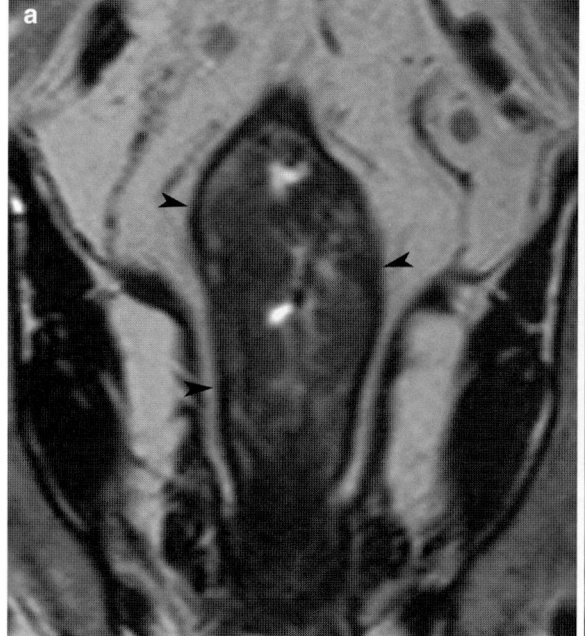

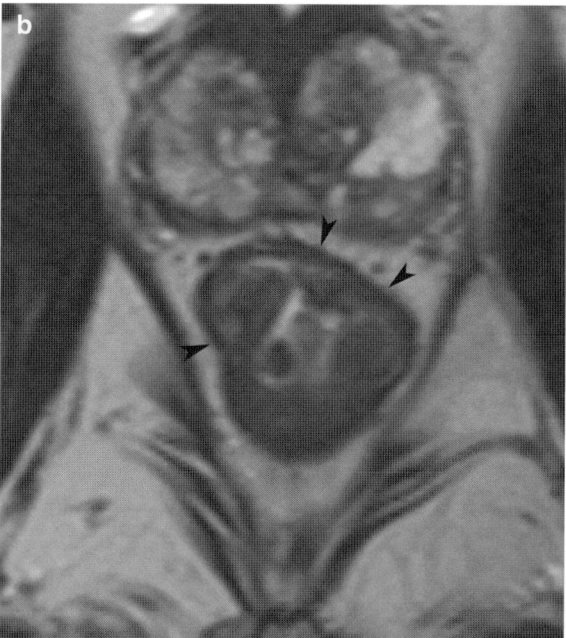

Fig. 13.14. Coronal (**a**) and axial (**b**) T2W FSE image of a male patient with rectal cancer. A hypointense line surrounds the tumor (*arrowheads*), indicating that the tumor is limited to the bowel wall. Further differentiation between a T1 and T2 tumor is not possible with standard MRI

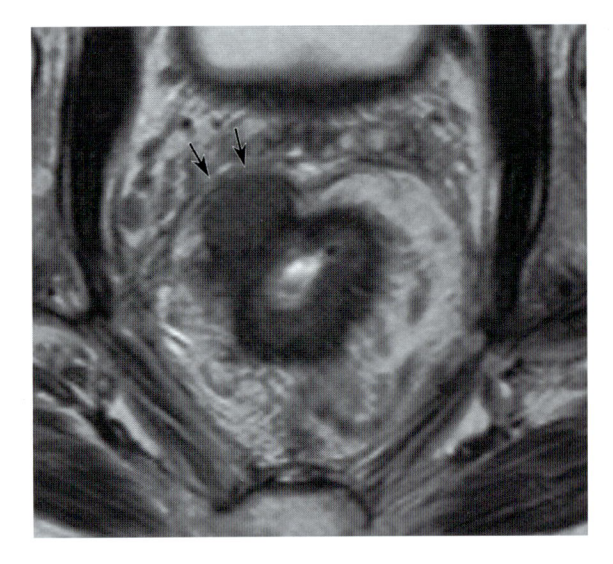

Fig. 13.15. Axial T2W FSE image of a male patient with a T3 tumor showing nodular ingrowth into the perirectal fat on the anterior side, where the tumor invades the mesorectal fascia (*arrows*)

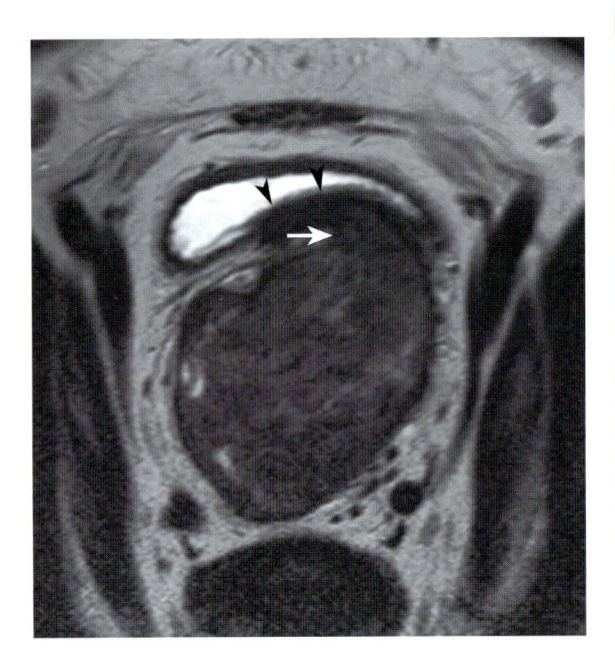

Fig. 13.16. Axial T2W FSE image of a male patient with a bulky T4 rectal tumor. The tumor invades the mesorectal fascia anteriorly (*white arrow*) and grows into the posterior bladder wall (*black arrowheads*)

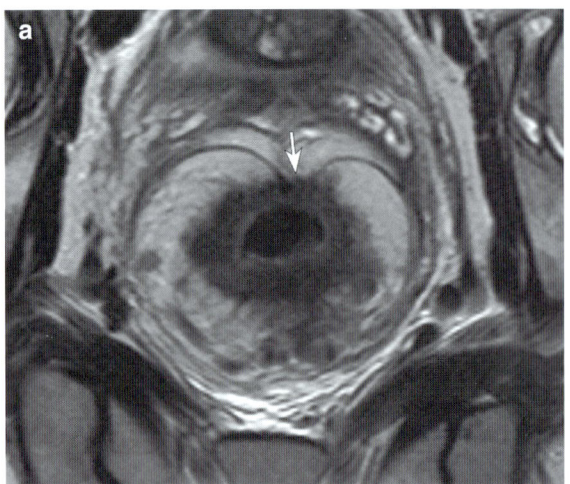

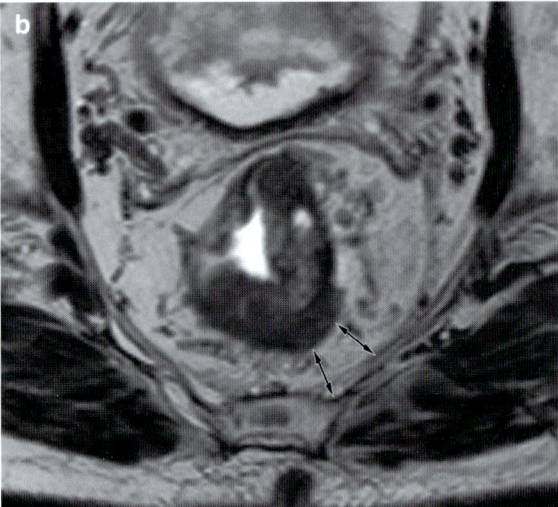

Fig. 13.17. Axial T2-weighted FSE images of two patients with a T3 rectal tumor. The first tumor (**a**) grows into the perirectal fat over the whole circumference. Anteriorly, the tumor invades the mesorectal fascia, which is retracted into the tumor (*white arrow*). The CRM is involved. The second tumor (**b**) penetrates the bowel wall and grows into the perirectal fat at the left dorsal site. The tumor stays at safe distance from the mesorectal fascia (*double arrows*) and the CRM is thus not threatened

involvement of the CRM. A meta-analysis of seven reports evaluated the accuracy of CT, MRI, and EUS for prediction of CRM involvement and found sensitivities of 60–88% and specificities of 73–100% (Lahaye et al. 2005). A large multicenter study in 408 patients reported an overall accuracy of 88%, PPV of 54%, and NPV of 94% for MRI prediction of CRM involvement, suggesting that MRI in staging rectal cancer is reproducible in general hands (Mercury Study Group 2006).

13.4.3
Lymph Nodes

Prediction of the nodal status by imaging methods has become essential due to the paradigm shift from adjuvant to neoadjuvant chemo- and/or radiation therapy. Accurate identification of involved nodes in- and outside the mesorectum allows for selection of patients at high risk for local recurrence, who benefit from intensive neoadjuvant treatment. None of the presently available modern imaging techniques, however, provides sufficient accuracy in assessing the exact nodal status – N0, N1 or N2 – for clinical decision-making. Although nowadays even nodes as small as 2 mm can be visualized using high-resolution MRI, discrimination between the benign and malignant lymph nodes remains a difficult task.

Traditionally, mainly size has been applied as a criterion to identify the malignant nodes, with the best cut-off size in pelvic nodes at 8 mm. Two meta-analyses exist that analyzed the pooled data from nodal imaging studies and showed that EUS and CT using size criteria are inaccurate for characterization of lymph nodes. MRI could not outperform the two other imaging methods, with sensitivities and specificities in the range of 55–78% (Bipat et al. 2004; Lahaye et al. 2005). The use of size criteria in rectal cancer nodes is furthermore limited, because in rectal cancer metastases frequently occur in small (<5 mm) nodes (Wang et al. 2005). When applying size as the only criterion, small metastatic nodes are thus understaged while overstaging occurs in the larger-sized nodes. Morphologic criteria in addition to size improve the nodal evaluation: nodes that are sharply delineated and homogeneous in signal often prove to be benign (Fig. 13.18a), while nodes showing an irregular border and heterogeneous signal pattern are more likely to be involved (Fig. 13.18b). With the use of these criteria, sensitivities of 36–85% and specificities of 95–100% were reported on a patient basis, where the existence of larger-sized nodes allowed accurate evaluation of the border and nodal heterogeneity (Kim et al. 2004; Brown et al. 2003). These criteria, however, are more difficult to evaluate in the very small nodes (2–3 mm). We can conclude that at present no imaging technique is sufficiently accurate for prediction of the nodal status and clinical decision-making based on it, unless of course when the presence of a large and suspicious metastatic node – like in the patient of Fig. 13.18b – gives no reason for doubt of the N+ status of the patient. Promising results were reported for nodal staging using lymph node specific MR contrast agents, such as Ultrasmall Particles of Iron Oxide (USPIO) (Wang et al. 2006; Lahaye et al. 2008). However, at the time of writing, USPIO contrast is not approved for clinical use and it remains unclear whether or when it will be available on the market.

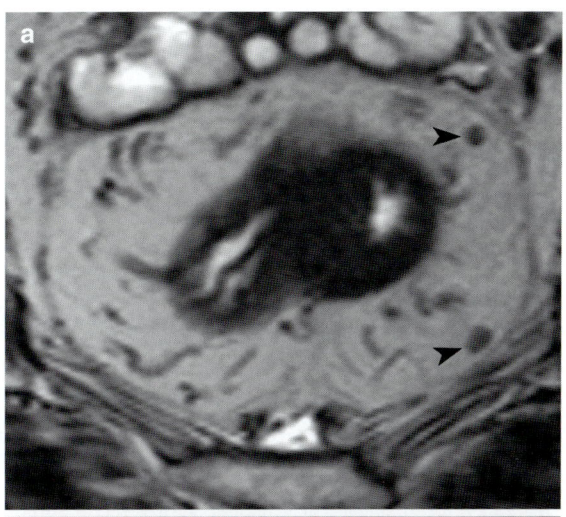

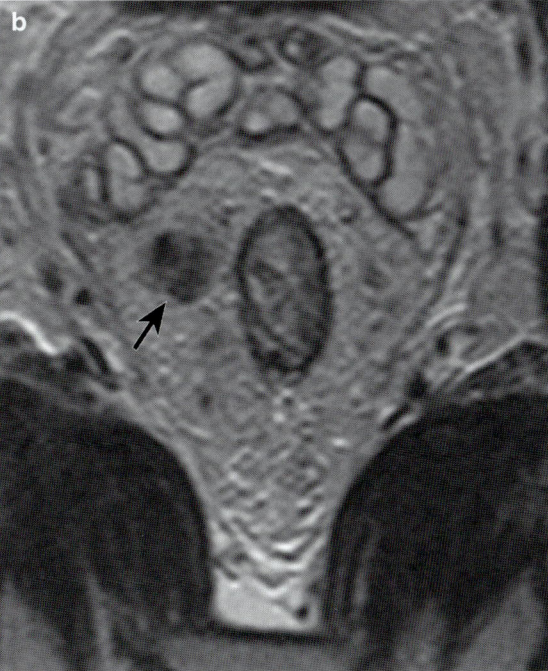

Fig. 13.18. Axial T2W FSE images of two patients with visible lymph nodes in the mesorectal fat. The two nodes in the first patient (*arrowheads* in **a**) show criteria for benignancy: oval shape in one of them, excentric white hilus in the other, sharp borders, and homogeneous signal in both. Both nodes were benign at histology. The node in the second patient (*arrow* in **b**) shows criteria for malignancy: irregular in border contour, heterogeneous in signal intensity, and larger than 8 mm in size. This node was confirmed to be malignant at histology

13.4.3.1
Extramesorectal Lymph Nodes

Evaluation of nodal disease on MRI should also include a careful search for suspicious lymph nodes

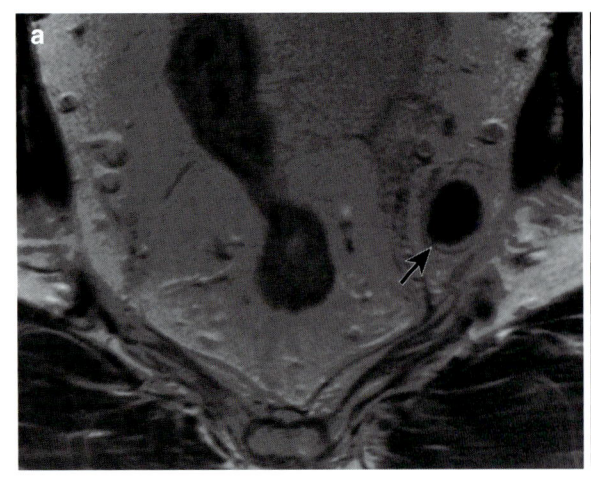

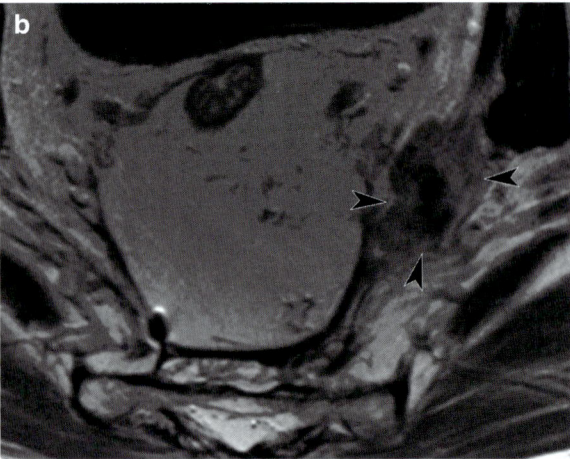

Fig. 13.19. Axial images of a patient with a rectal tumor before (**a**) and after (**b**) rectal cancer surgery. Note the enlarged suspicious node in the left lateral region (*black arrow*) that was misdiagnosed as a benign node. Two years after surgery, this patient developed a left lateral pelvic recurrence (*black arrowheads*), which probably originates from the extramesorectal node that was misinterpreted and left in situ after surgery

outside the mesorectum, in the lateral and inguinal regions. With a standard total mesorectal excision, these nodes remain in situ. When not identified preoperatively and removed at surgery, these nodes could harbor a serious risk for a local recurrence (Fig. 13.19). Nodes outside the mesorectum are evaluated on MRI using the same criteria of size, nodal border contour, and signal pattern. If on a restaging MRI after chemoradiation, an extramesorectal node remains suspicious for involvement, the surgeon would consider an extended lymphadenectomy.

13.5
Restaging Rectal Cancer

With the introduction of neoadjuvant chemoradiation for locally advanced rectal cancer, restaging of the cancer after neoadjuvant treatment can become a relevant issue if the surgeon would consider a less extensive resection or a local excision in the good responders.

Downsizing (shrinkage of tumor volume) and downstaging (a lower T- and/or N-stage when compared with pre-treatment imaging) of the tumor are increasingly encountered with nowadays intensive chemoradiation (CRT) schemes. A local excision has already been advocated for patients with minimal residual disease (yT1–2N0) after treatment without compromising local control (Borschitz et al. 2008; Lezoche et al. 2008). A complete response of the tumor and nodes is reported in 10–30% (Hughes et al. 2006; Valentini et al. 2002; Guillem et al. 2005; Habr-Gama et al. 2006) of patients treated with neoadjuvant chemoradiation. A "wait-and-see policy" (omission of surgery) in these ycT0N0 patients could then be considered. Although both minimal invasive strategies are still controversial at the time of writing, this probably is the way to go in the treatment management of rectal cancer patients: further tailoring of treatment and more organ preserving treatment options in the good/complete responders. This paradigm shift in treatment then puts MR imaging of rectal cancer in a new perspective: not only will the radiologist play a crucial role in the stratification of patients before treatment, but also will his role be important after CRT in the selection of the good and complete responders and in the surveillance of patients after a local excision or "wait-and-see policy."

A restaging MRI is best performed 6–8 weeks after completion of chemoradiation. Again, the previously mentioned risk factors (T-stage, CRM, and N-stage) need to be evaluated. In general, overstaging is the most encountered problem in restaging rectal cancer after chemoradiation. Because of chemoradiation effects, the tumor and nodes shrink and become fibrotic. This fibrosis cannot be distinguished from residual tumor with MRI and MRI cannot identify small residual tumor islets in fibrosis. This results in an increased rate of overstaging when compared with primary staging. Furthermore, studies show a variable interobserver agreement in the evaluation of postchemoradiation MR images, with Kappa's in the range of 0.33–0.64, which probably reflects the difficulty of discerning fibrosis from residual tumor (DRESEN et al. 2009; VLIEGEN et al. 2008a; KUO et al. 2005). Future studies and new techniques (such as molecular imaging) will have to provide a solution for this problem.

13.5.1
The yT-Stage

Low accuracies ranging from 43 to 60% are reported for restaging the yT stage after chemoradiation (KULKARNI et al. 2008; ALLEN et al. 2007). Overstaging is the main cause of errors with reported overstaging rates varying from 10 to 47%, while understaging occurs in 6–20% (CHEN et al. 2005; KUO et al. 2005). When after CRT, the bowel wall becomes thickened and dark on T2W FSE MR images, it suggests that the tumor has been replaced by scar tissue. The problem is that scar tissue, which is depicted as an area of hypo-intense signal on T2W-FSE MR images, cannot be discerned from scar tissue that harbors residual tumor or small tumor islets (Fig. 13.20). Thus, these interpretation difficulties with fibrosis lead to significant over and understaging errors. The same holds

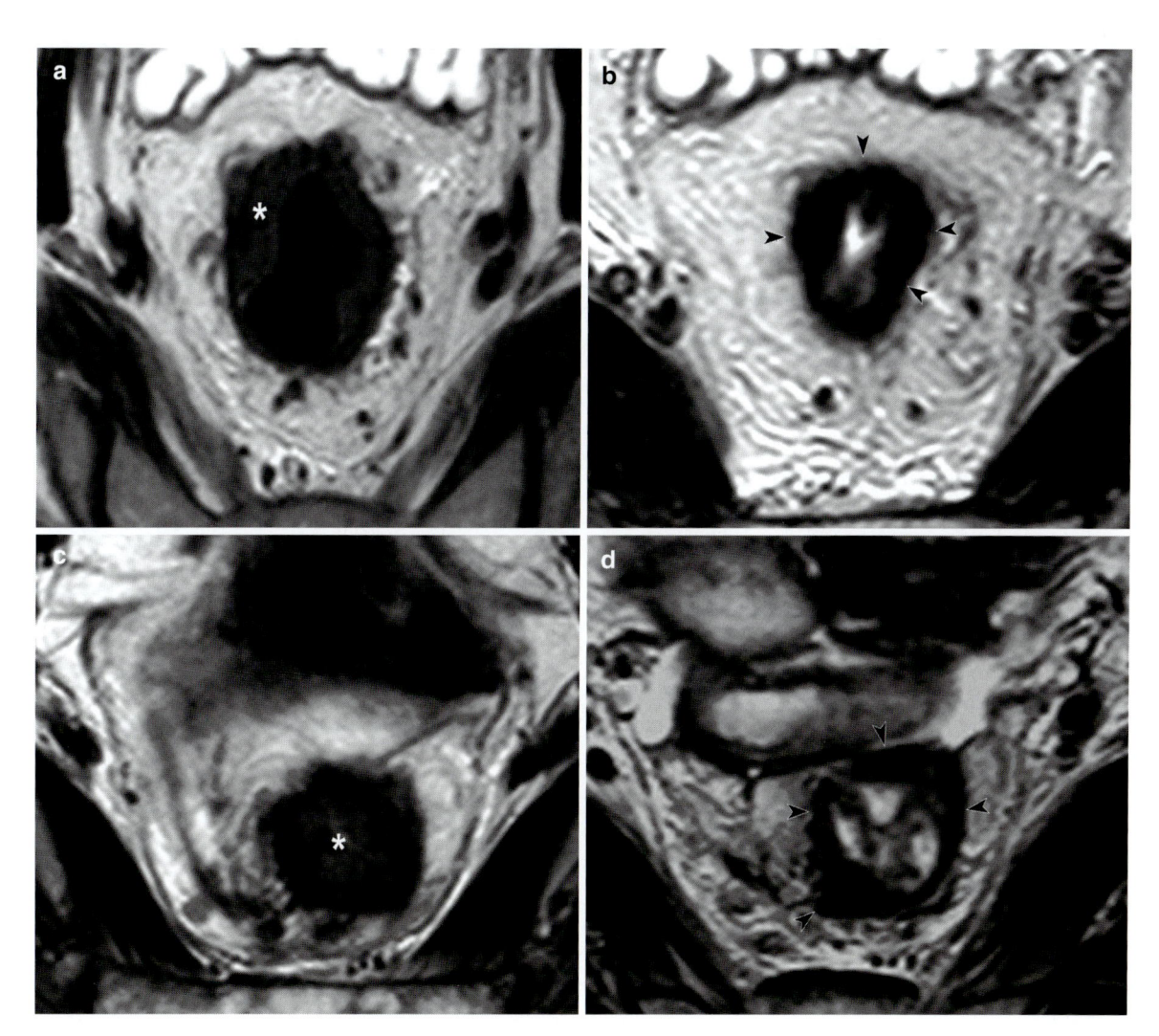

Fig. 13.20. Axial T2-weighted FSE MR images of two patients with locally advanced tumors (*asterisks*) before chemoradiation (**a, c**) and after chemoradiation (**b, d**). Both tumors responded well to the chemoradiation with remaining thickened and fibrotic bowel at the site of the previous tumor (*black arrowheads*). In the first patient (**a, b**), residual viable tumor was found at histologic examination, staged as yT3. In the second patient (**c, d**), no residual tumor was found and the patient was staged yT0. Note how the MR images of a yT3 tumor (**b**) fully mimic those of a yT0 tumor (**d**) when the bowel wall on post-CRT MRI appears thickened and fibrotic

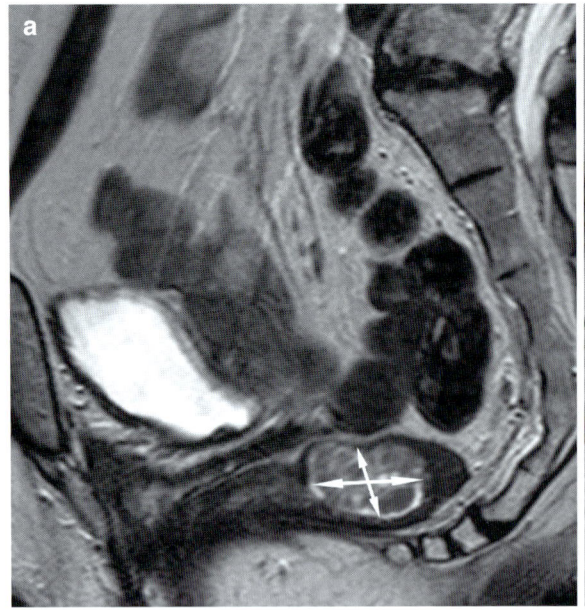

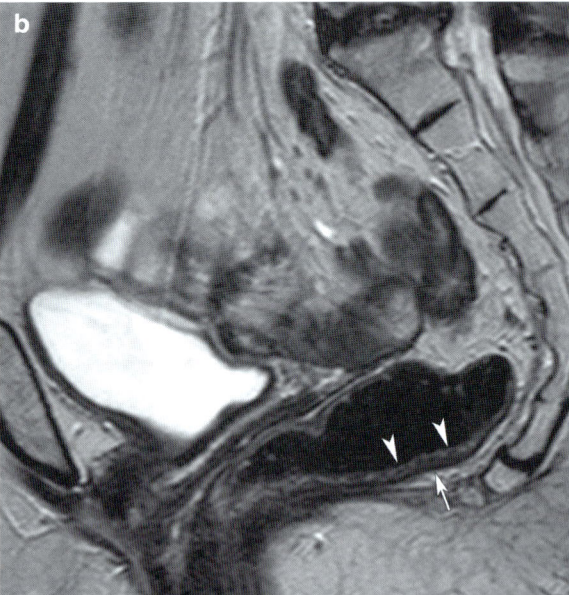

Fig. 13.21. Preoperative administration of chemoradiation to a small volume tumor (**a**, *double arrows*, 2.5 × 3 × 1.5 cm^3) resulted in a complete response at histologic examination. On the restaging MRI after chemoradiation (**b**), the tumor has disappeared and a normal rectal wall can be seen with a hyperintense inner mucosal layer (*white arrowheads*) and a hypointense outer layer (*white arrow*)

true for the identification of a pathologic complete responder (ypT0N0) after chemoradiation. One study reported that MRI did not identify any of the 12 pathologic complete responders in a group of 43 patients (MARETTO et al. 2007). Nevertheless, a recent study in 63 patients has shown that post CRT MRI can accurately predict tumors that are confined to the bowel wall (ypT0–2) with PPVs of 86–91% and NPVs of 70–75% for expert radiologists, non-expert radiologists, and surgeons (DRESEN et al. 2009). Furthermore, if the tumor on pre CRT MRI at the start of the treatment was ≤50 cm^3 and if the tumor volume shrinkage on post CRT MRI was measured ≥75%, tumors were likely to be downstaged to a tumor limited to the bowel wall (Fig. 13.21). Combining yT-stage prediction and volume reduction thus could improve the overall accuracy for yT prediction from 74 to 87%.

13.5.2
Tumor Regression from the Mesorectal Fascia

A multicenter study group reported an accuracy of 77% for CRM involvement prediction on post CRT MRI with a PPV of 45% and NPV of 98% (MERCURY STUDY GROUP 2006). Two single-center studies confirmed these findings with high NPVs of 91–100% and moderate PPVs of 44–68% (VLIEGEN et al. 2008a, KULKARNI et al. 2008). Again, these results reflect the difficulties of post CRT MRI in interpreting fibrosis. This is beautifully illustrated in Fig. 13.22. When a tumor before CRT shows massive invasion of the MRF and, after CRT, fibrotic scar tissue has replaced the tumor bed but has not regressed from the mesorectal fascia, the distinction between fibrosis with and without residual tumor remains a difficult task and again – to be on the safe side – the radiologist rather overstages than understages an involved mesorectal fascia. This results in overstaging errors as reflected by the low PPV. However, the high NPV tells us that when tumor regression is seen on post CRT MRI and the margin is uninvolved, this is almost always true. VLIEGEN et al. (2008a) proposed predictive patterns for CRM involvement after chemoradiation. They stratified 64 patients into four patterns: (A) fat pad larger than 2 mm between the residual tumor mass and MRF (Fig. 13.23), (B) development or persistence of spiculations invading the MRF, (C) development of diffuse hypointense "fibrotic" tissue infiltrating the MRF at the initial tumor site, and (D) persistence of diffuse iso- or hyperintense tissue infiltrating the MRF (Fig. 13.24). From pattern A to D, an increasing frequency of tumor invasion was found at matching with histology. Patterns A and B

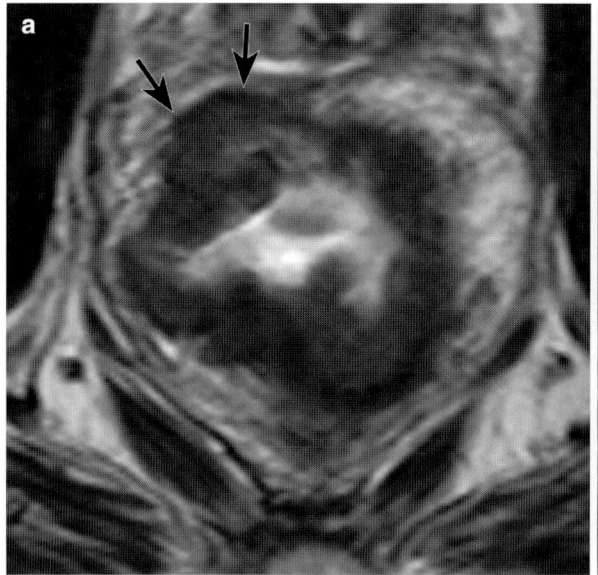

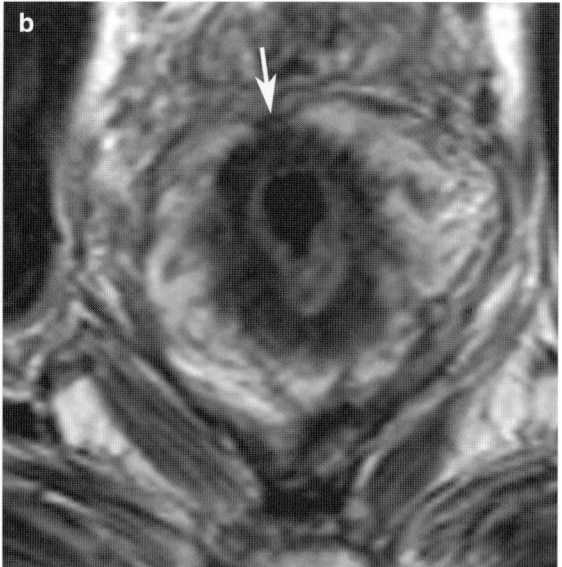

Fig. 13.22. Axial T2W FSE image of a rectal tumor before (**a**) and after (**b**) neoadjuvant chemoradiation treatment. Before treatment, there is a huge circumferential tumor that invades the MRF anteriorly (*black arrows*). After treatment, the tumor has become fibrotic. Anteriorly, the fibrotic tissue grows into the MRF (*white arrow*). It is not possible to discriminate tumor involvement of the MRF in these areas of fibrotic scar tissue. In this patient, the MRF turned out to be free of tumor involvement at histologic evaluation

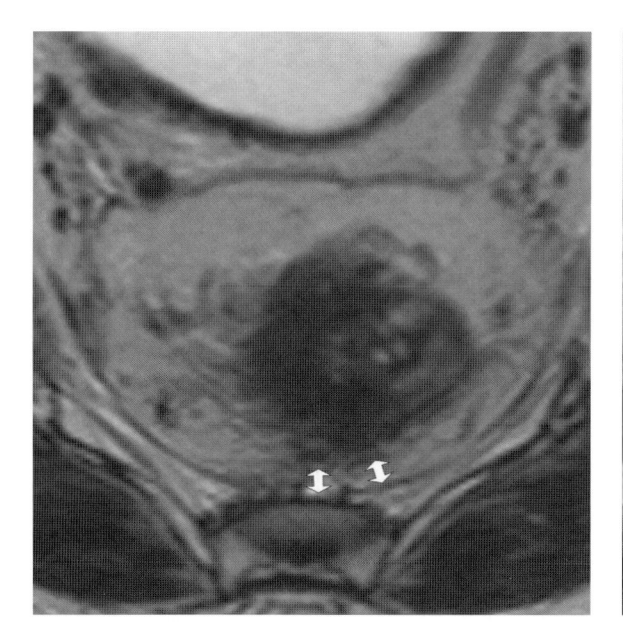

Fig. 13.23. Axial T2W FSE image of a male patient with rectal cancer after neoadjuvant chemoradiation treatment. The tumor area (from 6 to 12 o'clock) has become fibrotic. A clear fat pad can be visualized between the dorsal tumor area and the MRF (*double arrows*). The CRM is not involved

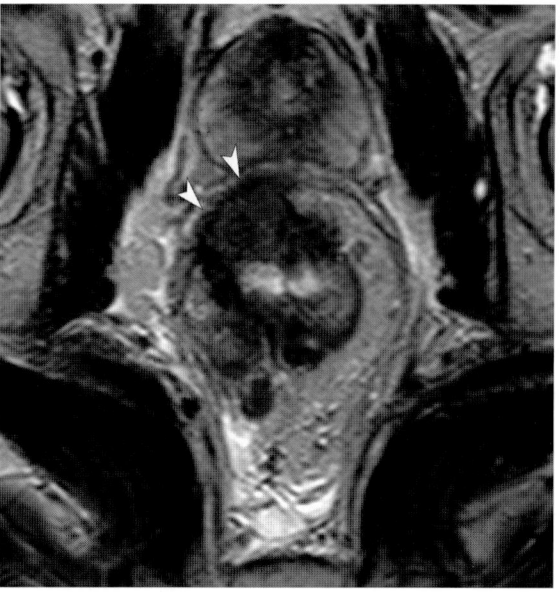

Fig. 13.24. Axial T2W FSE image of a male rectal cancer patient that was treated with neoadjuvant chemoradiation for a big T3N2 rectal tumor. After chemoradiation, a residual solid tumor mass with intermediate signal intensity invades the MRF on the anterior side (*arrowheads*). We can now state with certainty that the CRM is still involved

indicate an uninvolved CRM, pattern C reflects possible CRM involvement, and when pattern D is encountered, the CRM is definitely involved. Implementation of these patterns reduced overstaging from 54 to 34%, with an understaging rate of 0%. In clinical decision–making, the high overstaging rate means overtreatment in a significant proportion of patients that in fact have an uninvolved CRM, bringing about more morbidity than with standard surgery (TME). On the other hand, the gain is that R0 resections are often obtained.

13.5.3
The yN Stage

The most important issue in restaging nodal stage after chemoradiation is to evaluate whether pre-treatment suspected lymph nodes have become sterilized (non-malignant) as a result of the neoadjuvant treatment. Therefore, comparison of pre and post chemoradiation MRI is of crucial importance when interpreting nodes on post CRT MRI. Nodes can undergo a substantial volume reduction or even disappear after CRT. One study found a significant difference in lymph node retrieval after surgery with and without neoadjuvant chemoradiation treatment: 13 vs. 17 lymph nodes ($p < 0.001$) were retrieved per specimen, respectively (Rullier et al. 2008). The diagnostic performance of yN stage prediction with post chemoradiation MRI is reported equal or slightly better than with primary staging MRI, with accuracies varying from 64 to 88%. Overstaging is encountered slightly more often than understaging with overstaging rates from 4 to 28% and understaging rates from 4 to 19% (Kuo et al. 2005; Kulkarni et al. 2008; Vanagunas et al. 2004; Chen et al. 2005). One study evaluated whether the pre chemoradiation criteria for nodal staging with USPIO-MRI are re-applicable after chemoradiation. The results for lymph node evaluation with USPIO-MRI after chemoradiation were comparable with the pre chemoradiation evaluation with a PPV of 83% and NPVs from 99 to 100% for both the expert as well as the nonexpert reader. Furthermore, it was found that using standard T2W MR sequences, after chemoradiation size criteria were more reliable and nodal staging more accurate than before chemoradiation, probably because the number and size of lymph nodes decreased due to chemoradiation effects (Lahaye et al. 2009b).

13.6
Other Imaging Modalities

13.6.1
Endorectal Ultrasound (EUS)

Endorectal (or Endoluminal) ultrasound has traditionally been used for the local staging of rectal cancer. EUS is very accurate for assessment of tumor ingrowth in the bowel wall and is known to be the best imaging method to discriminate between tumors limited to the submucosa (T1) and tumors with ingrowth in the muscularis externa (T2). EUS also has a high sensitivity in predicting tumor penetration into the perirectal fat (T3) but specificity remains limited, because – like MRI – EUS has difficulties in discriminating normal desmoplastic stranding in T2 tumors from actual tumor penetration, causing mainly overstaging of T2 tumors. Because of the low contrast-resolution of EUS and the limited field of view of the ultrasound probe, the technique is less suitable for evaluation of the circumferential resection margin and tumor infiltration into neighboring organs in T4 tumors (Bipat et al. 2004). A prospective multicenter study reported that in 649 of 5,056 patients (13%) who underwent EUS for rectal cancer staging, EUS did not succeed in assessing the tumor lesion due to difficulties with the positioning of the ultrasound probe or limited visibility of the tumor, especially in patients with high or stenosing tumors (Ptok et al. 2006). Furthermore, the performance of EUS is limited by the investigator's experience. A definitive learning curve for EUS was shown with an improvement in accuracy from 58% at the baseline to 87.5% after the first 30 months of experience (Carmody and Otchy 2000). Like CT and MRI, EUS without additional fine-needle aspiration (FNA) is insufficiently accurate for the evaluation of lymph nodes. Furthermore, with EUS only nodes in the proximity of the probe are visualized while nodes in the drainage area of the superior rectal and inferior mesenteric arteries are not well captured.

13.6.2
CT

Multislice CT (MSCT) has often been proposed as a "one stop shop" technique for both the distant and local staging of rectal cancer. Although CT is routinely used for distant staging, there are some drawbacks to the use of CT for local staging. Reports have shown that CT is not a good method for evaluation of the nodal status. When predicting nodal involvement, CT can only rely on size criteria, while in rectal cancer lymph node metastases often occur in very small nodes (Wang et al. 2005). This will inherently lead to under- and overstaging errors when using CT for nodal evaluation. For the prediction of an involved circumferential resection margin, MSCT is reported to have moderate to poor accuracy (54–66%). Results were particularly poor in the low-anterior tumors, but improved for the mid and high located tumors (Vliegen et al. 2008b). This was again confirmed by a multicenter study in 250 patients, which found a low performance for 4–16 slice CT in the evaluation of CRM involvement in low rectal cancer. Results in mid and high rectal cancer were significantly better, with a PPV of 86% and NPV of 94%, suggesting that early generation multislice CT is able to select those tumors with free CRM and no visible nodes (Wolberink et al. 2009). At present, the role of newer generation (64) multislice CT is still undetermined and needs further investigation.

13.6.3
PET-CT

FDG PET-CT combines functional information with anatomic registration. PET-CT is known to be valuable for response monitoring in patients with locally advanced rectal cancer treated with neoadjuvant chemoradiation. A decrease of the standardized uptake value (SUV) during and after chemoradiation is a strong indicator for a good response (Capirci et al. 2007). At present, PET-CT is thus the most promising technique for early selection of the good responders, although as to date this selection would not alter treatment regimen. Whether PET will be able to identify the pathologic complete responders after CRT is yet to be proven. The value of PET-CT is reported to be limited for prediction of tumor clearance of the circumferential resection margin after CRT. In 20 patients, none of the tumor distances from the MRF measured at PET-CT corresponded with the tumor clearance that was verified at histological evaluation (Vliegen et al. 2008c). The detection level of FDG-PET at the time of writing is further limited for very small volume disease (<5–10 mm). PET-CT is unreliable for detection of mesorectal lymph node metastases and small residual tumor after neoadjuvant treatment, partly due to artifacts caused by intense uptake of the adjacent tumor and bladder void and partly because after chemoradiation uptake in acute inflammatory tissue causes confounding effects on PET images. In the longer run, during the early years surveillance of patients after treatment, PET has advantages over CT and MRI in differentiating scar tissue from viable tumor, making the technique more suitable for the (early) detection of tumor recurrence. Furthermore, PET-CT has proven its use for (whole body) screening for extrahepatic metastases in those patients with liver metastases on CT that are scheduled for curative liver resection or metastasectomy. A PET screening before liver surgery has shown to reduce the number of unnecessary laparotomies (Wiering et al. 2005). In the future, the introduction of hybrid PET MR techniques could bring us into a new era of "one stop shop" fast staging methods combining the superior soft tissue contrast resolution of MRI with the metabolic and functional information obtained with FDG PET.

13.7
Future Perspectives

With rapid technological developments, new imaging techniques are emerging. Improved image quality with higher resolution images allow for a more accurate evaluation of small volume disease. Faster image acquisition combined with advancing moving table techniques could expand the use of MRI from locoregional staging to whole body screening within an acceptable time frame. While the traditional techniques only provided morphological information, functional and quantifiable data can now be obtained. Diffusion-weighted MRI (DWI) is rapidly advancing in the field of oncology. DWI provides unique quantitative information reflecting tissue cellularity, without the need for exogenous contrast agents (Bammer 2003). While the use of DWI was initially limited to the brain, recent advances in MR techniques have made extracranial applications of DWI and even whole body DWI possible, creating a whole new window of opportunity for the noninvasive detection and functional assessment of tumors. Perfusion MRI techniques have been reported to be promising for response monitoring in rectal cancer (De Lussanet et al. 2005). Readers are referred to Chap. 4 for more technical details on DWI and MR perfusion. While none of the traditional imaging techniques have overcome the limitations in lymph node staging, MRI using lymph node specific contrast could be promising for more accurate characterization of lymph nodes (Will et al. 2006; Lahaye et al. 2008, 2009a). Specific molecular target agents are being investigated for tumor imaging at a microscopic and even molecular level, aiming at providing new insights in the pathologic tumor processes and developing new targeted treatment strategies. Extensive research will be required to further validate these new – and promising – MR imaging techniques and validate their use in clinical practice.

13.8
Conclusions and Recommendations for Rectal Cancer Management

Treatment strategies for rectal cancer have emerged from uniform treatment toward more tailored treatment, based on preoperative selection of different risk groups for local recurrence. The role of the radiologist in the multidisciplinary management of rectal cancer has thus evolved into a full discussant, a sparring partner for the clinicians providing them the relevant imaging findings necessary to stratify patients into the best treatment option. For the selection of low-risk patients (T1–2N0) who can be treated with surgery only, endorectal ultrasound remains the best imaging technique. For the assessment of larger (T3–4) tumors that will benefit from neoadjuvant treatment and to analyze involvement of the circumferential resection margins, MRI is the preferred imaging technique. Especially in low rectal tumors, MRI is more accurate than CT in assessing tumor invasion of the mesorectal fascia and adjacent organs and is therefore recommended. At present, no imaging technique is sufficiently accurate for exact nodal staging. New imaging techniques combining anatomical and functional information need to be investigated to solve this issue. The role of MRI in restaging rectal cancer after intensive neoadjuvant treatment is upcoming. When further tailoring of treatment, such as local excision or a "wait-and-see policy" for the good and complete responders, respectively, can be considered, this can only be realized when there is an accurate selection tool to identify these patients. Again, future research should indicate the role of imaging for this selection.

13.9
Anorectal Fistulas

An anorectal fistula is an abnormal tract between the anal canal (or occasionally the rectum) and the perianal skin. The disease has a tendency to recur despite curative surgery. Recurrence after surgery is almost always due to infection that is missed during surgical exploration and thus gone untreated. It is now recognized that pre-operative imaging, in specific MRI, is able to identify fistulas and associated abscesses in complex tracks that would otherwise have been missed by the surgeons. Pre-operative MRI has been shown to influence subsequent surgery and significantly diminish the chance of recurrent disease as a result. Because of this, pre-operative MRI has become a standard routine in the work-up of patients with complex fistulas.

Anorectal fistulas can exist as (1) a simple or primary track (Fig. 13.25) or (2) a complex track, consisting of a primary track and its secondary extensions including abscesses (Fig. 13.26). The latter are most often associated with perianal Crohn's disease and with recurrent fistulas. There have been a variety of

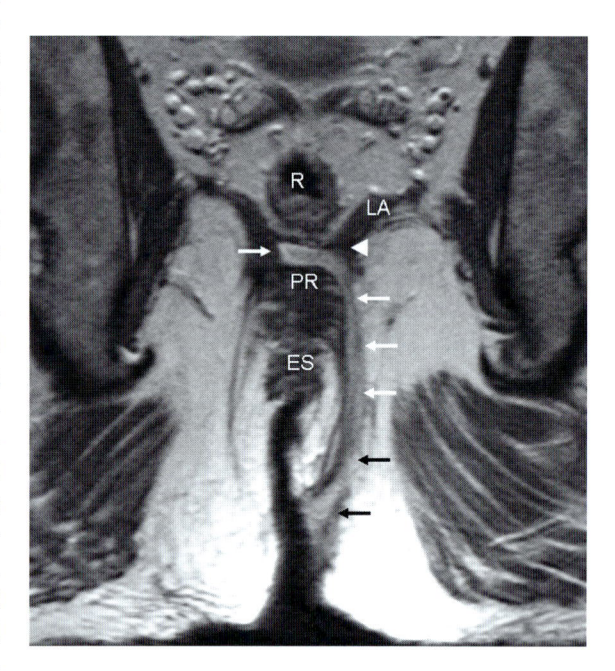

Fig. 13.25. Coronal T2-weighted turbo spin-echo in a male patient with a very high transsphincteric cryptoglandular fistula (*arrows*) extending to the level of the anorectal junction (*arrow head*). *R* rectum; *LA* levator ani plate; *PR* puborectalis; *ES* external sphincter (Fig. courtesy of Jaap Stoker MD)

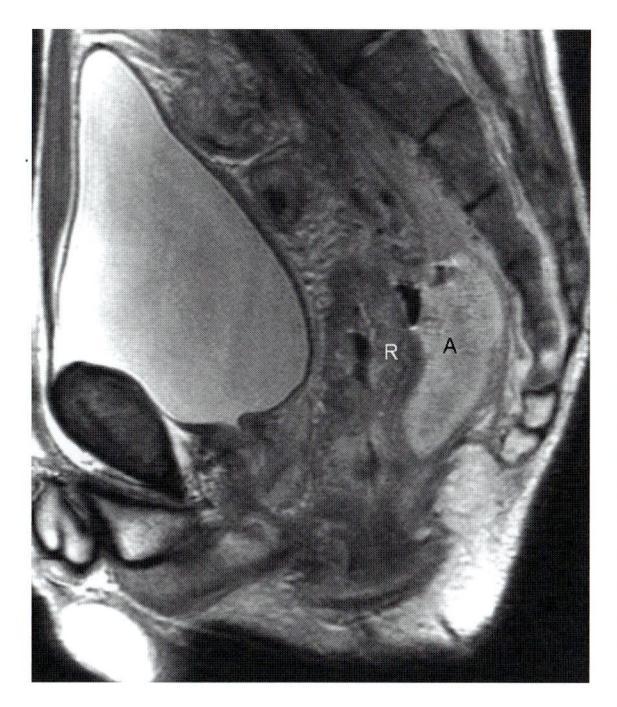

Fig. 13.26. Sagittal T2-weighted turbo spin-echo in a male patient with Crohn's disease. There is a large presacral abscess (*A*) with air fluid level and there is a thickened rectal wall (*R*) (Fig. courtesy of Jaap Stoker MD)

attempts to classify fistula-in-ano but by far the most widely used is that proposed by Parks et al. in 1976: intersphincteric, transsphincteric, suprasphincteric, and extrasphincteric fistulas. Intersphincteric and transsphincteric fistulas are with submucosal fistulas the most frequent type of fistulas. Suprasphincteric fistulas and extrasphincteric fistulas extend to the rectum.

For a more extensive description of the different classes and more detailed elaboration on the efficacy of MRI and the optimal standard MR imaging protocol as well as its influence on treatment, we refer to Chap. 19. With this subsection, we intend to briefly summarize the role of MR imaging with respect to other imaging methods for identifying and classifying anorectal fistulas.

The aim of anal fistula surgery is to eradicate all sepsis identified during exploration. While doing so, it is important for the surgeon to maintain the right balance between eradication of sepsis and preservation of anal function. To achieve this, two surgical questions need to be answered preoperatively by imaging:

1. What is the relationship between the fistula and the anal sphincter? (In other words, what would be the chance for post-operative incontinence when the track would be laid open?)
2. Are there any extensions from the primary track that need to be treated to prevent recurrence and if so, where are they located: supra- or infra levatoric, inter- or extrasphincteric?

Contrast fistulography was the first modality ever employed but has become obsolete since Kuijpers and Schulpen (1985) showed an accuracy for this method of only 16%. The major drawback of fistulography is that tracks behind stenosis and/or debris-plugs in complex fistulas cannot be filled. Furthermore, information on the relation of the track to the pelvic floor and anal sphincter complex is lacking. CT has never played an important role for anal fistulas imaging mainly due to its insufficient soft tissue contrast resolution for detailed visualization of the anal sphincter complex. Endoanal Sonography (EAS) was the first technique to directly visualize the anal sphincter complex in detail and to show effectiveness in the classification of fistula-in-ano. A study comparing EAS to digital evaluation and MRI in 108 primary tracks found that digital evaluation correctly classified 61%, EAS 81%, and MR imaging 90% (Buchanan et al. 2004). Although EAS was superior in identifying the site of the internal opening (97% vs. 91% for MRI), MRI was the most superior technique for providing all relevant information that surgeons want to know from imaging. This was again confirmed in a systematic review by Sahni et al. (2008) reporting a sensitivity, specificity, PPV, and NPV of 97, 96, 97, and 96% for MRI and 92, 85, 89, and 89%, respectively, for EUS. A further advantage of MRI is that it is less operator-dependent than US. While there is no doubt that EAS remains a valuable technique in experienced hands, MRI is generally more reproducible in general centers and thus preferred as a method in the preoperative standard work-up of patients with anorectal fistulas.

Studies in the mid-1990s have advocated the use of endoanal coils for MR imaging of anal fistulas and reported equal to superior results when compared with EAS (Stoker et al. 1996). Halligan and Bartram (1998) compared the endoanal MR technique with MRI using an external coil (a conventional body coil) and found 68 and 96%, concordance of MRI with surgery respectively, and concluded that endoluminal MR techniques are thus less preferred. Although endoanal MRI is superior to an external coil technique in detecting and classifying primary tracks (deSouza et al. 1998), it is less accurate in

13.10
Endometriosis

Endometriosis is the presence of ectopic functional endometrial tissue outside the uterus.

Endometriosis can present as different clinical entities, such as ovarian endometriosis (endometrioma), peritoneal endometriosis (early-stage endometriosis often occurring in the adolescent symptomatic patient) or deep endometriosis, an advanced stage of the disease that infiltrates the peritoneum in the Douglas pouch and invades the deep pelvic organs (rectum, bladder, etc.). The pathogenic mechanism of endometriosis has been described in several studies and is not fully understood yet. Endometriosis affects 10–15% of women during pre-menopause and, although it is a benign disorder, has a substantial social and professional impact because of its association with dyspareunia, dysmenorrhea, pelvic pain, and subfertility. In rare cases, endometriosis can undergo malignant transformation and give rise to epithelial ovarian cancer. Patients generally present with advanced disease that infiltrates deep pelvic structures such as the rectum and sigmoid, the sacro-uterine ligaments, the ureters, the bladder, the rectovaginal septum and the cervix and uterine body. This infiltrating "deep endometriosis" (as opposed to the earlier stage of "peritoneal endometriosis") mainly consists of massive fibrotic tissue (Fig. 13.27), encircling small hemorrhagic endometriotic nodules. Repeated cyclic bleeding of these small nodules causes the fibrosis to further extend – as reactive scar tissue – and to diffusely infiltrate the deep pelvis, which is the reason why patients who are diagnosed at this advanced stage may already have suffered years of chronic unexplained and disabling symptoms of pain. The correct diagnosis is known to be made only 8–11 years after the patient has reported the first complaints. The diagnosis for endometriosis currently only relies on clinical symptoms and exams and is confirmed by laparoscopy. Although laparoscopy reveals a good view of the extent of peritoneal endometriosis, it tends to underestimate the extent of deep endometriosis. Modern imaging techniques thus serve as a complementary tool to assess the extent of clinically confirmed deep endometriosis.

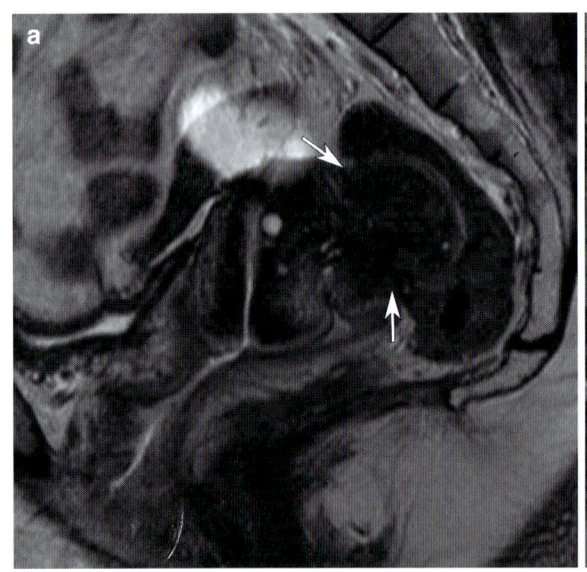

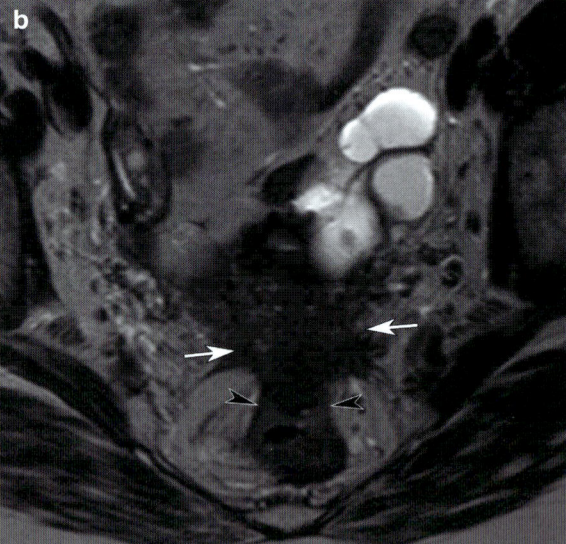

identifying abscesses outside the field of view of the endoanal probe, especially with complex fistulas associated with recurrences and with Crohn's disease. In these situations, a phased array body coil is preferred (STOKER et al. 2000; HALLIGAN and BARTRAM 1998). For further elaboration on the best MR protocol, we again refer to Chap. 19.

Fig. 13.27. Sagittal (**a**) and axial (**b**) T2W FSE images of a patient with deep endometriosis. The patient underwent a hysterectomy in the past, but the cervix was left in situ. There is a large hypointense signal area of endometriosis located at the dorsal cervix and fornix posterior (*white arrows*) that grows through the mesorectal fascia and invades the anterior rectal wall (*black arrowheads*)

Modern imaging techniques mainly used for this goal are transvaginal- and endorectal sonography and/or MRI. All are insufficiently sensitive for accurate diagnosis of the very early "peritoneal endometriosis," so for this laparoscopy ± biopsies remain the gold standard diagnostic tool. The focus of this subsection will mainly be on the role for MR imaging in evaluating the extent of deep endometriosis.

13.10.1
MRI of "Deep Endometriosis"

The hemorrhagic endometrial nodules as visualized on MRI of deep endometriosis have a high signal intensity on T1-weighted MRI and high signal intensity on T2-weighted MRI, reflecting the presence of blood degradation products. MRI may have difficulties in identifying these hemorrhagic implants among massive hypointense fibrotic tissues. Fat-suppression MR sequences have therefore in the past been advocated as very useful for accurate detection of these tiny lesions (SIEGELMAN et al. 1994). Although this may be true, the main question the gynecological surgeon wants answered with MRI is not whether the patient has deep endometriosis (this diagnosis is often already made at clinical exam and/or laparoscopy), but how far the deep endometriotic lesions have extended into pelvic structures such as the rectum, the ureters, etc.

Depending on the severity of the patient's symptoms, endometriosis may be managed expectantly, with hormonal therapy or surgically (REMORGIDA et al. 2007). Better information on involved deep pelvic structures would help the surgeon to anticipate resection of these structures together with the massive endometriotic pelvis mass, or in the case of hormonal treatment to have a baseline exam for monitoring treatment response.

BAZOT et al. (2007) reported a high sensitivity and specificity of 88 and 90% for MRI in identifying rectal involvement of deep endometriosis, figures similar to those for endorectal ultrasound (96 and 94%). Transvaginal Ultrasound (TVUS) is very accurate for diagnosing endometrioma, as TVUS is highly sensitive for excluding or confirming ovarian cystic lesions, even when small. MRI with its superior contrast resolution is more specific than endoluminal sonography for diagnosing endometrioma. The MR appearance of the "shading effect" on T2W MR images (hyperintense luminal content of the cysts on T1W, which turns hypointense on T2W images) is 100% predictive for endometrioma (Fig. 13.28). As most endometriomas are associated with deep endometriotic lesions in the posterior pelvis (the sacro-uterine ligament and the rectum), an MR exam additional to TVUS for confirming the sonographic diagnosis of endometrioma could at the same time efficiently assess the presence or absence of deep endometriotic lesions in the posterior pelvis.

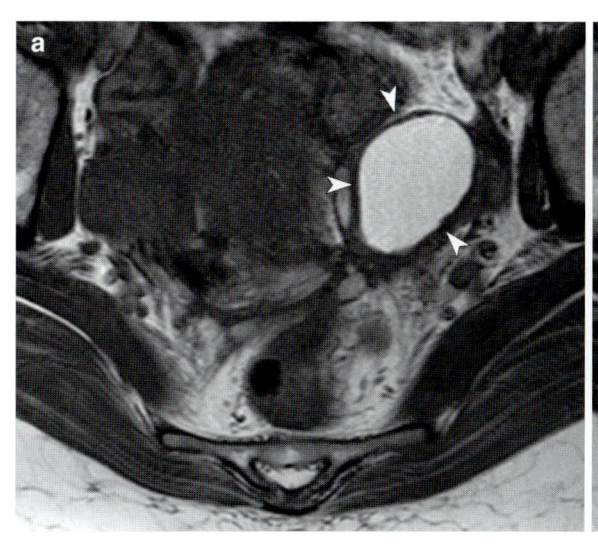

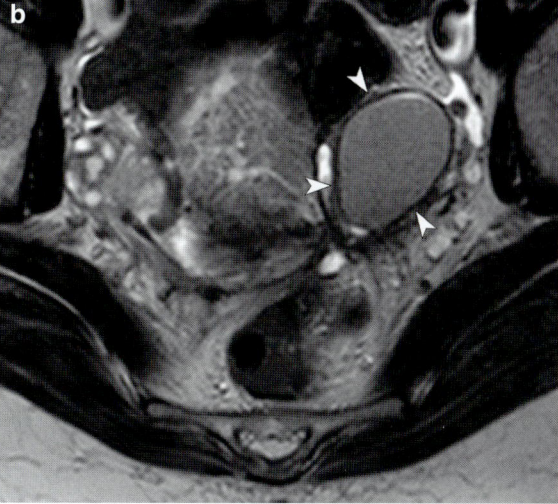

Fig. 13.28. Axial T1-weighted (**a**) and T2-weighted (**b**) image of a female patient showing an endometrioma located at the left ovary (*white arrowheads*). The content of the cyst is hyperintense on the T1-weighted image and turns hypointens ("shading") on the T2-weighted image; MR features that are 100% predictive for endometrioma

List of Abbreviations

CT	Computed tomography
CRM	Circumferential resection margin
CRT	Chemoradiation treatment
DWI	Diffusion weighted (MR) imaging
EAS	Endoanal ultrasound
EUS	Endorectal/endoluminal ultrasound
FSE	Fast spin echo
MDT	Multi-disciplinary team
MSCT	Multislice CT
MRF	Mesorectal fascia
MRI	Magnetic resonance imaging
NPV	Negative predictive value
PET	Positron emission tomography
PPV	Positive predictive value
T2W	T2-weighted
TME	Total mesorectal excision
TVUS	Transvaginal ultrasound
UK	United Kingdom

References

Allen SD, Padhani AR, Dzik-Jurasz AS, et al (2007) Rectal carcinoma: MRI with histologic correlation before and after chemoradiation therapy. Am J Roentgenol 188:442–451

Bammer R (2003) Basic principles of diffusion-weighted imaging. Eur J Radiol 45:169–184

Bazot M, Bornier C, Dubernard G, et al (2007) Accuracy of magnetic resonance imaging and rectal endoscopic sonography for the prediction of location of deep pelvic endometriosis. Hum Reprod 22:1457–1463

Beets-Tan RG, Beets GL, Vliegen RF, et al (2001) Accuracy of magnetic resonance imaging in prediction of tumour-free resection margin in rectal cancer surgery. Lancet 357:497–504

Bipat S, Glas AS, Slors FJ, et al (2004) Rectal cancer: local staging and assessment of lymph node involvement with endoluminal US, CT, and MR imaging–a meta-analysis. Radiology 232:773–783

Blomqvist L, Machado M, Rubio C, et al (2000) Rectal tumour staging: MR imaging using pelvic phased-array and endorectal coils vs endoscopic ultrasonography. Eur Radiol 10:653–660

Borschitz T, Wachtlin D, Mohler M, et al (2008) Neoadjuvant chemoradiation and local excision for T2–3 rectal cancer. Ann Surg Oncol 15:712–720

Brown G, Richards CJ, Bourne MW, et al (2003) Morphologic predictors of lymph node status in rectal cancer with use of high-spatial-resolution MR imaging with histopathologic comparison. Radiology 227:371–377

Buchanan GN, Halligan S, Bartram CI, et al (2004) Clinical examination, endosonography, and MR imaging in preoperative assessment of fistula in ano: comparison with outcome-based reference standard. Radiology 233(3):674–681

Capirci C, Rampin L, Erba PA, et al (2007) Sequential FDG-PET/CT reliably predicts response of locally advanced rectal cancer to neo-adjuvant chemo-radiation therapy. Eur J Nucl Med Mol Imaging 34:1583–1593

Carmody BJ, Otchy DP (2000) Learning curve of transrectal ultrasound. Dis Colon Rectum 43:193–197

Chen CC, Lee RC, Lin JK, et al (2005) How accurate is magnetic resonance imaging in restaging rectal cancer in patients receiving preoperative combined chemoradiotherapy? Dis Colon Rectum 48:722–728

De Lussanet, Backes WH, Griffïen AW, et al (2005) Dynamic contrast-enhanced magnetic resonance imaging of radiation therapy-induced microcirculation changes in rectal cancer. Int J Radiat Oncol 63:1309–1315

deSouza NM, Gilderdale DJ, Coutts GA, et al (1998) MRI of fistula-in-ano: a comparison of endoanal coil with external phased array coil techniques. J Comput Assist Tomogr 22:357–363

Dresen RC, Beets GL, Rutten HJ, et al (2009) Locally advanced rectal cancer: MR imaging for restaging after neoadjuvant radiation therapy with concomitant chemotherapy part I. Are we able to predict tumor confined to the rectal wall? Radiology 252:71–80

Guillem JG, Chessin DB, Cohen AM, et al (2005) Long-term oncologic outcome following preoperative combined modality therapy and total mesorectal excision of locally advanced rectal cancer. Ann Surg 241:829–836

Habr-Gama A, Perez RO, Proscurshim I, et al (2006) Patterns of failure and survival for nonoperative treatment of stage c0 distal rectal cancer following neoadjuvant chemoradiation therapy J Gastrointest Surg 10:1319–1328

Halligan S, Bartram CI (1998) MR imaging of fistula in ano: are endoanal coils the gold standard? AJR Am J Roentgenol 171:407–412

Heald RJ, Ryall RD (1986) Recurrence and survival after total mesorectal excision for rectal cancer. Lancet 28:1479–1482

Hughes R, Glynne Jones R, Grainger J, et al (2006) Can pathological complete response in the primary tumour following pre-operative pelvic chemoradiotherapy for T3-T4 rectal cancer predict for sterilisation of pelvic lymph nodes, a low risk of local recurrence and the appropriateness of local excision? Int J Colorectal Dis 21:11–17

Hünerbein M, Pegios W, Rau B, et al (2000) Prospective comparison of endorectal ultrasound, three-dimensional endorectal ultrasound, and endorectal MRI in the preoperative evaluation of rectal tumors. Preliminary results. Surg Endosc 14:1005–1009

Kapiteijn E, Marijnen CA, Nagtegaal ID, et al (2001) Preoperative radiotherapy combined with total mesorectal excision for resectable rectal cancer. N Engl J Med 30:638–646

Kim JH, Beets GL, Kim MJ, et al (2004) High-resolution MR imaging for nodal staging in rectal cancer: are there any criteria in addition to the size? Eur J Radiol 52:78–83

Kuijpers HC, Schulpen T (1985) Fistulography for fistula-in-ano. Is it useful? Dis Colon Rectum 28(2):103–104

Kulkarni T, Gollins S, Maw A, et al (2008) Magnetic resonance imaging in rectal cancer downstaged using neoadjuvant chemoradiation: accuracy of prediction of tumour stage and circumferential resection margin status. Colorectal Dis 10:479–489

Kuo LJ, Chern MC, Tsou MH, et al (2005) Interpretation of magnetic resonance imaging for locally advanced rectal carcinoma after preoperative chemoradiation therapy. Dis Colon Rectum 48:23–28

Lahaye MJ, Engelen SM, Nelemans PJ, et al (2005) Imaging for predicting the risk factors–the circumferential resection margin and nodal disease–of local recurrence in rectal cancer: a meta-analysis. Semin Ultrasound CT MR 26:259–268

Lahaye MJ, Engelen SM, Kessels AG, et al (2008) USPIO-enhanced MR imaging for nodal staging in patients with primary rectal cancer: predictive criteria. Radiology 246:804–811

Lahaye MJ, Beets GL, Engelen SM, et al (2009a) Gadovosfeset Trisodium (Vasovist®) enhanced MR lymph node detection: initial observations. Open Magn Reson J 2:1–5

Lahaye MJ, Beets GL, Engelen SM, et al (2009b) Locally advanced rectal cancer: MR imaging for restaging after neoadjuvant radiation therapy with concomitant chemotherapy part II. What are the criteria to predict involved lymph nodes? Radiology 252:81–91

Lezoche G, Baldarelli M, Guerrieri M, et al (2008) A prospective randomized study with a 5-year minimum follow-up evaluation of transanal endoscopic microsurgery versus laparoscopic total mesorectal excision after neoadjuvant therapy. Surg Endosc 22:352–358

MERCURY Study Group (2006) Diagnostic accuracy of preoperative magnetic resonance imaging in predicting curative resection of rectal cancer: prospective observational study. BMJ 14:333:779

National Cancer Institute United States, http://www.cancer.gov; website accessed at 14–04–09

Parks AG, Gordon PH, Hardcastle JD (1976) A classification of fistula-in-ano. Br J Surg 63(1):1–12

Ptok H, Marusch F, Meyer F, et al (2006) Feasibility and accuracy of TRUS in the pre-treatment staging for rectal carcinoma in general practice. Eur J Surg Oncol 32:420–425

Quirke P, Durdey P, Dixon MF, et al (1986) Local recurrence of rectal adenocarcinoma due to inadequate surgical resection. Histopathological study of lateral tumour spread and surgical excision. Lancet 2:996–999

Remorgida V, Ferrero S, Fulcheri E, et al (2007) Bowel endometriosis: presentation, diagnosis, and treatment. Obstet Gynecol Surv 62:461–470

Rullier A, Laurent C, Capdepont M, et al (2008) Lymph nodes after preoperative chemoradiotherapy for rectal carcinoma: number, status, and impact on survival. Am J Surg Pathol 32:45–50

Sahni VA, Ahmad R, Burling D (2008) Which method is best for imaging of perianal fistula? Abdom Imaging 33:26–30

Sauer R, Becker H, Hohenberger W, et al (2004) Preoperative versus postoperative chemoradiotherapy for rectal cancer. N Engl J Med 21:1731–1740

Sebag-Montefiore D, Stephens RJ, Steele R, et al (2009) Preoperative radiotherapy versus selective postoperative chemoradiotherapy in patients with rectal cancer (MRC CR07 and NCIC-CTG C016): a multicentre, randomised trial. Lancet 373:811–820

Siegelman ES, Outwater E, Wang T, et al (1994) Solid pelvic masses caused by endometriosis: MR imaging features. AJR Am J Roentgenol 163:357–361

Slater A, Halligan S, Taylor SA, et al (2006) Distance between the rectal wall and mesorectal fascia measured by MRI: effect of rectal distension and implications for preoperative prediction of a tumor-free circumferential resection margin. Clin Radiol 61:65–70

Stoker J, Hussain SM, van Kempen D, et al (1996) Endoanal coil in MR imaging of anal fistulas. AJR Am J Roentgenol 166(2):360–362

Stoker J, Rociu E, Wiersma TG, et al (2000) Imaging of anorectal disease. Br J Surg 87:10–27

Swedish Rectal Cancer Trial. Improved survival with preoperative radiotherapy in resectable rectal cancer. Swedish Rectal Cancer Trial. (1997) N Engl J Med 336:980–987

United Kingdom Cancer Research, http://info.cancerresearchuk.org/cancerstats/; website, accessed 14–04–09

Valentini V, Coco C, Picciocchi A, et al (2002) Does downstaging predict improved outcome after preoperative chemoradiation for extraperitoneal locally advanced rectal cancer? A long-term analysis of 165 patients. Int J Radiat Oncol Biol Phys 53:664–674

Vanagunas A, Lin DE, Stryker SJ (2004) Accuracy of endoscopic ultrasound for restaging rectal cancer following neoadjuvant chemoradiation therapy. Am J Gastroenterol 99:109–112

Vliegen RF, Beets GL, von Meyenfeldt MF, et al (2005) Rectal cancer: MR imaging in local staging–is gadolinium-based contrast material helpful? Radiology 234:179–188

Vliegen RF, Beets GL, Lammering G, et al (2008a) Mesorectal fascia invasion after neoadjuvant chemotherapy and radiation therapy for locally advanced rectal cancer: accuracy of MR imaging for prediction. Radiology 246:454–462

Vliegen R, Dresen R, Beets G, et al (2008b) The accuracy of Multi-detector row CT for the assessment of tumor invasion of the mesorectal fascia in primary rectal cancer. Abdom Imaging 33:604–606

Vliegen RF, Beets-Tan RG, Vanhauten B, et al (2008c) Can an FDG-PET/CT predict tumor clearance of the mesorectal fascia after preoperative chemoradiation of locally advanced rectal cancer? Strahlenther Onkol 184:457–464

Wallengren NO, Holtas S, Andren-Sandberg A, et al (2000) Rectal carcinoma: double-contrast MR imaging for preoperative staging. Radiology 215:108–114

Will O, Purkayastha S, Chan C, et al (2006) Diagnostic precision of nanoparticle-enhanced MRI for lymph-node metastases: a meta-analysis. Lancet Oncol 7:52–60

Wang C, Zhou Z, Wang Z, et al (2005) Patterns of neoplastic foci and lymph node micrometastasis within the mesorectum. Langenbecks Arch Surg 390:312–318

Wiering B, Krabbe PF, Jager GJ, et al (2005) The impact of fluor-18-deoxyglucose-positron emission tomography in the management of colorectal liver metastases. Cancer 15:2658–2670

Wolberink SVRC, Beets-Tan RGH, de Haas-Kock DFM, et al (2009) Multi slice computed tomography as a primary screening tool for the predicition of an involved mesorectal fascia and distant metastases in primary rectal cancer: a multicenter study. Dis Colon Rectum 52:928–934

MRI of Bowel Motility

14

Michael A. Patak, Constantin von Weymarn, Klaus-Ulrich Wentz, Radu Tutuja, Michael Wissmeyer, and Johannes M. Froelich

CONTENTS

14.1 Introduction 229
14.1.1 Physiology 229
14.1.2 Current Measuring Techniques 231
14.1.2.1 Scintigraphy 231
14.1.2.2 Manometry 232
14.1.2.3 Impedance Measurement 232
14.1.3 Magnetic Resonance Imaging 233

14.2 Technique 233
14.2.1 Preparation 233
14.2.2 Imaging 235
14.2.3 Data Analysis 237

14.3 In Vivo Results of Peristaltic Motion Using Dynamic MRI 240
14.3.1 Displaying Normal Motility with MRI 241
14.3.2 Postoperative Ileus and Its Recovery Phase 241
14.3.3 Impact of Drugs on Small Bowel Motility 241
14.3.4 Motility Changes in Inflammatory Bowel Diseases 242
14.3.5 Future MR Motility Imaging Applications 244

14.4 Motility Measurement: Which Technique for What Task? 245
14.4.1 Ultrasound 245
14.4.2 Scintigraphy 245
14.4.3 Manometry 245
14.4.4 MR Motility Imaging 245

14.5 Conclusion 246
References 246

Michael A. Patak, MD
Constantin Von Weymarn, PhD
Johannes M. Froelich, PhD
Institute of Diagnostic, Interventional and Pediatric Radiology, University Hospital, Inselspital Bern, Freiburgstrasse, Bern, Switzerland
Klaus-Ulrich Wentz, MD
Institute of Radiology, Kantonspital, Münsterlingen, Switzerland
Radu Tutuja, MD
Institute of Nuclear Medicine, University Hospitel, Geneva, Switzerland
Michael Wissmeyer, MD
Clinic for Visceral Surgery and Medicine, University Hospital, Inselspital Bern, Freiburgstrasse, Bern, Switzerland

KEY POINTS

This chapter gives an overview of small bowel motility imaging. A short summarization on the physiology of small bowel peristalsis is followed by the different techniques currently used to monitor small bowel function such as manometry and scintigraphy. Until now, no technology has been available that is able to visualize bowel motility. For MRI, the techniques to acquire motility images are described as well as the analysis of motility and the interpretation of the data. Some clinical applications of small bowel motility changes are demonstrated to indicate the possibilities of monitoring bowel function with MRI.

14.1
Introduction

14.1.1
Physiology

The physiologic task of bowel motility is composed of different aspects. The bowel wall contractions mix and homogenize the food, disperse digestive enzymes, optimize the extraction of nutrition by churning the bowel content, and propel the food through the gastrointestinal (GI) tube from the mouth to the rectum. This peristaltic system is based on the coordinated contractions of smooth muscle cell layers within the bowel wall, the muscularis propria. These contractions are independently coordinated within the bowel by the plexus myentericus of Auerbach, also called the "brain in the gut" (Fig. 14.1). The smooth muscle cell layers are arranged in a circular and longitudinal layer. The interface between the two layers is formed by the myenteric plexus, which contains nerve cells and the interstitial cells of Cajal (ICC). The ICC serve as electrical pacemakers generating slow waves in the Auerbach plexus of the stomach and the small intestine, helping to define the contraction rate of the circular smooth muscle layer characterized by dominating radial shortenings, torsion, and shear (Deetjen et al. 2006).

The motility itself is created by a coordination of the two peristaltic reflex phases. The oral phase consists of the contraction of the circular muscle layer with concomitant relaxation of the longitudinal layer. The second phase, the so-called caudate phase of the peristaltic reflex, corresponds to the relaxation of the circular muscle in conjunction with the contraction of the longitudinal muscle. The coordination of these phases produces the actual propagation of the bowel content from the pylorus to the terminal ileum and cecum (Husebye 1999).

Many factors have a direct influence on either the ICC or smooth muscle layers, including the locally secreted hormones acetylcholine, tachykinin nitric oxide, glucagon-like protein, and vasoactive intestinal peptide (VIP). Bowel motility is also influenced by extrinsic hormones such as insulin and adrenalin. Another factor impacting motility is the content of the food. Unabsorbed fat or protein in the ileum delays the passage of the chyme through the small intestine, the so-called ileal brake. Glucose by contrast is a strong stimulant to the peristalsis. Changes in intestinal pH also have a clear influence on peristalsis and the transit time in the small bowel. Theoretically, pathological changes such as the neuropathy of diabetic patients may alter motility, contraction frequency, and contraction strength of the small bowel wall. There are also reports of decreased motility with advancing age, a phenomenon that may be indirectly related to an age-related shift in pH as well as other functional concomitants of aging.

Overall, the "brain in the gut" is a complex system with many contributing factors, making structured research and clear diagnosis very difficult (Thomson et al. 2003a, b).

Normal values for a well distended small bowel average around 8–11 contractions per minute, for the large bowel 1–3 contractions per minute, these usually grouped in series of five contractions followed by a period of "silence" (Bassotti et al. 2005). Contraction frequency is not the only general parameter of function; the transit time is also a marker of overall function. Normal transit time for the small bowel is a nearly constant 30–60 min for liquids and 4–5 h for solid food (Gryback et al. 2002; Rauch et al. 2009). The transit time for the colon is much longer, varying widely from 1 hour to as long as 3 days.

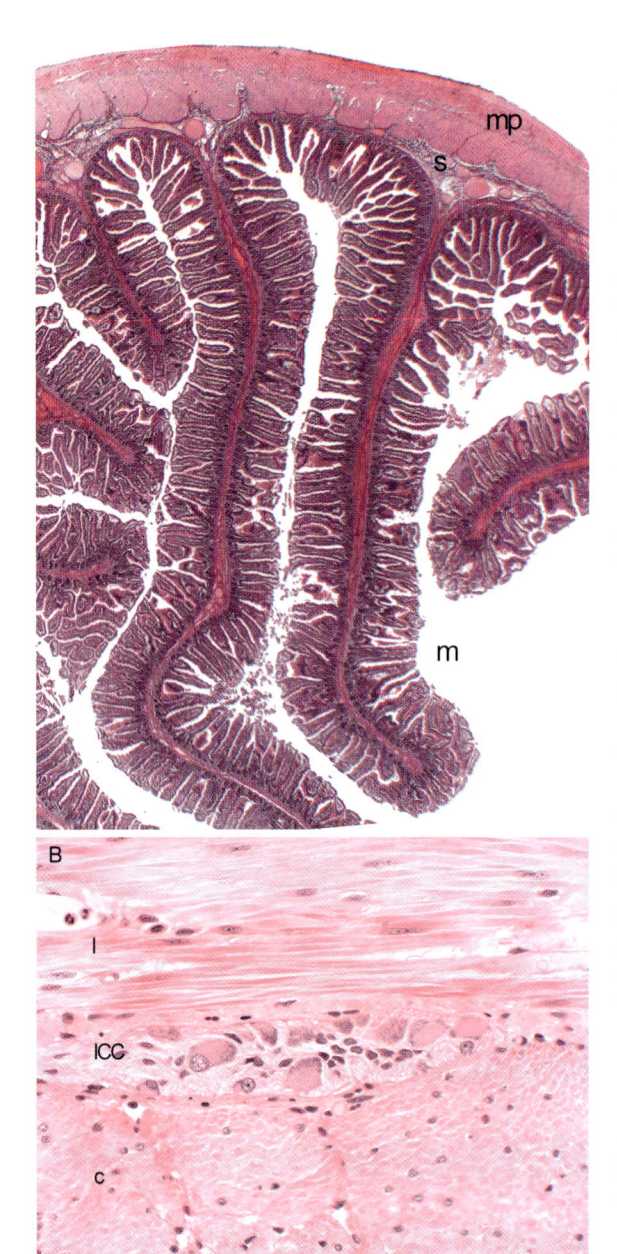

Fig. 14.1. Anatomy of the small bowel wall. Cross-sectional anatomy of the small bowel wall overivew (**A**) showing the 3 layers of mucosa (m) submucosa (s) and muscularis propria (mp). The muscularis propria (**B**) itself is separated into two layers of smooth muscle cells, the longitudinal (l) and the circular (c). Between these two layers lies the myenteric plexus containing the intestinal cells of Cajal (ICC), which form the central unit for the coordination of motility of the small bowel. The ICC is an independent pacemaker for smooth muscle contraction that is regulated by hormones and by vagal or sympathetic nerve stimulation

Intestinal function is normally measured indirectly by assessing the transit time as a surrogate marker. Although visualization and quantification of small bowel wall motion are still not done clinically on a routine basis, the results of initial experience and first clinical studies are highly promising. Further investigation is needed to better understand the clinical importance and therapeutic consequences of small bowel motility. This chapter will therefore focus on the various modalities for characterization and measuring of small bowel motility, with special emphasis on the possibilities of MR motility imaging.

14.1.2
Current Measuring Techniques

Small bowel function is currently measured using scintigraphy, manometry, and assessment of the impedance of smooth muscle contractions.

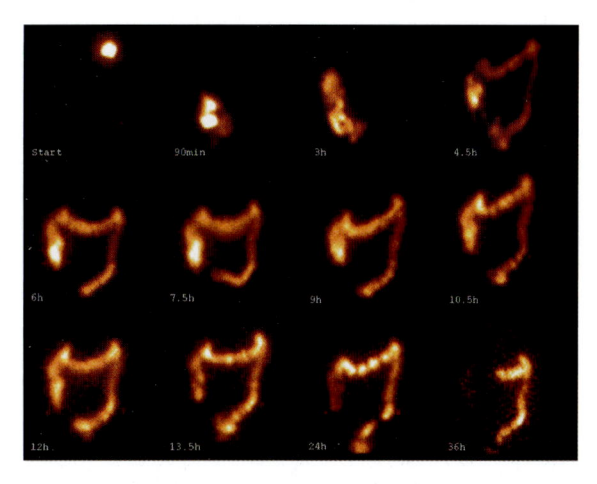

Fig. 14.2. Normal gut transit scintigraphy. Normal whole gut transit scintigraphy in a healthy male subject shown by repetitive planar anterior scintigraphic images of the abdomen up to 36 h after ingestion of a gastric acid resistant capsule containing 3.7 MBq of In-111. The small bowel transit time (SBT) is 81%, the CTI after 4 h (CTI4) 2.07 and the CTI after 24 h (CTI24) 2.8

14.1.2.1
Scintigraphy

Scintigraphy is an inexpensive, simple, and noninvasive method to track and measure small bowel transit velocity using radio-labeled solid and/or liquid food. Typically, scintigraphy evaluates gastric emptying and small bowel and colonic transit (ZIESSMAN 1992). Patients are therefore usually required to fast overnight prior to receiving a standardized meal radiolabeled with a small amount of Tc-99m (half-life: 6 h). The normal dosage is 37 MBq for gastric and small bowel emptying studies or 3.7 MBq of In-111 (half-life: 2.8 days) for small bowel, colon transit, or whole gut transit studies (MULLAN 1996). For whole gut transit studies, gastric acid resistant capsules can be administered. After ingestion, the movement of the radiation-emitting bowel content is tracked by repetitive gamma camera measurements over 6 h for gastric and small bowel-transit studies and 24–48 h for whole gut transit studies (MULLAN 1996). The transit times for the small bowel and the colon are obtained by detecting when the tip of the radio-labeled bowel content reaches the terminal ileum and the rectum, respectively. Since this requires a high frequency of image acquisitions, semi-quantitative measurement of the small bowel and colon transit times, is usually performed at predefined time points after ingestion of the radioactive material (MADSEN et al. 2000). Using the region of interest technique, different clearance indices are calculated for the small bowel and colon. For the small bowel, the percentage of radioactivity cleared to the colon at 6 h is calculated. If more than 41% of the radioactivity is emptied to the colon by this time, then the small bowel transit is considered as normal (Fig. 14.2). Since the colonic transit takes longer and the colonic frame with its different segments is easy to detect even on planar scintigraphic images, colonic transit is evaluated semi-quantitatively by dividing the colon into four segments, the ascending colon, transverse colon, descending colon, and recto-sigmoid, ending with the loss of radioactivity with the stool. The radioactivity loss is calculated by subtracting the decay-corrected residual bowel radioactivity from the ingested dose at 24 h postadministration. The colon transit index (CTI) is calculated at 4 (CTI4) and 24 (CTI24) hours as the geometric center of the count percentages in the four segments and the stool (only at CTI24). Colon transit is considered as normal, if the CTI4 is between 0.8 and 1.4 and the CTI24 between 1.7 and 4.0 (Fig. 14.3). In general, no gender or age-specific differences have been demonstrated, although considerable intra-individual differences are noted when repeated examinations are performed (ARGENYI et al. 1995).

The scintigraphic techniques just described are well established and have been used for decades. They are easy to apply and patient-friendly. The patient is only exposed to minimal irradiation (effective doses: 0.2 mGy/37 MBq for Tc-99m; 0.3 mGy/3.7 MBq for In-111) (MULLAN 1996). The spatial and temporal resolutions of planar scintigraphic images are very

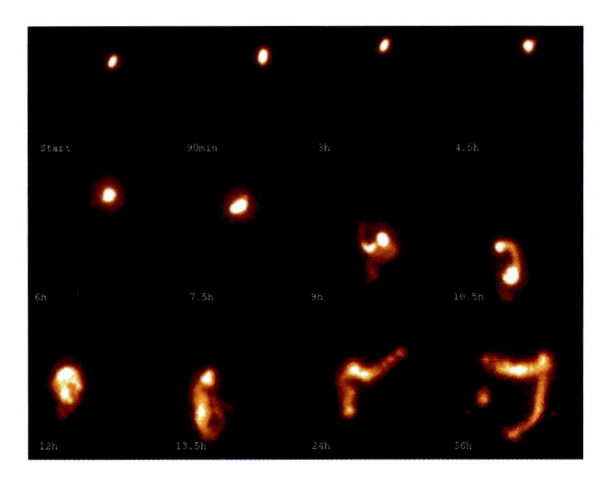

Fig. 14.3. Delayed small bowel transit. The same healthy male under morphine medication. The images show clearly delayed whole gut transit. The small bowel transit time (SBT) is 0%, the CTI after 4 h (CTI4) 0.05 and the CTI after 24 h (CTI24) 2.07

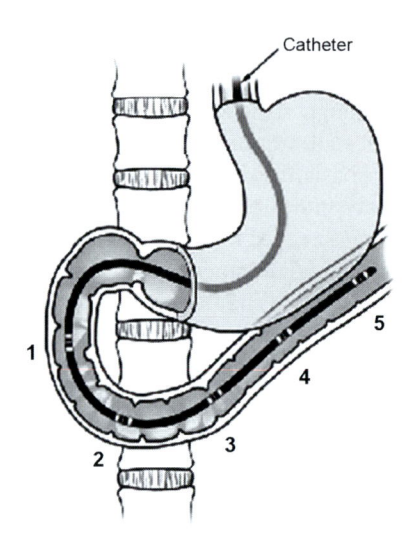

Fig. 14.4. Small bowel (duodenal) manometry. The catheter is placed across the pylorus into the duodenum and proximal jejunum. Pressure transducers spaced 5-10 cm apart are used to measure intraluminal pressure changes. The numbers 1-5 indicate measuring points, representing the location of measuring for the plots in Fig 14.5

low, and there are no anatomical landmarks to reliably localize pathologic changes within the bowel. The scintigraphic method is a typical transit measuring tool that allows no direct statements regarding the actual motility of the bowel wall or the detailed segmental propagation of the bowel content.

14.1.2.2
Manometry

Manometry evaluates GI function by measuring pressure changes within segments of the GI tract. In clinical practice, esophageal and anorectal manometries are routinely used to study patients with dysphagia, chest pain, or reflux symptoms, and fecal incontinence or obstructive defecation, respectively (PANDOLFINO and KAHRILAS 2005). Easy accessibility explains why manometry is mainly implemented in the esophagus and rectum, other segments of the GI tract (stomach, small and large intestine) being more difficult to access. Motility testing of these segments is frequently limited to monitoring their contractile activity (BARNETT et al. 1999).

For the small intestine the majority of clinical experience has been with multichannel pressure catheters (solid-state or water perfused) positioned across the antrum, through the pylorus into the duodenum and proximal jejunum (Fig. 14.4). The catheter is positioned either with endoscopic assistance or by attaching a small balloon to the tip of the catheter, inserting the tube the night before the examination and hoping that the GI activity will advance the balloon distally. Correct positioning is usually verified radiologically (MALAGELADA and STANGHELLINI 1985).

Recently, combined wireless pressure and pH capsules were used to obtain information on the amplitude of contractions as they traverse the stomach and small intestine (CAMILLERI et al. 2008).

Small bowel motility is evaluated by quantifying peristaltic activity in the inter-prandial period (Fig. 14.5). In addition to meals, breathing, body position, and any activity that increases intra-abdominal pressure (e.g., coughing, sneezing, laughing) lead to artifacts in small bowel manometry that may hamper evaluation and diagnosis. Despite these challenges and its relative invasiveness, small bowel manometry is regarded as the gold standard for evaluating small bowel motility. It complements scintigraphy as it provides information on the contractility of defined segments of the small intestine.

14.1.2.3.
Impedance Measurement

A further technique only used for basic physiological studies is the measurement of impedance on the surface of the small bowel wall. The electrical current of smooth muscle depolarization is measured as a function of its contraction. This technique can be compared to electrocardiography, but since the small bowel possesses only a small layer of smooth muscle

Fig. 14.5. Plot of small bowel manometry. Small bowel manometry recording depicting migrating motor complexes (MMCs) as measured by individual pressure transducers in the duodenum (D1–5)

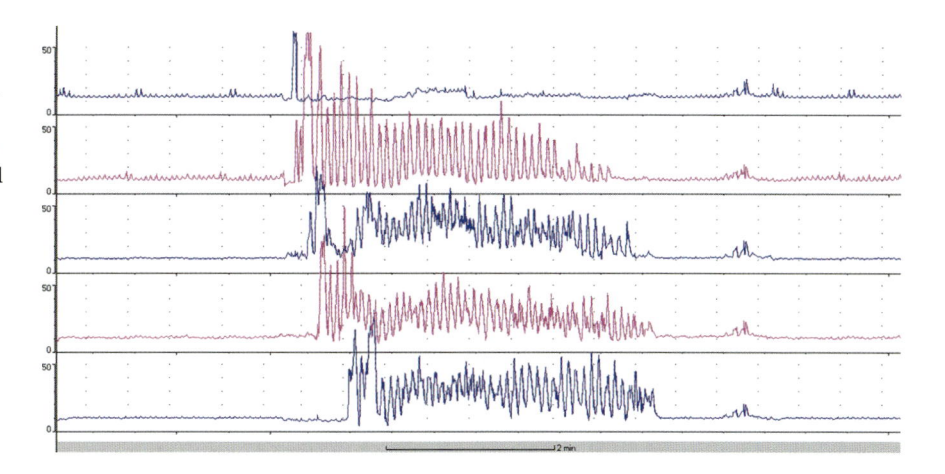

cells the measurement has to be done directly on the surface of the organ. This technique is therefore not applicable to human subjects and will presumably never be used in clinical practice (SOYBEL 1994).

14.1.3. Magnetic Resonance Imaging

The application of MRI as a tool to depict and monitor small bowel motility is quite a new concept, but could have a clear impact on the understanding of small bowel physiology and the diagnosis of small bowel pathologies. In this chapter we will introduce the technique of MRI of bowel wall motion, its current application in routine clinical practice, and provide an overview of possible future applications.

14.2 Technique

14.2.1 Preparation

To achieve high-quality MR images of the small bowel and its motility the patient must be properly prepared. Distention is achieved either by applying the agent through a naso-duodenal catheter (MR enteroclysis; see Chap. 9) or by oral ingestion (MR enterography; see Chap. 8). For oral preparation, the patient typically abstains from eating any solid food for at least 4 h prior to the exam. One hour prior to MRI, the patient is asked to drink a solution that properly distends the small bowel (see also Chap. 3). In the literature various preparation techniques are described for small bowel imaging, differing in the distension mechanism using gelifiers, osmotic acting, or macromolecular solutions. Contrast enhancers such as ferumoxsilum, barium sulfate, or paramagnetic liquids such as gadolinium or various fruit juices may be added as needed (DEBATIN and PATAK 1999). A standardized, homogenous, and good distention of the small bowel lumen facilitates differentiation of the individual bowel wall layers and thus the assessment of motility. It is also an important prerequisite for diagnosis of wall pathologies. It must be borne in mind, however, that the degree of filling itself might be an indirect inducer of small bowel motility. In fact, the intraluminal filling, its chemical composition, and its potential breakdown by intestinal bacteria might well influence peristaltic motion (SPILLER et al. 1987).

Various distending agents are applied in clinical routine for MR enterography. Like the methylcellulose gels used in enteroclysis, they assure a standardized and well reproducible distention together with a homogenous intraluminal signal quality. In practice, the choice of distender depends on factors such as patient compliance, availability and approval, adverse events, cost, and experience. To achieve comparability and reproducibility of results, it is advantageous for each institution to employ a uniform distention scheme. No data have yet been published assessing the influence of these various distenders on motility itself.

One of the most frequently used agents is a mannitol solution containing 30 g of the sugar alcohol monomer mannite dissolved in 1,000 mL of tap water (3% M/V) (SCHUNK et al. 2000). The white crystalline powder is simply dissolved in water shortly before starting preparation. This hypoosmolar solution has a slightly sweet flavor and is well appreciated by patients; it poses no compliance problems. Because mannitol is not absorbed, it slightly impedes water absorption and thus has the advantage of not increasing diuresis. Other agents are aqueous polyethylene glycol (PEG)-solutions, psyllium seed husks such as Metamucil or locust bean gum gels (Lauenstein et al. 2003). Each of these distending agents presents specific advantages, but also drawbacks regarding their practicability and clinical feasibility. All of these oral distenders should be taken continuously over a period of 45–60 min, the patient being asked to drink the agent one glass at a time every 5–10 min. Optimal preparation ends with the last glass being taken on the MRI table. This should help to optimally distend the stomach and duodenum for the MRI examination.

Positive and negative luminal contrast enhancers can be used in MRI of the GI tract, but are not essential for motility studies. The choice will depend on various factors such as the preferred image weighting, ability to distinguish the lumen from the bowel wall, the labeling of luminal content, or to improve the demarcation of the GI tract from surrounding tissue. Typically on T1-weighted sequences the lumen is rendered with a negative contrast agent to allow the use of i.v. gadolinium for the wall enhancement. On T2-weighted sequences water or even normal GI liquid will appear signal intensive towards a rather negative wall.

If the scheduled exam is specifically dedicated to motility imaging using ultra-fast T1-weighted pulse sequences the oral solution should be spiked with 10 mL of gadolinium-DOTA (Dotarem, Guerbet, Aulnay sur Bois, France) per liter. The oral application constitutes off-label-use, but has been proven to be safe without dissociation of any gadolinium (Schwizer et al. 1994). A strong and homogenous T1-contrast is achieved in the MRI by adding oral gadolinium to the intraluminal contents, improving the cutoff between bowel wall and bowel content (Patak et al. 2001). Nevertheless, in the case of wall abnormalities it should not be used in combination with i.v. contrast. The combined use of oral and i.v. gadolinium lowers the contrast and the delineation of the bowel wall and diminishes the diagnostic quality of both motility imaging and standard MR enterography of the small bowel (Fig. 14.6). Negative contrast enhancers such as ferumoxsil (Lumirem®, Guerbet, Aulnay sur Bois, France or Covidien, Mansfield, MA) lead to a signal decrease both on T1- and T2-weighted pulse sequences. The signal decrease within the lumen usually exceeds that of the bowel wall. Nevertheless, ferumoxsil might impede the visualization of subtle mucosal changes due to susceptibility artifacts, which may obscure the interfaces in PD or T2-weighted pulse sequences (Maccioni et al. 2006).

Once the contrast agent has been administered, the patient is then preferably placed into the magnet in the prone position, which reduces displacement of the bowel out of the image slice of interest. Even in case of prolonged motility measurements and despite respiration, the bowel loops remain stable in their original location thus improving reproducibility.

Another important practical aspect of preparation is to train the patient for the breath hold phases. An effective and easy way to substantially prolong

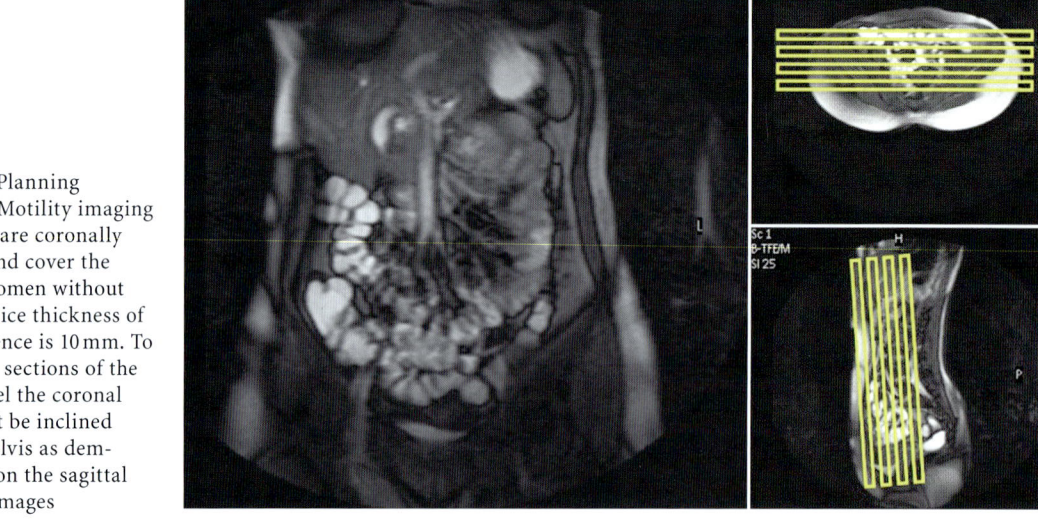

Fig. 14.6. Planning sequence. Motility imaging sequences are coronally oriented and cover the entire abdomen without gap. The slice thickness of each sequence is 10 mm. To include all sections of the small bowel the coronal plane must be inclined into the pelvis as demonstrated on the sagittal planning images

the apnea phases is to have the patient prepare for the breath hold by hyperventilating. When the patient is ready for the breath hold sequence, he simply presses the alarm knob as a sign to start. As is true for virtually all MRI examinations, it is important for the success of this procedure that it is explained to the patient prior to the exam.

14.2.2 Imaging

The details of the mentioned sequences are described in Table 14.1, for a detailed discussion of the sequences see Chap. 1 also. The best way to start MRI after the survey is to use coronal imaging to get an overview of the entire abdomen and pelvis (Fig. 14.6). Preferable for this purpose is a so-called rapid 2D T2-weighted single-shot fast-spin echo (FSE) pulse sequence that is almost unaffected by bowel motion (haste, single-shot turbo spin echo, single-shot free precession (SSFP)) (Fig. 14.7). This imaging sequence allows planning of a range of stacks within the abdomen to cover the entire small bowel. The essential sequence to assess small bowel motility is a fast cine sequence using either fast T1-weighted gradient echo or fast T2-weighted SSFP or echo planar imaging sequences with a maximum repetition time of one second. These sequences allow the repeated acquisition of images every 500–1,000 ms on the same plane for one breath hold period (Fig. 14.8). The apnea training should allow the dynamics to be acquired over 25 s per imaging plane. With a slice thickness of 10 mm, the whole abdomen can be covered in repetitive coronal planes without gaps. Depending on the patient's size, the number of required imaging planes, each representing a cine sequence, lies between 10 and 25. The total required imaging time for specific motility imaging is about 10–15 min. In most cases, this will be combined with a standard MR enterography of the small bowel (Fig. 14.9) (see also Chap. 8). It is important to note that motility images must be acquired prior to execution of a standard small bowel imaging protocol so as to avoid interference with the administration of a spasmolytic drug such as glucagon or *n*-hyoscine (Buscopan®, Boehringer Ingelheim, Basel, Switzerland).

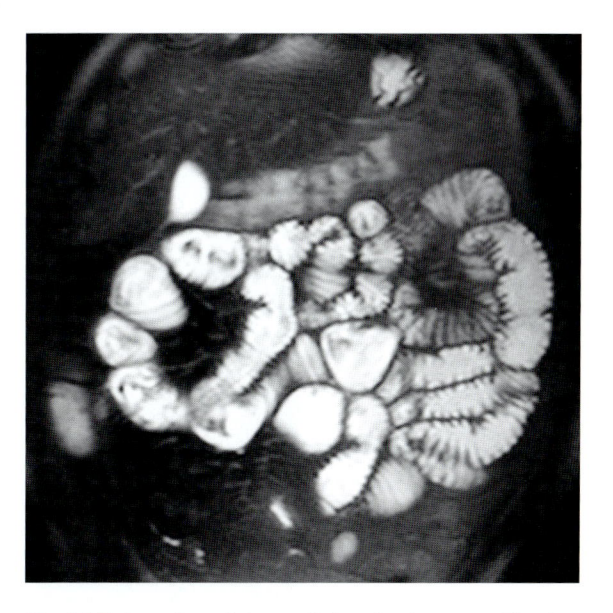

Fig. 14.7. Overview of the small bowel prior to motility imaging. Coronal T2-weighted single-shot fast spin echo image covering the whole abdomen. This sequence gives an overview prior to small bowel motility imaging. Rapid image acquisition reduces movement artifacts generated by small bowel motility. It is therefore ideal as a sequence for planning the actual motility imaging and to obtain a complete overview

Table 14.1 List of MR-parameters for small bowel motility imaging for different vendors

Vendor	Sequence acronym	Parameters						
		Plane	TR	TE	Flip	Matrix	Slice thickness	Parallel factor
Philips	3D bFFE	Cor	4.4	1.3	20	512 × 512	5	2
	2D FFE	Cor	3.4	1.4	25	256 × 256	10	
Siemens	Haste	Cor	1010	80	90	512 × 512	6	
	TruFisp	Cor	283	1.9	55	256 × 256	10	

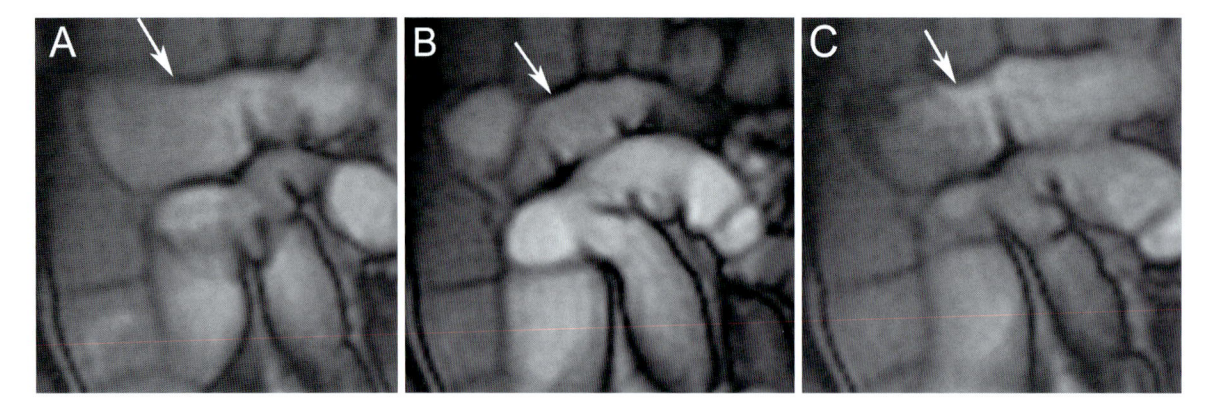

Fig. 14.8. Display of motility. Coronal cine steady-state free precession images of small bowel motility (*arrow*) acquired on the same imaging plane with a slice repetition time of one second. Magnified section of the upper right abdomen showing a normally distended (**A**) small bowel segment shortly after a contraction (**B**) followed by renewed distention (**C**)

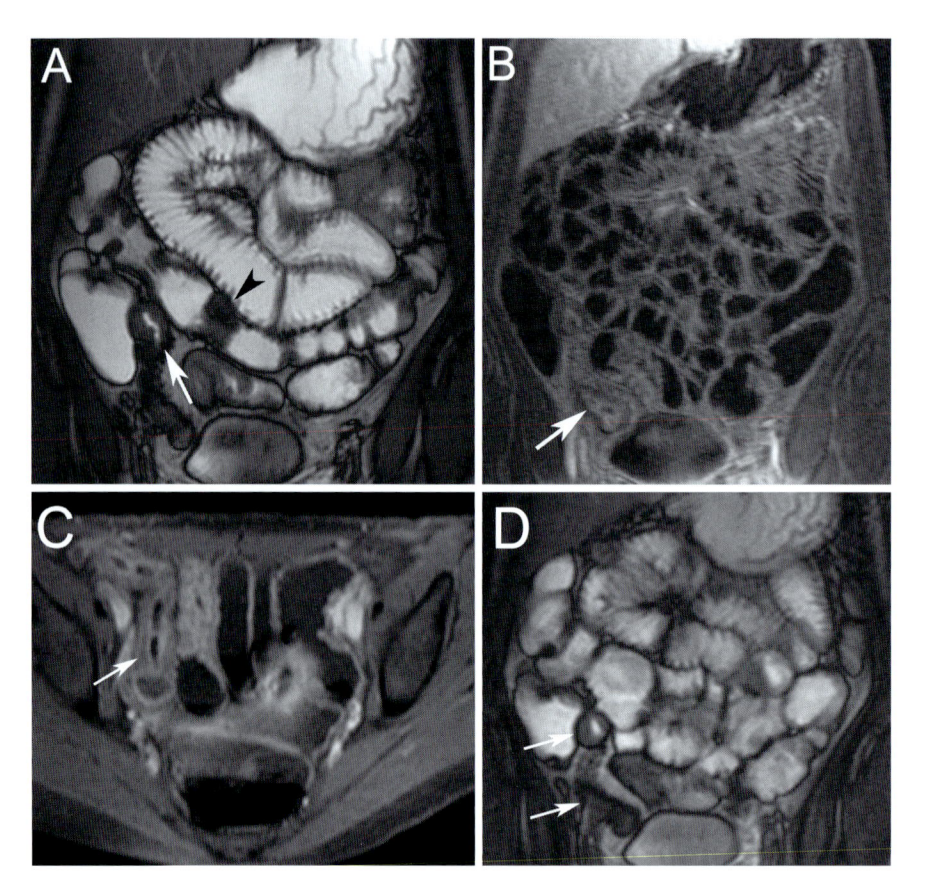

Fig. 14.9. Standard MR enterography. MR enterography of a 28-year-old female suffering from Crohn's disease. The coronal SSFP images show wall thickening in the terminal ileum (*arrow*) as well as in sections of the preterminal ileum and transverse colon (*arrowhead*) (**a**). The corresponding dynamic contrast enhanced 3D T1-weighted fat-saturated coronal images show strong and early enhancement in the wall of the terminal ileum (*arrow*) indicating active disease (**b**). The corresponding 2D T1-weighted transversal fat satuarated images confirm the marked wall enhancement and the strong multi-layered contrast enhancement of the small bowel wall, which is strongest in the submucosa (*arrow*), indicating active disease (**c**). Motility images (coronal cine steady-state free precession sequence) are acquired routinely prior to the standard MR enterography showing thickened bowel wall of the terminal ileum (*arrows*) (**d**). The affected small bowel showed no motility in the cine sequences

14.2.3
Data Analysis

Once the dynamic images have been acquired the two-stage review or postprocessing phase begins. The first, qualitative, stage consists of visual assessment of the acquired sequences as cine loops to obtain an overview of the small bowel motility (Fig. 14.10). The best way to review motility is to display the cine images about two to three times faster than they were actually acquired. Using the cine loops, the reviewer compares the different sections of the displayed small bowel segments on the various imaging planes. The aim of this phase is to identify segments with apparent normal motility and segments with disturbed motility. Usually most of the displayed segments present with approximately the same bowel wall motion pattern consisting of regular contractions. There may also be segments which stand still, move slower, or much faster. The direct comparison of segments displaying normal motility with abnormal segments is especially helpful in providing an overview perspective. Segments that display a comparably diminished or absent motility are usually indicative of pathologic changes in the bowel wall. In our experience, the body generally reacts to a pathologic stimulus on the bowel wall with a reduction of motility. Inflammatory processes can lead to a concomitant bowel wall thickening, the two in combination being capable of generating a stenotic process. Most of the time such stenoses are readily depicted by motility imaging because they do not display any motion on the cine sequences. Segments that are upstream are usually dilated and produce a more intense motility with a higher frequency and amplitude close to the stenoses.

The second, quantitative, stage consists in assessing the bowel wall motion and peristalsis by measuring the cross-section diameter change over time (FROEHLICH et al. 2005). A well-distended, seemingly "normal" segment is selected within the plane to serve as the standard of reference. Abnormally moving segments are selected as well. If no normally moving segment is

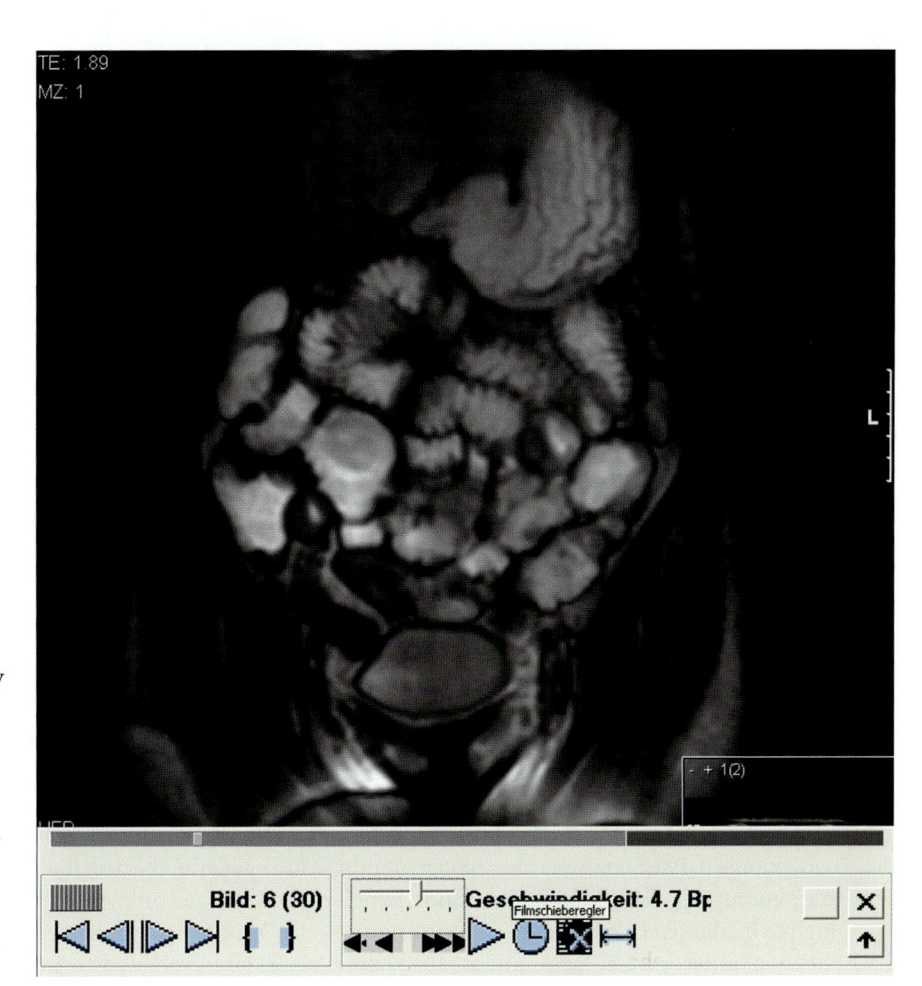

Fig. 14.10. Cine display mode. The acquired cine MR images can be displayed on our PACS workstation in cine display mode. The qualitative analysis of each imaging plane in this mode helps to differentiate between normal and abnormal loops. The images are usually displayed 2–3 times faster than acquired to emphasize motility differences between normal and pathologic sections

Fig. 14.11. Defining measuring points for quantitative analysis. Several small bowel segments are identified to quantitatively assess small bowel motility in the cine mode display. On each of these measuring points, a cross-sectional diameter is placed perpendicularly to the long axis of the selected small bowel section. These measuring lines have to be propagated throughout the complete imaging stack and then manually adjusted on every image to reproduce motility

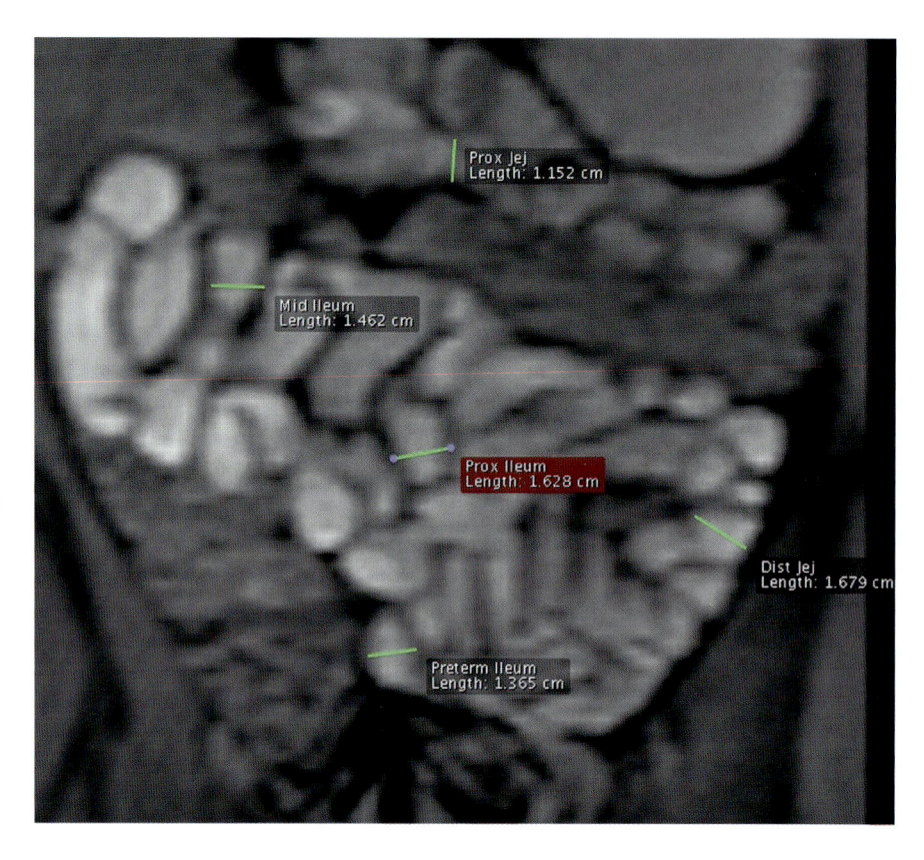

detectable, best would be to select standardized group of segments from different regions of the small bowel such as proximal and distal jejunum and ileum. On these normal and abnormal segments a cross-sectional diameter is placed at a right angle to the long axis of the respective small bowel segment (Fig. 14.11). These cross-sectional measurement lines must be propagated throughout the whole series within that image plane and adjusted manually on each image to represent the cross-sectional diameter variations on the particular segment. Alternatively, cross-section areas of the lumen may also be used on certain workstations and measured over time (Fig. 14.12).

These diameter measurements are then exported and plotted over time using normal spreadsheet programs (Fig. 14.13). These plots allow the differentiation of normal motility from abnormal as discussed below.

The part of data analysis, from image to the plot is the most challenging part of small bowel motility imaging. Qualitative analysis can be easily done on a workstation directly after the examination has taken place. All modern PACS stations or reconstruction workstations provide a cine loop display mode, which is enough to qualitatively validate small bowel motility. The qualitative phase takes about 10–15 min review time. The quantitative measurement is something completely different. It has to be done off-site and off-hours. The measurement is extremely time consuming and is at the moment only applicable in research centers with specialized infrastructure. To evaluate one measuring point on one image series of about 30 acquisitions takes about 5 min, the export of data, import into Excel and display the measurements as a plot takes another 5–10 min. Both analyzing methods, the qualitative and the quantitative, need some experience, but the learning curve is steep and differences between normal and abnormal are obviously distinguishable most of the time.

Measurement by hand is very time consuming, limits exploitation, and places a point of error in the assessment of small bowel motility. Software has, therefore, been developed to automatically measure these small bowel diameter variations and display them as a plot over time (Fig. 14.14). Dedicated software not only greatly speeds up the second stage of reviewing motility images, but also guards against user generated error. It also enables structured, well-standardized analysis of small bowel motility.

Once the plot is drawn several additional parameters are evaluated to interpret the motility curves

Fig. 14.12. Cardiac software for small bowel motility analysis. Another option for measuring small bowel motility is to use a vessel analysis program that automatically measures a cross-sectional area over time. Instead of applying this algorithm to a vessel the software is applied to cross-sectional small bowel images. These images are usually acquired in a sagittal plane to ease the display of cross-sectional small bowel

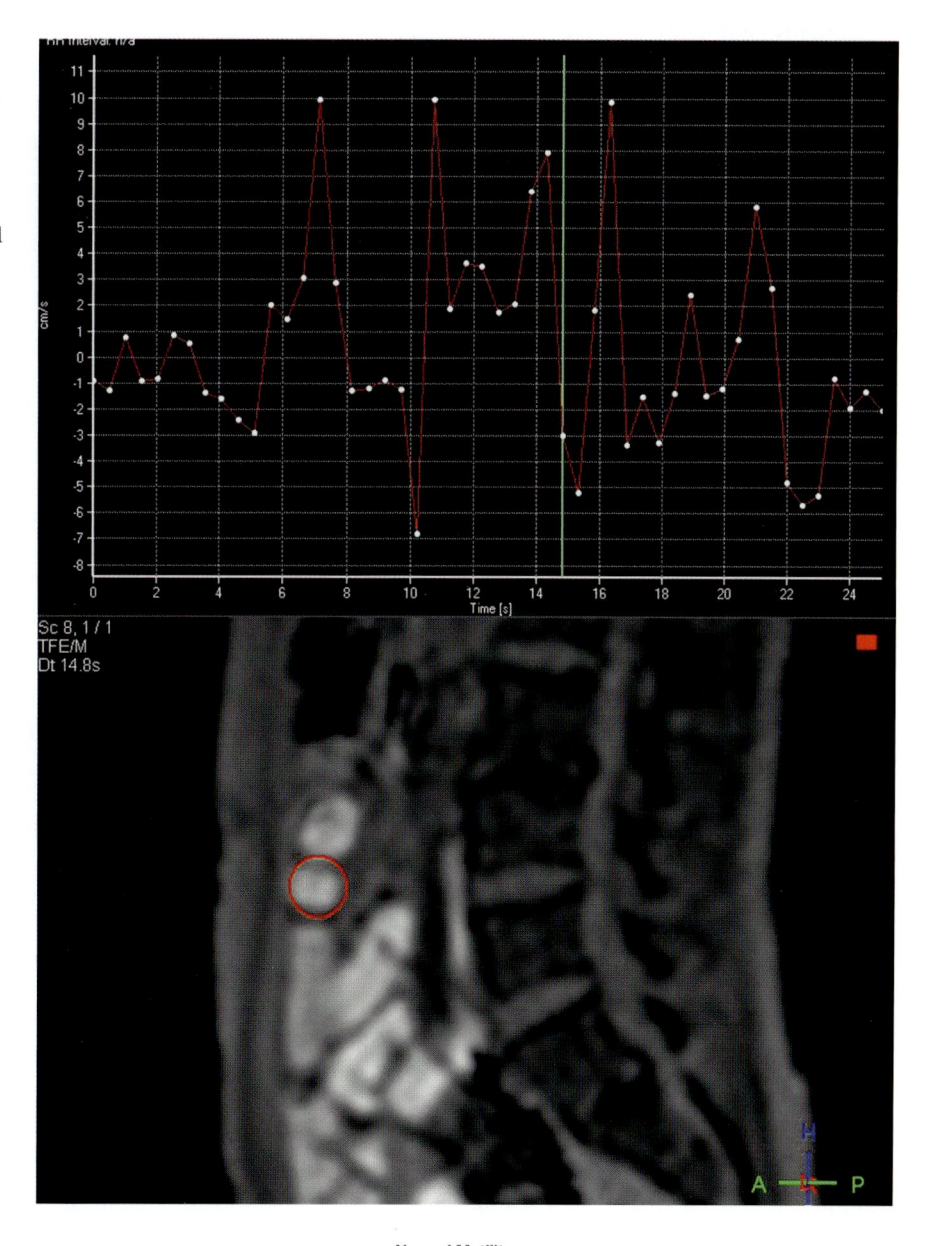

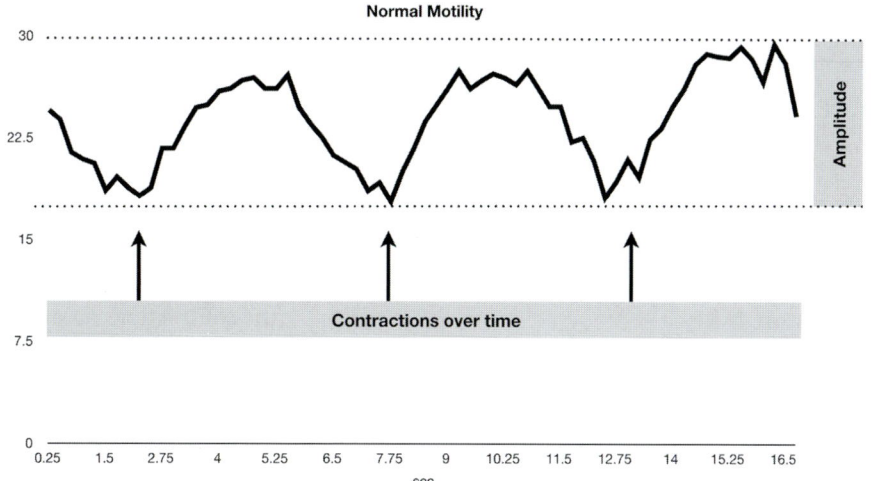

Fig. 14.13. Normal small bowel contraction curve. Plot of a small bowel cross-section diameter measured over time. The plot is characterized by regular contractions (*arrows*) and a quite constant amplitude (*grey block*). The rhythmic wave-like form of the curve resembles a sinusoidal form

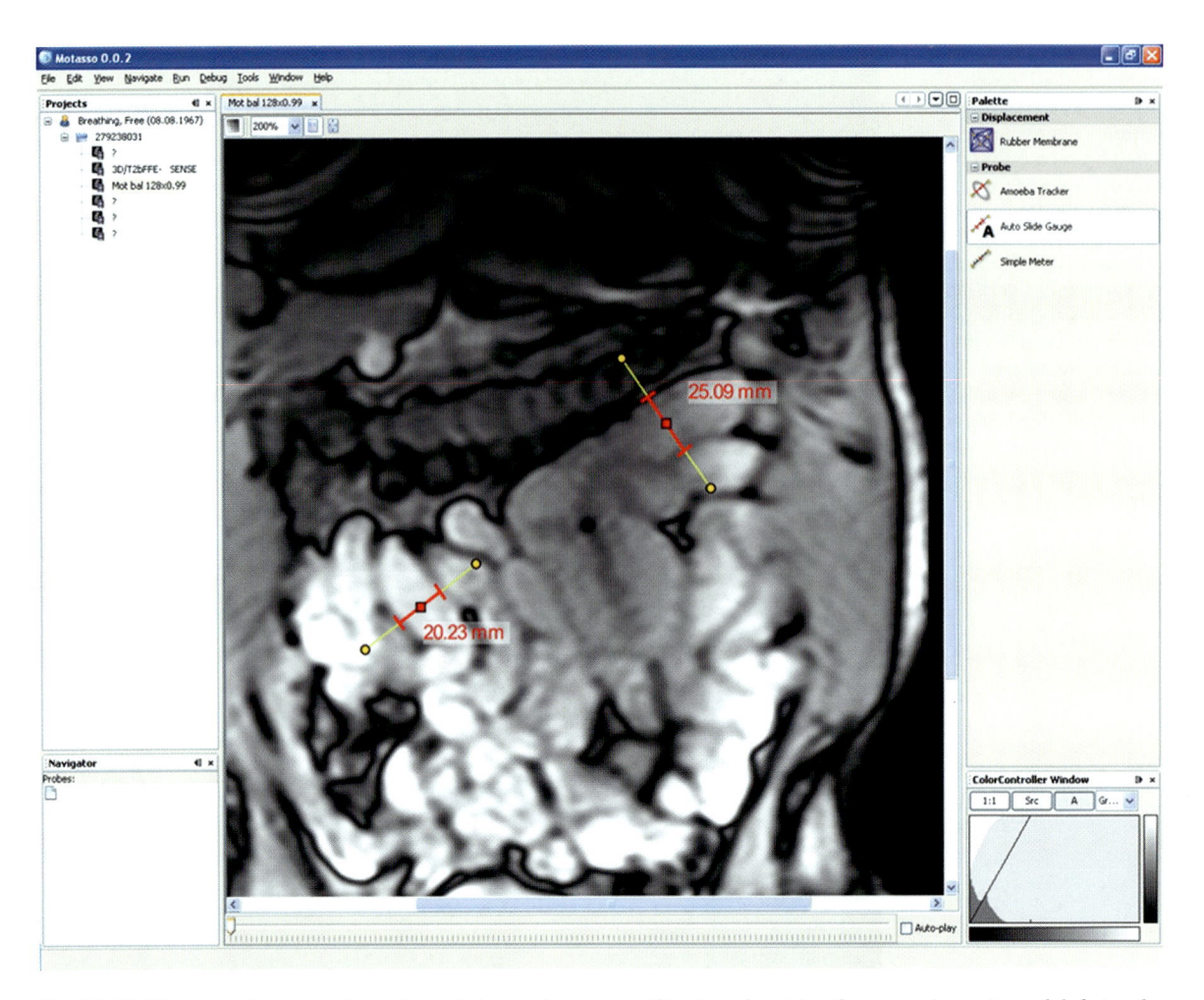

Fig. 14.14. Motasso software analysis. Quantitative analysis is important for small bowel motility imaging. Measuring by hand is enormously time consuming and impedes implementing these methods in clinical practice. A new program is being developed to semi-automatically analyze small bowel motility. By only setting the measuring point and defining the measuring direction the program can automatically assess small bowel diameter changes and display them as a plot over time. For more information refer to: www.motasso.ch

leading to a possible diagnosis. The four parameters commonly extracted from these plots are the mean cross-section diameters, the wave amplitudes, the contraction frequencies over time, and the overall wave forms of the curves (Fig. 14.13). These four parameters will form the basis for our discussion of the different pathologies in the following.

14.3
In Vivo Results of Peristaltic Motion Using Dynamic MRI

Many pathologies of the small bowel can alter small bowel motility (diabetes, obstipation, functional dyspepsia, irritable bowel syndrome, and visceral inflammatory neuropathies) (JONES and BRATTEN 2008). Some of them have already been examined with dynamic MRI in studies that show this imaging technique to be very promising for visualization and quantification of motility changes. Nevertheless, manometry remains the gold standard for motility quantification. As described above, MRI motility interpretation is based on bowel wall motion-plots over time, the basic display method for quantitative motility measurement. Furthermore, the cine loop images allow qualitative assessment by displaying the contractions as short movie sequences.

It has to be emphasized, though, that this technique is still undergoing early clinical evaluation so that a deeper understanding and practical interpretation of the various alterations need still to be established.

14.3.1
Displaying Normal Motility with MRI

Normal motility has been visualized, described qualitatively and quantitatively, and reproduced in several studies (Froehlich et al. 2005, 2009)

The plot of normal motility closely resembles a sinusoidal curve with a base line frequency between 9 and 11 contractions per minute, amplitudes between 15 and 30 mm, and mean diameters of roughly 5–35 mm (Fig. 14.13). Especially the cross-section diameters can show a wide variability depending on the filling status and local activity. In our experience, the general form of the curve, the mean diameter, and the frequency are the most important parameters to explore for diagnosis.

14.3.2
Postoperative Ileus and Its Recovery Phase

Postoperative ileus is a common problem without a clearly defined underlying physiological mechanism (Behm and Stollman 2003). Until the introduction of MRI motility measurements, little data had been published on the recovery phase of small bowel motility. Thirty patients were included in a prospective study of small bowel motility 3–5 days post major abdominal surgery (colectomy or rectum resection) (Patak et al. 2007a). They were placed in the magnet in a supine position without any specific oral preparation or distending agent. Standard imaging was done as mentioned above. In each patient four measurement points from the proximal jejunum to distal ileum were assessed (Fig. 14.11). Based on the data of these 30 patients, four distinct postoperative patterns of small bowel motility could be defined: (1) absent motility corresponding to ileus, (2) shivering, (3) uncoordinated contractions, and finally (4) wavelike normal motility (Fig. 14.15). It seems that the recovery phase of small bowel motility has a standard and distinguishable evolution. The known temporal course of the recovery phase after abdominal surgery starts with an ileus represented in the plot as a strongly dilated lumen without any amplitude that denotes complete cessation of motility (Fig. 14.15a). The first step of recovery seems to be a slight contraction of the lumen as a sign of initial smooth muscle cell activity. During this early phase there is hardly any bowel wall motion except some slight shivering (Fig. 14.15b). Slowly bowel wall motion starts to develop, but does not present a regular, rhythmic contraction pattern and therefore the amplitude appears to vary from contraction to contraction (Fig. 14.15c). Once this irregular phase has passed a normal sinusoidal curve ensues with regular contractions and constant amplitudes that correspond to normal motility (Fig. 14.15d). This study was the first to describe the phases of small bowel motility both visually and quantitatively following various abdominal surgical interventions 3–5 days after the surgical procedure.

It should be emphasized that patients in the study received no oral preparation or any other interventions or drugs during the procedure. Imaging without preparation extends the utility of the tool to be used without preparation being completely noninvasive. As shown in this study, it should be possible to obtain motility measurements and to visualize motility by simply placing the patient into the magnet without any specific oral preparation phase or intervention.

14.3.3
Impact of Drugs on Small Bowel Motility

MRI can be used to monitor motility changes after administration of a pharmaceutical compound. Both spasmolysis and prokinetic effects are of particular interest. The advent of MRI has made it possible to localize pharmacologic activity. Several studies have demonstrated its utility by injecting *n*-hyoscine butyl bromide (Buscopan). One study on ten volunteers compared the impact of hyoscine versus that of glucagon at 60-min follow up (GlucaGen Novo Nordisk, Küsnacht, Switzerland) (Fig. 14.16) (Froehlich et al. 2009). They underwent two separate MR examinations, one with Buscopan and one with glucagon as paralyzing agent. Intravenous injection of an antiperistaltic agent produces a rapid onset of aperistalsis for both drugs. Glucagon induced complete aperistalsis within 25 s in all subjects, hyoscine was in only 50% of the volunteers. The most important parameter of these drugs is the duration of the complete arrest or aperistalsis they induce, which is significantly longer for Glucagon (18.3 ± 7 min) than for hyoscine (6.8 ± 5.3 min). Further studies are warranted to explore these results in larger clinical trials or with other administration routes such as the intramuscular one.

In another study a prokinetic agent (Metoclopramid, Paspertin®, Solvay Pharma, Bern, Switzerland) used to monitor motility changes showed increased amplitudes and frequency about 30 s after administration, whereas the wash-out of the prokinetic (Fig. 14.17) (Froehlich et al. 2005).

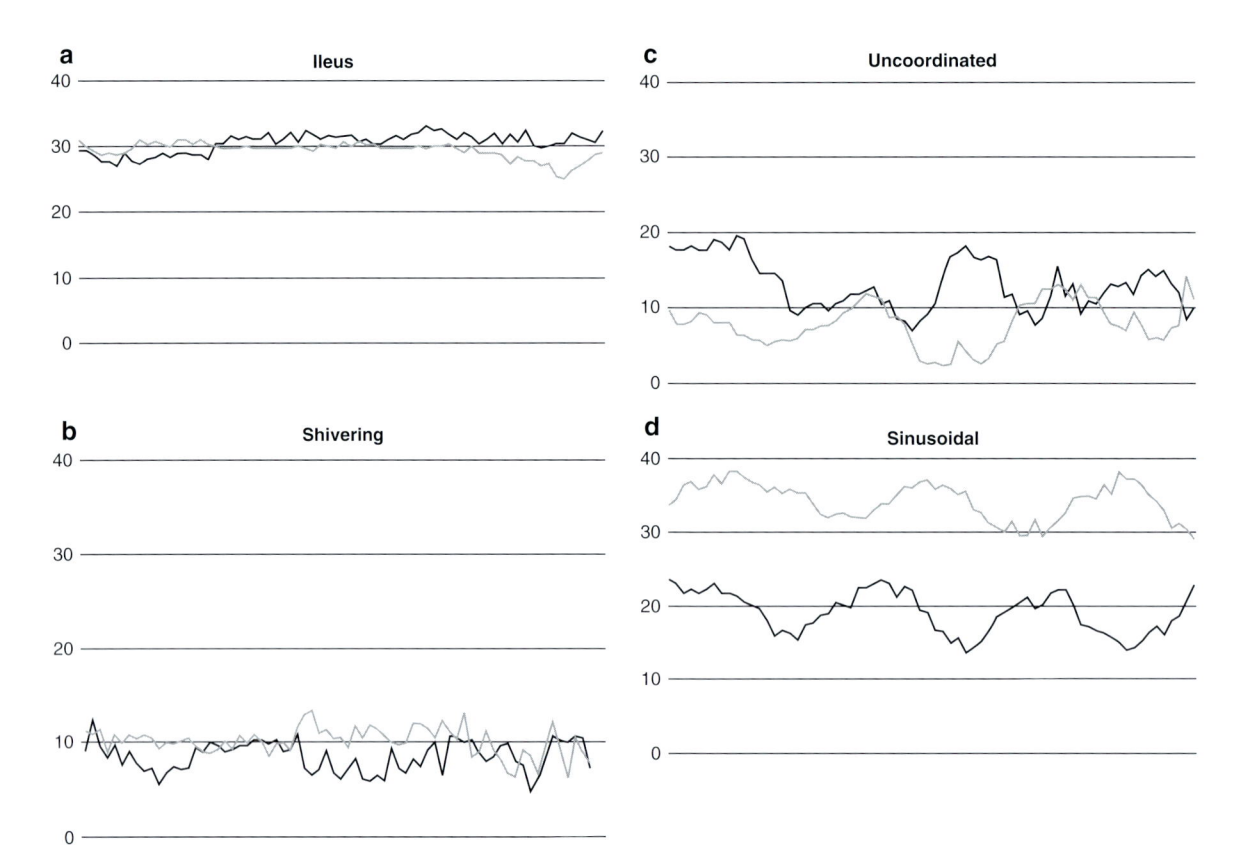

Fig. 14.15. Postoperative motility plots. MRI measurement after colorectal surgery presents with four distinguishable motility patterns occurring over time. Immediately after surgery the curve represents the postoperative ileus with a dilated lumen diameter and almost no contractions (**a**). The first movement of the bowel is a contraction indicated by the reduced diameter; this phase is defined as "shivering" (**b**). In a third phase, uncoordinated contractions are developing with an irregular amplitude and irregular frequency (**c**). The last phase represents complete recovery. Similar to the normal motility pattern sinusoidal contraction waves are produced (**d**)

These three drugs exemplify the possibilities for measuring and closely monitoring the impact of any given drug on small bowel motility or related adverse events. Drugs that are known to induce nausea, constipation, or diarrhea might be examined to determine the exact origin of the side effect and whether it is related to the GI system. Again this knowledge could help to eliminate or minimize such side effects by tailoring administration of the drug.

14.3.4 Motility Changes in Inflammatory Bowel Diseases

Roughly 30 years ago conventional enteroclysis was introduced (ANTES and LISSNER 1983; MAGLINTE et al. 1987). Its main advantage over the existing small bowel follow-through was its controlled distension and its ability to perform combined evaluation of the bowel mucosal surfaces and motility. A whole classification system was developed around the new technique and remained in use for decades (SELLINK and ROSENBUSCH 1981). Step by step though conventional enteroclysis was replaced by computed tomography (CT) and MR enteroclysis and MR enterography. CT evaluation of the small bowel completely lacks the possibility of displaying motility. MRI was not initially able to display motility due to its low temporal resolution, but recent speed-up techniques have considerably extended its potential. Thus, standard MR enterography and MR enteroclysis are increasingly used for diagnosis or follow-up in small bowel disease, especially Crohn's disease (CD) (GOURTSOYIANNIS et al. 2006) (see also Chaps. 8–10). MRI seems to be ideally suited for small bowel imaging because it has a high soft tissue contrast and lacks ionizing radiation, which is important for the usually young CD patient

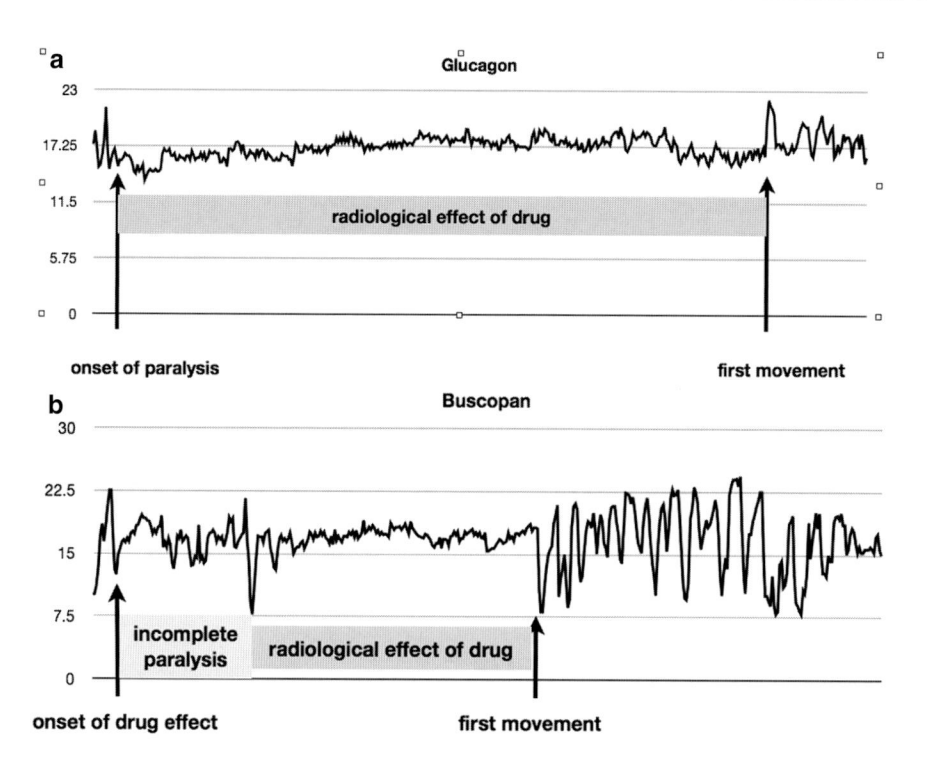

Fig. 14.16. Motility plots after injection of a spasmolytic drug. Small bowel contractions over time after i.v. injection of either 1 mg glucagon (**a**) or 40 mg n-hyoscine butyl bromide (HBB, Buscopan®) (**b**). Both drugs show a rapid onset (*first arrow*) in about 20–30 s. For HBB, only 50% of the volunteers showed a complete paralysis. In radiology, the time period with almost no measured contraction is the preferred one from the diagnostic point of view. The effect of Glucagon lasts significantly longer than that of HBB (*dark grey block*)

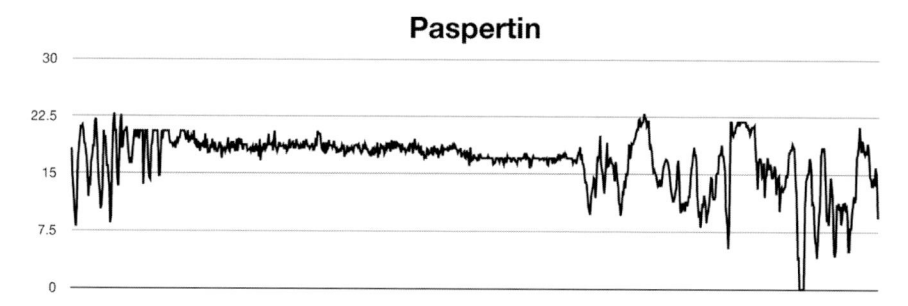

Fig. 14.17. Impact of paspertin. This plot represents normal motility in the first phase, followed by i.v. administration of n-hyoscine butyl bromide (Buscopan®) (*arrow*), then 10 min later by the administration of metoclopramide (Paspertin®) (*arrow head*). The impact of the prokinetic metoclopramide is indicated by wider amplitudes and a higher frequency compared to normal motility

and for repeated exams. Several studies have shown that CD-affected small bowel segments present with altered motility, a phenomenon known from fluoroscopy. The use of MR motility imaging as an additional screening method for CD-related disease manifestations produced a significant increase in the number of detected lesions as well as a significant increase in the number of patients presenting with lesions at all. Forty patients were included in a study where total of 26 CD-related lesions were found by standard MRE, whereas 35 lesions could be detected with the use of motility imaging as screening method ($p = 0.001$) (PATAK et al. 2007b). Only 25 patients were found to have CD by standard imaging compared to 34 patients identified with the help of motility changes ($p = 0.007$). Clearly, MR motility imaging in patients with inflammatory bowel disease has improved the diagnosis of CD (Fig. 14.18).

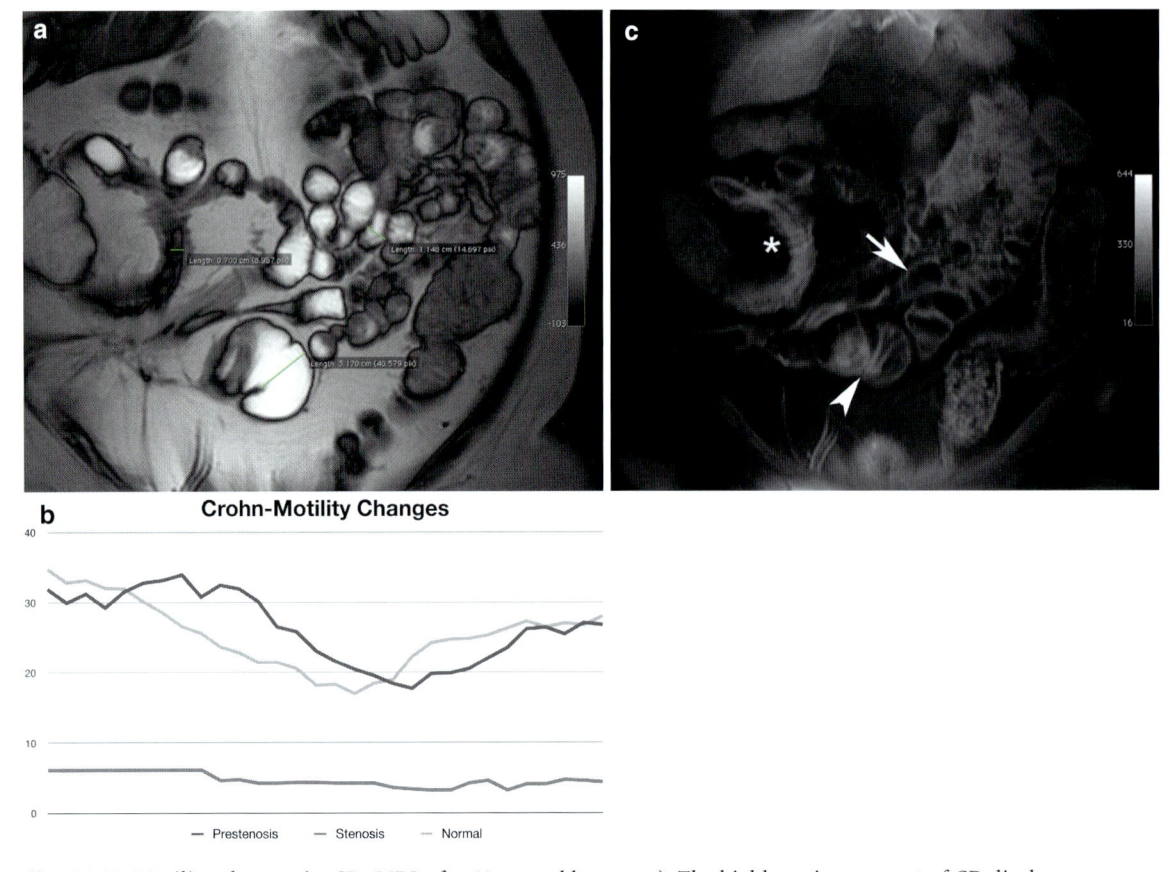

Fig. 14.18. Motility changes in CD. MRI of a 32-year-old female suffering from CD. The patient has several affected bowel segments between normal bowel segments visualized at this coronal steady-state free precession images of small bowel. Comparable measurements were done at a location with highly active disease (*asterisk*), a prestenotic segment (*arrow head*), and a normal segment (*arrow*). Displaying the plots over time the normal segments exhibit a nearly sinusoidal curve with a medium diameter of 13 mm (*dark grey curve*). The highly active segment of CD displays no movement at all (*light grey curve*), whereas the prestenotic segment shows an increased amplitude with a higher frequency (*black curve*) compared to normal motility. These motility plots may indicate affected small bowel sections in patients with CD. The coronal 2D T1-weighted postcontrast image correlates well with a highly active segment (*asterisk*). The prestenotic segment (*arrow head*) and the normal appearance of small bowel wall (*arrow*)

14.3.5
Future MR Motility Imaging Applications

Several pathologies of the GI tract have not yet been studied by MR motility imaging. Foremost among the future targets for MR imaging is irritable bowel syndrome (IBS). Studies with manometry suggest that aspects of the IBS symptom complex can be explained by motility alterations (GASBARRINI et al. 2008). About one third of IBS patients present with delayed gastric emptying. These patients have no interdigestive small bowel abnormalities, but they do have clear abnormalities in the manometry in the post meal phase. IBS has an enormous impact on the everyday life of these patients and on health care costs in general. There are estimates that approximately one third of every consultation in a general gastroenterologist is attributable to IBS. Millions work hours per year are lost in industry because of sick leave of these patients and billions are spent on diagnosing and treating IBS patients (MAXION-BERGEMANN et al. 2006). It is unfortunate, therefore, that a standardized diagnosis and a targeted therapy have yet to be established. Hopefully, MRI and specifically MR motility imaging can at least in part fill this diagnostic deficit. Large studies are needed to assess motility changes in IBS patients and eventually develop a classification that can be used for targeted therapy.

Other functional diseases of the small bowel should be amenable to assessment by MRI. From our point of view, this technique gives a welcome boost to the examination, localization, and interpretation of motility disorders that was not possible before.

14.4 Motility Measurement: Which Technique for What Task?

Different techniques to measure motility have been introduced and compared with one another. The clear technical differences between the techniques lead to different indications. This part of the chapter attempts to delineate the ideal measurement tool for a dedicated clinical request.

14.4.1 Ultrasound

The use of ultrasound in evaluation of small bowel motility is often used in a qualitative way obtaining information during abdominal ultrasound. Only a few studies use ultrasound to monitor small bowel motility (Dell'Aquila et al. 2005; Gimondo and Mirk 1997). Imaging motility and evaluation frequency and amplitude seems feasible with ultrasound. The limitation of the technique clearly lies in the limited coverage and its user dependency. Therefore, the use of ultrasound is mostly to provide a general overview of the visible segments, but should not be used as a dedicated technique to display overall small bowel motility.

14.4.2 Scintigraphy

The low resolution of scintigraphic imaging does not allow localization of an anatomical point of interest. It does, however, allow easy tracking of the tip of a radio-labeled meal and its propagation through the GI tract. It can produce an overview and measure the transit time in the small bowel and colon. MRI on the other hand is not very cost-effective for measuring transit time.

As mentioned above, the strength of scintigraphy lies in its overall display of bowel function, which enables ready diagnosis of diffuse or systemic diseases associated with an overall prolonged transit time. Diseases such as diabetic neuropathy or hormonal imbalances can be diagnosed with scintigraphy.

14.4.3 Manometry

Because manometry involves insertion of a tube into the GI tract to measure pressure changes, it has clear advantages in proximal GI systems such as the esophagus or the stomach. The placement of a longer tube (sometimes 2–3 m long) to monitor bowel motility beyond the ligament of Treitz is extremely unpleasant for the patient and cumbersome for the examiner. For this reason, manometry for bowel segments beyond the ligament of Treitz is performed by only a few centers worldwide. The migratory motor complex (MMC) produces a wave-like propagation of contractions starting from the duodenum and continuing through the entire small bowel system. Manometry can be a useful diagnostic tool for evaluating the MMC and its changes in the jejunum or ileum.

Compared to MRI, manometry is able to scan a larger section of small bowel in a single measurement, but only incrementally. There is an ongoing discussion as to whether the insertion of the measuring tool alters motility, thus creating a technical bias. The recording of pressure waves as applied in manometry has not yet been correlated with the peristaltic small bowel wall movement observed with dynamic MRI.

14.4.4 MR Motility Imaging

MRI is an easily applicable tool for the assessment of small bowel motility. There is no ionizing radiation and it can be applied totally noninvasively. It is the only tool that can visualize small bowel wall motion and analyze small bowel motility at virtually any given point within the small bowel. Its high-resolution imaging of the abdomen enables evaluation not only of selected segments of the small bowel, but also of virtually the whole organ. The greatest obstacle to its general adoption should be removed with the introduction of software-assisted quantitative measurements. We recommend performing motility measurements prior to any MRI exam on the small bowel especially for the detection of CD-related changes and other pathologies. MR motility imaging can be used as a tool for basic physiological research or in drug research to evaluate the impact of the administered drug on small bowel motility and function. Thus, visualization and quantification of small bowel motility using MRI promise to improve the diagnostics of small bowel pathologies or related problems.

14.5 Conclusion

Until now no technology has been available that could be applied noninvasively to assessment of small bowel motility. The introduction of MR motility imaging could fill this gap. The appropriate MRI sequences can be implemented on almost every MR system and are easy to execute. There is clear evidence that the evaluation of motility alterations may help to increase the sensitivity and specificity of MRI of the small bowel. Further studies are needed to establish fundamental classifications of motility disorders as assessed by MRI.

Acknowledgment We want to thank Barbara LeBlanc and Susanne Furrer for their great work in producing and editing the manuscript.

References

Antes G and Lissner J (1983). Double-contrast small-bowel examination with barium and methylcellulose. Radiology 148(1): 37–40.

Argenyi EE, Soffer EE, Madsen MT, et al. (1995). Scintigraphic evaluation of small bowel transit in healthy subjects: inter- and intrasubject variability. Am J Gastroenterol 90(6): 938–42.

Barnett JL, Hasler WL and Camilleri M (1999). American Gastroenterological Association medical position statement on anorectal testing techniques. American Gastroenterological Association. Gastroenterology 116(3): 732–60.

Bassotti G, de Roberto G, Castellani D, et al. (2005). Normal aspects of colorectal motility and abnormalities in slow transit constipation. World J Gastroenterol 11(18): 2691–6.

Behm B and Stollman N (2003). Postoperative ileus: etiologies and interventions. Clin Gastroenterol Hepatol 1(2): 71–80.

Camilleri M, Bharucha AE, di Lorenzo C, et al. (2008). American Neurogastroenterology and Motility Society consensus statement on intraluminal measurement of gastrointestinal and colonic motility in clinical practice. Neurogastroenterol Motil 20(12): 1269–82.

Debatin JF and Patak MA (1999). MRI of the small and large bowel. Eur Radiol 9(8): 1523–34.

Deetjen P, Speckmann EJ and Heschler J (2006). Physiologie. München, Urban&Schwarzberg.

Dell'Aquila P, Pietrini L, Barone M, et al. (2005). Small intestinal contrast ultrasonography-based scoring system: a promising approach for the diagnosis and follow-up of celiac disease. J Clin Gastroenterol 39(7): 591–5.

Froehlich JM, Daenzer M, von Weymarn C, et al. (2009). Aperistaltic effect of hyoscine N-butylbromide versus glucagon on the small bowel assessed by magnetic resonance imaging. Eur Radiol 19(6): 1387–93.

Froehlich JM, Patak MA, von Weymarn C, et al. (2005). Small bowel motility assessment with magnetic resonance imaging. J Magn Reson Imaging 21(4): 370–5.

Gasbarrini A, Lauritano EC, Garcovich M, et al. (2008). New insights into the pathophysiology of IBS: intestinal microflora, gas production and gut motility. Eur Rev Med Pharmacol Sci 12 Suppl 1: 111–7.

Gimondo P and Mirk P (1997). A new method for evaluating small intestinal motility using duplex Doppler sonography. AJR Am J Roentgenol 168(1): 187–92.

Gourtsoyiannis NC, Grammatikakis J, Papamastorakis G, et al. (2006). Imaging of small intestinal Crohn's disease: comparison between MR enteroclysis and conventional enteroclysis. Eur Radiol 16(9): 1915–25.

Gryback P, Blomquist L, Schnell PO, et al. (2002). [Scintigraphic assessment of the small intestine transit. Diagnostic investigation of dysmotility with 99mTc-HIDA]. Lakartidningen 99(14): 1556–8, 1561–2.

Husebye E (1999). The patterns of small bowel motility: physiology and implications in organic disease and functional disorders. Neurogastroenterol Motil 11(3): 141–61.

Jones MP and Bratten JR (2008). Small intestinal motility. Curr Opin Gastroenterol 24(2): 164–72.

Lauenstein TC, Schneemann H, Vogt FM, et al. (2003). Optimization of oral contrast agents for MR imaging of the small bowel. Radiology 228(1): 279–83.

Maccioni F, Bruni A, Viscido A, et al. (2006). MR imaging in patients with Crohn disease: value of T2- versus T1-weighted gadolinium-enhanced MR sequences with use of an oral superparamagnetic contrast agent. Radiology 238(2): 517–30.

Madsen JL, Graff J and Fugisang S (2000). A simplified method for processing dynamic images of gastric antrum. Nucl Med Commun 21(11): 1037–41.

Maglinte DD, Lappas JC, Kelvin FM, et al. (1987). Small bowel radiography: how, when, and why? Radiology 163(2): 297–305.

Malagelada JR and Stanghellini V (1985). Manometric evaluation of functional upper gut symptoms. Gastroenterology 88(5 Pt 1): 1223–31.

Maxion-Bergemann S, Thielecke F, Abel F, et al. (2006). Costs of irritable bowel syndrome in the UK and US. Pharmacoeconomics 24(1): 21–37.

Mullan BP (1996). Gastric Emptying, Small Bowel Transit, and Colonic Transit Studies. The Mayo Clinic Manual Of Nuclear Medicine. M. K. O'Connor. Rochester, Churchill Livingstone: 303–316.

Pandolfino JE and Kahrilas PJ (2005). AGA technical review on the clinical use of esophageal manometry. Gastroenterology 128(1): 209–24.

Patak MA, Froehlich JM, von Weymarn C, et al. (2007a). Noninvasive measurement of small-bowel motility by MRI after abdominal surgery. Gut 56(7): 1023–5.

Patak MA, Froehlich JM, von Weymarn C, et al. (2001). Noninvasive distension of the small bowel for magnetic-resonance imaging. Lancet 358(9286): 987–8.

Patak MA, Waldherr C, Stoupis C, et al. (2007b). Improved diagnosis of Crohn's disease by peristaltic motion assessment: a comparison of standardized MRE with and without cine

TrueFISP sequence. European Society of Gastrointestinal and Abdominal Radiology (ESGAR), 18th Annual Meeting and postgraduate Course, Lisbon, Portugal.

Rauch S, Krueger K, Turan A, et al. (2009). Determining small intestinal transit time and pathomorphology in critically ill patients using video capsule technology. Intensive Care Med 35(6): 1054–9.

Schunk K, Kern A, Oberholzer K, et al. (2000). Hydro-MRI in Crohn's disease: appraisal of disease activity. Invest Radiol 35(7): 431–7.

Schwizer W, Fraser R, Maecke H, et al. (1994). Gd-DOTA as a gastrointestinal contrast agent for gastric emptying measurements with MRI. Magn Reson Med 31(4): 388–93.

Sellink JL and Rosenbusch G (1981). ["The ten commandments" for enteroclysis or ten golden rules for proper enteroclysis technique (author's transl)]. Radiologe 21(8): 366–76.

Soybel DI (1994). Applications of electrophysiology in studies of ion transport by gut mucosa. J Surg Res 57(4): 510–26.

Spiller RC, Brown ML and Phillips SF (1987). Emptying of the terminal ileum in intact humans. Influence of meal residue and ileal motility. Gastroenterology 92(3): 724–9.

Thomson AB, Drozdowski L, Iordache C, et al. (2003a). Small bowel review: Normal physiology, part 1. Dig Dis Sci 48(8): 1546–64.

Thomson AB, Drozdowski L, Iordache C, et al. (2003b). Small bowel review: Normal physiology, part 2. Dig Dis Sci 48(8): 1565–81.

Ziessman HA (1992). Scintigraphy in the gastrointestinal tract. Curr Opin Radiol 4(3): 105–16.

MRI of the Peritoneum

Russell N. Low

CONTENTS

15.1 Introduction *249*

15.2 Technical Considerations and Protocols for Peritoneal MRI *250*
15.2.1 Intraluminal Contrast Material *250*
15.2.2 Intravenous Contrast Agents *251*
15.2.3 Antiperistaltic Agents *251*
15.2.4 MRI Protocol *251*
15.2.5 MR Image Interpretation *252*

15.3 Peritoneal Anatomy *253*

15.4 Benign Diseases of the Peritoneum *256*
15.4.1 Mesenteric Paniculitis *256*
15.4.2 Mesenteric Adenitis *257*
15.4.3 Peritonitis *257*
15.4.4 Tuberculous Peritonitis *257*
15.4.5 Sclerosing Encapsulating Peritonitis *258*

15.5 Malignant Diseases of the Peritoneum *259*
15.5.1 Mechanisms of Peritoneal Tumor Spread *259*
15.5.1.1 Intraperitoneal Tumor Dissemination *259*
15.5.1.2 Direct Spread of Tumors Along Peritoneum Pathways *260*
15.5.1.3 Hematogenous Tumor Dissemination to the Peritoneum *261*
15.5.2 Ovarian Cancer *261*
15.4.3 Gastrointestinal Cancers *263*
15.5.4 Pseudomyxoma Peritonei *263*
15.5.5 Mesothelioma *265*
15.5.6 Primary Peritoneal Cancer *266*

15.6 Conclusion *267*

References *267*

Russell N. Low, MD, PhD
Sharp and Children's MRI Center, 7901 Frost Street, San Diego, CA 92123, USA

KEY POINTS

The peritoneum forms an extensive network of serous membranes that line the abdominal cavity and coat the abdominal viscera. Involvement of the peritoneum by inflammatory and neoplastic diseases can be exceedingly challenging to image. The high contrast resolution of MR imaging makes it uniquely suited for depicting peritoneal disease. Abnormal peritoneal enhancement and thickening are extremely sensitive indicators of peritonitis or peritoneal tumor. Delayed gadolinium-enhanced MR images are most sensitive for depicting peritoneal inflammation and carcinomatosis owing to their slow accumulation of contrast material. Peritoneal disease also shows restricted diffusion and is displayed as areas of high signal intensity on diffusion-weighted MR imaging. Compared to helical CT and PET, MR imaging is a more sensitive test for depicting small volume peritoneal tumors and carcinomatosis.

15.1 Introduction

The peritoneum is a serous membrane that lines the abdominal cavity and is composed of mesothelial cells and connective tissue with a rich intervening network of vessels and lymphatics. The parietal and visceral layers of the peritoneum line the abdominal cavity, cover the internal organs and viscera, and form numerous mesenteries and ligaments that connect organs to the abdominal wall and to each other (Meyers 2000). In the adult, this extensive network covers over two square meters of peritoneal tissue. The peritoneum plays an important role in the dissemination of tumor throughout the intraperitoneal cavity. Intraperitoneal seeding of tumor cells resulting in peritoneal carcinomatosis or directing the spread of tumors along peritoneal reflections and ligaments occurs with many malignancies. The peritoneum is thus closely involved in the spread of tumor throughout the intraperitoneal cavity. A thorough understanding of the peritoneal anatomy and its potential role in tumor dissemination is vital for the radiologist interpreting cross-sectional imaging studies of the abdomen and pelvis.

Imaging the peritoneum and peritoneal tumors poses several significant challenges (Coakley and Hricak 1999). Tumor involving the peritoneum may be only a few cells thick and present as a thin coating of tumor that can be very difficult to detect. In addition, the peritoneum by nature is folded and convoluted as it lines spaces, coats the intestines and other organs, and forms numerous mesenteries. Depicting subtle small tumors involving this folded membrane is challenging at best. Multidetector CT scans have excellent spatial resolution and speed of acquisition. However, CT's limited contrast resolution limits its ability to detect subtle peritoneal tumor. Coakley et al. noted that the sensitivity of helical CT for peritoneal tumors <1 cm was only 25–50% when compared with 85–93% for all tumors (Coakley et al. 2002). Ultrasound is of limited value for depicting peritoneal disease. PET can depict moderate to large peritoneal tumors but is of limited value for demonstrating small volume peritoneal tumors or carcinomatosis. On the other hand, MR imaging is uniquely suited to depict small peritoneal tumors and carcinomatosis (Low 2007). Excellent soft tissue contrast combined with high spatial resolution allows MR to demonstrate small peritoneal tumors and peritonitis that is not visible with other imaging examinations. Delayed gadolinium-enhanced MR imaging has been described as a sensitive imaging sequence for demonstrating slowly enhancing peritoneal tumors (Low and Sigeti 1994; Low et al. 1997; Low 2001). More recently, diffusion-weighted imaging has been reported as a new tool for showing peritoneal tumors. In our experience, MR imaging with gadolinium and diffusion-weighted imaging is the examination of choice for depicting benign and malignant peritoneal disease (Low and Gurney 2007; Low et al. 2009).

15.2
Technical Considerations and Protocols for Peritoneal MRI

Patients are asked not to eat or drink for 4 h prior to their MR appointment. If rectal water is to be administered, patients self-administer a Fleet's enema prior to the examination.

15.2.1
Intraluminal Contrast Material

Water-soluble intraluminal contrast material is administered to distend the stomach, small bowel, and colon. Collapsed bowel loops can mask subtle peritoneal tumors or inflammation involving the bowel serosa, mesentery, or adjacent peritoneum. Alternatively, non-distended segments of the small bowel can be mistaken for an abdominal mass. Adequate bowel distention is, therefore, an essential element in the peritoneal MR imaging protocol that improves the accuracy and confidence in image interpretation (Low et al. 1997).

Water-soluble contrast material is administered orally beginning 45 min before the start of the MR examination. Water-soluble contrast materials are biphasic on MR images producing high intraluminal signal on T2-weighted images and low signal intensity on T1-weighted, and gadolinium-enhanced SGE images. Patients drink 1.0–1.5 L of oral contrast material of sufficient volume to distend the small bowel and stomach. There are a number of different oral contrast agents available that can be used for MR imaging. While their use for MR imaging is off label, they have proven to be safe and effective for bowel distention. These oral contrast agents are predominantly water with some other agents added to decrease absorption of the material through the small bowel wall. We currently use dilute barium sulfate suspension CT contrast material, which is 98% water. E-Z-EM Readi-CAT2® (Bracco) has been well tolerated and effective in our practice when used to distend the small bowel for MR imaging. Fruit-flavored versions of the oral contrast material are available, which may improve patient compliance. Chilling the oral contrast material is also preferred by some patients. A bottle of this oral agent can also be administered at home to increase the transit and distension of the distal small bowel. Another oral agent that has been adopted for gastrointestinal MR imaging is VoLumen® Barium Sulfate Suspension, 0.1% w/v, 0.1% w/w, 450 mL (Bracco). VoLumen was designed as a negative CT intraluminal contrast agent and is composed of sorbitol, bean gum, and water. For the purposes of MR imaging, it is predominantly water and appears as a biphasic intraluminal agent that is identical to dilute barium sulfate suspension products.

Distention of the rectum and colon can be accomplished with 1 L of tap water administered through a balloon tipped barium enema catheter. The balloon should be filled with water and not air to decrease the susceptibility artifact that the air would create. While rectal water is not an absolute requirement, it can improve the depiction of subtle serosal and peritoneal tumor involving the colon and rectum. In other patients, one may find that the colon is adequately distended with stool so that rectal water is not required.

15.2.2
Intravenous Contrast Agents

Intravenous gadolinium chelate is administered using a power injector at an injection rate of 2 mL/s through an angiocatheter. In the past, we have used a double dose of intravenous gadolinium to increase the degree of enhancement of peritoneal tumors and inflammation. We currently use a single dose of MultiHance® (gadobenate dimeglumine) (Bracco), which due to its higher relaxivity may show greater enhancement of peritoneal tumors. To our knowledge, a comparison of Multihance and other gadolinium chelates for depicting peritoneal disease has not been performed.

15.2.3
Antiperistaltic Agents

A medication should be administered to decrease bowel peristalsis on the gadolinium-enhanced images. The 3D FSPGR and 2D SGE images are sensitive to bowel motion and image quality is improved by administering an antiperistaltic pharmacologic agent. Available agents include Glucagon for injection (Eli Lilly and Company, Indianapolis, IN) 1 mg administered intravenously at the time of gadolinium injection, Buscopan® (hyoscine-N-butylbromide), and Levsin® (Hyoscyamine sulfate Injection) 0.25 mg administered intravenously 5 min prior to the gadolinium injection. Package inserts should be carefully reviewed for all of these medications prior to their use to understand contraindications and potential drug interactions.

15.2.4
MRI Protocol

Our protocol for peritoneal imaging is optimized for depicting small peritoneal tumors (Low 2007). All images are obtained during suspended respiration to minimize breathing artifact that can obscure subtle peritoneal tumors or inflammation. Faster pulse sequences that facilitate breath-hold imaging also decrease the overall examination time, which is essential when using intraluminal contrast material to distend to small bowel and colon. Other key elements that improve tumor depiction are fat suppression and high spatial resolution. Fat suppression is utilized for T2-weighted imaging, diffusion-weighted imaging (DWI), and all gadolinium-enhanced images. By suppressing the high signal intensity fat, small peritoneal tumors and inflammation become more conspicuous. To depict small tumors, a reasonably high in-plane resolution must be balanced against the requirements for times short enough to allow for breath-hold imaging. Our current post-contrast imaging is performed with 3D FSGPR images obtained with an in-plane resolution of 320 × 192. Increasing the resolution further may have diminishing returns. In our experience, peritoneal tumors often present as sheets for tumor cells lining the peritoneal surfaces rather than as solitary discrete small tumor nodules. In this setting, high contrast resolution is probably more essential to distinguish thin sheets of tumor from normal anatomic structures.

Table 15.1 lists the specifying imaging parameters for our current peritoneal MRI protocol. In summary, the examination includes axial dual echo T1 SGE images, fat suppressed T2-weighted FSE imaging, and breath-hold DWI using an intermediate b-value of 400–500 s/mm^2 (ICHIKAWA et al. 1999). Following injection of intravenous gadolinium, we obtain fat-suppressed 3D FSPGR images in the axial plane twice through the abdomen and pelvis. Coronal and sagittal 3D FSPGR imaging is performed. The final set of images is the axial 2D SGE with fat suppression. We find that these images are less sensitive to breathing and motion artifact and provide very sharp anatomic detail. The fat-suppressed 2D SGE images are

Table 15.1 Peritoneal MR imaging protocol (GE system)

Pulse Sequence	TR	TE	Matrix	NSA	Thick	Gap	ASSET	Angle	Plane	Note	Time
T1 SGE dual echo	140	4.4 2.1	256 × 224	1	7	3	2	80	A		:24
T2 FRFSE	2,050	88	320 × 192	1	7	3	2	90	A	fat sat	:24 × 2
DWI SSEPI	3,000	min	192 × 224	3	8	1	2	90	A	B 400	:22
3D FSPGR	min	min	320 × 192	1	4.4	−2.2	2	12	A×2	Fat sat	:24
3D FSPGR	min	min	320 × 192	1	4.4	−2.2	2	12	A/C	fat sat	:24
2D SGE	140	2.1	256 × 192	1	8	1	2	70	A	fat sat	:24 × 2

Table shows imaging parameters for complete MR examination
SGE spoiled gradient-echo; *FRFSE* fast recovery fast spin echo; *DWI SSEPI* diffusion weighted single shot echo planar imaging; *LAVA* liver acceleration volume acquisition; *3D FSPGR Dixon* 3D fast spoiled gradient-echo with Dixon water reconstruction (LAVA-FLEX); *SGE* spoiled gradient echo; *ASSET* array spatial sensitivity encoding technique
Times listed are the breath-hold times for the abdomen or pelvis

obtained about 5 min after the injection of gadolinium when slowly enhancing peritoneal tumors are most conspicuous.

15.2.5 MR Image Interpretation

Unenhanced T1- and T2-weighted images may show larger peritoneal tumor nodules and masses, but are relatively insensitive for the depiction of small peritoneal tumors, carcinomatosis, and peritonitis (Low and Sigeti 1994). Following the intravenous injection of extracellular gadolinium chelates, peritoneal inflammation and peritoneal tumors enhance slowly. Peritoneal enhancement is thus best visualized on delayed images obtained 5 min after gadolinium injection. Normal peritoneal tissues are relatively thin measuring <3 mm in thickness and typically show only mild enhancement that is less than or equal to that of the liver parenchyma. Moderate to marked peritoneal enhancement and associated thickening is abnormal and is the hallmark of peritonitis or peritoneal carcinomatosis. In our experience, small peritoneal tumors a few millimeters in size can be routinely detected. In some instances, sheets of very subtle peritoneal tumor depicted on MRI may not be visible or palpable at laparotomy but microscopic can be confirmed by biopsy or peritoneal washings. It should be noted that the distinction between peritoneal inflammation and peritoneal tumor is based on the clinical presentation since the MR imaging findings can be identical. Peritoneal thickening from tumors may be thin and regular, nodular, or mass-like. Peritonitis usually presents as smooth and regular peritoneal thickening and enhancement without dominant masses or nodules (Low 2001).

Diffusion-weighted (DW) MR images are also very useful for depicting peritoneal diseases (Low 2009; Fuji et al. 2008). Single-shot EPI DW images using an intermediate b-value of 500 s/mm^2 show restricted diffusion with peritoneal tumors and inflammation. On DW images, ascites and bowel contents are suppressed while peritoneal and serosal tumors show restricted diffusion and are depicted as areas of high signal intensity. Suppression of ascites and bowel contents improves the conspicuity of peritoneal and serosal tumors on DW images. We evaluate the magnitude of DW image, which has contributions from diffusion and T2 signal. ADC maps could be used to further suppress the T2 signal from bowel contents, ascites, and other fluid-containing structures. We have found that the most accurate examination for detecting peritoneal tumors is the combination of DWI and delayed gadolinium-enhanced MRI (Low et al. 2009). The DW images are more easily interpreted when viewed in conjunction with the conventional MR images, which provided better depiction of anatomic landmarks. Mesenteric tumors, bowel serosa tumors, and tumors involving the peritoneal reflections around the liver and pancreas were usually better seen on the DW images owing to the high contrast of peritoneal tumors on these images (Fig. 15.3). When comparing the B0 and B500 DW images, one may see an interesting reversal of signal intensity. On the B0 images, bowel contents are hyperintense while the bowel wall and serosal tumors are of low signal intensity. On the corresponding B500 image, the bowel contents are suppressed and the serosal and peritoneal tumor becomes hyperintense. The DW images are also useful to demonstrate associated lymphadenopathy, hepatic, and osseous metastases (Koh and Collins 2007).

15.3 Peritoneal Anatomy

The peritoneum is a serous lining of mesothelial cells that lines the abdominal cavity and covers the abdominal organs. The peritoneum consists of a parietal layer lining the inner surface of the abdominal and pelvic cavity and the visceral peritoneum that covers the organs (Fig. 15.1). Peritoneal reflections form the ligaments and mesenteries that connect organs and secure organs to the abdominal wall. In the anterior abdomen, the omentum is composed of four layers of peritoneum (Meyers et al. 1987). A mesentery is a double layer of peritoneum that results from the invagination of an organ into the peritoneum. Examples of mesenteries include the small bowel mesentery, the transverse mesocolon, the mesoduodenum, and the sigmoid mesentery (Hamrick-Turner et al. 1992) (Fig. 15.1).

The peritoneal ligaments connect abdominal organs. The coronary ligament represents peritoneal reflections, which firmly attach the liver to the diaphragm and retroperitoneum. The liver surface between the leaves of the coronary ligament is not covered by serosal or visceral peritoneum and is referred to as the bare area of the liver. The gastrohepatic ligament also known as the lesser omentum extends from the lesser curvature of the stomach to the left lobe of the liver (Fig. 15.2). On the liver surface, the gastrohepatic ligament extends into the fissure for the ligamentum venosum, which separates the caudate lobe from the left hepatic lobe. The hepatoduodenal ligament is located along the free margin of the gastrohepatic ligament. It extends from the porta hepatis to the duodenal sweep and contains the components of the portal triad: the portal vein, hepatic artery, and bile ducts. An opening posterior to the gastrohepatic ligament known as the Foramen of Winslow provides an important communication between the greater and lesser sacs of the peritoneal cavity. The falciform ligament extends from the left intersegmental fissure between the medial and lateral segments of the left hepatic lobe to the adjacent anterior abdominal wall. The falciform ligament encases the ligamentum teres representing the obliterated umbilical vein, which in utero connect the umbilicus to the left portal vein (Vikram et al. 2009) (Fig. 15.3).

The greater omentum is formed by four layers of peritoneum. Two layers arise from the greater curve of the stomach, which fuse with the two layers of the transverse mesocolon to form the four-layered greater omentum. Ligaments associated with the greater omentum include the gastrocolic, gastrosplenic, splenorenal, gastrophrenic ligaments. The phrenicocolic ligament connects the diaphragm to

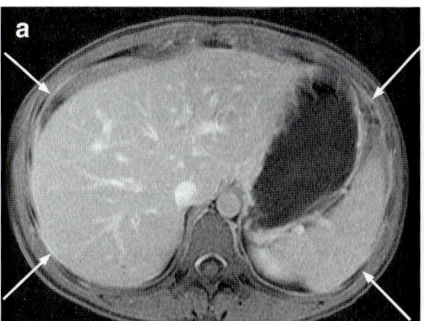

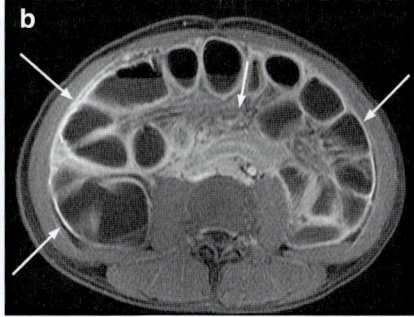

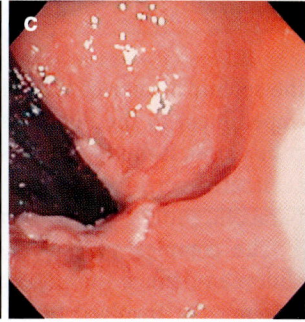

Fig. 15.1. Bacterial peritonitis – 19-year-old with abdominal pain. Equilibrium phase fat-suppressed, gadolinium-enhanced SGE image (a) shows diffuse abnormal enhancement of the right and left subphrenic peritoneum (arrows) indicating peritonitis.
Equilibrium phase fat-suppressed, gadolinium-enhanced SGE image through the middle abdomen (b) shows diffuse abnormal peritoneal and bowel serosal enhancement (*arrows*) indicating peritonitis. Associated mesenteric infiltration and enhancement (*small arrow*) represents additional evidence of peritonitis.
Laparoscopic view (c) confirms diffuse peritoneal inflammation and peritonitis

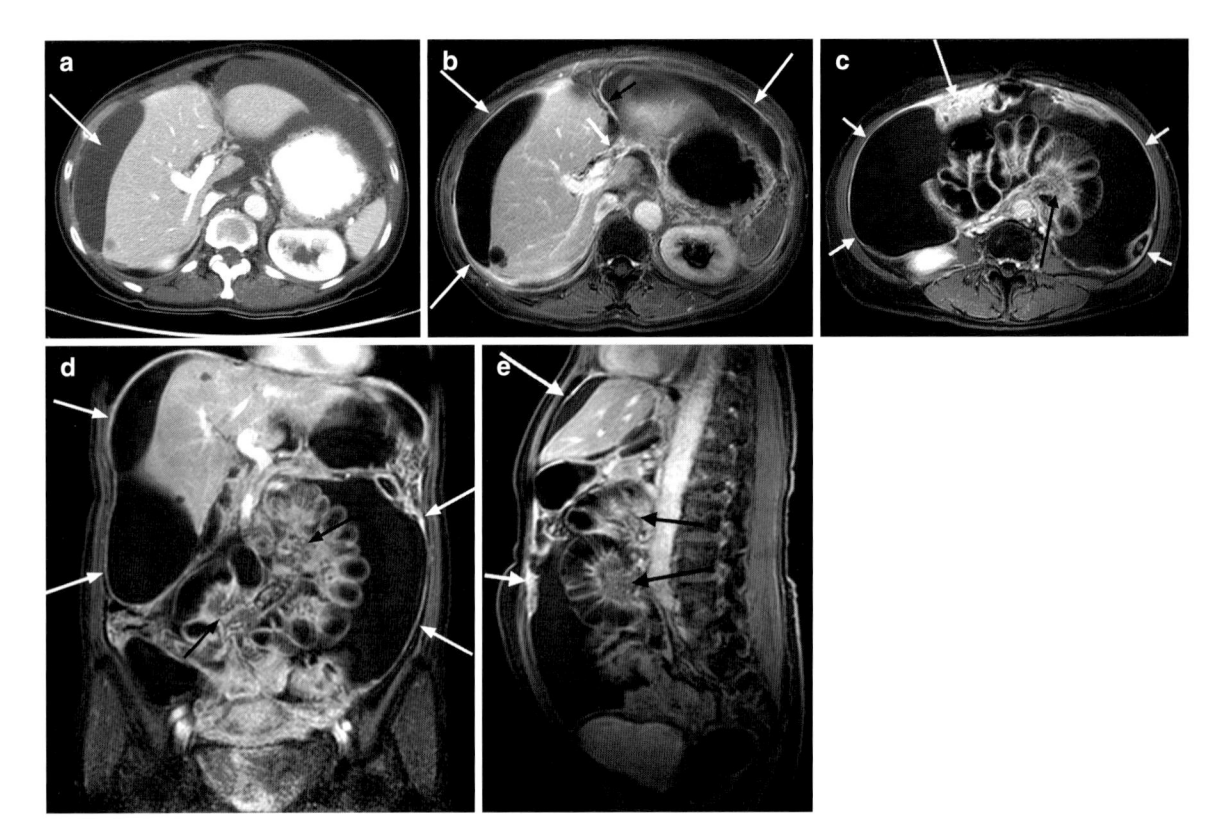

Fig. 15.2. (a) Primary ovarian cancer – 67-year-old woman presenting with abdominal distension. Multidetector CT shows ascites (*arrow*) but no evidence of peritoneal tumor. (b) Delayed gadolinium-enhanced fat-suppressed SGE MR image confirms peritoneal carcinomatosis with abnormal enhancement of the subphrenic peritoneum (*long white arrows*). Enhancement of the peritoneum in the left intersegmental fissure and falciform ligament (*black arrow*) represents additional peritoneal tumor. Tumor also extends into transverse fissure and periportal space anterior to the main portal vein (*short white arrow*). (c) Axial delayed gadolinium-enhanced SGE image through the middle abdomen depicts bulky omental tumor (*long white arrow*), bilateral paracolic parietal peritoneal tumor (*short white arrows*), and mesenteric tumor (*black arrow*). (d) Coronal gadolinium-enhanced 3D FSPGR image confirms peritoneal carcinomatosis (*white arrows*) involving the right and left subphrenic peritoneum and the paracolic gutter. Infiltration and enhancement of the small bowel mesentery (*black arrows*) represents additional metastatic peritoneal tumor. Laparotomy confirmed primary ovarian cancer. (e) Sagittal gadolinium-enhanced 3D FSPGR image (d) confirms peritoneal carcinomatosis with tumor involving the omentum (*short white arrow*), subphrenic peritoneum (*long white arrow*), transverse mesocolon (*short black arrow*), and small bowel mesentery (*long black arrow*)

the splenic flexure of the colon and is an important impediment to the flow of ascites up the left paracolic gutter. It thus serves to redirect ascites and disseminated peritoneal tumor cells to the larger right paracolic gutter (MEYERS et al. 1987) (Fig. 15.3).

The complex peritoneal anatomy of the upper abdomen defines the potential spaces and surfaces that may be involved by peritoneal malignancy or inflammation. The visceral peritoneum covering the liver surface invaginates into the liver parenchyma creating anatomic fissures including the fissures of the ligamentum teres, ligamentum venosum, gallbladder, and the transverse fissure. The peritoneal reflections surrounding the hepatic pedicle as it enters the liver parenchyma form the transverse fissure. The transverse fissure contains the horizontal portions of the right and left portal veins. The fissure is continuous with the periportal space, which is a potential space surrounding the intrahepatic portal vein branches. The periportal space is a common site for direct tumor spread in patients with ovarian carcinoma or pancreatic carcinoma (Fig. 15.3). The peritoneal reflections in the upper abdomen define the spaces that may be involved by peritoneal tumor. The right subphrenic space is a large, continuous space separating the right lobe of the liver from the adjacent right hemidiaphragm. The right subphrenic space is the most common site for peritoneal tumor

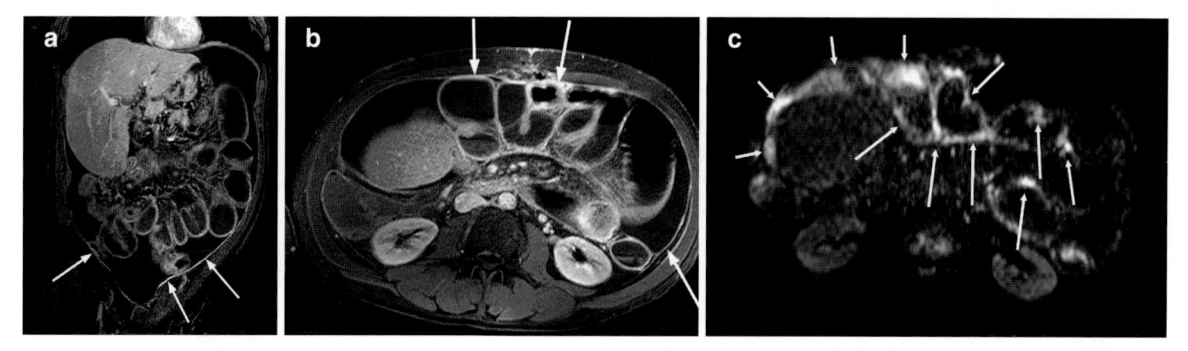

Fig. 15.3. Gastric cancer – 62-year-old man with treated gastric cancer presenting with nausea and vomiting. Coronal gadolinium-enhanced 3D FSPGR image (**a**) shows dilated fluid filled small bowel and abnormal thickening and enhancement of the paracolic peritoneum (*arrows*) and ascites. Axial delayed 2D gadolinium-enhanced SGE image (**b**) confirms peritoneal carcinomatosis (*arrows*) involving the parietal peritoneum, omentum, and bowel serosa. Malignant bowel obstruction and peritoneal carcinomatosis was confirmed at laparotomy. (**c**) Axial diffusion weighted image (b) 500 s/mm2 confirms the right subphrenic tumor (*short arrows*). Serosal and mesenteric tumors (*long arrows*) are also depicted as linear soft tissue showing restricted diffusion

involvement in patients with peritoneal carcinomatosis (Fig. 15.3). The left subphrenic space in the left upper quadrant forms one continuous space that freely communicates (Fig. 15.3). The perihepatic spaces surrounding the left lobe of the liver freely communicate with the adjacent perigastric and perisplenic spaces in the left upper quadrant of the abdomen. When involved by inflammation or tumor, this large potential space in the left upper abdomen may be compartmentalized by the splenorenal ligament, gastrosplenic ligament, and lesser omentum (MEYERS et al. 1987).

The lesser sac is bounded anteriorly by the stomach, lesser omentum, and gastrocolic ligament and posteriorly by the pancreas. Inferiorly the lesser sac is delimited by the transverse colon and the mesocolon. On the left, the lesser sac is delimited by the splenorenal ligament and the gastrosplenic ligament. On the right, the lesser sac communicates with the greater sac via the Foramen of Winslow, an opening behind the free edge of the lesser omentum.

The right subhepatic space is separated into an anterior right subhepatic space and a posterior right subhepatic space. The anterior compartment is delimited inferiorly by the transverse mesocolon. The posterior right subhepatic space separates the right lobe of the liver and the right kidney and is known as Morrison's pouch or the hepatorenal fossa. The right subhepatic space communicates with the adjacent right subphrenic space and the right paracolic gutter (Fig. 15.3).

In the middle abdomen, parietal and visceral peritoneum covers the inner surface of the abdominal wall and the small intestine and colon (Fig. 15.4).

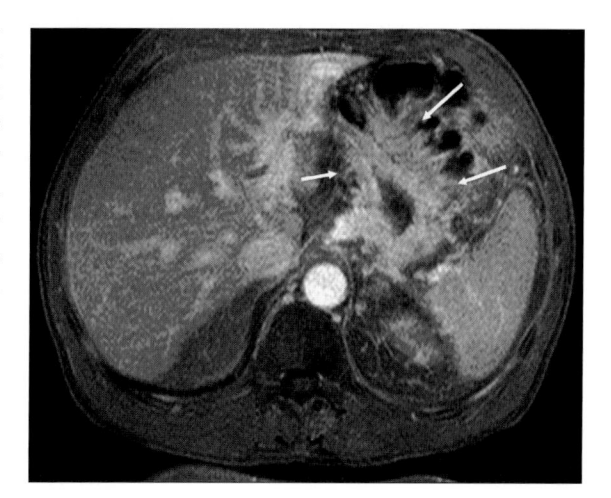

Fig. 15.4. Gastric cancer – 55-year-old woman with nausea. Gadolinium-enhanced SGE image shows marked diffuse gastric mural thickening representing gastric cancer with a pattern of linitis plastica. Note the direct extension of the gastric tumor into the gastrohepatic ligament (*short arrow*) and lateral extension from the greater curvature (*long arrows*) to involve the gastrocolic ligament and hepatic flexure of the colon

In the middle abdomen, the four-layered greater omentum arises from the greater curvature of the stomach and drapes over the small bowel, colon, and other abdominal viscera (Fig. 15.3). The transverse mesocolon, attaching the transverse colon to the posterior abdominal wall, is best depicted on sagittal MR images (Fig. 15.3). Below its colonic attachment, the transverse mesocolon fuses with the posterior portion of the omentum inferiorly, forming the posterior two layers of the four-layered omentum. Much of the middle abdomen is dominated by small intestine and the small bowel mesentery that attaches the jejunum and the ileum to the posterior abdominal wall. The fan-shaped folds of the small bowel mesentery are well depicted on axial, coronal, or sagittal MR images. The small bowel mesentery is a common site for peritoneal tumor deposition (Fig. 15.3). As ascites pools in the folds of the small bowel mesentery, it flows to the most dependent section, which is the mesentery of the distal ileum in the right lower quadrant. The mesentery of the terminal ileum is, therefore, a common first site of peritoneal tumor deposition. The attachments of the ascending and descending colon to the posterior abdominal wall define the paracolic gutters and serve to help direct the flow of ascites and peritoneal tumor deposition. Because the phrenicocolic ligament blocks flow of ascites up the left paracolic gutter, there is preferential flow of ascites and disseminated peritoneal tumor cells up the wider right paracolic gutter (Hamrick-Turner et al. 1992) (Fig. 15.3).

Within the pelvis, the parietal peritoneum covers the inner surface and the abdominal and pelvic wall. The peritoneum reflects over the bladder, rectum, and uterus placing these structures in an extraperitoneal location (Fig. 15.3). The inferior extent of the pelvic peritoneal reflections forms the Pouch of Douglas or rectovaginal pouch in the female and the rectovesicle pouch in the male. As the most dependent portions of the peritoneal cavity, the rectovaginal pouch and rectovesicle pouch are the first sites to accumulate ascitic fluid. The dome of the bladder is covered by the visceral peritoneum and may be involved by peritoneal tumor or inflammation. The sigmoid mesentery attaching the sigmoid colon to the posterior abdominal wall is another important site of peritoneal tumor deposition.

15.4
Benign Diseases of the Peritoneum

15.4.1
Mesenteric Paniculitis

Mesenteric paniculitis is an inflammatory and fibrotic disease involving the fatty tissues of the mesentery. Histopathologically, one sees a combination of mesenteric fibrosis, inflammation, and fat necrosis. The term retractile mesenteritis has been used when the fibrotic reaction predominates. Mesenteric lipodystrophy is the term used when the mesenteric fat necrosis is the predominant feature. Mesenteric

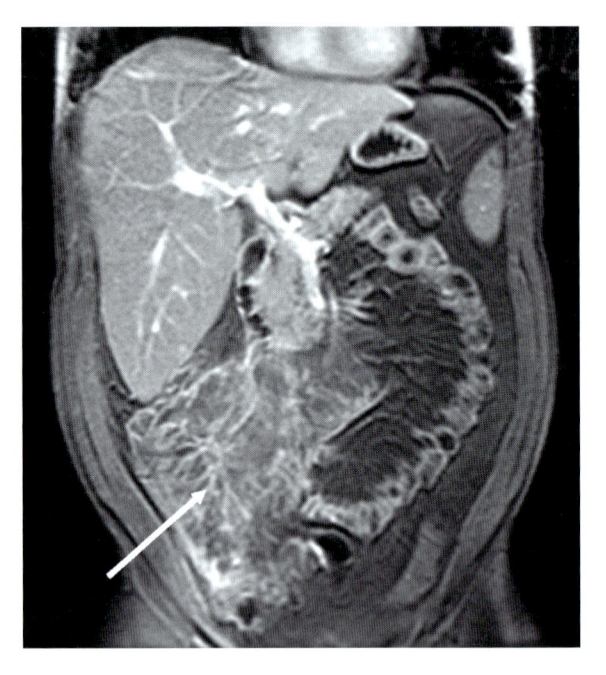

Fig. 15.5. Mesenteric paniculitis – 66-year-old woman with abdominal pain. Coronal gadolinium-enhanced 3D FSPGR image demonstrates diffuse abnormal infiltration and enhancement of the small bowel mesentery

paniculitis is usually idiopathic. The clinical presentation includes long-standing abdominal pain, nausea, vomiting, fever, and weight loss. The small bowel mesentery is involved most frequently by a solitary large dominant mass averaging 10 cm in diameter (Emory et al. 1997). Less commonly, one may see multiple smaller mesenteric masses, or diffuse mesenteric thickening. Other inflammatory and infectious diseases can lead to mesenteric inflammation and retractile mesenteritis.

MR imaging may demonstrate a single or multiple enhancing soft tissue mass in the small bowel mesentery with tethering and distortion of adjacent bowel loops (Kronthal et al. 1991) (Fig. 15.5). The mass may contain regions of fat demonstrated as high signal on T1-weighted images or as areas of low signal on fat-suppressed images. In the diffuse form of mesenteric adenitis, one will see ill-defined areas of soft tissue infiltration of the mesentery representing inflammation and fibrosis. On T1-weighted MR images, this will be depicted as low signal intensity stands infiltrating the small bowel mesentery. On fat-suppressed, gadolinium-enhanced images, the mesentery will be infiltrated with enhancing soft tissue (Fujiyoshi et al. 1997; Kobayashi et al. 1993; Kobayashi et al 1993).

15.4.2
Mesenteric Adenitis

Mesenteric adenitis is an uncommon inflammatory process involving the mesenteric lymph nodes. It is most frequently caused by a viral infection but may also be associated with bacterial infections secondary to *Yersinia enterocolitica*, *Helicobacter jejuni*, *Campylobacter jejuni*, and *Salmonella* or *Shigella* species. It most commonly involves the lymph nodes near the terminal ileum and is, therefore, often misdiagnosed as acute appendicitis. It is a self-limited disease that presents with right lower quadrant abdominal pain, nausea, vomiting, fever, and occasionally diarrhea. The MR features of mesenteric adenitis include enlarged mesenteric lymph nodes in the right lower quadrant. Strandy infiltration and enhancement of the adjacent mesentery may also be seen. Absence of an enlarged and inflamed appendix excludes the diagnosis of acute appendicitis.

15.4.3
Peritonitis

Peritonitis is an inflammation of the peritoneal lining of the abdomen cavity. Peritonitis may be spontaneous, secondary, or a complication of catheter peritoneal dialysis. Spontaneous bacterial peritonitis is seen in patients with chronic liver disease or renal failure in which ascites accumulates in the peritoneal cavity (Kanematsu et al. 1997). Infection of the ascitic fluid may occur as a result of hematogenously borne bacteria that spread to the peritoneal cavity. Secondary peritonitis may occur as a result of bowel perforation with subsequent leak of intestinal fluids and bacteria into the peritoneal cavity.

Patients with peritonitis present with abdominal pain and tenderness, distension, nausea, vomiting, fever, chills, and leukocytosis. Because of the nonspecific nature of these symptoms, patients with peritonitis may be misdiagnosed with other infectious or inflammatory abdominal diseases. Complications of peritonitis include development of an intra-abdominal abscess and sepsis.

MR imaging is an effective and very sensitive examination in patients with suspected peritonitis (Elsayes et al. 2006). There have been no direct comparisons of helical CT and MR imaging for depicting peritonitis. In our experience, MR imaging with its superior soft tissue contrast is better suited to depict subtle changes of peritonitis when compared with helical CT (Low 2001). Inflammation of the peritoneum leads to increased vascularity and subsequent abnormal enhancement with intravenous gadolinium. As with peritoneal carcinomatosis, peritonitis shows slow gradual enhancement of the peritoneum. For this reason, the findings of peritonitis are most evident on 5 min delayed gadolinium-enhanced SGE images (Fig. 15.1). The presence of delayed enhancement of ascitic fluid has been noted in patients with peritoneal disease. Kanematsu et al. noted delayed gadolinium enhancement of ascites in spontaneous bacterial peritonitis. Other authors have noted that delayed enhancement of ascites on MR imaging is nonspecific finding that correlates with the presence of exudative ascites and increased peritoneal permeability that may be due to benign or malignant peritoneal disease (Arai et al. 1993).

Fat suppression is used to eliminate the competing high signal of adjacent abdominal or pelvic fat. On these gadolinium-enhanced images, one may see abnormal peritoneal enhancement with peritoneal thickening. In some mild cases of peritonitis, the abnormally enhancing peritoneum may be normal in thickness. In our experience, the degree of thickening of the peritoneum with peritonitis is less than that often seen with peritoneal tumor. Also, in our experience the peritoneum tends to be smoothly thickened without the nodular thickening and peritoneal masses seen with carcinomatosis. Fat-suppressed T2-weighted images or SSRARE images are also useful to depict associated ascites. To depict serosal inflammation, the addition of oral contrast material can be used to distend and separate loops of intestine. Collapsed segments of bowel can mask or mimic peritoneal and serosal disease. Adequate luminal distension allows one to depict bowel wall thickening and abnormal enhancement, which can be signs of serosal peritonitis.

15.4.4
Tuberculous Peritonitis

Tuberculous peritonitis is a rare extra pulmonary manifestation of tuberculosis caused by Mycobacterium tuberculosis (Manohar et al. 1990). The disease is fairly insidious with slow onset, nonspecific symptoms that typically lead to a delay in diagnosis of several months. Risk factors include cirrhosis, CAPD, diabetes mellitus, underlying malignancy, use of systemic corticosteroids, and AIDS. Infection usually occurs from reactivation of a latent focus of peritoneal infection that had previously spread to the peritoneum hematogenously from a primary lung infection. Less common primary hematogenous spread from an active pulmonary TB may seed the peritoneum or rarely transmural spread from gastrointestinal tuberculosis can occur. Peritoneal involvement by tuberculosis may rarely occur in isolation or more commonly is present in association with gastrointestinal tuberculosis (Hossein et al. 1997).

Three forms of tuberculous peritonitis have been described (Leder and Low 1995; Pereira et al. 2005). The wet-type characterized by large volume ascites is the most common form with 90% of patients presenting with ascites at the time of diagnosis. The fibrotic-mixed type is characterized by large omental masses, with matted intestines, and mesentery. The dry or plastic type is uncommon and is characterized by caseous nodules and fibrous peritoneal reaction. This latter form is indistinguishable from peritoneal carcinomatosis.

As the disease progresses, tubercles seed the parietal and visceral peritoneum and produce an exuadative ascites. Nonspecific peritoneal thickening, peritoneal nodules, and enhancement are noted combined with nonenhancing ascites (Ha et al. 1996) (Fig. 15.6). Features that favor the presence of tuberculous peritonitis include the presence of associated abdominal and retroperitoneal tuberculous lymphadenitis. Nodal masses will show peripheral enhancement with low signal intensity centers. This appearance is due to lymph nodes with peripheral inflammation and central caseous necrosis and corresponds with the low-density lymph nodes seen on helical CT in patients with abdominal tuberculosis. Other authors have noted mass-like cystic lesions in patients with tuberculous lymphadenitis (Kim et al. 2000). Inflammation that extends through the peritoneum to involve the abdominal wall is also been described as a feature of abdominal tuberculosis (Akhan and Pringo 2002).

15.4.5
Sclerosing Encapsulating Peritonitis

Sclerosing peritonitis is a rare but serious complication of continuous ambulatory peritoneal dialysis with an incidence of 20% after 8 years of peritoneal dialysis (Slim et al. 2005). The small bowel becomes encased in sheets of fibrous tissue, which comprise myofibroblastic spindle cells, and chronic inflammatory cells. Dense adhesions and mural fibrosis is pres-

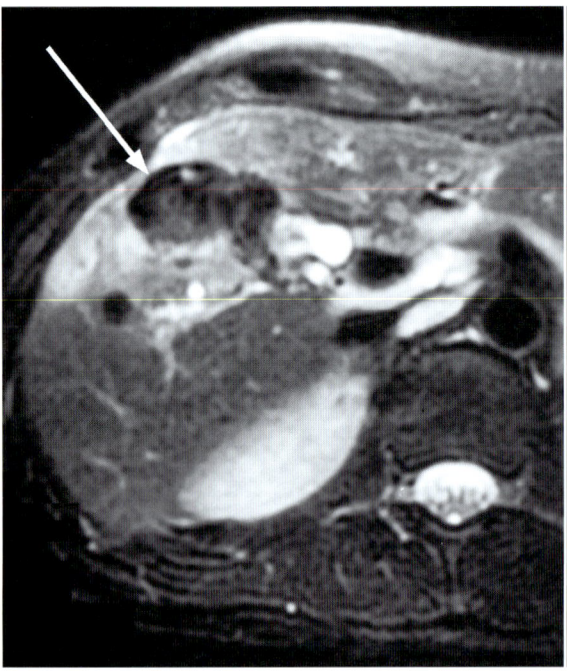

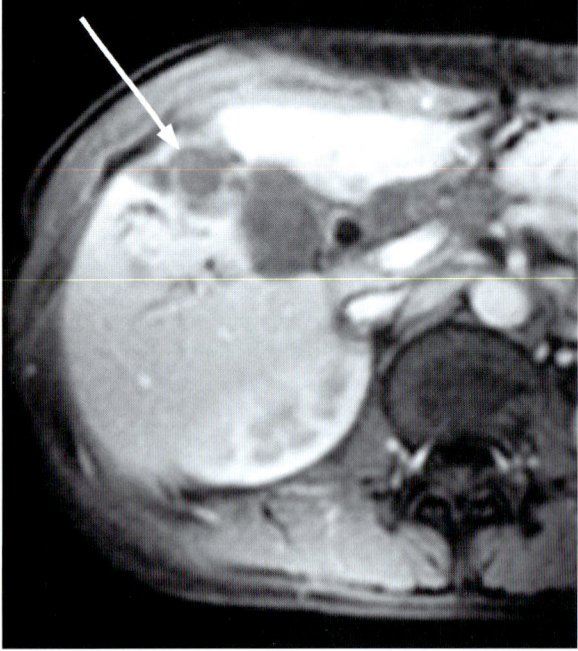

Fig. 15.6. Tuberculous peritonitis – 52-year-old man with abdominal discomfort: T2-weighted (*left*) and fat-suppressed gadolinium-enhanced (*right*) MR images depict a nonenhancing mass (*arrow*) in the gallbladder fossa with surrounding edema. Findings are that of an intraperitoneal tuberculoma and associated peritonitis

ent. Patients present with abdominal pain, weight loss, anorexia, and small bowel obstruction. Sclerosing peritonitis may be associated with bacterial or fungal peritonitis. Complications of long-term sclerosing peritonitis include small bowel necrosis and enterocutaneous fistulas (CHOI et al. 2004) with rare cases of associated colonic obstruction. In one study (RIGBY and HAWLEY 1998), the overall prevalence was 0.7%, which increased progressively with the duration of peritoneal dialysis being 1.9, 6.4, 10.8, and 19.4% for patients on dialysis for more than 2, 5, 6, and 8 years, respectively. In some patients, the cessation of peritoneal dialysis and initiation of hemodialysis appears to serve as a trigger for sclerosing encapsulating peritonitis. Overall mortality is as high as 50–80% with mortality increasing with the length of time the patient is on peritoneal dialysis. Medical therapy may consist of treatment with steroids, tamoxifen, and or immunosuppression. Surgical intervention with laparotomy and peritonectomy has been performed with the intention to resect all diseased and thickened peritoneal membranes.

Imaging findings of sclerosing encapsulating peritonitis at CT and MRI include peritoneal calcification, bowel distribution , bowel wall thickening, and bowel dilation, bowel tethering, loculation of ascites, and peritoneal thickening (TARZI et al. 2008; HUSER et al. 2006). In one study, peritoneal calcifications and bowel tethering were the most specific findings (TARZI et al. 2008). On MR imaging, one may see similar intestinal findings with sheets of thickened and enhancing peritoneum encasing dilated and distorted small bowel (MENASSA-MOUSSA et al. 2006) (Fig. 15.7). Visualization of the peritoneal findings on CT is much more limited.

15.5
Malignant Diseases of the Peritoneum

15.5.1
Mechanisms of Peritoneal Tumor Spread

15.5.1.1
Intraperitoneal Tumor Dissemination

Intraperitoneal dissemination is an important mechanism of tumor spread that occurs when tumor cells break off from the primary cancer and are shed into the peritoneal cavity (Figs. 15.3 and 15.4). As described in the seminal work of Dr. Morton Meyers, these tumor cells then spread throughout the peritoneal cavity in a pattern determined by established pathways of ascitic flow (Meyers). Ascites accumulates in the most dependent areas of the peritoneal cavity. In the pelvis, ascites initially accumulates in the dependent pouch of Douglas and then fills the paravesical spaces bilaterally. The mesentery of the sigmoid colon helps to direct fluid around the sigmoid colon making this another common location for peritoneal tumor deposition.

Flow of ascites into the abdominal cavity is directed by the peritoneal reflections, ligaments, and the attachments of the mesenteries to the posterior abdominal wall. The mesenteries attaching the ascending and descending colon to the posterior abdominal wall form the paracolic gutters that channel fluid from the pelvis superiorly into the abdomen. Flow up the left paracolic gutter is blocked by the phrenicocolic ligament. Therefore, pelvis ascites preferentially flows up the wider right paracolic gutter. From the right paracolic gutter, ascites flows into the right subhepatic space and right subphrenic space. The attachments of the transverse mesocolon and the small bowel mesentery to the posterior abdominal wall similarly help to redirect ascites and tumor cells within the peritoneal cavity (Fig. 15.3). Fluid trapped in the multiple folds of the small bowel mesentery forms pools that cascade from the left upper quadrant to the right lower quadrant near the terminal ileum. The terminal ileum and right lower quadrant small bowel mesentery is thus another important area for peritoneal tumor deposition.

Based on these mechanisms of ascitic flow, tumor cells deposit and multiply in areas of stasis. Highly predictable areas for tumor deposition include the pouch of Douglas, the sigmoid colon and its mesentery, the terminal ileum, the right paracolic gutter, the posterior right subhepatic space, and the right subphrenic space. Eventually, all peritoneal surfaces and spaces may be involved by peritoneal carcinomatosis. However, the earliest tumor deposition will occur at the peritoneal tumor "hot spots" listed above. Each of these anatomic areas should be evaluated carefully for evidence of peritoneal metastases. The tumors that most commonly spread via intraperitoneal dissemination can be remembered by the mnemonic "SCOPE," standing for primary tumors of the Stomach, Colon, Ovary, Pancreas, and Endometrium. Another "C" tumor is Cholangiocarcinoma and a couple of additional "P" tumors include *Primary Peritoneal Cancer*, and *Pseudomyxoma Peritonei*.

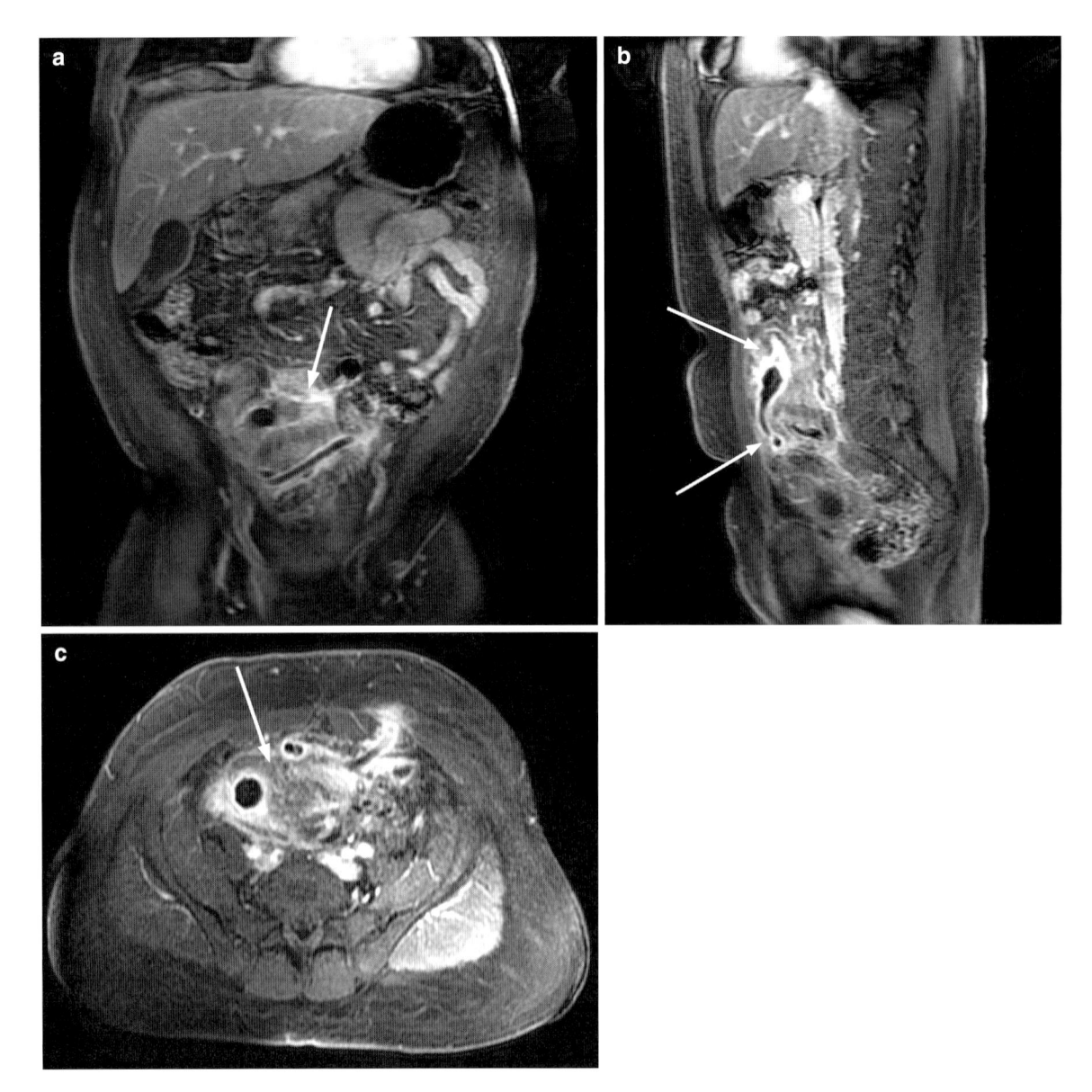

Fig. 15.7. Sclerosing encapsulating peritonitis – 44-year-old male peritoneal dialysis patient presents with abdominal pain and bowel obstruction. Coronal (a) and sagittal (b), and axial (c) fat-suppressed gadolinium-enhanced 3D FSPGR image shows a sheet of enhancing soft tissue (*arrow*) the mesentery, bowel, and the peritoneal dialysis catheter

15.5.1.2
Direct Spread of Tumors Along Peritoneum Pathways

The peritoneal reflections, ligaments, and mesenteries can also serve as pathways for direct spread of abdominal and pelvic tumors (Fig. 15.2) ARENAS et al 1994. The peritoneum interconnects the solid abdominal and pelvic organs, the hollow visceral organs or the gastrointestinal tract, and the adjacent abdominal wall. A primary malignancy of one organ can use the extensive peritoneal pathways to directly spread to contiguous and noncontiguous structures.

In the upper abdomen, the peritoneum interconnects the liver, stomach, spleen, pancreas, colon, small intestine, and abdominal wall. The nine major upper abdominal peritoneal reflections include the gastrohepatic ligament, the hepatoduodenal ligament, the gastrocolic ligament, the transverse mesocolon, the duodenal ligament, the gastrosplenic ligament, the splenorenal ligament, the phrenicocolic ligament, and the small bowel mesentery. Gastric cancers commonly spread to involve the gastrohepatic ligament or lesser omentum with subsequent spread to the hepatoduodenal ligament located along its free edge (Fig. 15.2). From this location, the tumor may extend cephalad into the liver through the fissure for the ligamentum venosum separating the caudate lobe from the left hepatic lobe. Once tumor enters the liver, it may extend along the periportal space following the branches of the portal vein. Tumor may eventually reach the left intersegmental fissure and track along the falciform ligament to reach the anterior abdominal wall. Alternatively, gastric cancers located along the greater curvature may spread inferiorly along the gastrocolic ligament to reach the transverse colon and the transverse mesocolon, which is its attachment to the posterior abdominal wall (Fig. 15.2). Tumor may then involve the greater omentum formed from the fused layers of the gastrocolic ligament and the transverse mesocolon. Using the same peritoneal pathway, transverse colon cancers may extend cephalad along the gastrocolic ligament to reach the greater curvature of stomach.

These same peritoneal pathways also connect extraperitoneal organs with intraperitoneal organs. The classic example of pancreatic cancer spreading superiorly along the hepatoduodenal ligament to reach the liver and periportal space was described above. Pancreatic cancer can also spread inferiorly into the retroperitoneal attachment of the transverse mesocolon or small bowel mesentery to reach the transverse colon or small intestines. Pancreatic tail cancers can spread laterally into the splenorenal, gastrosplenic, or phrenicocolic ligaments. In fact, malignancy originating in any of the upper abdominal organs can track along the peritoneal reflections and ligaments to reach contiguous and noncontiguous organs. A thorough knowledge of the upper abdominal peritoneal anatomy will assist the radiologist in interpreting cross-sectional abdominal examinations in the oncology patient with disseminated tumor.

In the pelvis, the peritoneal reflections and mesenteries similarly connect the uterus, ovaries, bladder, gastrointestinal tract, and pelvic sidewalls. Ovarian cancer may spread along the broad ligament to involve the serosal surface of the uterus or may spread laterally to involve the peritoneum of the pelvic sidewall. Adenocarcinoma of the left ovary may extend into the sigmoid mesentery to involve the sigmoid colon. A sigmoid colon cancer may spread to involve the sigmoid mesentery and the adjacent pelvic sidewall. Rectal and prostate cancers may directly spread to involve adjacent organs and the intervening peritoneal reflections of the pelvis.

15.5.1.3
Hematogenous Tumor Dissemination to the Peritoneum

Blood borne metastases to the peritoneum, mesentery, omentum, and bowel occur in patients with widely metastatic tumor. Hematogenous peritoneal metastases most commonly occur with primary tumors of the breast, lung, and metastatic melanoma (Fig. 15.8). Patients may present with bowel obstruction, gastrointestinal bleeding, ascites, or increasing abdominal girth. In some cases, these signs of abdominal metastases may be the initial presentation prior to diagnosis of the primary malignancy. Metastatic melanoma to the gastrointestinal tract results in the classic target appearance with multiple centrally ulcerated submucosal nodules. In our experience, metastatic breast cancer often presents with a scirrhous appearance owing to sheets of poorly defined tumor coating the peritoneum and gastrointestinal tract. Diffuse involvement of the stomach may produce a linitus plastica appearance with a nondistensible stomach encased in tumor. Bronchogenic carcinoma may produce metastases to the peritoneum, mesentery, and bowel, most commonly occurring in the setting of widely metastatic tumor.

15.5.2
Ovarian Cancer

Epithelial carcinoma of the ovary is one of the most common gynecologic malignancies and the fifth most frequent cause of cancer death in women, with 50% of all cases occurring in women older than 65 years. Widespread tumor dissemination at the time of diagnosis is common with more than 60% of patients presenting with Stage III or IV disease (American Cancer Society 2008). Most of these women have peritoneal metastases to abdomen and pelvis. Intraperitoneal tumor spread occurs with ovarian cancer as tumor cells are shed into the peritoneal cavity followed by implantation on the peritoneum in areas of stasis. Local invasion of bowel, bladder, and other organs also commonly occurs. The incidence of malignant lymph nodes at primary surgery has been reported to be as much as 24% in patients with stage I disease, 50% in patients with stage II disease, 74% in patients

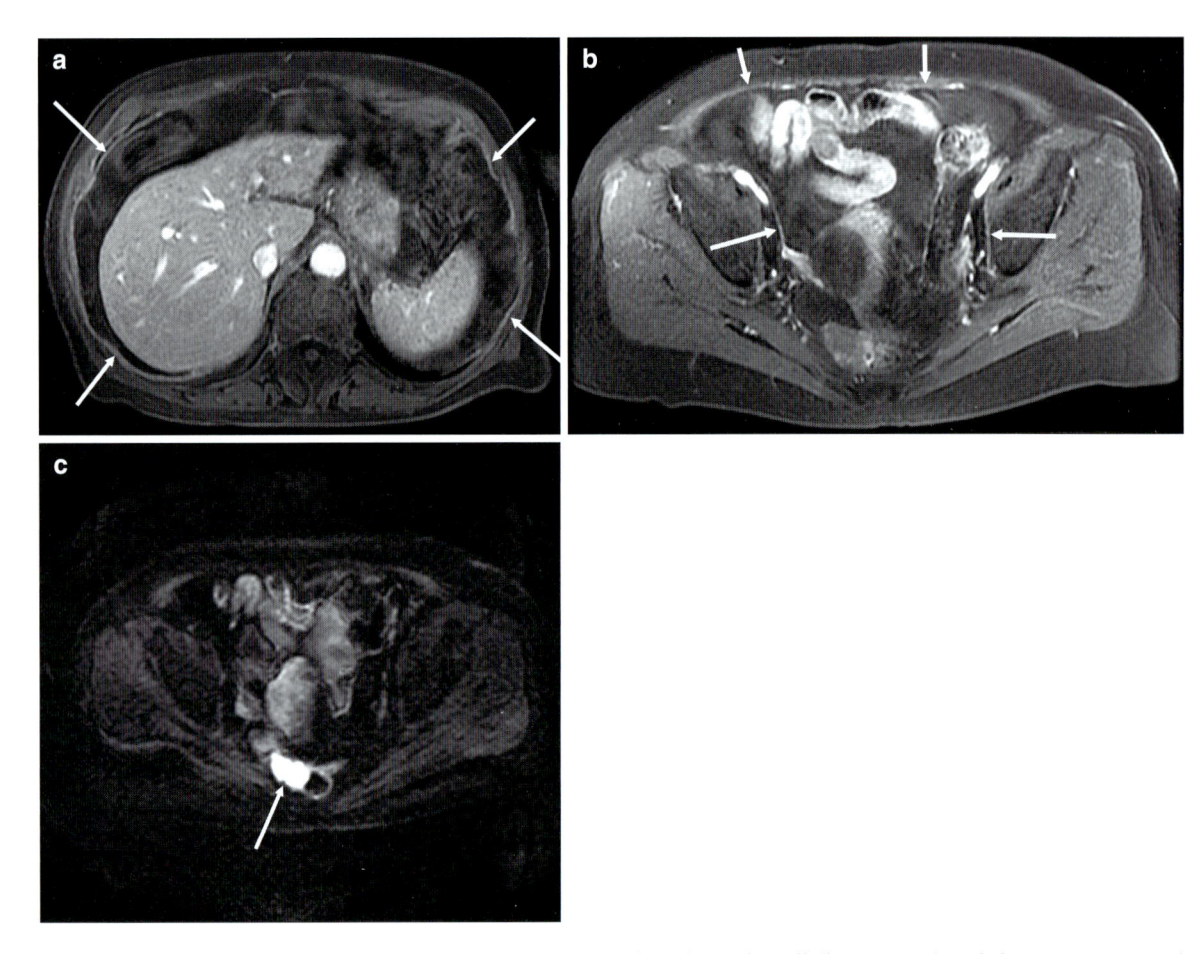

Fig. 15.8. Hematogenous peritoneal metastases – 60-year-old woman with breast cancer and abdominal distension. (**a**) Delayed gadolinium-enhanced SGE image shows ascites and abnormal perionteal enhancement (*arrows*) indicating peritoneal carcinomatosis. (**b**) Delayed gadolinium-enhanced SGE image shows subtle peritoneal metastases involving the pelvic side wall (*long arrows*) and the anterior parietal peritoneum (*short arrows*). (**c**) DW image *b*-value 400 s/mm^2 shows a 3-cm perirectal tumor (*arrow*) that was not prospectively identified on the gadolinium-enhanced images. The high tumor to background contrast of the DW images can improve the depiction of peritoneal and serosal tumors

with stage III disease, and 73% in patients with stage IV disease (Burghradt et al. 1991).

In patients with primary ovarian cancer, accurate preoperative MR imaging and CT can assist the oncologist in making treatment decisions (Qayyum et al. 2005). Patients with bulky abdominal tumor are often treated with several cycles of chemotherapy to reduce the tumor burden prior to surgical staging and cytoreduction (NIH 1995). Surgical understaging occurs frequently. Preoperative cross-sectional imaging is useful to improve surgical staging by directing the location of intraoperative biopsies. In patients with treated ovarian cancer, the value of accurate imaging studies is even more important. Following chemotherapy, the serum CA-125 tumor marker is an unreliable indicator or residual tumor. A normal serum CA-125 level following treatment has a low negative predictive value for the presence of residual tumor. In some studies, over one half of women with a normal CA-125 level following treatment for ovarian cancer have residual tumor. Second-look laparotomy is rarely performed as surgical reassessment has very little effect on outcome. In this clinical setting, accurate imaging assessment of residual tumor is critical to make treatment decisions.

The accuracy of gadolinium-enhanced MR imaging in depicting peritoneal metastases in ovarian cancer is well established and is superior to that of CT (Low et al. 1999; Ricke et al. 2003) (Fig. 15.3). In 16 patients with primary ovarian cancer, MR imaging depicted 81% of peritoneal metastases when compared with 51% for helical CT (Low et al. 1995). The difference was most notable for small (<1 cm) metastases with MR imaging depicting 71% of subcentimeter tumors compared with 32% for helical CT. In a recent study, we compared MR imaging and laparotomy reassessment in 76 women with treated ovarian cancer using clinical outcome at 1 year as the gold standard. MR imaging and surgical reassessment were equally accurate for depicting residual tumor following treatment. MR imaging had a 90% sensitivity, 88% specificity, and 89% accuracy when compared with laparotomy (88%, 100%, 89%). The positive predictive values for MR imaging and laparotomy were 98% and 100% while the corresponding negative predictive values were 50% for both tests (Low et al. 2005). In our current practice, surgical reassessment in women with treated ovarian cancer is rarely performed. The results of serial MR examinations are combined with those from serial CA-125 values to make treatment decisions regarding the need for additional chemotherapy or surveillance. In a prospective evaluation of peritoneal spread in primary or recurrent ovarian cancer, Ricke et al. found that fat-suppressed gadolinium-enhanced MRI improved planning of cytoreduction preceding chemotherapy in advanced primary or relapsed ovarian carcinoma. Sensitivity for tumor was high in the lower pelvis (73–83%) and for the bowel and mesentery (73–77%) and was lower for the bladder (40%), omentum (38%), and pelvic lymph nodes (28%) (Ricke et al. 2003). In our experience, the addition of DW imaging will significantly improve these results for peritoneal, serosal, and nodal metastases in patients with ovarian cancer (Low 2009).

15.4.3
Gastrointestinal Cancers

Primary tumors of the stomach, small intestine, colon, and rectum often metastasize to the peritoneum via intraperitoneal tumor dissemination. In a study of 458 patients with gastric cancer, 28% showed tumor cells within peritoneal lavage fluid. Sixteen percent of patients undergoing curative resection for gastric cancer showed positive peritoneal lavage cytologic evaluation (Nakajima et al. 1978). Similarly, Stage IV primary colorectal cancer may present with peritoneal metastases involving the pelvis, free peritoneal surfaces, omentum, mesentery, and bowel serosa. Recurrence of gastrointestinal cancers also often involves the peritoneum. It is estimated that 20–50% of recurrences of colon cancer involves the peritoneum and is thus a major source of treatment failure for patients with colorectal cancer (Bleiberg). The use of adjuvant heated intraperitoneal chemotherapy at the time of initial surgical resection of the gastric or colorectal cancer has been advocated to decrease the likelihood of subsequent peritoneal recurrence.

MR imaging detects the primary gastric or colorectal cancer as well as the intraperitoneal metastases (Beets-Tan and Beets 2004). Primary intestinal cancers are depicted as focal areas of mural thickening or mural masses (Fig. 15.2). These findings are demonstrated on unenhanced T1- and T2-weighted images and on the fat-suppressed gadolinium-enhanced images (Brown et al. 1999). DW images are also particularly useful as these primary gastrointestinal tumors demonstrate restricted water diffusion and are markedly hyperintense on magnitude DW images (Ichikawa et al. 2006). The conspicuity of the primary tumor on DW images makes them one of the most useful MR images to confirm the location of a primary intestinal malignancy (Low et al. 2007). Peritoneal metastases from gastric and colorectal cancers are shown on MR imaging as peritoneal thickening, nodules, or masses, which may be focal or widely disseminated. As with peritoneal metastases from other tumors, they are best demonstrated on delayed, fat-suppressed gadolinium-enhanced images (Low et al. 2007) (Fig. 15.4). Larger masses such as Krukenberg ovarian metastases from gastric cancer will be easily depicted on all MR images. However, more subtle peritoneal tumors and carcinomatosis are typically seen only because of their enhancement with gadolinium chelates. DW images using an intermediate b-value are a very useful adjunct for showing peritoneal and serosal tumor as areas of restricted diffusion (Low et al. 2009). Nodal metastases from intestinal cancers are almost always best demonstrated on DW imaging. The ability of MR imaging to accurately depict peritoneal metastases in patients with gastrointestinal malignancy is critical in determining patient management at initial diagnosis. For the patient in remission, MR imaging effectively delineates sites of local and distant tumor recurrence, which may involve the peritoneum.

15.5.4
Pseudomyxoma Peritonei

Mucinous appendiceal neoplasms with peritoneal spread are often clinically referred to as pseudomyxoma peritonei syndrome. It is a rare condition with a reported incidence of one per million per year, which is characterized by accumulation of copious gelatinous

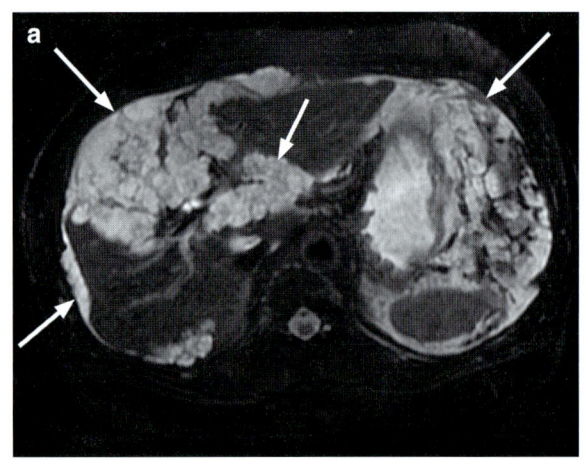

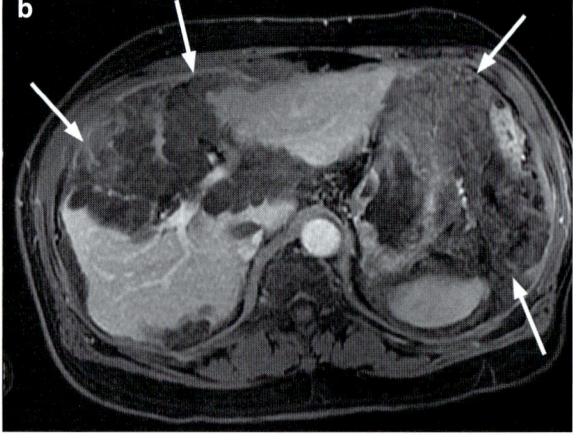

Fig. 15.9. Pseudomyxoma peritonei – 70-year-old woman with increasing abdominal distension. Axial fat suppressed T2-weighted image (**a**) shows confluent bulky tumor (*arrows*) in the upper abdomen surrounding the liver, stomach, and spleen. Delayed gadolinium-enhanced 2D SGE image (**b**) confirms the bulky upper abdominal peritoneal tumors. The degree of tumor enhancement is less than that of the liver, which indicates a DPAM (disseminated peritoneal adenomucinosis) or intermediate grade mucinous peritoneal tumor. Findings were confirmed by biopsy and histopathologic evaluation

masses throughout the peritoneal cavity. Mucinous appendiceal neoplasms may be associated with appendiceal mucin-producing adenomas or adenocarcinomas. Mucin-producing tumor cells escape from the appendix and distribute throughout the peritoneal cavity. The peritoneal lesions contain varying amounts of benign mucin and cellular material composed of mucinous epithelium and adenocarinoma. The spectrum of disease of pseudomyxoma peritonei syndrome may be separated into three clinical pathologic categories as described by Ronnett and colleagues (1995). Disseminated peritoneal adenomucinosis (DPAM) is a benign condition arising from appendiceal adenomas while peritoneal mucinous carcinomatosis (PMCA) is characterized by architectural and cytological features of adenocarinoma. PMCA arises from appendiceal or intestinal mucinous adenocarcinomas. An intermediate category occurs with features in between those of DPAM and PMCA. The classification of pseudomyxoma peritonei determines the clinical course and long-term survival. The age adjusted 5-year survival for DPAM is 84% when compared with 37.5% for patients with intermediate features, and 6.7% for those with PMCA (Cerame 1988).

Surgical cytoreduction with intraperitoneal chemotherapy form the foundation of treatment for mucinous appendiceal neoplasm with peritoneal spread. Successful cytoreduction requires removal of all gross peritoneal tumors (Glehen et al. 2004). However, complete surgical cytoreduction cannot be achieved in all patients. Careful patient selection is essential because of the potential high postoperative morbidity and mortality of the procedure.

Preoperative MR evaluation of patients with pseudomyxoma peritonei can be used to determine the location and extent of peritoneal tumor, to predict successful surgical resection, and to predict the histologic tumor grade. MR findings that predict suboptimal cytoreduction included a large >5 cm mesenteric mass, diffuse mesenteric tumor, tumor encasement of mesenteric vessels, or diffuse serosal tumor (Low et al. 2008). The mucinous component is well demonstrated on T2-weighted images. DW images are useful to distinguish high signal intensity tumor with its restricted diffusion from ascites, which is suppressed. Histologic classification of tumor is accurately predicted by the degree of tumor enhancement with intravenous gadolinium. Lower grade DPAM and intermediate tumors display only mild enhancement that is typically equal to or less than that of the liver parenchyma on delayed images (Fig. 15.9). High-grade PMCA tumors exhibit marked gadolinium enhancement that is more than that of the liver parenchyma and often equal to that of intravascular gadolinium in the aorta or IVC (Fig. 15.10). Quantitatively, Tumor: Liver contrast for DPAM and Intermediate tumors was $0.67 + 0.13$ when compared with $1.53 + 0.28$ for PMCA ($p < 0.0001$) (Low et al. 2008). The information obtained from preoperative

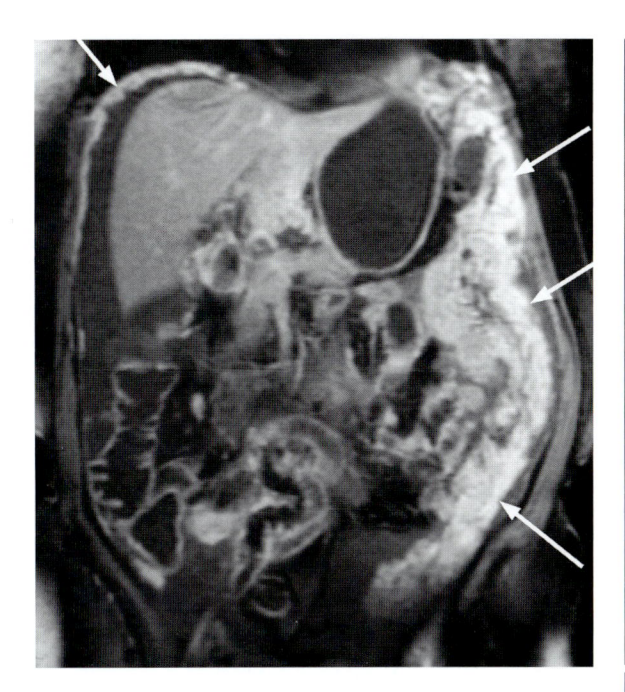

Fig. 15.10. Pseudomyxoma peritonei – 70-year-old woman with abdominal fullness. Coronal gadolinium-enhanced MR image demonstrates bulky enhancing peritoneal tumor (*arrows*) in the upper and middle abdomen. The tumors show marked gadolinium enhancement, which is greater than that of the liver. The degree of tumor enhancement indicates a high-grade PMCA tumor (peritoneal mucinous carcinomatosis). Laparotomy confirmed metastatic intraperitoneal tumor from a primary mucinous appendiceal adenocarcinoma

MR imaging can assist the surgeon in selecting patients for surgical resection. Patients with lower grade tumors and those with less extensive mesenteric and serosal tumor involvement are better candidates for laparotomy and tumor debulking.

15.5.5
Mesothelioma

Malignant peritoneal mesothelioma is a rare aggressive tumor of the peritoneum with mean survival of 6–12 months (Sugarbaker et al. 2003) (Fig. 15.11). Peritoneal mesothelioma is much less common than pleural mesothelioma with only 20–30% of mesotheliomas arising from the peritoneum. The incidence of peritoneal mesothelioma is one per 1,000,000. Risk factors include asbestos exposure, which can be documented in 50% of patients with peritoneal mesothelioma (Raptopoulos 1985). Patients present with nonspecific symptoms including abdominal pain, distention, anorexia, weight loss, and ascites. Imaging

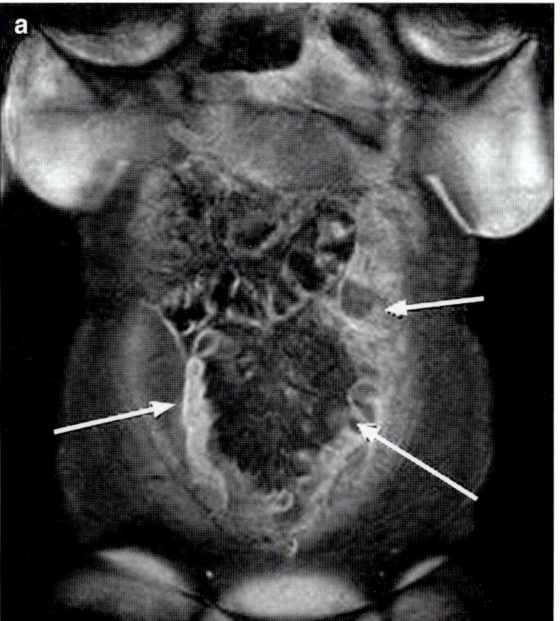

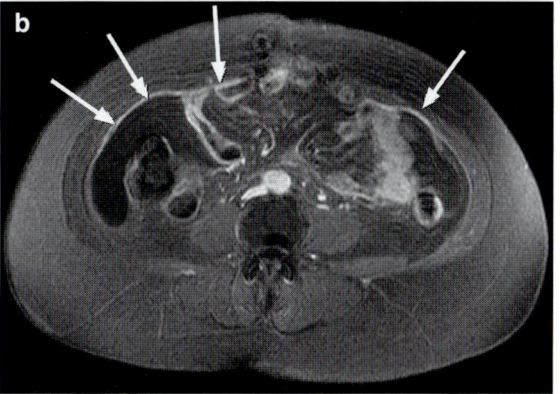

Fig. 15.11. Peritoneal mesothelioma – 59-year-old woman with and abdominal distension. Coronal fat-suppressed, gadolinium-enhanced 3D FSPGR image shows moderately bulky omental and peritoneal tumor (*arrows*). (b) Axial fat-suppressed, gadolinium-enhanced 2D SGE image shows diffuse peritoneal thickening and enhancement (*arrows*) and nonenhancing ascites. Surgery and histopathologic exam confirmed peritoneal mesothelioma

findings are also nonspecific so that definitive diagnosis of peritoneal mesothelioma depends on histologic and immunohistochemical examination. Optimal treatment consists of cytoreductive surgery and intraperitoneal chemotherapy, which can prolong median survival to 50–60 months (Mohamed and Sugarbaker 2002).

Peritoneal mesothelioma can be classified into three categories. "Dry-painful" type is the most common demonstrating a single large mass or multiple small peritoneal masses without ascites. The "wet" type is

MR imaging of peritoneal mesothelioma demonstrates peritoneal thickening and enhancement with or without associated ascites (Puvaneswary et al. 2002) (Fig. 15.11). To date, MR descriptions of peritoneal mesothelioma have been limited to case reports with one or two examples. As tumors progress, single or multiple abdominal and pelvic tumor masses will be demonstrated involving the peritoneum, omentum, or mesentery. Subsequent bowel obstruction produces focally dilated loops of bowel and an obstructing tumor mass. Mesenteric mesothelioma may produce a desmoplastic effect with encasement of bowel and mesenteric vessels. Cystic mesothelioma is depicted on MR imaging as multiple thin walled fluid containing cystic masses (Fig. 15.12).

15.5.6
Primary Peritoneal Cancer

Primary peritoneal carcinoma (PPC) is a rare cancer closely related to papillary serous epithelial ovarian cancer in its clinical presentation, histologic appearance, and response to chemotherapy. It may account for up to 10% of cases presumptive ovarian cancer. Unlike ovarian cancer, primary peritoneal carcinoma develops within cells of the peritoneal lining of the pelvis and abdomen. These cells closely resemble the epithelial cells on the surface of the ovaries. It is thought that primary peritoneal cancer may develop from remnants of ovarian tissue that remain from fetal development or may occur following metaplasia of peritoneal cells into ovarian epithelial cells (Piver et al. 1993).

- This cancer occurs almost exclusively in postmenopausal women who present with anorexia, abdominal pain, distension, changes in bowel and bladder habits, and unexplained weight gain. At diagnosis, patients have widespread multifocal peritoneal tumors with minimal or no ovarian involvement. Similar to other cancers undergoing intraperitoneal dissemination, PPC tends to spread along the peritoneal surfaces of the abdomen and pelvis with eventual tumor dissemination to involve all peritoneal, serosal, and omental surfaces. At laparotomy, PPC is identical in appearance to Stage III or IV epithelial ovarian cancer that has spread throughout the intraperitoneal cavity. Histologically and clinically, PPC closely resembles epithelial ovarian cancer. Other names for this cancer include extra-ovarian primary peritoneal carcinoma or serous surface papillary carcinoma. Primary

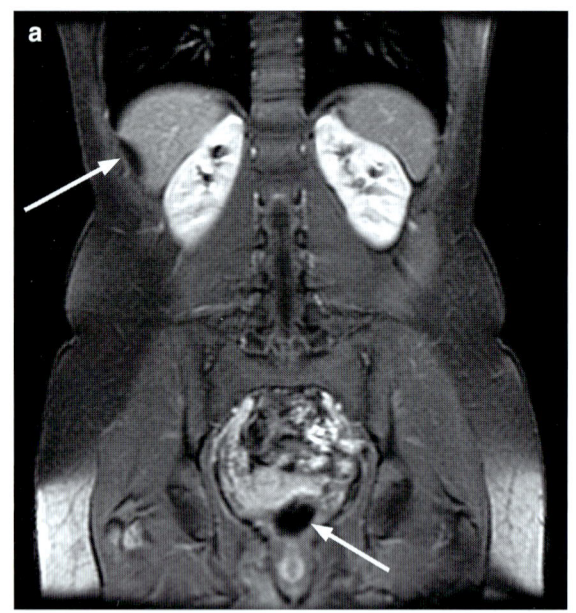

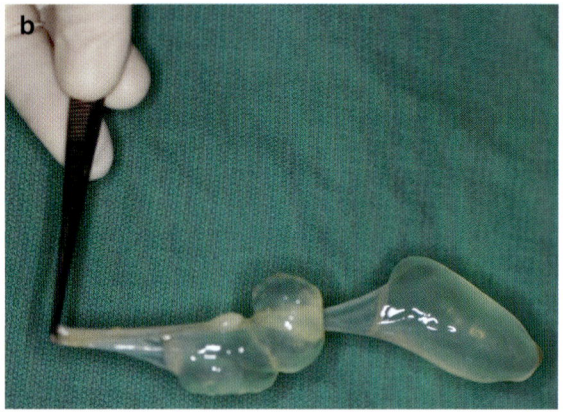

Fig. 15.12. Cystic mesothelioma – 23-year-old woman presenting with right lower quadrant pain. Coronal gadolinium enhanced 3D FSPGR image (**a**) shows nonenhancing cystic masses (*arrows*) adjacent to the liver and within the pelvis. Laparotomy-confirmed cystic mesothelioma. Surgical specimen (**b**) shows one of the gelatinous masses

characterized by ascites and intestinal distension with extensive small nodules and plaques, and no solid masses. The third type of peritoneal mesothelioma is the "mixed" form with a combination of findings.

Cystic mesothelioma is a rare intermediate-grade tumor with a predilection for surfaces of the pelvis. Lesions consist of multiple grapelike clusters of mesothelial-lined cysts separated by fibrous tissue (Fig. 15.12). Cystic mesothelioma is a tumor commonly occurring in young to middle-aged women who present with nonspecific abdominal pain, tenderness, or abdominal distension (Cunha et al. 2002).

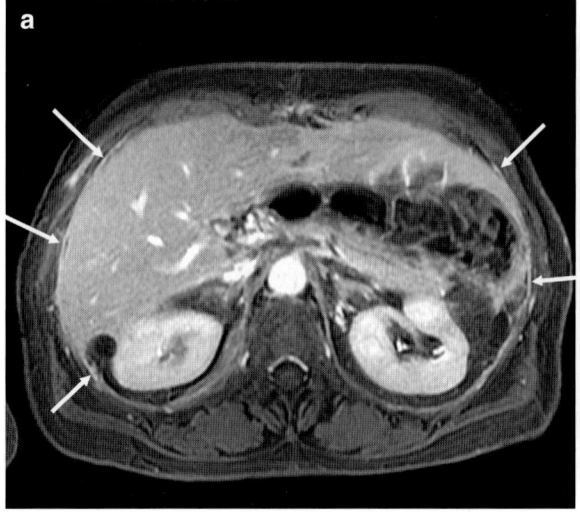

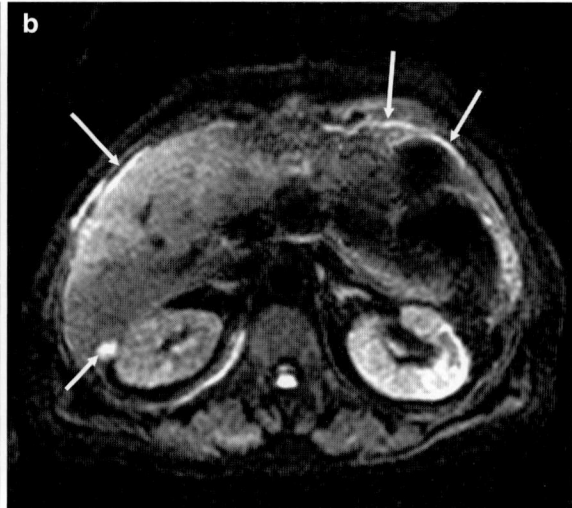

Fig. 15.13. Primary peritoneal cancer – 67-year-old woman with hip pain and abdominal discomfort. Delayed gadolinium-enhanced SGE image (a) demonstrates subtle abnormal peritoneal enhancement indicating peritoneal carcinomatosis. Diffusion-weighted MRI image b-value 400 s/mm^2 (b) shows a thin rim of peritoneal tumor involving the right and left subphrenic peritoneum (*long arrows*). A small right subhepatic peritoneal tumor (*short arrow*) is also noted

peritoneal cancer may occur years after salpingo-oophorectomy and may eventually develop in up to 5% of women who have previously undergone oophorectomy for benign disease or prophylaxis (Eltabbakh and Piver 1998).

- On MR images, PPC is depicted as peritoneal carcinomatosis with an appearance identical to metastatic epithelial ovarian cancer. Absence of an ovarian mass or other primary malignancy is critical to diagnosis of PPC. Other features of PPC include omental caking and peritoneal calcifications. There have been no formal reports of the use of MR imaging for patients with PPC. As with other types of peritoneal tumor, delayed fat suppressed gadolinium-enhanced MR imaging and DW imaging should be the most sensitive MR images for depicting PPC (Fig. 15.13).

15.6
Conclusion

MR imaging is uniquely suited for evaluation of benign and malignant peritoneal diseases. With its unmatched contrast resolution and excellent spatial resolution, MRI can routinely depict small volume peritoneal tumors and carcinomatosis as well as benign inflammatory peritoneal diseases. Gadolinium-enhanced MR imaging combined with newer imaging techniques including DW imaging affords a level of sensitivity for peritoneal diseases that makes MRI the examination of choice.

References

Akhan O, Pringo J (2002) Imaging of abdominal tuberculosis. Eur Radiol 12:312–323
American Cancer Society (2008) Cancer Facts and Figures 2008. Atlanta, Ga: American Cancer Society
Arai K, Makino H, Morioka T, et al. (1993) Enhancement of ascites on MRI following intravenous administration of Gd-DTPA. J Comput Assist Tomogr 17:617–622
Arenas AP, Sanchez LV, Albilklos JM, et al. (1994) Direct dissemination of pathologic abdominal processes through perihepatic ligaments: identification with CT. Radiographics 14:515–528
Beets-Tan RGH, Beets GL (2004) Rectal cancer: review with rmphasis on MR imaging. Radiology 232:335–346
Burghardt E, Girardi F, Lahousen M, et al (1991) Patterns of pelvic and paraaortic lymph node involvement in ovarian cancer. Gynecol Oncol 40:103–106
Brown G, Richards CJ, Newcombe RG, et al. (1999) Rectal carcinoma: thin-section MR imaging for staging in 28 patients. Radiology 211:215–222
Cerame MA (1988) A 25-year review of adenocarcinoma of the appendix: a frequently perforating carcinoma. Dis Colon Rectur 31:143–150
Choi JH, Kim JH, Kim JJ, et al. (2004) Large bowel obstruction caused by sclerosing peritonitis: contrast-enhanced CT findings. Br J Radiol 77:344–346
Coakley FV, Hricak H (1999) Imaging of peritoneal and mesenteric disease: key concepts for the clinical radiologist. Clin Radiol 54:563–574

Coakley FV, Choi, PH, Gougoutas CA, et al.(2002) Peritoneal metastases: detection with spiral CT in patients with ovarian cancer. Radiology 223:495–499

Cunha P, Luz Z, Seves I, et al. (2002) [Malignant peritoneal mesothelioma – diagnostic and therapeutic difficulties]. Acta Med Port 15:383–386

Elsayes KM, Staveteig PT, Narra VR, et al. (2006) MRI of the peritoneum: spectrum of abnormalities. AJR Am J Roentgenol 186:1368–1379

Eltabbakh GH, Piver MS (1998) Extraovarian primary peritoneal carcinoma. Oncology 12:813–819

Emory TS, Monihan JM, Carr NJ, et al. (1997) Sclerosing mesenteritis, mesenteric panniculitis and mesenteric lipodystrophy: a single entity? Am J Surg Pathol 21:392–398

Fuji S, Matsusue E, Kanasaki Y, et al. (2008) Detection of peritoneal dissemination in gynecological malignancy: evaluation by diffusion-weighted MR imaging. Eur Radiol 18:18–23

Fujiyoshi F, Ichinari N, Kajiya Y, et al. (1997) Retractile mesenteritis: small-bowel radiography, CT, and MR imaging. AJR Am J Roentgenol 169:791–793

Glehen O, Kwiatkowski F, Sugargaker PH, et al. (2004) Cytoreductive surgery combined with perioperative intraperitoneal chemotherapy for the management of peritoneal carcinomatosis from colorectal cancer: a Multi-Institutional Study. J Clin Oncol 22:3284–3292

Ha HK, Jung JI, Lee MS, et al. (1996) CT differentiation of tuberculous peritonitis and peritoneal carcinomatosis. AJR Am J Roentgenol 167:743–748

Hamrick-Turner JE, Chiechi MV, Abbitt PL, et al. (1992) Neoplastic and inflammatory processes of the peritoneum, omentum, and mesentery: diagnosis with CT. Radiographics 12:1051–1068

Hossein J, Bindelzun RE, Olcott EW, et al. (1997) Still the great mimicker: abdominal tuberculosis. AJR Am J Roentgenol 168:1455–1460

Hüser N, Stangl M, Lutz J, et al. (2006) Sclerosing encapsulating peritonitis: MRI diagnosis. Eur Radiol 16:238–239

Ichikawa T, Erturk SM, Motosugi U, et al. (2006) High-B-value diffusion weighted MRI in colorectal cancer. AJR Am J Roentgenol 187:181–184

Ichikawa T, Haradome HH, Hachiya J, et al. (1999) Diffusion-weighted MR imaging with single-shot echo-planar imaging in the upper abdomen: preliminary clinical experience in 61 patients. Abdom Imag 24:456–461

Kanematsu M, Hoshi H, Murakami T, et al. (1997) Spontaneous bacterial peritonitis in cirrhosis: enhancement of ascites on delayed MR imaging. Radiat Med 15:185–187

Kim SY, Kim MJ, Chung JJ, et al. (2000) Abdominal tuberculous lymphadenopathy: MR imaging findings. Abdom Imaging 25:627–632

Kobayashi S, Takeda K, Tanaka N, Hirano T, Nakagawa T, Matsukmoto K (1993) Mesenteric panniculitis: MR findings. J Comput Assist Tomogr 17:500–502

Koh DM, Collins DJ (2007) Diffusion-weighted MRI in the body: applications and challenges in oncology. AJR Am J Roentgenol 188:1622–1635

Kronthal AJ, Kang YS, Fishman EK, et al. (1991) MR imaging in sclerosing mesenteritis. AJR Am J Roentgenol 156:517–519

Leder RA, Low VHS (1995) Tuberculosis of the abdomen. Radiol Clin North Am 33:691–705

Low RN (2001) Gadolinium-enhanced MR imaging of liver capsule and peritoneum. Magn Reson Imaging Clin N Am 9:803–819

Low RN (2007) MR imaging of the peritoneal spread of malignancy. Abdom Imaging 32:267–283

Low RN, Gurney J (2007) Diffusion-weighted MRI (DWI) in the oncology patient: value of breath hold DWI compared to unenhanced and gadolinium-enhanced MRI. J Magn Reson Imaging 25:848–858

Low RN, Sigeti JS (1994) MR imaging of peritoneal disease: comparison of contrast-enhanced fast multiplanar spoiled gradient-recalled and spin-echo imaging. AJR Am J Roentgenol. 163:1131–1140

Low RN, Barone RM, Gurney JM, et al. (2008) Mucinous appendiceal neoplasms: preoperative mr staging and classification compared with surgical and histopathologic findings. AJR Am J Roentgenol 190:656–665

Low RN, Barone RM, Lacey C, et al. (1997) Peritoneal tumor: MR imaging with dilute oral barium and intravenous gadolinium-containing contrast agents compared with unenhanced MR imaging and CT. Radiology 204:513–520

Low RN, Barone R, Sebrechts C, et al. (2009) Diffusion weighted MR imaging of peritoneal tumor: comparison with conventional MR imaging, and surgical and histopathologic findings. Am J Roentgenol AJR 193:461–470

Low RN, Carter WD, Saleh F, et al. (1995) Ovarian cancer: comparison of findings with perfluorocarbon-enhanced MR imaging, In-111-CYT-103 Immunoscintigraphy, and CT. Radiology 195:391–400

Low RN, Duggan B, Barone RM, et al. (2005) Treated ovarian cancer: MR imaging, laparotomy reassessment, and serum CA-125 values compared with clinical outcome at 1 year. Radiology 235:918–926

Low RN, Saleh F, Song SY, et al. (1999) Treated ovarian cancer: comparison of MR imaging with serum CA-125 level and physical examination–a longitudinal study. Radiology 211:519–528

Manohar A, Simjee AE, Haffejee AA, et al. (1990) Symptoms and investigative findings in 145 patients with tuberculous peritonitis diagnosed by peritoneoscopy and biopsy over a five year period. Gut 31:1130–1132

Menassa-Moussa L, Bleibel L, Sader-Ghorra C, et al. (2006) MRI findings in intestinal cocoon. AJR Am J Roentgenol 186:905–906

Meyers MA (2000) Dynamic radiology of the abdomen. normal and pathologic anatomy, 5th edn. Springer, New York

Meyers MA et al. (1987) The peritoneal ligaments and mesenteries: pathways of intra abdominal spread of disease. Radiology 163:593–604

Mohamed F, Sugarbaker PH (2002) Peritoneal mesothelioma. Curr Treat Options Oncol 3:375–386

Nakajima T, Harashima S, Hirata M, et al. (1978) Prognostic and therapeutic values of peritoneal cytology in gastric cancer. Acta Cytol 22:225–229

NIH consensus conference (1995) Ovarian cancer. Screening, treatment, and follow-up. NIH Consensus Development Panel on Ovarian Cancer. JAMA 273:491–497

Pereira J, Madureira A, Vieira A, et al. (2005) Abdominal tuberculosis: imaging features. Eur J Radiol 55:173–180

Piver MS, Jishi MF, Tsukada Y, et al. (1993) Primary peritoneal carcinoma after prophylactic oophorectomy in women with a family history of ovarian cancer. A report of the gilda radner familial ovarian cancer registry. Cancer Cytopathol Cancer 71:2751–2755

Puvaneswary M, Chen S, Proietto T (2002) Peritoneal mesothelioma: CT and MRI findings. Australas Radiol 46:91–96

Qayyum A, Coakley FV, Westphalen AC, et al. (2005) Role of CT and MR imaging in predicting optimal cytoreduction of newly diagnosed primary epithelial ovarian cancer. Gynecologic Oncol 96:301–306

Raptopoulos V (1985) Peritoneal mesothelioma. Crit Rev Diagn Imaging 24:293–328

Ricke J, Sehouli J, Hach C, et al. (2003) Prospective evaluation of contrast-enhanced MRI in the depiction of peritoneal spread in primary or recurrent ovarian cancer. Eur Radiol 13:943–949

Rigby R, Hawley C (1998) Sclerosing peritonitis: the experience in Australia. Nephrol Dial Transplant 13:154–159

Ronnett RM, Zahn CM, Kurman RJ, et al. (1995) Disseminated peritoneal adenomucinosis and peritoneal mucinous carcinomatosis: a clinicopathologic analysis of 109 cases with emphasis on distinguishg features, site of origin, prognosis, and relationship to "Psedumyxoma Peritonei." Am J Surg Pathol 19:1390–1408

Slim R, Tohme C, Yaghi C, et al. (2005) Sclerosing encapsulating peritonitis: a diagnostic dilemma. J Am Coll Surg 200: 974–975

Sugarbaker PH, Welch LS, Mohamed F, et al. (2003) review of peritoneal mesothelioma at the Washington Cancer Institute. Surg Oncol Clin N Am 12:605–621

Tarzi RM, Lim A, Moser S, et al. (2008) Assessing the validity of an abdominal CT scoring system in the diagnosis of encapsulating peritoneal sclerosis. Clin J Am Soc Nephrol 3: 1702–1710

Vikram R, Balachandranm A, Bhosale PR, et al. (2009) Pancreas: peritoneal reflections, ligamentous connections, and pathways of disease spread. RadioGraphics (Published Online Only). http://radiographics.rsnajnls.org/cgi/content/abstract/e34v1

MRI of Adhesions and Small Bowel Obstruction

Andreas Lienemann and Sonja Kirchhoff

CONTENTS

16.1 Introduction 271

16.2 MR Imaging Protocols 272
16.2.1 Functional Cine MRI 272
16.2.1.1 Method 272
16.2.1.2 Imaging Criteria 273

16.3 Bowel Obstruction 275
16.3.1 General Considerations 275
16.3.2 Extrinsic Causes 276
16.3.2.1 Intraabdominal Adhesions 276
16.3.2.2 Hernia 276
16.3.2.3 Extrinsic Masses 278
16.3.3 Intrinsic Causes 279
16.3.3.1 Adenocarcinoma 279
16.3.3.2 Crohn's Disease 279
16.3.3.3 Radiation Enteropathy 279
16.3.3.4 Intramural Intestinal Hemorrhage 280
16.3.3.5 Intussusception 280
16.3.4 Intraluminal Causes 280
16.3.4.1 Bezoars 280
16.3.4.2 Other Intraluminal Causes 280
16.3.5 Developmental Causes 280
16.3.5.1 Malrotation 280

16.4 Conclusion 281

References 281

Andreas Lieneman, MD
Radiologie Mühleninsel, Mühlenstrasse 4, 84028 Landshut, Germany
Sonja Kirchhoff, MD
Klinikum der Universität München, Campus Großhadern, Institut für Radiologie, Marchioninistrasse 15, 81377 München, Germany

KEY POINTS

Among the various causes of bowel obstruction, adhesions are most likely to be found and can be a disastrous alliance. The first-line modality in an acute emergency with pending ileus is CT. Nevertheless, MRI can provide superior information. Besides the classical signs of obstruction with distended bowel loops and transition points, its potential to detect visceral slide using functional cine MRI has been proven.

16.1 Introduction

Intraabdominal adhesions are the most common cause of bowel obstruction at least in the industrialized countries, accounting for approximately 65–75% of cases (Menzies and Ellis 1990). There is a wide range of values reported in the literature for the risk of developing adhesive bowel obstruction after surgery. In general, procedures in the lower abdomen, pelvis, or both and those resulting in damage to a large peritoneal surface area tend to put patients at a higher risk (Dijkstra et al. 2000). It is estimated that the risk of bowel obstruction is 1–10% after appendectomy (Ahlberg et al. 1997; Zbar et al. 1993), 6.4% after open cholecystectomy (Zbar et al. 1993), and 10–25% after intestinal surgery (Beck et al. 1999; Nieuwenhuijzen et al. 1998).

The presence of adhesions and possibly resulting obstruction is usually suspected on the basis of clinical signs and symptoms and patients' history. Acute or chronic pain is most often the only symptom.

To manage the treatment properly, it is mandatory to establish a correct diagnosis and even prognosis prior to surgery. This means that the imaging modality used has to determine the site, level, and cause of bowel obstruction with high accuracy.

Obstruction can be caused by extrinsic, intrinsic, intraluminal, and developmental causes. Computed tomography is used in the acute setting, but MRI including cine sequences can be a valuable alternative. In this chapter, we outline the role of MRI in imaging of the various causes of obstruction with the main focus on peritoneal adhesions.

16.2
MR Imaging Protocols

MR imaging protocols should be tailored to the patient's clinical condition, and image acquisition time should be minimized.

Looking into the literature, MR imaging protocols are not standardized. The use of oral contrast material is optional. A combination of ferumoxsil and dilute barium has been reported to provide excellent depiction on both T1-weighted and T2-weighted images without causing magnetic susceptibility artifacts (Pedrosa and Rofsky 2003). Gadolinium-based contrast agents are routinely used intravenously except in pregnant women and patients with marked renal impairment. Either a free-breathing protocol or a breath-hold protocol can be used. The use of a free-breathing protocol is preferable for patients who are unable to hold their breath for longer than 20 s (Semelka et al. 1999). When using the free-breathing technique, the most reproducible position for triggering is end expiration using a navigator technique.

A typical MR imaging protocol for evaluation of the abdomen may include:

1. Axial and coronal T2-weighted images obtained with a half-Fourier single-shot spin echo (acronym: HASTE), or a half-Fourier rapid acquisition with relaxation enhancement. Insensitivity to susceptibility or black boundary artifacts and high contrast between the lumen and the bowel wall are the main advantages of the HASTE sequence. In addition, the T2-weighted images provide excellent depiction of the pancreaticobiliary tree, ascites, pleural effusion, hydronephrosis, and fluid-filled bowels.
2. T1-weighted breath-hold gradient-echo sequences including dual-echo sequences that produce both in-phase and out-of-phase images. These sequences can be used to define hemorrhagic collections.
3. Axial and coronal unenhanced or contrast-enhanced breath-hold 3D interpolated T1-weighted imaging with fat-saturation (acronyms: VIBE, THRIVE, FAME, and LAVA). The high in-plane resolution allows for MPR reconstructions and simplifies evaluating the course of anatomical structures. Owing to the fast acquisition time, several contrast enhancement phases are possible.
4. Coronal images of coherently balanced steady-state free precession sequences (acronyms: TrueFISP, FIESTA), which are sensitive to the T2/T1 ratio. Such sequences play a role in visualization of the anatomy before organ transplantation or for evaluation of vessels for thrombosis or dissection.

16.2.1
Functional Cine MRI

16.2.1.1
Method

Functional cine MRI can be explained as obtaining consecutive MRI images during respiration with freezing of motion. It should not be confused with dynamic MRI using intravenous or arterial contrast media.

At present, imaging sequences do not allow a sufficient depiction of motion using true 3D techniques. To overcome this limitation, we developed a special MR imaging protocol to visualize extrinsic or intrinsic movements within the abdomen (Lienemann et al. 2000).

The basic principle consists in the acquisition of multiple single slices at the same slice position. This approach allows for a high temporal resolution (one image/0.7–1 s) and can thus analyze intrinsic (e.g., bowel motility) or extrinsic motion (e.g., straining) continuously in more detail at a given anatomical position. The duration of a single measurement has to be less than the expected frequency of the motion itself. Disadvantages are the limited overview and the thickness of a single slice. Therefore, to cover the whole region of interest (e.g., abdomen) the slice position has to be changed repeatedly.

For the functional MRI examination, high-field MRI systems of at least 1.5 T are used. The examination is carried out with the patient being in a supine position, using a body-array surface coil. No premedication or opacification of any organs is necessary.

A coronal localizer with a superimposed grid (Fig. 16.1) is used as reference for screening the whole

Table 16.1. Functional cine MRI: parameters

Type of sequence	True FISP
TR (ms)	5.8
TE (ms)	2.5
Flip angle (degree)	70
Matrix	228 × 256
Number of acqusitions	1
Field of view (mm)	400
Slice thickness (mm)	7
Time of acquisition (s)	1.0

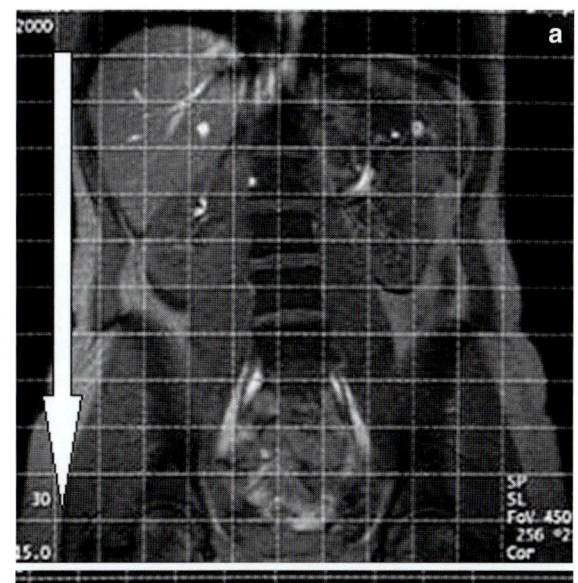

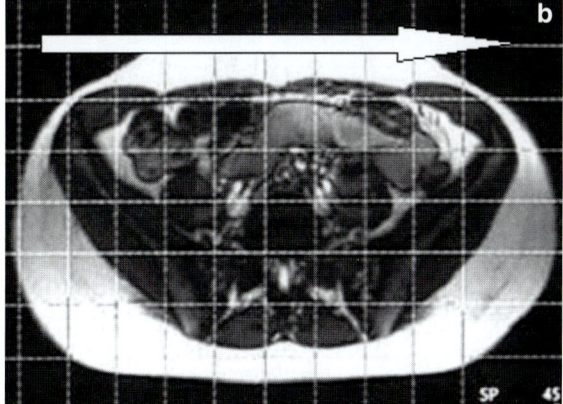

Fig. 16.1. MRI, coronal (**a**) and axial (**b**) scout. The superimposed grid allows for precise positioning of the slices. During the entire procedure, the patient's abdomen is scanned from right to left and from cranial to caudal (*arrows*) with an interslice gap of 3 cm

abdomen in a sagittal and axial direction from right to left and from the diaphragma to the pelvic floor. For sequence details, see Table 16.1.

One cycle consists of 10 consecutive measurements in the same position. During each cycle, the patients are asked to increase the intraabdominal pressure by straining and to subsequently relax again, thus inducing a visceral slide.

The above-mentioned cycle is repeated in sequence until both axial and sagittal images were acquired of the whole abdomen. The average distance (= gap) between two consecutive slice positions is 3 cm. A total of 300–400 images of the whole abdomen were acquired. The overall examination time is on average 30 min, which makes this type of examination suitable for everyday work.

16.2.1.2
Imaging Criteria

To facilitate the evaluation of the MR imaging data, the entire abdomen is divided into nine segments with bilateral vertical lines along the lateral border of the rectus abdominis muscle, and transverse lines across the inferior costal margins and across the iliac crest as initially described by us (LIENEMANN et al. 2000) (Fig. 16.2).

MRI criteria for the diagnosis of adhesions can be best explained figurative when compared with a pair of swings (see Fig. 16.3). They represent two independent bowel loops, whereas the scaffold symbolizes the border of the peritoneal cavity. The freedom of movement back and forth of the two swings stands for the movement induced by the Valsalva-maneuver (Fig. 16.4).

Without adhesions, a single bowel loop will move back and forth in a mainly cranio-caudal direction during the Valsalva maneuver (Fig. 16.4). The presence of adhesions will substantially alter this movement. First, this bowel loop will no longer move in and out of an image plane perpendicular to the direction of the movement (Fig. 16.5). Second, there will be an impediment of the movement next to nonvarying structures like the peritoneal border. Third, if two or more adjacent structures (e.g., other bowel loops) are involved, no separation between the single organs will occur. This may account for pseudo-ramification of bowel loops (Fig. 16.6). In addition, the typical boundary artifact, which normally can be seen on

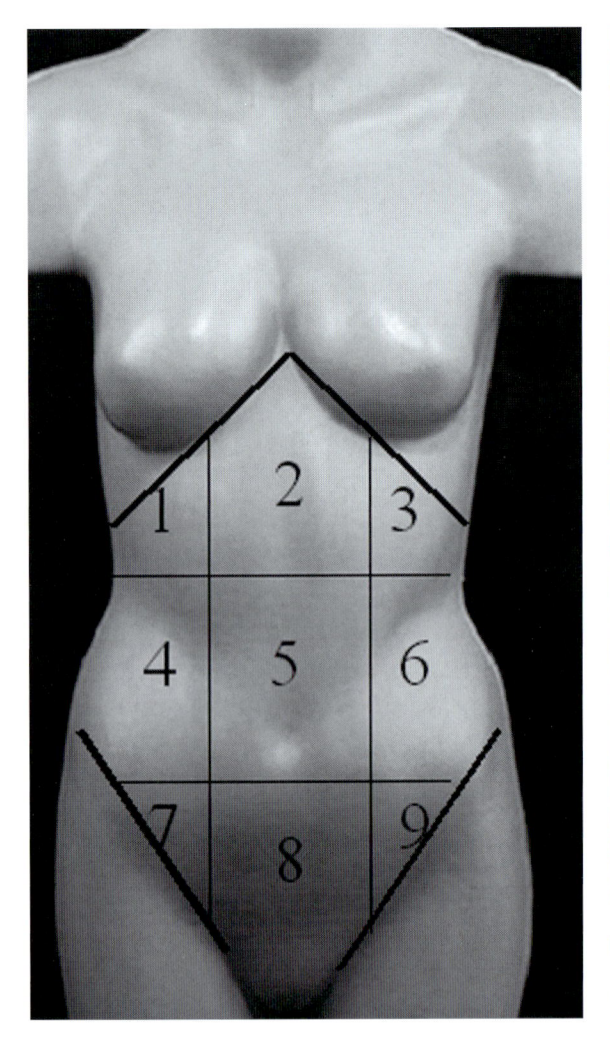

Fig. 16.2. This scheme shows the 9-field map of the abdomen for locating adhesions throughout the abdomen

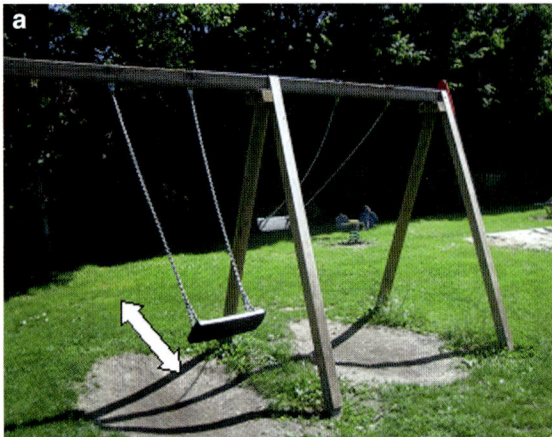

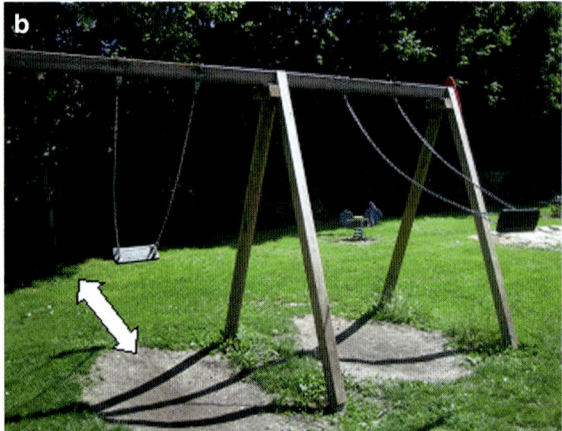

Fig. 16.4. If no adhesions are present, there will be no restriction of movement in between two adjacent bowel loops or between bowel loops and the parietal peritoneum. Thus, the swings can independently move forth (**a**) and back (**b**) as shown in the two images (*arrows*)

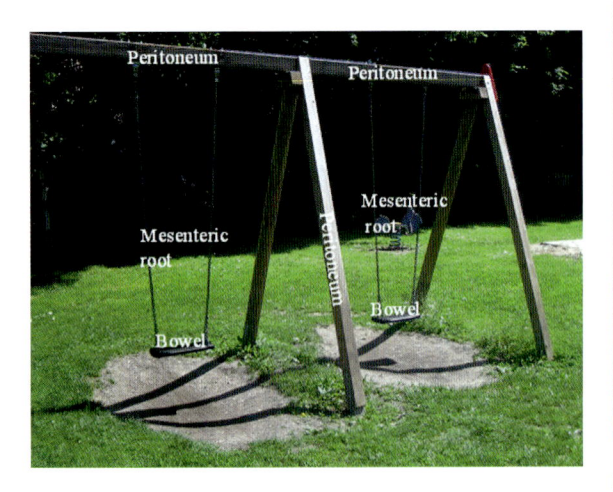

Fig. 16.3. The concept of functional cine MRI using the detection of visceral slide can be best explained using a pair of swings for comparison. Details given in the text

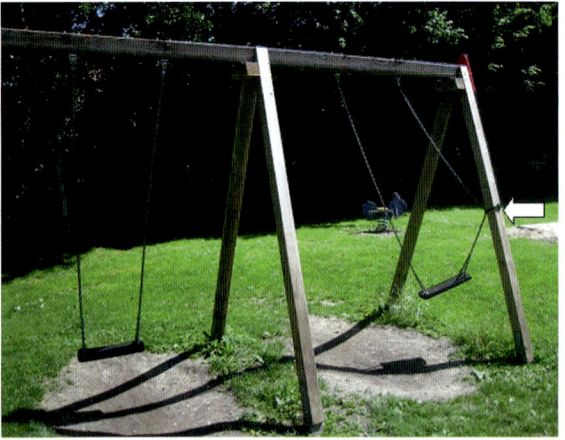

Fig. 16.5. Formation of adhesions between a bowel loop and the peritoneal border will show an adherent structure, which exhibits no or only partial movement on a Valsalva maneuver

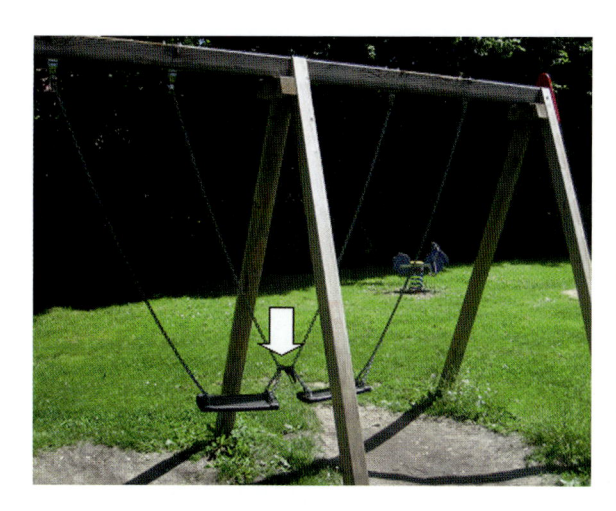

Fig. 16.6. Adhesions in between two bowel loops (*arrow*) will alter the degree of movement. The bowel loops stick together and no longer move independently of each other

tissue interfaces on True FISP sequences, will disappear. Direct signs like a distortion of adjacent organs or obstructive, dilated bowel loops with fluid levels may also be noticed.

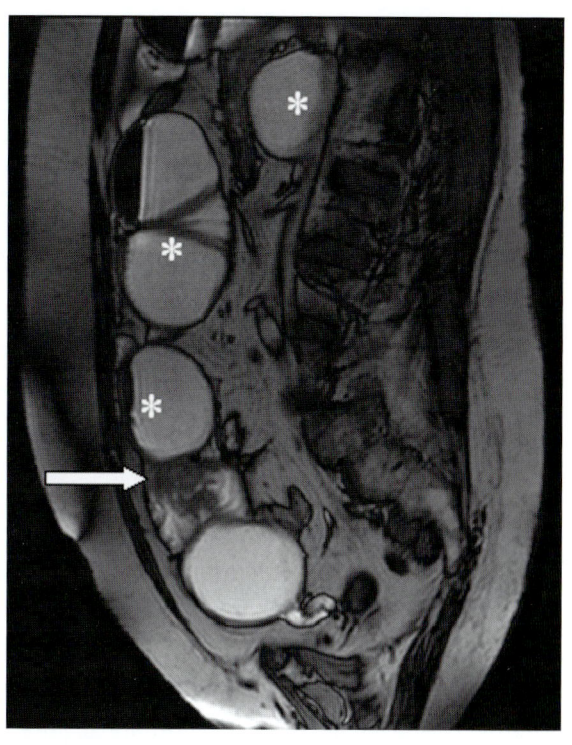

Fig. 16.7. Functional cine MRI, sagittal plane at rest: the image reveals signs of obstruction with fluid-filled and overdistended small loops and ascending colon (*asterisks*). In addition, a stenotic tumor is depicted (*arrow*), representing a carcinoma

16.3
Bowel Obstruction

16.3.1
General Considerations

Two major signs have been reported in the literature to be encountered in almost all cases of bowel obstruction:

The identification of dilated, fluid-filled bowel loops throughout the whole abdomen or within a segment of the abdomen should alert to the diagnosis of bowel obstruction (BALTHASAR 1994; GAZELLE et al. 1994). A small bowel loop with a diameter greater than 2.5–3.0 cm is considered dilated (FUKUYA et al. 1992). However, the degree of bowel dilatation alone is not a reliable criterion for distinguishing bowel obstruction from an adynamic ileus (BALTHAZAR 1994). If, in contrast, distension of the entire small bowel is observed without colonic collapse, the most probable diagnosis is an adynamic ileus.

Identification of dilated proximal and collapsed distal bowel segments is another important sign to diagnose bowel obstruction. This so-called bowel transition point can be found anywhere in the abdomen (Fig. 16.7) (SANDHU et al. 2007).

Other signs reported at computed tomography are the small bowel feces sign and the whirl sign. Both signs are less common but reliable indicators of small bowel obstruction. In the small bowel feces sign, gas bubbles are mixed with particulate matter in dilated small bowel loops proximal to an obstruction (MAYO-SMITH et al. 1995). The whirl sign is related to volvulus and has been defined as either a counterclock or clockwise swirl extending for at least 90° and including both bowel and vessels (FISHER 1981). Both signs, the small bowel feces sign and the whirl sign, can also be recognized on abdominal MRI.

In general, there is difference in the cause of obstruction of the small bowel and the large bowel. For small bowel obstruction, adhesions present the most common cause, whereas cancer is the most common cause for large bowel obstruction.

The level of obstruction is determined by identifying the site of the transition zone and comparing the relative lengths of dilated vs. collapsed bowel in case of small bowel obstruction. Indicating the level of small bowel obstruction based on the expected position of small bowel loops (e.g., distal jejunum in the left lower abdomen) can be misleading.

Complete vs. partial obstruction of the small bowel is determined by the degree of collapse and the amount of the residual contents in the portion of the bowel distal to the obstructed site. Passage of the contrast material through a transition point always indicates incomplete obstruction.

16.3.2
Extrinsic Causes

16.3.2.1
Intraabdominal Adhesions

Peritoneal adhesions are the most frequent cause of small bowel obstruction. Peritoneal adhesions can be defined as abnormal fibrous bands between organs or tissues or both in the abdominal cavity that are normally separated (Sulaiman et al. 2002; Vrijland et al. 2002; Vrijland et al. 2003). Adhesions may be acquired or congenital. However, most are acquired as a result of peritoneal injury, the most common cause of which is abdomino-pelvic surgery (Dijkstra et al. 2000). It is estimated that 93–100% of patients who undergo transperitoneal surgery will develop postoperative adhesions (Menzies and Ellis 1990).

Fortunately, most patients with adhesions do not experience any overt clinical symptoms. For others, adhesions may be the cause of significant morbidity and mortality (Ellis et al. 1999). To this day, no clinical standard exists for any preventive measure, to control the formation of postoperative adhesions.

The correct diagnosis of the presence and extent of adhesions in patients with bowel obstruction is of great importance regarding indication as well as planning of an operation (Freys et al. 1994). Plain film radiography of the abdomen may only reveal distended air-filled bowel loops with or without air-fluid levels. Real-time ultrasonography is able to detect a restriction of the movement of abdominal viscera (visceral slide) next to the abdominal wall. Small bowel enteroclysis occasionally will show fibrous bands with luminal narrowing. In addition, externally applied manual pressure to the abdomen may fail to show separation of adjacent bowel loops (Bartram 1980).

Bowel obstruction is considered to be present at CT when distended bowel loops are seen proximal to collapsed loops. When a point of transition from dilated to normal-caliber bowel loops without apparent cause is identified, adhesions are to be presumed.

Our own results suggest that the best modality for the detection of intraabdominal adhesions is functional cine MRI (Lang et al. 2008). In a recent study, 89 consecutive patients with adhesion-related complaints after previous abdominal surgery underwent preoperative workup including functional cine-MRI. The results were correlated to the findings on 59 laparotomies and 30 laparoscopies. The use of functional cine-MRI scan for the detection of adhesions showed an overall accuracy of 90%, a sensitivity of 93%, and a positive predictive value of 96%. The more restricted movement due to adhesions, the more accurate scan findings resulted. There were no common causes for discordant findings. The MRI images revealed most adhesions to involve the small intestines (75%), large intestines (35%), or abdominal cavity (42%).

In addition to the aforementioned criteria of bowel obstruction (Fig. 16.7), functional cine MRI provides additional signs. Large adhesive fibrous bands can be seen as homogeneous tissue of low signal intensity in all sequences (Fig. 16.8). These bands may interconnect and/or cross adjacent small bowel loops. The distorsion of neighboring organs including bowel loops during Valsalva maneuver is considered to be another direct sign for the presence of adhesions (Fig. 16.8). Next, one should look for a hampered visceral slide of adjacent structures to each other or along the peritoneal layer and/or a missing separation between them (Fig. 16.9). If the omentum or other parts of the mesenteric fat stick to the peritoneal layer, the hypointense vessels within the hyperintense mesenteric fat may exhibit a perpendicular angle with the abdominal wall and show a cut-off-like appearance. In addition, vanishing susceptibility artifacts suggest an obliteration of the mostly fatty tissue between two adjacent bowel loops. This may lead to a pseudo-branching or star-like appearance of bowel loops (Fig. 16.10).

16.3.2.2
Hernia

Hernia is the second most frequent cause of small bowel obstruction, with a reported prevalence of approximately 10% (Bizer et al. 1981). Based on the anatomic origin of its orifice, hernias can be classified into external (e.g., inguinal, femoral, obturator) and internal (e.g., paraduodenal, foramen of winslow, intersigmoid) hernia.

Most often, the orifice of an external hernia is located in specific sites of congenital weakness or

Fig. 16.8. Functional cine MRI, sagittal plane at rest (a) and during Valsalva maneuver (b) of a 45-year-old woman suffering from unspecific abdominal pain following previous appendectomy: Two small bowel loops are adherent to the ventral abdominal wall (*arrow*). During a Valsalva maneuver, one can notice a lack of separation and excursion of the bowel loops alongside the peritoneal border. At the most cranial end of the adhesion, there is a steep angle (*curved arrow*), indicating a nonadhesive portion of a small bowel loop

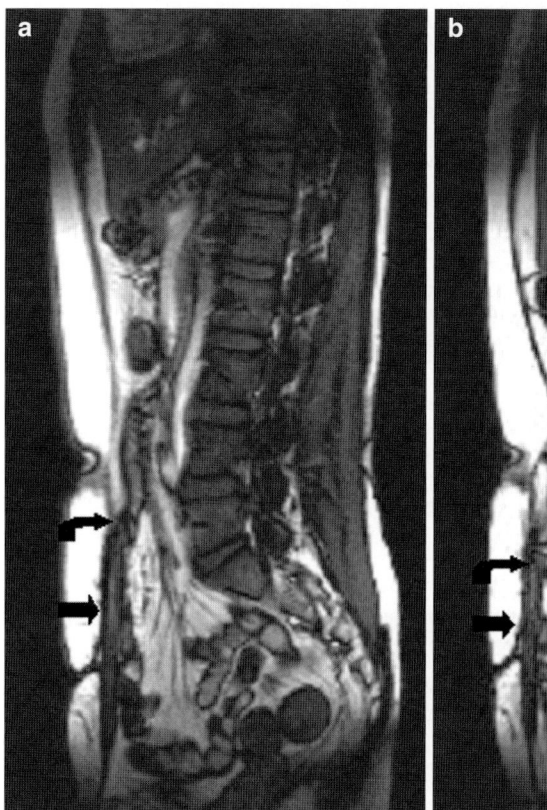

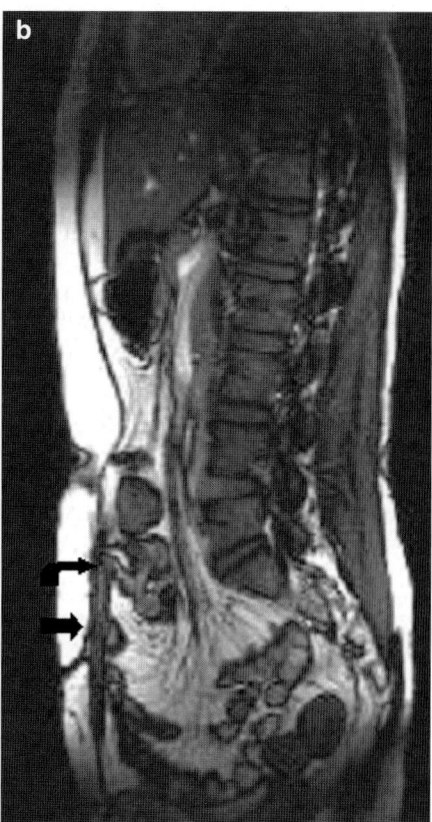

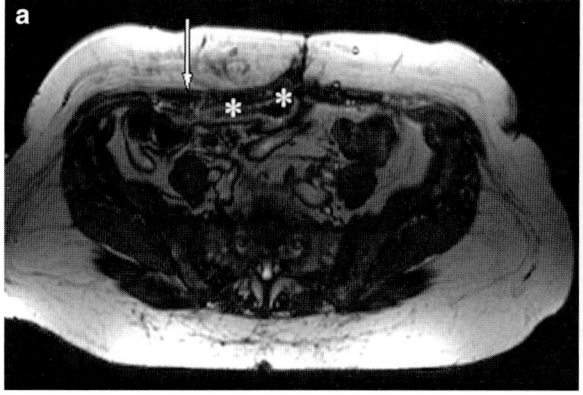

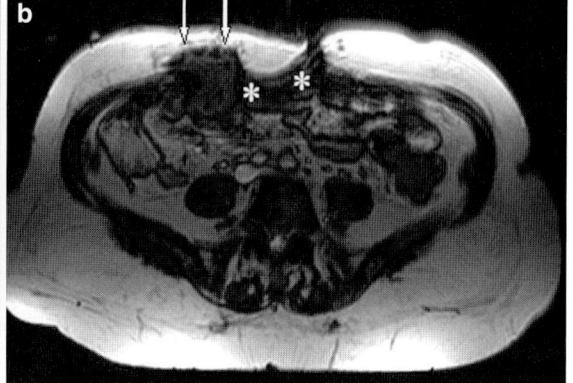

Fig. 16.9. Functional cine MRI, axial plane at rest (a) and during Valsalva maneuver (b): next to a postoperative scar several small bowel loops can be noticed (*asterisk*). They show no excursion during Valsalva maneuvers. There is also an abdominal wall hernia (*arrows*) with bowel entering the hernial sac

previous surgery. Therefore, defects in the abdominal or pelvic wall account for most external hernias (Fig. 16.11), with inguinal hernias being the most common abdominal wall hernias.

An internal hernia is a herniation of the bowel loops through a developmental or surgically created defect of the peritoneum, omentum, or mesentery. They are less common than external hernias. Diagnosis is always based on radiological findings alone.

Functional cine MRI is useful in detecting hernias in unsuspected sites, in obese patients, or after

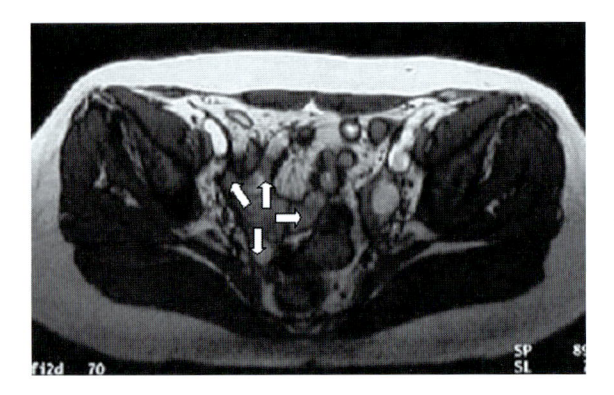

Fig. 16.10. Functional cine MRI, axial plane at rest of a 37-year-old female with a history of adhesions and pain in the lower abdomen. In the lesser pelvis, adhesions between multiple small bowel loops and the right adnexial region can be noticed. This leads to a star-like or pseudo-branching appearance (*arrows*)

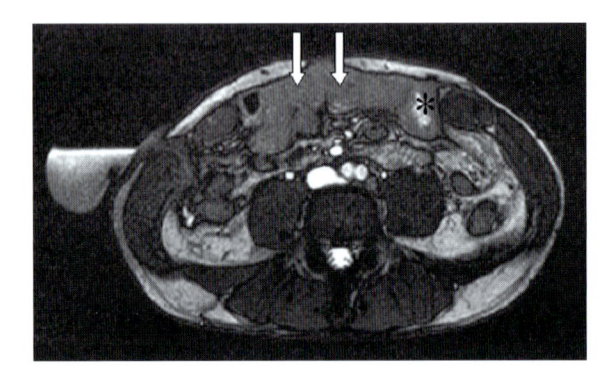

Fig. 16.11. Functional cine MRI, axial plane of a 61-year-old male patient after laparoscopic hernia repair: postoperative diastasis of the rectum muscle with formation of a broad hernia (*arrows*). Multiple adhesions of small bowel loops next to the peritoneum are present. In addition, one fluid-filled bowel loop shows a thickening of the wall (*asterisk*)

surgery (Fig. 16.9). In a study with 43 patients, we were able to reliably detect and evaluate implanted meshes and reveal typical complications like mesh defects and dislocation, adhesions, and abdominal wall dysmotility (Kirchhoff et al. 2009).

Complications include strangulation and the formation of a closed loop.

The reported prevalence of strangulating small bowel obstruction ranges from 5 to 42% with a mortality rate ranging from 20 to 37% (Bizer et al. 1981; Sarr et al. 1983). In cases of a strangulated hernia, compromise of the blood supply is present. This results in a circumferential bowel wall thickening, referred to as the target sign. Adjacent inflammatory changes with local mesenteric edema due to congestion and pathological uptake of contrast media can be seen on MRI in association with small bowel obstruction. Eventually, ascites and pneumatosis intestinalis may develop.

A closed small bowel loop presents as a mechanical obstruction in which a segment of bowel together with its mesentery is occluded at two points along its course by a single constrictive lesion. The closed loop is able to rotate along its axis, thereby producing a small bowel volvulus.

Depending on the length, degree of distention, and orientation of the closed loop, sometimes MRI is able to depict a U- or C-shaped configuration on the images with stretched mesenteric vessels converging toward the site of torsion. At the site of obstruction, a fusiform tapering of the involved small bowel segment (beak sign) or a volvulus with a whirl sign may be noticed.

16.3.2.3
Extrinsic Masses

A wide variety of neoplastic, inflammatory, and vascular lesions may also cause bowel obstruction, either by direct luminal compression or by initiating a desmoplastic reaction of the bowel wall through the serosa.

Peritoneal Carcinomatosis

Advanced peritoneal carcinomatosis is the most common cause of bowel obstruction. On MRI, multiple transition zones of nodular wall thickening are demonstrated (Megibow 1994).

Ovarian carcinoma is the most frequent cause of metastatic disease to the peritoneal cavity and omentum. Other tumors that frequently spread to the omentum include carcinoma of the colon, stomach, pancreas, breast, and endometrium. Carcinoid tumors and desmoid tumors may have radiographic features similar to those of peritoneal carcinomatosis.

Lymphoma

Primary non-Hodgkin's lymphomas of the small bowel rarely cause obstruction, even when they are annular, because they are soft lesions that infiltrate the bowel wall and tend to produce early cavitation. However, nodal non-Hodgkin's lymphomas may arise in the mesentery and grow to invade small bowel segments, causing obstruction by compression, kinking, and infiltration. MRI findings include polycyclic masses within the mesenteric root with infiltration of adjacent bowel loops and signs of obstruction.

Appendicitis and Diverticulitis

In appendicitis and diverticulitis, small bowel obstruction may occur when complications such as phlegmon, abscess, and peritonitis develop. This might be due to the anatomic proximity to the sigmoid colon or appendix, which makes portions of the small bowel vulnerable to pericolic inflammatory processes. The bowel loops become trapped within the inflammatory processes, resulting in fixation and narrowing. Thus, a pericolic process may directly affect adjacent small bowel loops, resulting in obstruction (KIM et al. 1998).

16.3.3
Intrinsic Causes

Intrinsic lesions such as neoplasms, inflammatory or vascular lesions, and hematoma lead to bowel wall thickening. Because of the liquid content, small bowel obstruction occurs only when lesions grow large enough to cause significant luminal narrowing.

Adenocarcinoma and Crohn's disease are the most frequent intrinsic lesions to cause small bowel obstruction. However, Crohn's disease is the more frequent one. Radiation enteropathy and intramural hematoma are other, rare causes. Most intrinsic bowel lesions causing obstruction are seen at the transition zone and manifest as localized mural thickening on MRI.

16.3.3.1
Adenocarcinoma

Adenocarcinoma of the small bowel is seen more frequently in the duodenum and proximal jejunum than in the ileum (LEVINE et al. 1987). The tumor is usually detected at an advanced stage. The tumor itself usually manifests as mural thickening with luminal narrowing and possible invasion of adjacent structures (Figs. 16.7 and 16.12). Besides depicting local anatomy, MRI can provide useful information of metastatic lesions and lymphadenopathy.

16.3.3.2
Crohn's Disease

In advanced stages of Crohn's disease, patients frequently present with recurrent episodes of partial small bowel obstruction (Fig. 16.13). MRI performed as MR enterography or MR enteroclysis is extremely

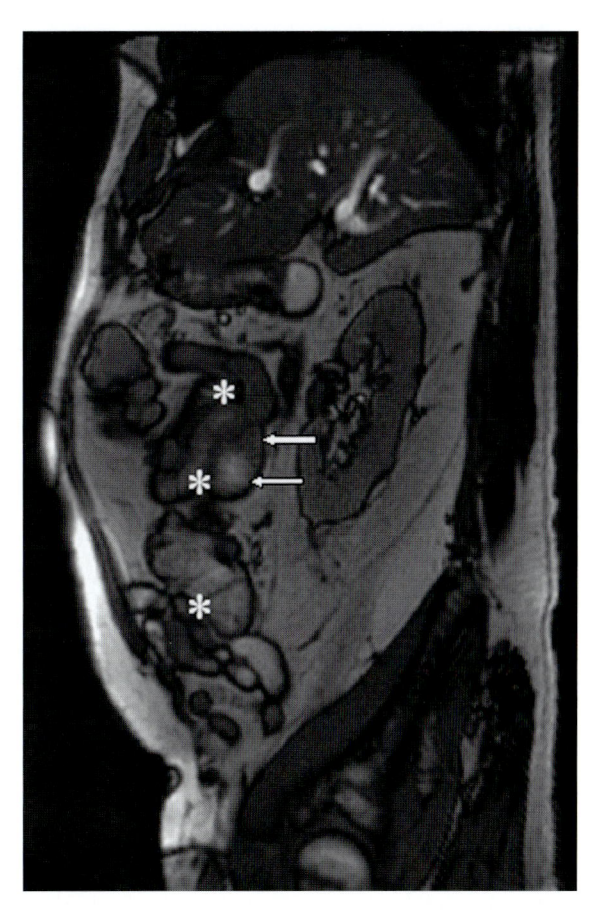

Fig. 16.12. Functional cine MRI, sagittal plane at rest: ventral to the right kidney a group of small bowel loops is visible (*asterisk*). Some of these small bowel loops stick together and show a luminal distention. The underlying cause is a tumor mass (*small arrows*) being a histological proven carcinoma of the small bowel

useful to determine the site, level, and cause of small bowel obstruction secondary to Crohn's disease (see Chaps. 8–10). In the acute phase, images may show a wall thickening and luminal narrowing together with an increased uptake of contrast media in the wall of the affected bowel segments. Even a mural stratification and a target-like or "double halo" appearance can be seen. During the chronic phase, mural stratification disappears. In addition, fat deposition in the bowel wall in Crohn's disease indicates inactive disease.

16.3.3.3
Radiation Enteropathy

Radiation enteropathy may cause small bowel obstruction (DEITEL VASIC 1979). The changes are mainly restricted to the irradiated area. In such cases,

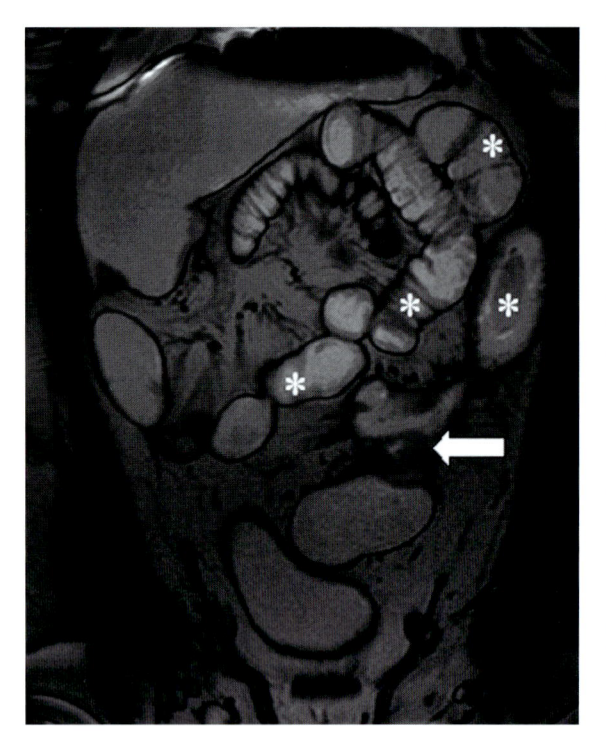

Fig. 16.13. Functional cine MRI, coronal plane at rest: Within the abdominal cavity multiple distended and fluid-filled small bowel loops are present (*asterisk*). The transition point is in the midabdomen (*arrow*). On laparoscopy, an intusussception with a midgrade stenosis was found due to underlaying Crohn's disease with an adherent neighboring small bowel loop

16.3.3.5
Intussusception

Various extrinsic, intrinsic, or intraluminal processes may result in small bowel intussusception (ABIRI et al. 1986). Polypoid tumors are the most common cause of small bowel intussusception in adults (Fig. 16.13). Intussusception may occur in extrinsic disorders such as adhesions or duplications. The mechanism consists of an invagination of an entire proximal small bowel loop and part of its mesentery into the lumen of a more distal small bowel.

Although diagnosis on MRI alone may be difficult, on CT three patterns depending on the severity and duration of the disease have been described (MERINE et al. 1987): a sausage-shaped mass with a wall-in-wall appearance, a target sign, and a reniform mass.

16.3.4
Intraluminal Causes

16.3.4.1
Bezoars

Bezoars are an unusual cause of acute abdomen due to small bowel obstruction. Complete mechanical bowel obstruction is the most frequent clinical manifestation of bezoars. The obstruction caused by small bowel phytobezoars frequently occurs in the jejunum. One may find an intraluminal mass in the transition zone causing obstruction. Fluid in the small bowel helps to outline the mass, which has an inhomogeneous signal intensity with air retained in the interstices. An important differential diagnosis may be the small bowel feces sign in patients with high-grade small bowel obstruction.

16.3.4.2
Other Intraluminal Causes

Gallstones, foreign bodies, retained meconium, or tangles of ascarides may cause obstruction.

16.3.5
Developmental Causes

16.3.5.1
Malrotation

Intestinal malrotation is defined as an anomaly of rotation and fixation of the midgut. It is usually an isolated abnormality, but can be associated with

obstruction is caused by adhesions and by a luminal narrowing and dysmotility related to radiation mucositis and serositis. MRI may show the extent of mural thickening and mesenteric fibrosis.

16.3.3.4
Intramural Intestinal Hemorrhage

In adults, intramural intestinal hemorrhage may involve any portion of the small bowel and is usually a complication of anticoagulation therapy. However, it may also be secondary to any condition that predisposes to bleeding or result from trauma or biopsy.

Intramural intestinal hemorrhage most often involves the duodenum and jejunum. Detection on MRI depends on the "age" of the hematoma in view of the sequence used. The perception of the hematoma may also be impaired by a similar signal intensity of the bowel content.

congenital heart disease or situs problems (Balthasar 1976).

Intestinal malrotation in adults is usually an incidental finding. To underline the diagnosis, it is extremely helpful to identify and follow the entire small and large bowel pathway on all consecutive slices on MRI and CT. Findings include right-sided small bowel, left-sided colon, abnormal relationships between superior mesenteric vessels, and aplasia of the uncinate process.

Small bowel volvulus is usually secondary to various conditions such as malrotation, congenital bands, postoperative adhesions, and internal hernias.

If a u-shaped configuration or radial distribution of distended loops converging toward the point of torsion or a mesentery tightly wound around the point of torsion (whirl sign) is present, one should consider the diagnosis of a volvulus. The whirl sign of mesenteric vessels is not a very specific sign and may also be identified without volvulus.

16.4
Conclusion

The diagnosis of bowel obstruction and establishing the cause of obstruction is based on a comprehensive approach that includes clinical background, patient history, and results of physical examination.

Imaging modalities have to provide correct information on level, degree, and cause of the obstruction. In an acute setting, CT mainly is the modality of choice. MRI and especially functional cine MRI has potential as alternative techniques. Although until now, data are relatively limited, MRI proved to be correct in the detection of adhesions.

References

Abiri S, Baer J, Abiri M (1986) Computed tomography and sonography in small bowel intussusception: a case report. Am J Gastroenterol 81:1076–1077

Ahlberg G, Bergdahl S, Rutqvist J, et al (1997) Mechanical small-bowel obstruction after conventional appendectomy in children. Eur J Pediatr Surg 7:13–15

Balthazar EJ (1976) Intestinal malrotation in adults. AJR Am J Roentgenol 126:358–367

Balthazar EJ (1994) CT of small-bowel obstruction. AJR Am J Roentgenol 162:255–261

Bartram CI (1980) Radiologic demonstration of adhesions following surgery for inflammatory bowel disease. Br J Radiol 53:650–653

Beck DE, Opelka FG, Bailey HR, et al (1999) Incidence of small-bowel obstruction and adhesiolysis after open colorectal and general surgery. Dis Colon Rectum 42:241–248

Bizer LS, Liebling RW, Delany HM, et al (1981) Small bowel obstruction: the role of non-operative treatment in simple intestinal obstruction and predictive criteria for strangulation obstruction. Surgery 89:407–413

Deitel Vasic V (1979) Major intestinal complications of radiotherapy. Am J Gastroenterol 72:65–70

Dijkstra FR, Nieuwenhuijzen M, Reijnen MM, et al (2000) Recent clinical developments in pathophysiology, epidemiology, diagnosis and treatment of intra-abdominal adhesions. Scand J Gastroenterol Suppl 232:52–59

Ellis H, Moran BJ, Thompson JN, et al (1999) Adhesion-related hospital readmissions after abdominal and pelvic surgery: a retrospective cohort study. Lancet 353:1476–1480

Fisher JK (1981) Computed tomographic diagnosis of volvulus in intestinal malrotation. Radiology 140:145–146

Freys SM, Fuchs KH, Heimbucher J, et al (1994) Laparoscopic adhesiolysis. Surg Endosc 8:1202–1207

Fukuya T, Hawes D, Lu C, et al (1992) CT diagnosis of small-bowel obstruction: efficacy in 60 patients. Am J Roentgenol 158:765–769

Gazelle GS, Goldberg MA, Wittenberg J, et al (1994) Efficacy of CT in distinguishing small-bowel obstruction from other causes of small-bowel dilatation. Am J Roentgenol 162: 43–47

Kim AY, Bennett GL, Bashist B, et al (1998) Small bowel obstruction associated with sigmoid diverticulitis: CT evaluation in 16 patients. Am J Roentgenol 170:1311–1313

Kirchhoff S, Ladurner R, Kirchhoff C, et al (2009) Detection of recurrent hernia and intraabdominal adhesions following incisional hernia repair: a functional cine MRI-study. Abdom Imaging online first 29.03.09

Lang RA, Buhmann S, Hopman A, et al (2008) Cine-MRI detection of intraabdominal adhesions: correlation with intraoperative findings in 89 consecutive cases. Surg Endosc 22:2455–2461

Levine MS, Drooz AT, Herlinger H (1987) Annular malignancies of the small bowel. Gastrointest Radiol 12:53–58

Lienemann A, Sprenger D, Steitz HO, et al (2000) Detection and mapping of intraabdominal adhesions by using functional cine MR Imaging: preliminary results. Radiology 217:421–425

Mayo-Smith W, Wittenberg J, Bennett GL, et al (1995) The CT small bowel faeces sign: description and clinical significance. Clin Radiol 50:765–767

Megibow AJ (1994) Bowel obstruction: evaluation with CT. Radiol Clin North Am 32:861–870

Menzies D, Ellis H (1990) Intestinal obstruction from adhesions–how big is the problem? Ann R Coll Surg Engl 72:60–63

Merine D, Fishman EK, Jones B, et al (1987) Enteroenteric intussusception: CT findings in nine patients. AJR Am J Roentgenol 148:1129–1132

Nieuwenhuijzen M, Reijnen MM, Kuijpers JH, et al (1998) Small bowel obstruction after total or subtotal colectomy: a 10-year retrospective review. Br J Surg 85:1242–1245

Pedrosa I, Rofsky NM (2003) MR imaging in abdominal emergencies. Radiol Clin North Am 41:1243–1273

Sandhu PS, Joe BN, Coakley FV, et al (2007) Bowel transition points: multiplicity and posterior location at CT are associated with small-bowel volvulus. Radiology 245:160–167

Sarr MG, Bulkley GB, Zuidema GD (1983) Preoperative recognition of intestinal strangulation obstruction: prospective evaluation of diagnostic capability. Am J Surg 145:176–182

Semelka RC, Balci NC, Op de Beeck B, et al (1999) Evaluation of a 10-minute comprehensive MR imaging examination of the upper abdomen. Radiology 211:189–195

Sulaiman H, Dawson L, Laurent GJ, et al (2002) Role of plasminogen activators in peritoneal adhesion formation. Biochem Soc Trans 30:126–131

Vrijland WW, Tseng LN, Eijkman HJ, et al (2002) Fewer intraperitoneal adhesions with use of hyaluronic acid-carboxymethylcellulose membrane: a randomized clinical trial. Ann Surg 235:193–199

Vrijland WW, Jeekel J, van Geldorp HJ, et al (2003) Abdominal adhesions: intestinal obstruction, pain, and infertility. Surg Endosc 17:1017–1022

Zbar RI, Crede WB, McKhann CF, et al (1993) The postoperative incidence of small bowel obstruction following standard, open appendectomy and cholecystectomy: a six-year retrospective cohort study at Yale-New Haven Hospital. Conn Med 57:123–127

MRI of Acute Conditions of the Gastrointestinal Tract

Karen S. Lee and Ivan Pedrosa

CONTENTS

17.1 Introduction 283
17.2 Imaging Protocols 284
17.3 Specific Acute Conditions of the Gastrointestinal Tract 287
17.3.1 Acute Inflammatory Conditions of the Gastrointestinal Tract 287
17.3.1.1 Acute Appendicitis 287
17.3.1.2 Inflammatory Bowel Disease 293
17.3.1.3 Primary Epiploic Appendagitis 298
17.3.1.4 Colonic Diverticulitis 300
17.3.1.5 Peptic Ulcer Disease 301
17.3.1.6 Ectopic Pancreas 304
17.3.2 Acute Neoplastic Conditions of the Gastrointestinal Tract 304
17.3.3 Ischemia and Obstruction of the Gastrointestinal Tract 305
17.3.4 Infection of the Gastrointestinal Tract 308

17.4 Conclusion 309

References 311

KEY POINTS

Magnetic resonance imaging (MRI) has often been considered a second-line, alternative imaging modality for the evaluation of patients with suspected acute gastrointestinal tract pathology because of its limited availability, cost, and relatively long imaging times. The multiplanar capability and excellent soft-tissue contrast of MRI, combined with the advent of ultrafast MRI techniques, however, have increased the utilization of MRI in more recent years for the imaging assessment of acute conditions of the gastrointestinal tract. Furthermore, because of its lack of ionizing radiation, MRI not only plays an especially critical role in the imaging evaluation of pregnant patients presenting with acute abdominal symptoms, but also is evolving to become a principal imaging modality for the evaluation of young patients with inflammatory bowel disease. This chapter presents the general principles regarding the imaging protocols for the evaluation of appendicitis in pregnant and nonpregnant patients, and discusses the MRI appearances of a variety of common and uncommon acute conditions of the gastrointestinal tract.

17.1
Introduction

Traditionally, computed tomography (CT) has served as the primary imaging modality for the evaluation of patients presenting with acute abdominal pain and clinically suspected intestinal pathology, with MRI relegated as a second-line, problem-solving modality. The limited availability, expense, and long

Karen S. Lee, MD
Ivan Pedrosa, MD
Department of Radiology, Beth Israel Deaconess Medical Center, 330 Brookline Avenue, Boston, MA 02215, USA

acquisition times associated with MRI have hampered the widespread adoption of this modality in acute settings. Furthermore, in the past, MRI evaluation of the gastrointestinal tract, in particular, was challenging due to artifacts related to peristalsis and respiratory motion. In more recent years, however, MRI has come to be used increasingly to evaluate acute abdominal pain, especially in pregnant patients where ionizing radiation exposure from CT is undesirable, and in those patients allergic to iodinated contrast. Additionally, the multiplanar capability and excellent soft-tissue contrast of MRI, combined with the development of ultrafast MRI techniques, have enabled MRI to be increasingly employed for the diagnosis of acute gastrointestinal conditions. These particular characteristics of MRI are especially advantageous in patients in whom intravenous contrast is to be avoided, such as those with renal insufficiency or allergies to intravenous contrast agents. In this chapter, the imaging protocols used by the authors for the evaluation of suspected appendicitis in both pregnant and nonpregnant patients are presented, and the MRI appearance of a variety of common and rare acute conditions related to the gastrointestinal tract is discussed.

17.2 Imaging Protocols

The MRI protocol should be tailored for the specific indication and patient population. Previous chapters (Chaps. 1, 8, 9, and 11) in this book had discussed the protocols used for the targeted evaluation of the small bowel and large bowel. The protocol used by the authors to evaluate for suspected appendicitis both in pregnant (Table 17.1) and nonpregnant individuals will be specifically presented.

For all pregnant patients, informed consent is obtained prior to imaging. MRI is considered safe in pregnancy, and can be performed regardless of the trimester if the data obtained from the examination could potentially affect the care of the patient (KANAL et al. 2007). Patients are imaged in a supine position, and a body phased-array coil is recommended whenever possible because of its higher signal-to-noise ratio compared to the built-in body coil. The authors routinely administer oral contrast for improved distention and visualization of the bowel. An oral contrast preparation containing 450 mL of ferumoxsil (Gastromark, Mallinckrodt Medical, St Louis, MO)

Table 17.1. MRI protocol for pregnant patients with suspected appendicitis

	Pulse sequences					
	Coronal single-shot FSE	Axial single-shot FSE	Sagittal single-shot FSE	Axial 2D FS single-shot FSE	In phase and out of phase 2D T1W GRE	2D TOF
Repetition time (ms)	800–1,100	800–1,100	800–1,100	800–1,100	205	5,500
Echo time (ms)	60	60	60	60	2.2/4.5	100
Flip angle (degrees)	130–155	130–155	130–155	130–155	80	45
Section thickness (mm)	4	4	4	4	5	3
Gap (mm)	1	1	1	1	2	1
Field of view (mm)	350	350	350	350	350	350
Number of partitions or sections	20	20	20	20	32	24
Phase × frequency steps	192 × 256	192 × 256	192 × 256	192 × 256	160 × 256	128 × 256
Rectangular field of view	No	0.75	0.75	0.75	0.75	0.75
Bandwidth (kHz)[a]	62.5	62.5	62.5	62.5	62.5	31.25

FSE fast spin echo; *FS* fat-saturated; *IP* in-phase; *OP* opposed-phase; *T1W* T1-weighted; *TOF* time of flight
[a] 62.5 kHz = 488 Hz/pixel, 31.25 kHz = 244 Hz/pixel

combined with 300 mL of barium sulfate (Readi-Cat 2, E-Z-Em, Lake Success, NY) is administered 1–1.5 h prior to the MRI study. This iron-containing oral preparation acts as a negative contrast agent, therefore providing dark signal intensity on both T1- and T2-weighted sequences, without creating considerable susceptibility artifact (Liebig et al. 1993). In order to decrease bowel peristalsis, 1 mg of glucagon (Glucagen, Bedford Laboratories, Bedford, OH) is administered intramuscularly in nonpregnant patients immediately prior to the initiation of imaging. When butyl scopalaminebromide (Buscopan, Boehringer, Ingelheim, Germany) is allowed as bowel relaxant (not in the USA), this is preferred over glucagon. Imaging is obtained at suspended end expiration with each acquisition lasting approximately 20–24 s long.

The use of oral contrast in pregnant patients with suspected appendicitis is controversial. MRI without oral contrast has been used successfully to evaluate acute appendicitis in pregnancy (Cobben et al. 2004; Birchard et al. 2005; Oto et al. 2005; Israel et al. 2008; Oto et al. 2009), with excellent reported appendiceal visualization rates (Oto et al. 2005). Some authors have suggested that the lower visualization rate of the normal appendix in some of these studies, however, may be attributable to the absence of oral contrast material (Israel et al. 2008). A recent study comparing the visualization of the appendix in 26 pregnant patients without and with oral contrast found an improvement in interreader agreement for visualization of the appendix when oral contrast was used (Woodfield and Lazarus 2008). In the authors' experience, the increased confidence in the visualization of the appendix with oral contrast likely results in optimal negative laparotomy and perforation rates in the pregnant population (Pedrosa et al. 2009). The potential impact of oral contrast in the diagnosis of acute appendicitis in this particular patient population, however, requires further investigation.

Axial T1-weighted in-phase and opposed-phase gradient echo (GRE) imaging is useful for the characterization of soft-tissue lesions by enabling the detection of lipid, hemorrhagic, and proteinaceous contents (Pedrosa and Rofsky 2003). Additionally, magnetic susceptibility from air, calcium, or hemosiderin can be easily detected as a blooming effect on the longer echo time sequence (in-phase sequence on 1.5 T magnets) compared to the shorter echo time sequence (opposed-phase sequence on 1.5 T magnets) (Pedrosa et al. 2007).

Axial, sagittal, and coronal T2-weighted fast spin echo (FSE) or single-shot FSE imaging is performed for localization of anatomic structures and for identifying pathology. The addition of frequency-selective fat saturation pulse to these T2-weighted sequences allows for areas of edema, inflammation, and fluid to be highlighted. When compared to single-shot techniques, T2-weighted FSE techniques have higher in-plane resolution and higher signal-to-noise ratio due to multiple excitations, but are more sensitive to motion artifacts (Regan et al. 1998; Pedrosa et al. 2007). Therefore, in pregnant patients who may have a limited breath-hold capability and in whom fetal motion can cause substantial image degradation, motion-insensitive single-shot FSE techniques are essential for accurate evaluation (Eyvazzadeh et al. 2004; Oto et al. 2005; Pedrosa et al. 2007). Additionally, the use of respiratory-triggered single-shot sequences can not only be helpful in patients with limited breath-hold capability, but also to ensure that sequential imaging of the bowel is obtained. The sensitivity of single-shot FSE acquisitions for the detection of lesions and inflammatory changes can be improved by optimizing the dynamic range of these images with the addition of a frequency-selective fat saturation pulse.

In nonpregnant patients, pre- and dynamic post-contrast 3D fat-saturated T1-weighted spoiled GRE are routinely acquired in patients presenting with suspected appendicitis without renal failure (estimated glomerular filtration rate greater than 30 mL/min). Compared to 2D acquisitions, 3D sequences provide higher signal-to-noise ratio, and allow for thinner sections and multiplanar reformations to be generated (Rofsky et al. 1999; Pedrosa et al. 2007). A 0.1 mmol/kg dose of gadopentetate dimeglumine (Magnevist; Berlex Laboratories, Wayne, NJ) is administered at a rate 2 mL/s followed by a 20-mL dose of saline at the same rate. A 2-mL test bolus of the gadolinium-based contrast agent is injected at 2 mL/s to appropriately time the arterial phase (Earls et al. 1997). Arterial phase, portal venous phase (20 s after the arterial phase), and delayed venous phase (60 s after the arterial phase) imaging is then obtained.

Gadolinium-based contrast agents are not considered safe in pregnancy (Shellock and Crues 2004). In pregnant patients where the use of gadolinium-based contrast agents is contraindicated, axial 2D time-of-flight GRE T2*-weighted images are useful for differentiating the appendix from mimickers, primarily pelvic venous varices, which are common in

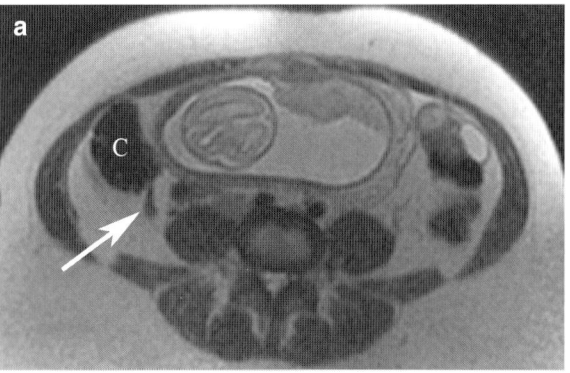

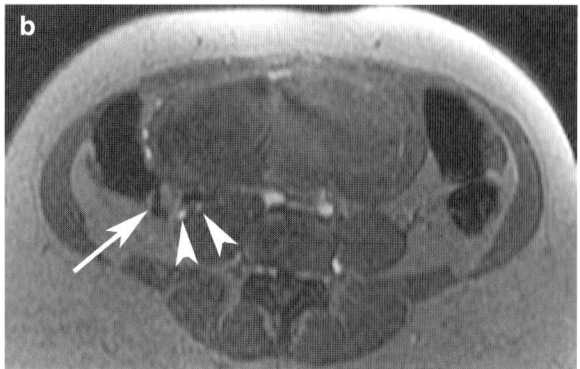

Fig. 17.1. (a) Axial T2-weighted single-shot FSE image of the pelvis in a pregnant patient at 14-week gestational age demonstrates both the cecum (*C*) and the normal appendix (*arrow*) to be filled with negative oral contrast material, thereby appearing as low signal intensity structures. **(b)** Axial time-of-flight GRE image at the same level shows the appendix (*arrow*) to be mildly enlarged and decreased in signal intensity when compared with the T2-weighted single-shot FSE image, compatible with the blooming effect. Pelvic veins (*arrowheads*) are seen as high signal intensity structures, aiding differentiation from the normal appendix

pregnant patients, particularly in their third trimester. An appendix containing either air or the iron-containing oral contrast material within its lumen (i.e. normal appendix) exhibits susceptibility effect on this sequence, appearing as a low signal intensity structure with a blooming effect (Fig. 17.1) (Pedrosa et al. 2007). Venous varices, in distinction, will appear as high signal intensity structures on the time-of-flight sequences due to the presence of flow (Pedrosa et al. 2007).

Diffusion-weighted imaging (DWI) has become increasingly used in a variety of abdominal applications because of its ability to highlight areas of neoplastic involvement (Ichikawa et al. 2007; Parikh et al. 2008; Zhang et al. 2008) and acute inflammatory and infectious conditions without the need for intravenous contrast material administration (Chan et al. 2001; Verswijvel et al. 2002; Fattahi et al. 2009). Potentially, DWI may serve as an alternative to contrast material-enhanced sequences in those patients in whom gadolinium-based contrast agents are contraindicated, such as in pregnant patients, and those patients with renal insufficiency at risk for developing nephrogenic systemic fibrosis (Sadowski et al. 2007; Kim et al. 2009; Taouli et al. 2009). The authors have now begun to use DWI in pregnant patients presenting with acute abdominal pain. For this application, the authors use a respiratory-triggered, axial, single-shot echo-planar diffusion-weighted sequence with the following parameters: slice thickness, 5 mm with no gap; repetition time, one respiratory cycle; echo time, 60–85 ms; matrix, 64 × 64; field of view, 30–35 cm; b values, 0 and 1,000 s/mm^2. The use of respiratory triggering improves anatomic co-registration and minimizes artifacts related to respiratory motion. The use of respiratory bellows, however, may be challenging in pregnancy due to the protuberance of the abdomen from the gravid uterus, particularly in the third trimester, which may result in respirations too shallow for triggering image acquisition. Respiratory triggering using navigator techniques may be more optimal for this particular application; however, this requires further investigation. Anecdotally, the authors have found that DWI may have value in diagnosing different acute conditions resulting in abdominal pain, including genitourinary conditions such as pyelonephritis and degenerating fibroids, and acute conditions of the gastrointestinal tract including acute flares of inflammatory bowel disease and acute appendicitis (Fig. 17.2). The use of DWI in the diagnosis of acute gastrointestinal tract conditions in the abdomen, however, remains in the early stages of validation.

In order for MRI to become more generalized for use in nonpregnant patients presenting with acute abdominal pain, shorter imaging protocols need to be developed. The lack of anatomic distortion in nonpregnant patients may facilitate the implementation of a simpler and shorter MRI protocol for the evaluation of acute appendicitis (Cobben et al. 2009). Additionally, the use of alternative sources of image contrast such as DWI may further enhance the implementation of such protocols in the general population.

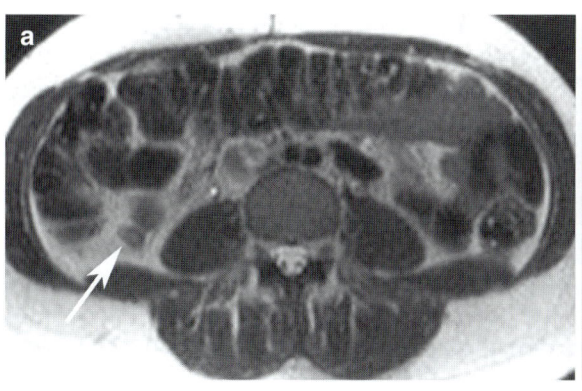

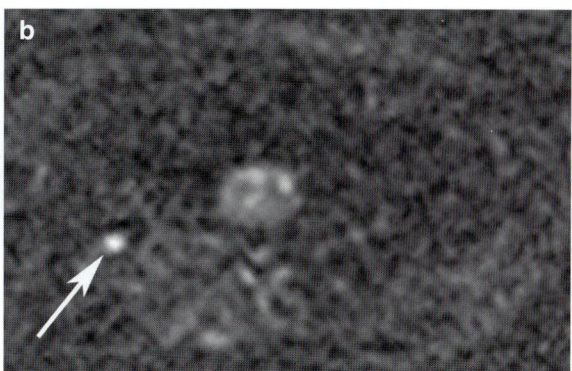

Fig. 17.2. (a) Axial T2-weighted single-shot FSE image in a pregnant patient at 11-week gestational age demonstrates a thick-walled, fluid-filled, dilated appendix measuring 9 mm, compatible with early, uncomplicated, acute appendicitis (*arrow*). (b) Diffusion-weighted image ($b=1,000\,s/mm^2$) obtained at the same level shows markedly high signal within the appendix (*arrow*). Acute appendicitis was confirmed at surgery and pathologic analysis

17.3
Specific Acute Conditions of the Gastrointestinal Tract

In the following sections, the MRI appearances of a variety of common and uncommon GI conditions that manifest as acute abdominal pain will be presented and organized by etiology, including inflammatory, neoplastic, ischemic, and infectious causes.

17.3.1
Acute Inflammatory Conditions of the Gastrointestinal Tract

Various acute inflammatory conditions of the GI tract will be addressed in the following section, including appendicitis, inflammatory bowel disease, epiploic appendagitis, colonic diverticulitis, peptic ulcer disease, and ectopic pancreas.

17.3.1.1
Acute Appendicitis

Because of their widespread availability, relatively low cost, and excellent accuracy rates, CT and ultrasound serve as the primary imaging modalities used to diagnose acute appendicitis in adults (Van Randen et al. 2008). In more recent years, however, MRI has become increasing utilized for the evaluation of appendicitis, particularly in children and in pregnant patients, where exposure to ionizing radiation is an important consideration (Incesu et al. 1997; Cobben et al. 2004; Birchard et al. 2005; Oto et al. 2005; Pedrosa et al. 2006, 2007; Oto et al. 2009). MRI has demonstrated excellent performance in diagnosing acute appendicitis both in nonpregnant and pregnant patients. In 60 consecutive nonpregnant patients, Incesu and colleagues (1997) showed gadolinium-enhanced MRI was superior to ultrasound in identifying acute appendicitis with a sensitivity of 97%, specificity of 92%, positive predictive value of 94%, negative predictive value of 96%, and accuracy of 95%. More recently, Pedrosa et al. (2006) in a study of 51 consecutive pregnant patients demonstrated noncontrast-enhanced MRI to have an overall sensitivity of 100%, specificity of 93.6%, prevalence-adjusted positive predictive value of 1.4%, prevalence-adjusted negative predictive value of 100%, and accuracy of 94% in the diagnosis of acute appendicitis. While ultrasound remains the first-line imaging study of choice for evaluating for acute appendicitis in pregnancy, MRI is an important adjunctive study for excluding appendicitis in pregnant patients with inconclusive ultrasound results (Pedrosa et al. 2006, 2007; Patel et al. 2007).

A recent report by Cobben et al. (2009) has demonstrated the feasibility of noncontrast-enhanced MRI in the initial assessment of nonpregnant patients with suspected acute appendicitis with excellent sensitivity and specificity for the diagnosis of acute appendicitis. Using a protocol consisting of axial and coronal T1-weighted FSE imaging, and T2-weighted FSE imaging with and without fat suppression, MRI was able to diagnose appendicitis with a sensitivity and specificity of 100% and 99%, respectively (Cobben et al. 2009). Furthermore, in those patients without appendicitis, MRI was able to provide an alternative diagnosis in 55% of the remaining patients (Cobben et al. 2009).

Imaging Features of the Normal Appendix

The normal appendix is a blind-ending tubular structure, typically arising from the medial base of the cecum, approximately 3 cm inferior to the ileocecal valve, averaging 10 cm in length with a wall thickness less than 2 mm (Birnbaum and Wilson 2000). The normal appendix is either collapsed, or partially filled with air, fluid, or oral contrast (Birnbaum and Wilson 2000). The appendix appears as a cord-like structure, which is intermediate in signal intensity on both T1- and T2-weighted images, similar in signal to muscle (Nitta et al. 2005; Pedrosa et al. 2006). When the appendix contains oral contrast (using ferumoxsil combined with barium sulfate as routinely prepared at our institution) and/or air, low signal is seen within the appendiceal lumen on both T1- and T2-weighted imaging with the blooming effect identified on T2* time-of-flight (Fig. 17.1) or T1-weighted in-phase (longer echo time) GRE sequences (Pedrosa et al. 2006, 2007). The normal appendix has a diameter measuring 6 mm or less on single-shot FSE imaging (Pedrosa et al. 2006). The visualization rate of the normal appendix on MRI ranges from 86 to 90% in nonpregnant individuals (Hormann et al. 2002; Nitta et al. 2005) and 87 to 89% in pregnant patients (Oto et al. 2005; Pedrosa et al. 2006). Recently, the rate of visualization of the normal appendix in pregnant patients on MRI has been shown to be significantly higher than that of ultrasound (<2%) (Pedrosa et al. 2009). Furthermore, identification of the normal appendix in pregnant patients virtually excludes the presence of appendicitis and may avoid unnecessary laparotomies. In their series of 148 pregnant patients presenting with suspected appendicitis, Pedrosa et al. (2009) demonstrated a normal appendix with MRI in 87% (116/134) of their patients, which resulted in a negative predictive value of 100%. In this series, a negative laparotomy rate of 7% would have been achievable without incurring an increased perforation rate (21%), if the decision to avoid surgical exploration was based on a negative MRI (i.e. normal appendix seen, or nonvisualization of the appendix without inflammatory changes or secondary signs of appendicitis seen on MRI) (Pedrosa et al. 2009).

In pregnancy, identification of the appendix may be challenging due to alterations in anatomy from the enlarging, gravid uterus. While the appendix is superiorly displaced with increasing gestational age, the gestational age has been found to be a poor predictor of the location of the appendix on an individual basis (Lee et al. 2008b). The authors have found that when the cecum is superiorly tilted 90° or higher with respect to the plane of the imaging table on sagittal MR images, the appendix can be localized to the right upper quadrant of the abdomen (i.e. above the fourth lumbar vertebral body) with a specificity of 98%, irrespective of gestational age (Lee et al. 2008b).

Imaging Features of Acute Appendicitis

In acute appendicitis, the inflamed appendix typically appears as a dilated fluid-filled structure, which is hyperintense on T2-weighted imaging and hypointense on T1-weighted imaging, and measures 7 mm or greater on single-shot FSE sequences (Fig. 17.3) (Hormann et al. 2002; Cobben et al. 2004; Birchard et al. 2005; Oto et al. 2005; Pedrosa et al. 2006, 2007). As the material within the appendiceal lumen becomes more purulent, the signal intensity within the lumen decreases on T2-weighted imaging, appearing slightly hypointense relative to fluid. In these cases, the diagnosis of appendicitis on MRI is usually unequivocal because of associated marked appendiceal enlargement (Fig. 17.4). Periappendiceal inflammation may appear as band-like areas of high signal intensity on T2-weighted images, which is highlighted with fat suppression techniques (Pedrosa et al. 2007). In cases of early appendicitis, the presence of periappendiceal edema may precede dilation of the appendix (Fig. 17.5) (Pedrosa et al. 2007). The wall of the inflamed appendix is thickened and edematous, which is hypointense on T1-weighted images and slightly hyperintense on T2-weighted imaging (Pedrosa et al. 2006, 2007). Single-shot FSE images are particularly valuable for contrasting the thickened wall of the inflamed appendix from the hyperintense signal within the lumen of the appendix and the edema within the surrounding periappendiceal fat (Fig. 17.6) (Pedrosa et al. 2007). On contrast-enhanced fat-suppressed T1-weighted sequences, the appendix demonstrates marked mural enhancement (Fig. 17.7) (Incesu et al. 1997; Singh et al. 2009). While CT is considered superior for the

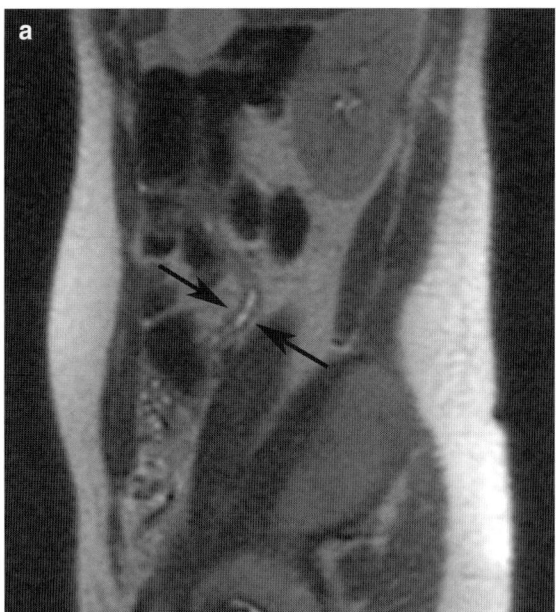

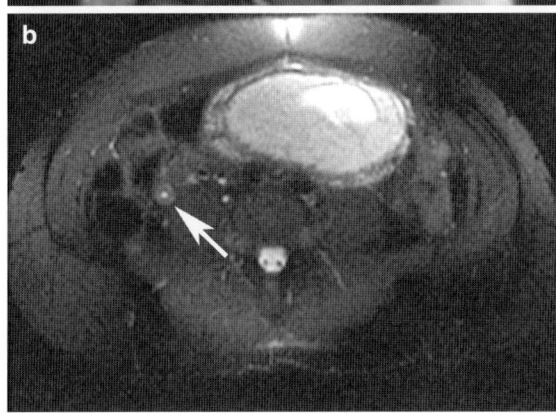

Fig. 17.3. (a) Sagittal T2-weighted single-shot FSE image of the pelvis in a pregnant patient at 14-week gestational age shows a thick-walled, fluid-filled tubular structure dilated to 8 mm (*arrows*) compatible with early, uncomplicated acute appendicitis. Note the surrounding bowel contains negative oral contrast material. (b) On axial T2-weighted, fat-suppressed, single-shot FSE image, the appendix demonstrates marked circumferential mural edema (*white arrow*) with a high-signal intensity, fluid-filled lumen centrally

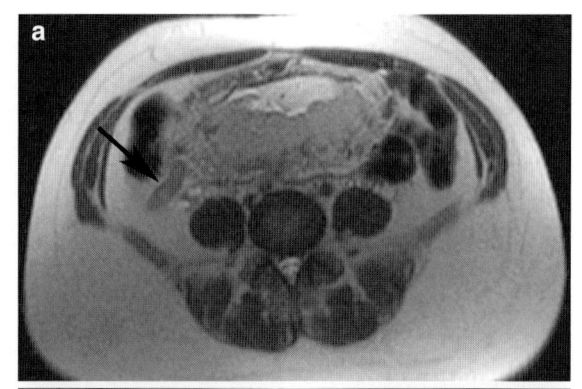

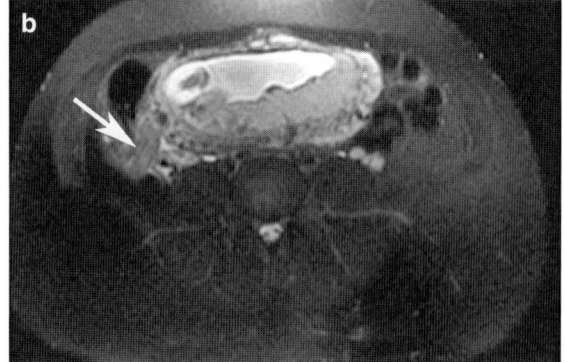

Fig. 17.4. (a) Axial T2-weighted single-shot FSE image of the pelvis in a pregnant patient at 16-week gestational age demonstrates a diffusely dilated appendix (*arrow*) measuring up to 10 mm, which is mildly increased in signal intensity and not filled normally with air or oral contrast material, compatible with uncomplicated acute appendicitis. (b) Axial T2-weighted fat-suppressed single-shot FSE of the pelvis shows the dilated appendix (*arrow*) with high signal in the surrounding periappendiceal fat compatible with edema

depiction of appendicoliths, when visible on MRI, appendicoliths appear as low signal intensity foci on all imaging sequences (Fig. 17.8) (PEDROSA et al. 2007). Although the appearance of appendicoliths on MRI may mimic air, the presence of obstruction, such as dilation of the appendix distally, suggests that an intraluminal low signal intensity focus within the appendix may be an appendicolith.

MRI can depict complications from appendicitis including appendiceal rupture with periappendiceal phlegmon and abscess formation. Phlegmons typically present as ill-defined heterogeneous periappendiceal masses, which are moderately high in signal intensity on T2-weighted images (Fig. 17.9), and demonstrate increased enhancement on postcontrast T1-weighted fat-suppressed sequences (INCESU et al. 1997; PEDROSA et al. 2007; SINGH et al. 2009). Abscesses appear as periappendiceal fluid-filled collections which are hyperintense on T2-weighted imaging and contain a well-demarcated, enhancing wall (Fig. 17.10) (INCESU et al. 1997; PEDROSA et al. 2007).

An appendix that measures 6–7 mm and does not contain air or oral contrast material within its lumen is considered indeterminate (PEDROSA et al. 2006). In these cases, careful evaluation for secondary findings including periappendiceal fat stranding, appendiceal wall thickening, phlegmon, and abscess formation can help determine the proper diagnosis

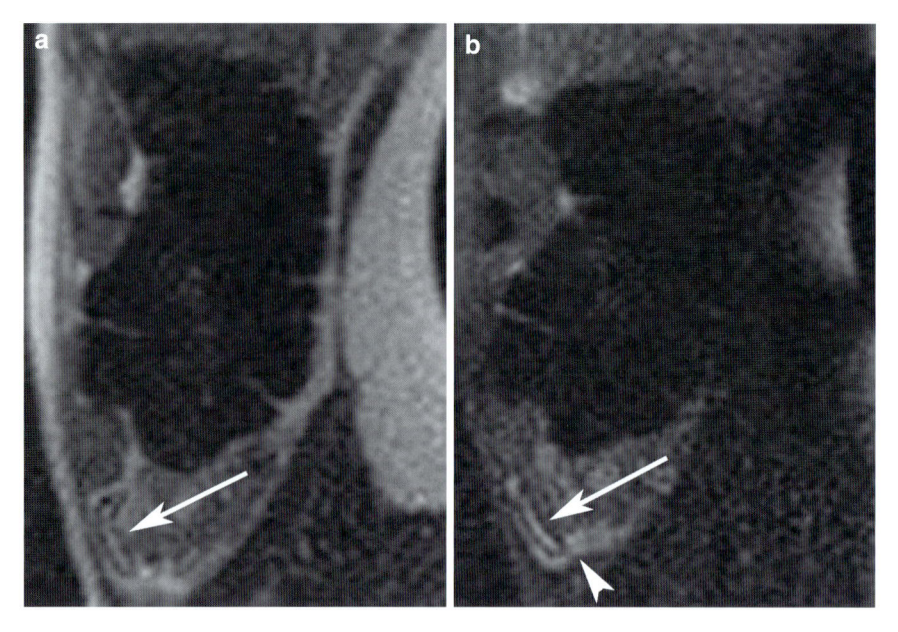

Fig. 17.5. (a) Sagittal T2-weighted single-shot FSE image in a 25-year-old pregnant patient at 31-week gestational age demonstrates a fluid-filled, normal-caliber appendix (*arrow*) measuring 6 mm. (b) On the sagittal T2-weighted single-shot FSE image with fat suppression obtained at the same level, the fluid-filled appendix is re-demonstrated (*arrow*), with high signal within the periappendiceal region indicating edema and inflammation (*arrowhead*). Acute appendicitis was confirmed at surgery and pathologic analysis

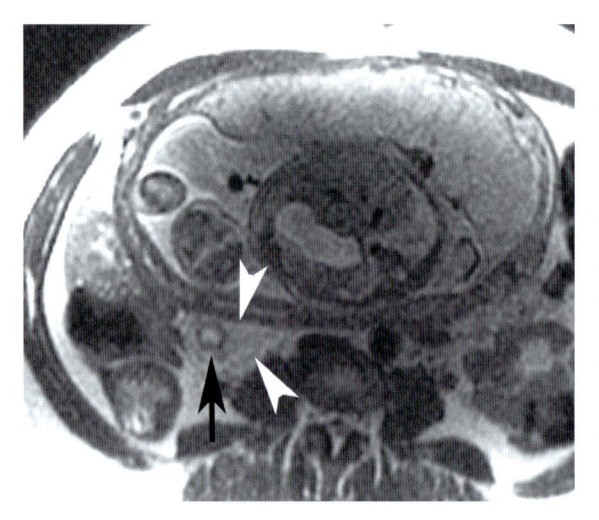

Fig. 17.6. Axial T2-weighted single-shot FSE image in a 30-year-old pregnant patient at 31-weeks gestational age presenting with right lower quadrant abdominal pain demonstrates a dilated, thick-walled appendix containing high signal within the lumen compatible with fluid, measuring up to 15 mm (*black arrow*). High signal within the periappendiceal fat is compatible with inflammatory stranding (*arrowheads*). Findings were compatible with acute appendicitis, which was confirmed at surgery and pathologic analysis

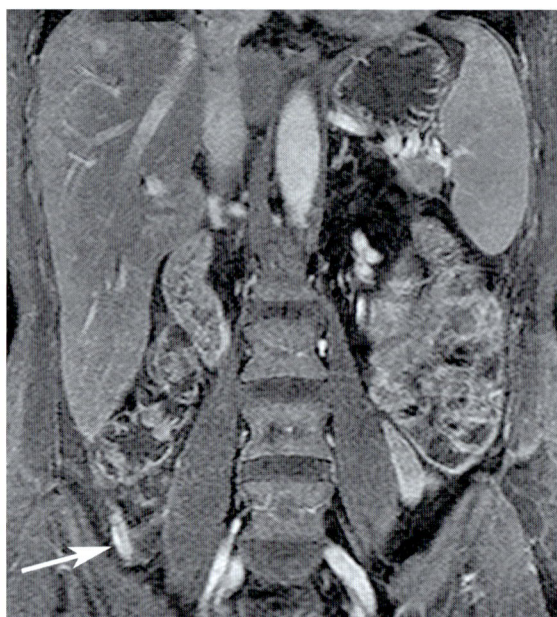

Fig. 17.7. Coronal, contrast-enhanced, fat-saturated, spoiled GRE T1-weighted image of the abdomen and pelvis in a 60-year-old woman with right lower quadrant pain demonstrates a mildly dilated appendix with hyperenhancing walls (*arrow*) compatible with acute appendicitis

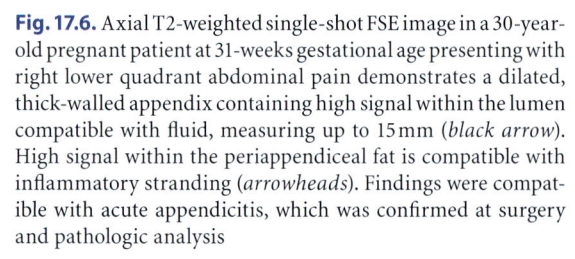

(Pedrosa et al. 2007). Close clinical observation combined with follow-up MRI is often advised for these uncertain situations. Similar to CT, nonvisualization of the appendix on MRI without the presence of secondary inflammatory findings can be used to exclude the presence of acute appendicitis (Ganguli et al. 2006; Garcia et al. 2009; Pedrosa et al. 2009).

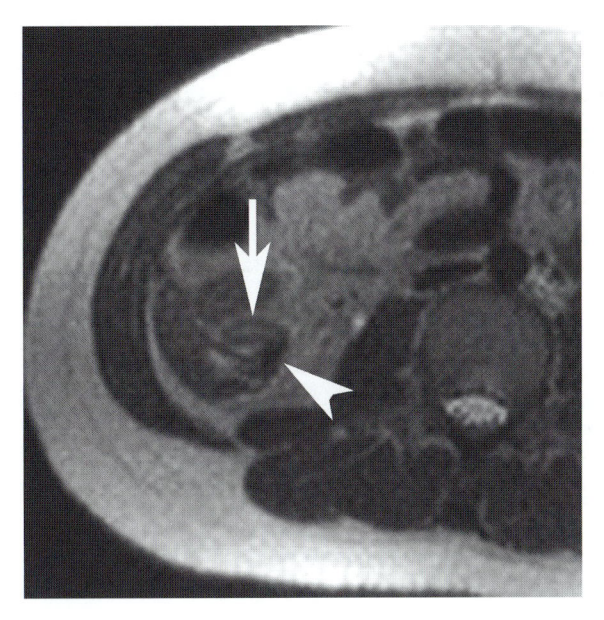

Fig. 17.8. Axial T2-weighted single-shot FSE image in a 25-year-old pregnant woman at 16-week gestational age with acute appendicitis demonstrates a dilated appendix containing high signal within its lumen (*arrow*) with mild surrounding periappendiceal fat stranding, and a low signal intensity focus within the lumen compatible with an appendicolith (*arrowhead*)

Alternative Diagnoses

Appendiceal mucoceles are an important mimicker of acute appendicitis on MRI. A mucocele is an abnormal intraluminal accumulation of mucus within a dilated appendix (CARR et al. 1995). The prevalence of mucoceles at appendectomy is low, reportedly ranging from 0.2 to 0.3% (AHO et al. 1973; HIGA et al. 1973). Four histologic subtypes of mucoceles have been described, ranging from benign to malignant: postobstructive mucous retention cyst (simple mucocele); mucosal hyperplasia; mucinous cystadenoma; and mucinous cystadenocarcinoma (HIGA et al. 1973; QIZILBASH 1975). Mucoceles usually are found incidentally or present with chronic right lower quadrant abdominal pain. When mucoceles become acutely inflamed or rupture, these lesions present with acute right lower quadrant pain and are clinically indistinguishable from acute appendicitis (PICKHARDT et al. 2002; BENNETT et al. 2009).

A mucocele typically appears as a well-circumscribed, spherical or tubular mass arising from the base of the cecum, containing mucinous material which appears as hyperintense signal on T2-weighted imaging (Fig. 17.11) (MADWED et al. 1992; PICKHARDT et al. 2003; PEDROSA et al. 2007). While both acute

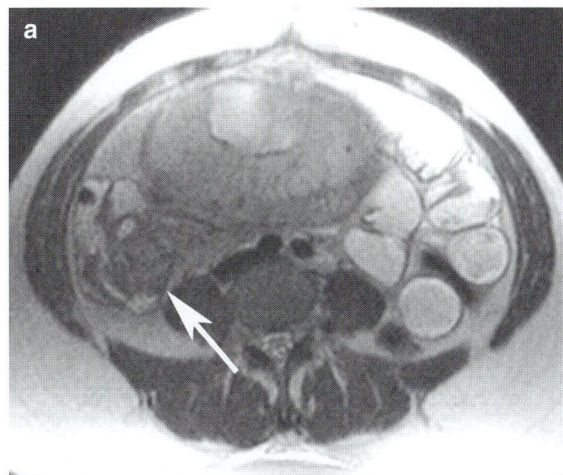

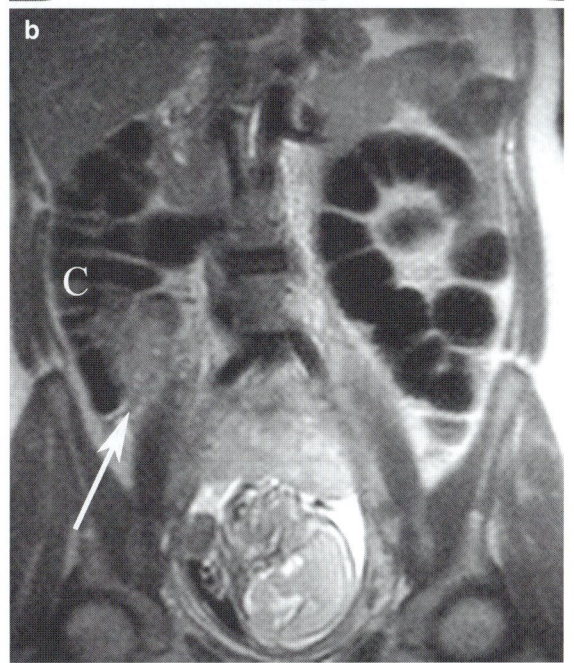

Fig. 17.9. (a) Axial T2-weighted single shot FSE image of the pelvis in a pregnant patient at 22-week gestational age with right lower quadrant pain and perforated appendicitis shows fluid-filled, dilated loops of small bowel in the left hemiabdomen compatible with a small bowel obstruction, with a transition point in the right lower quadrant at the level of an ill-defined heterogeneous mass, compatible with a periappendiceal phlegmon (*arrow*). (b) Follow-up study in the same patient with negative oral contrast agent now reaching the ascending colon confirms the presence of a periappendiceal phlegmon (*arrow*) exerting mass effect upon the adjacent cecum (*C*)

appendicitis and appendiceal mucoceles appear as dilated appendices containing intraluminal high signal on T2-weighting imaging, mucoceles often lack the associated periappendiceal fat stranding and

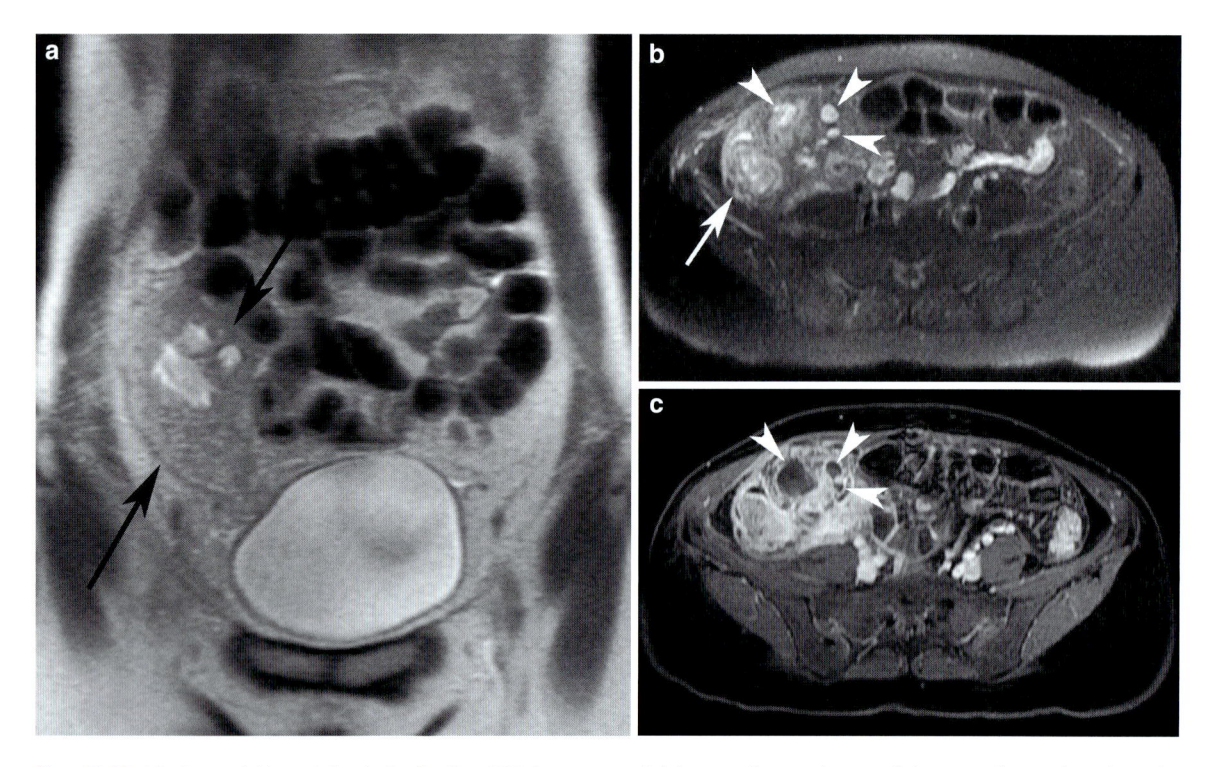

Fig. 17.10. (a) Coronal T2-weighted single-shot FSE image obtained in a 46-year-old female with perforated appendicitis after an inconclusive CT examination demonstrates a large, heterogeneous, ill-defined region of signal abnormality in the right lower quadrant of the abdomen (*arrows*) compatible with an extensive area of inflammation and phlegmonous change. Several small focal areas of increased signal intensity within this area of signal abnormality are compatible with abscesses. (b) Axial T2-weighted fat-suppressed axial image shows abnormal increased signal within the right lower quadrant including the cecum (*arrow*), compatible with edema and inflammation, with small abscesses (*arrowheads*) depicted as small, well-delineated round collections of high signal. (c) Axial, contrast-enhanced, fat-saturated, spoiled GRE T1-weighted image demonstrates extensive abnormal enhancement of the phlegmonous changes within the right lower quadrant, with rim-enhancement of the small abscesses (*arrowheads*)

mural thickening seen with acute appendicitis (PEDROSA et al. 2007). In addition, the degree of appendiceal dilation seen with a mucocele is often disproportionate to the extent of periappendiceal inflammatory changes, except when mucocele has ruptured or become inflamed (PICKHARDT et al. 2002; PEDROSA et al. 2007; BENNETT et al. 2009). Specifically, an appendiceal diameter of greater than 15 mm suggests the presence of a mucocele or appendiceal neoplasm (PICKHARDT et al. 2003; BENNETT et al. 2009). Visualization of a focal enhancing mass can suggest the presence of mucinous cystadenoma or cystadenocarcinoma (PICKHARDT et al. 2002; PEDROSA et al. 2007).

Mucocele perforation can lead to spillage of mucinous contents into the peritoneal cavity, resulting in focal or diffuse pseudomyxomatous peritonei (QIZILBASH 1975; LANDEN et al. 1992). On imaging, a perforated mucocele may be virtually indistinguishable from perforated acute appendicitis (BENNETT et al. 2009). A ruptured mucocele may appear as cystic dilation of the appendix with an abnormally thickened and enhancing wall with surrounding periappendiceal inflammatory stranding and fluid (Fig. 17.12).

Inflammation of residual appendiceal tissue left after an inadvertent, incomplete appendectomy is extremely rare, a condition known as stump appendicitis (MANGI and BERGER 2000; TRUTY et al. 2008). A potential increased risk of stump appendicitis has been reported with the use of laparoscopic techniques (GREENBERG and ESPOSITO 1996; WALSH and ROEDIGER 1997). Stump appendicitis can appear similar to acute appendicitis at CT if the remnant appendiceal stump is long, with mural enhancement and adjacent pericecal fat stranding (SHIN et al. 2005). Additionally, the arrowhead sign has been described in stump appendicitis where inflammation

These imaging findings, however, are nonspecific and other inflammatory and infectious conditions can cause similar findings within the appendiceal base (Fig. 17.13). Other differential diagnoses are in the following sections.

17.3.1.2
Inflammatory Bowel Disease

With its multiplanar capability, excellent soft-tissue contrast, the development of ultrafast imaging pulse sequences, and lack of ionizing radiation, MRI is ideally suited for the imaging evaluation of inflammatory bowel disease, particularly in chronic relapsing conditions such as Crohn's disease and ulcerative colitis where repeated imaging examinations are needed to assess disease status. Several reports have shown MRI to have sensitivities greater than 90% for the detection of active inflammation in Crohn's disease (Low et al. 2000; Koh et al. 2001; Gourtsoyiannis et al. 2002). A recent study by Lee and colleagues comparing CT and MR enterography with small bowel follow through found the three modalities equally accurate in the detection of active inflammation in the small bowel in patients with Crohn's disease (Lee et al. 2009). Additionally, extraenteric complications of inflammatory bowel disease, including fistulas, sinus tracts, and abscesses, are well depicted with MRI (Furukawa et al. 2004; Bernstein et al. 2005; Lee et al. 2009). When compared with small bowel follow through, Lee and colleagues showed MR enterography to have an improved detection rate, equivalent to that of CT enterography, in the detection of extraenteric complications (Lee et al. 2009).

The MRI findings in inflammatory bowel disease are extensively discussed in separate chapters in this book (Chaps. 8 and 9). Here we emphasize the role of MRI in evaluating acute complications in inflammatory bowel disease. With active inflammatory bowel disease, the bowel wall is thickened more than 3 mm, with bowel wall edema appearing as high signal within the wall on T2-weighted imaging (Furukawa et al. 2004). On T2-weighted single-shot FSE imaging, mural stratification is often seen in active, inflamed bowel segments where a central layer of high signal intensity is sandwiched on both sides by a layer of intermediate signal intensity within the bowel wall (Furukawa et al. 2004; Siddiki and Fidler 2009). Postcontrast administration, marked mural enhancement, and mural stratification can be seen within actively diseased bowel loops, with the intensity of

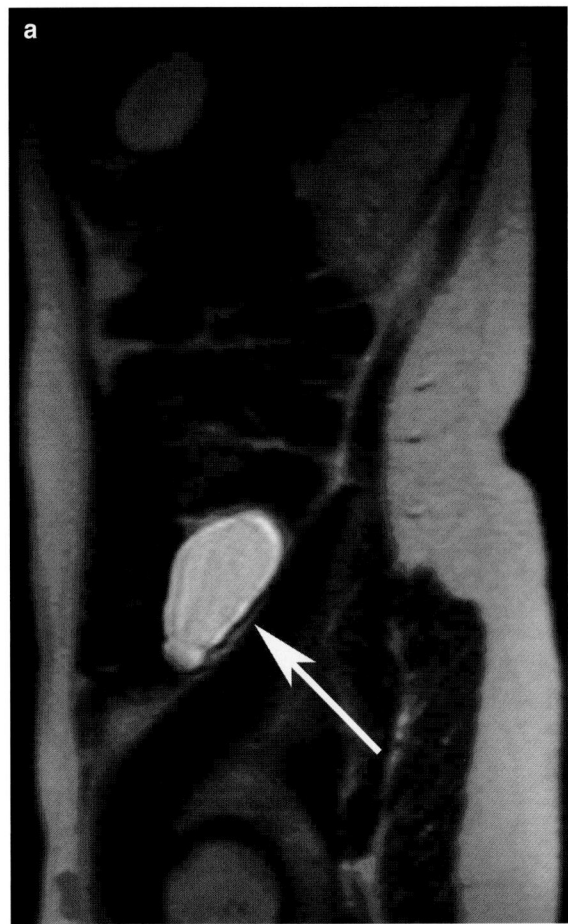

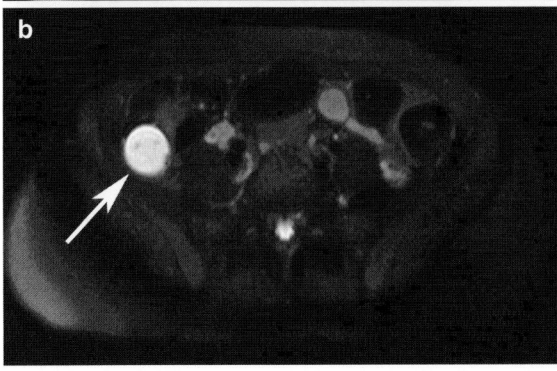

Fig. 17.11. (a) Sagittal T2-weighted single-shot FSE image of a woman with an appendiceal mucinous cystadenoma demonstrates a dilated, bulbous appendix (*arrow*) with a diameter greater than 3 cm, containing high signal within its lumen, compatible with mucin. (b) On the axial, T2-weighted, fat-suppressed image, wall thickening and periappendiceal inflammatory changes are noted to be absent about the appendiceal mucinous cystadenoma

at the cecal base and origin of the appendiceal orifice results in a funneling of oral contrast material in the cecum in the shape of an arrowhead (Rao et al. 1998).

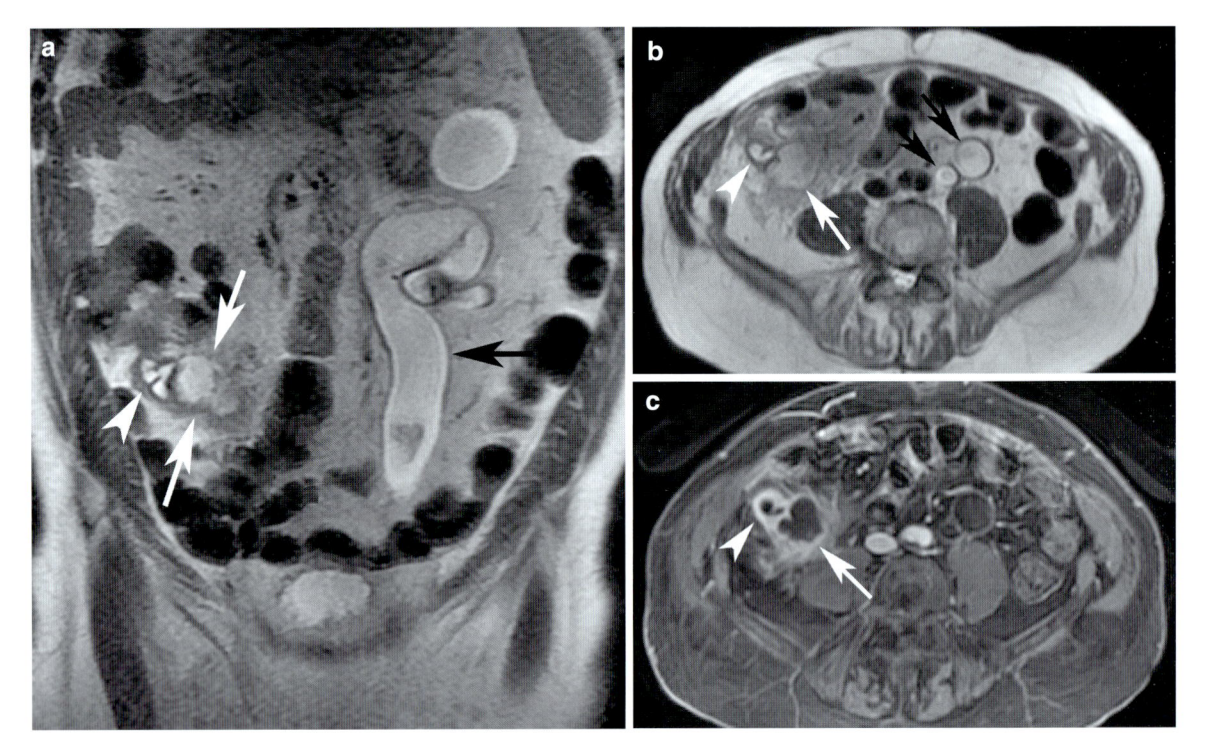

Fig. 17.12. (**a**) Coronal, and (**b**) axial, T2-weighted single-shot FSE images in a 76-year-old-male with a ruptured mucocele demonstrates a dilated, thick-walled, tubular structure arising from the cecal base containing high signal material, compatible with an appendiceal mucocele (*arrowhead*). An adjacent periappendiceal fluid collection is present with inflammatory stranding (*white arrows*). Incidental note was made of left hydroureter (*black arrow* in **a**) and duplicated collecting system (*black arrows* in **b**). (**c**) Axial, contrast-enhanced, fat-saturated, spoiled GRE T1-weighted image shows marked mural enhancement of the appendiceal mucocele (*arrowhead*) and the adjacent abscess with phlegmonous change (*arrow*)

enhancement reflective of the degree of disease activity (Figs. 17.14 and 17.15) (Maccioni et al. 2000, 2006; Siddiki and Fidler 2009).

MRI readily and accurately depicts the number and extent of diseased bowel segments, the presence of skip lesions, pseudo-diverticulae formation, and areas of luminal caliber change, including stenosis, and bowel dilation (Furukawa et al. 2004; Siddiki and Fidler 2009). Ulcerations may be depicted on MRI as areas of mural irregularity on T2-weighted and contrast-enhanced sequences (Siddiki and Fidler 2009).

MRI is particularly useful for depicting the extramural manifestations of active inflammatory bowel disease. Balanced steady-state free precession (TrueFISP or FIESTA), and gadolinium-enhanced, fat-suppressed, spoiled GRE T1-weighted sequences are especially helpful for delineating the increased vascularity and engorgement of the vasa recta within areas of mesenteric fatty proliferation, a finding known as the comb sign (Figs. 17.14 and 17.15). Areas of edema and inflammation within the mesenteric and perienteric fat appear as high signal intensity regions on T2-weighted imaging, which is more conspicuous with fat-suppression, and demonstrate enhancement on contrast-enhanced sequences (Fig. 17.15) (Furukawa et al. 2004; Siddiki and Fidler 2009). Sinus and fistula tracts appear as fluid-filled linear areas of signal abnormality with peripheral enhancement (Fig. 17.16). Tracts with a primarily inflammatory component demonstrate homogeneous enhancement without central fluid as the tract is filled with enhancing granulation tissue (Siddiki and Fidler 2009). Complex internal tracts may demonstrate a stellate configuration, radiating from a central point with associated bowel retraction and tethering (Herrmann et al. 2006). Phlegmons appear as ill-defined soft-tissue masses with heterogeneous, mildly increased signal on T2-weighted imaging, and demonstrate avid enhancement Postcontrast administration (Fig 17.17). Abscesses appear as fluid-filled collections, which may contain air, with well-defined, enhancing walls (Fig. 17.18) (Pedrosa et al. 2007; Siddiki and Fidler 2009).

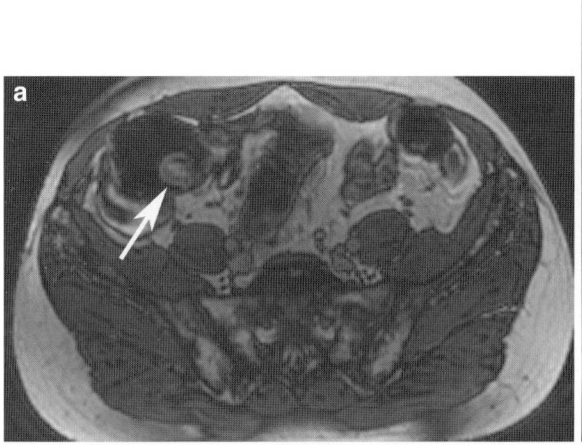

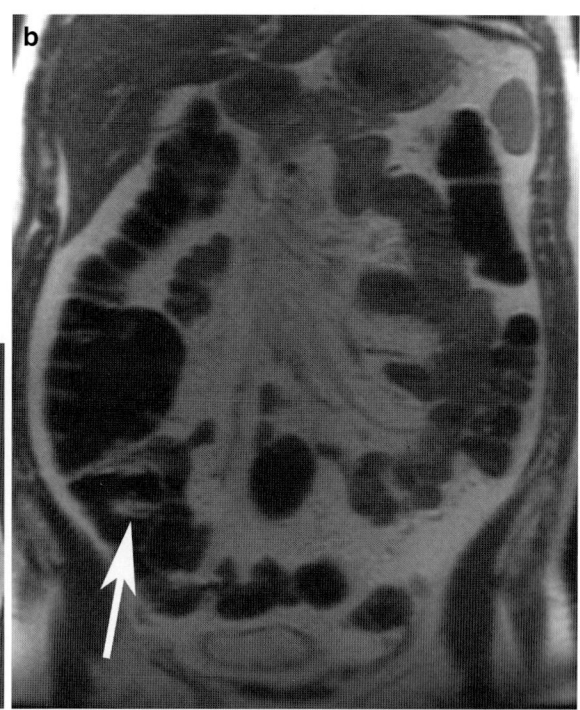

Fig. 17.13. (a) Axial, 2D fast imaging employing steady-state acquisition (FIESTA) image in a 47-year-old male with prior appendectomy demonstrates a heterogeneous round mass arising from the medial wall of the cecum in the region of the appendiceal orifice (*arrow*). (b) Coronal, T2-weighted, single-shot FSE image shows increased signal within this intraluminal cecal mass (*arrow*). While the imaging findings suggested stump appendicitis within an inverted appendiceal remnant, the patient had recently traveled to Central America and his strongyloides serology was elevated. The patient received antiparasitic medication and his symptoms improved. Follow-up MRI demonstrated decreased size and enhancement of the cecal lesion, and a presumptive diagnosis of strongyloides was made

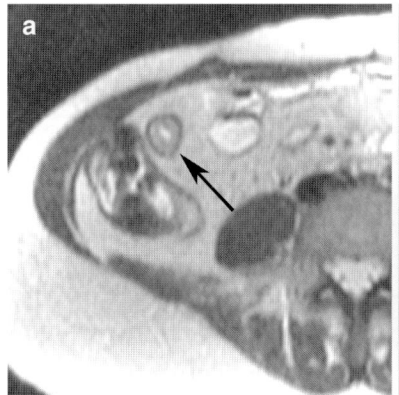

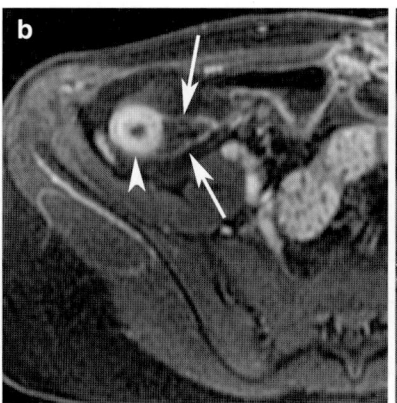

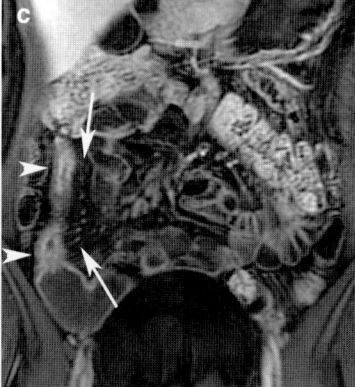

Fig. 17.14. (a) Axial T2-weighted single-shot FSE image in a woman with Crohn's disease and prior ileocecectomy demonstrates mural thickening and stratification (*arrow*) within the neoterminal ileum, indicative of active disease. (b) Axial and (c) coronal contrast-enhanced, fat-saturated, spoiled GRE T1-weighted images show marked mural hyperenhancement (*arrowheads*) and luminal narrowing within the neoterminal ileum. Dilatation and prominence of the vasa recta within areas of proliferative mesenteric fat is compatible with the comb sign (*arrows*)

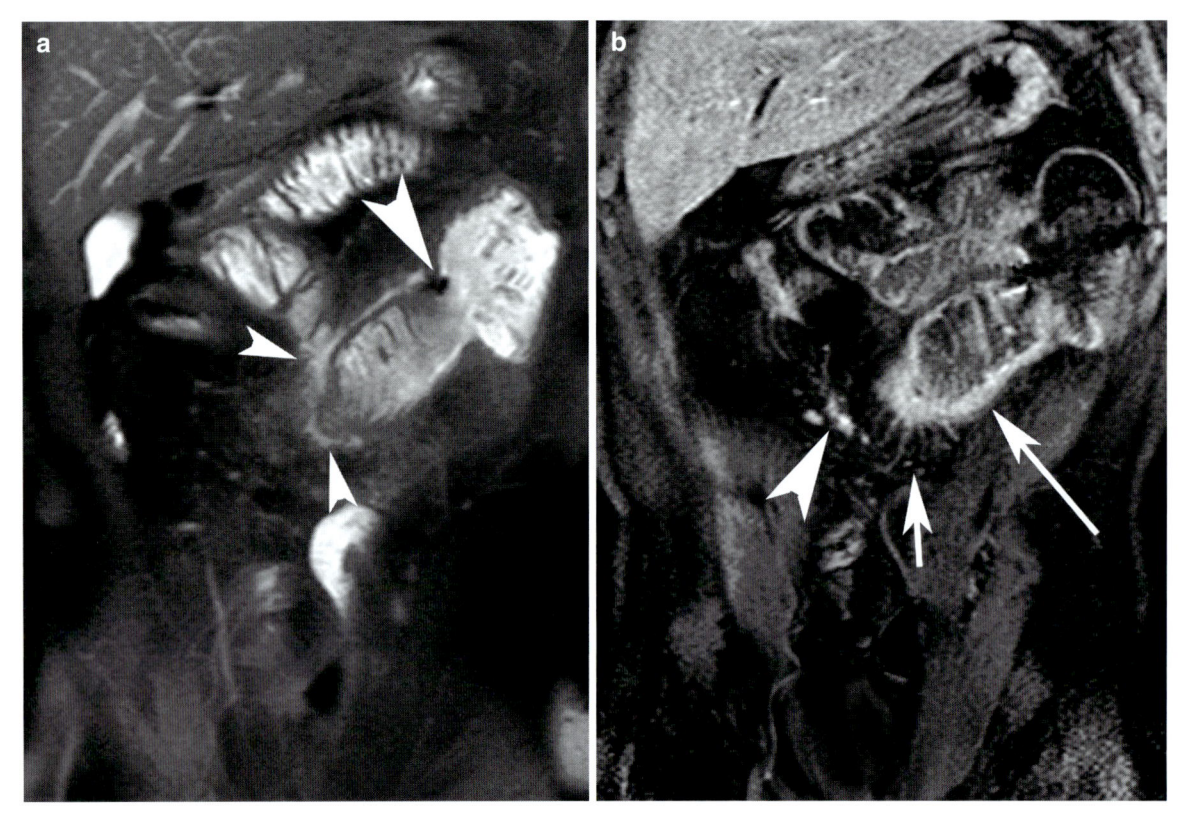

Fig. 17.15. (a) Coronal, fat-suppressed, T2-weighted single-shot FSE image in this patient presenting with acute abdominal pain and history of Crohn's disease with prior proctocolectomy and small bowel resection depicts a mildly dilated loop of jejunum in the mid-abdomen, just distal to a small bowel anastamosis (*large arrowhead*), with high signal within the wall and surrounding perienteric fat (*small arrowheads*) compatible with edema and inflammation. (b) Coronal, contrast-enhanced, fat-saturated, spoiled GRE T1-weighted image shows mural wall thickening and hyperenhancement within the diseased loop of jejunum (*long arrow*), and the comb sign with engorgement of the vasa recta (*short arrow*). Note marked enhancement of nonpathologically enlarged mesenteric nodes (*large arrowhead*)

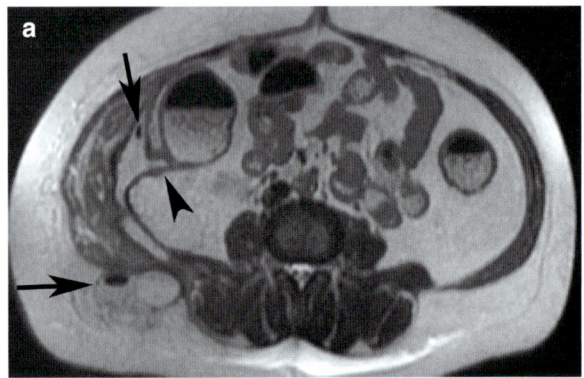

Fig. 17.16. (a) Axial T2-weighted single-shot FSE image in a 45-year-old female with Crohn's disease depicts a fistula between the ascending colon (*arrowhead*) and an extensive, complex, phlegmonous area of multiple fluid collections within the right abdominal wall which track into the deep subcutaneous fat posteriorly. Nondependent areas of low signal intensity within the fluid collections (*black arrows*) denote air within these abscesses. (b) Axial, gadolinium-enhanced, 3D fat-saturated, spoiled GRE T1-weighted image at the same level demonstrates extensive enhancement of the fistula (*arrowhead*) between the ascending colon and the complex right abdominal wall collections, as well as intense enhancement of the walls of the multiple abscesses (*white arrows*)

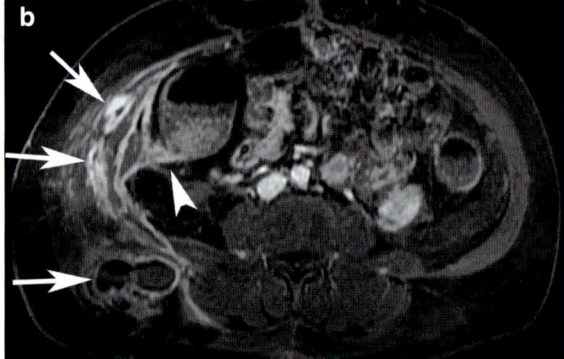

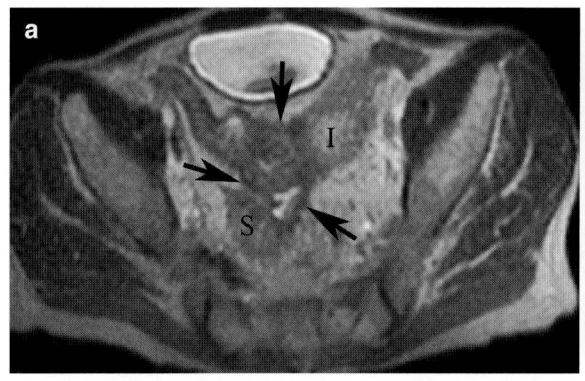

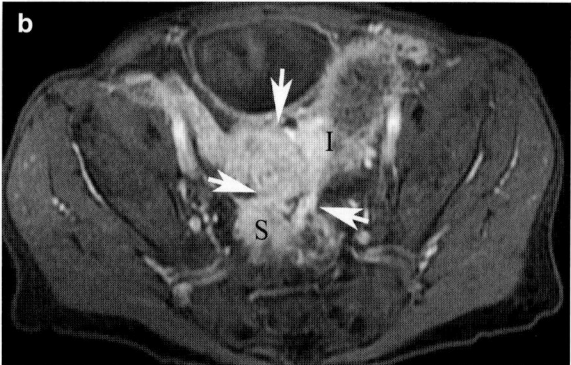

MRI of Acute Conditions of the Gastrointestinal Tract 297

Fig. 17.17. (a) Axial, T2-weighted single-shot FSE image of the pelvis in a 75-year-old man with Crohn's disease demonstrates a heterogeneous, ill-defined mass-like area of mildly increased signal intensity, compatible with a phlegmon, with fistulous tracts (*arrows*) identified between the inflamed distal ileum (*I*) and the rectosigmoid junction (*S*). (b) Axial, gadolinium-enhanced, 3D fat-saturated, T1-weighted GRE image depicts marked enhancement of the phlegmon (*arrows*) and enterorectal fistulous tracts

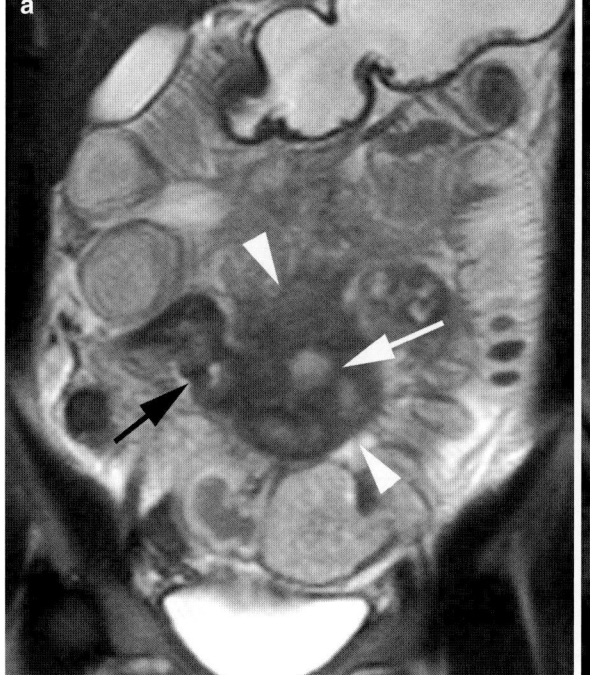

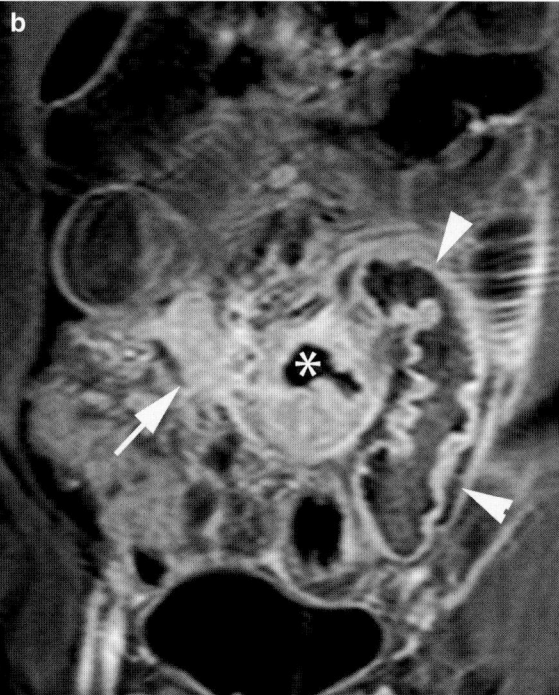

Fig. 17.18. (a) Coronal, T2-weighted single-shot FSE image in a 38-year-old female with Crohn's disease, prior ileocolectomies, and ileo-sigmoid anastomosis presenting with abdominal pain, fever, and mild leukocytosis shows diffuse hypointense thickening of the terminal ileum (*black arrow*) with upstream bowel dilatation, findings suggestive of fibrostenotic disease. A large phlegmonous region (*white arrowheads*) with a focal area of increased signal (*white arrow*) consistent with an abscess indicates a superimposed active flare of Crohn's disease. (b) Coronal, 3D fat-saturated, T1-weighted GRE image during the portal venous phase shows diffuse wall thickening and enhancement in the sigmoid colon (*white arrowheads*) and terminal ileum (*white arrow*). The abscess is confirmed as a focal area without enhancement (*asterisk*) within the area of phlegmonous change

As in pregnant patients with suspected acute appendicitis, MRI plays an important role in the assessment of pregnant patients presenting with acute abdominal pain and known or suspected inflammatory bowel disease. The authors use the same imaging protocol in this patient population as the one described for patients with suspected acute appendicitis. T2-weighted single shot FSE techniques play an essential role in determining the extent of bowel involvement as well as extraluminal complications (Fig. 17.19). At the authors' institution, MRI is commonly used in pregnant patients with a known history of Crohn's disease and new onset of acute right lower quadrant pain to distinguish between acute appendicitis and an acute flare of Crohn's disease, as these two conditions are managed differently. The presence of inflammatory changes primarily affecting the terminal ileum and/or colon with or without secondary involvement of the appendix are indicative of Crohn's disease. In the absence of extraluminal acute complications (i.e. abscess, perforation), these patients are managed conservatively (Fig. 17.20). Extraluminal complications secondary to inflammatory bowel disease like intraabdominal abscesses can be managed as in nonpregnant patients, although the use of MRI can prevent the patient and the fetus from repeated exposure to ionizing radiation (Fig. 17.21). In contrast, inflammatory changes centered in the appendix without involvement of the terminal ileum and/or colon are suspicious for acute appendicitis and should prompt surgical exploration.

17.3.1.3
Primary Epiploic Appendagitis

The epiploic appendages are peritoneal pouches composed of adipose tissue and blood vessels, which arise from the colonic serosal surface, ranging from 0.5 to 5 cm in length (Singh et al. 2005). The epiploic appendages extend from the cecum to the rectosigmoid junction, and number about 100, arranged in two rows along the free tenia and tenia omentalis (Rioux and Langis 1994; Singh et al. 2005). Primary epiploic appendagitis is a condition that arises when these structures torse or undergo spontaneous venous thrombosis, resulting in infarction and inflammation (Barbier et al. 1998; Sirvanci et al. 2002; Singh et al. 2005). Primary epiploic appendagitis presents with acute abdominal pain and is a self-limiting condition, necessitating only conservative management (Singh et al. 2005).

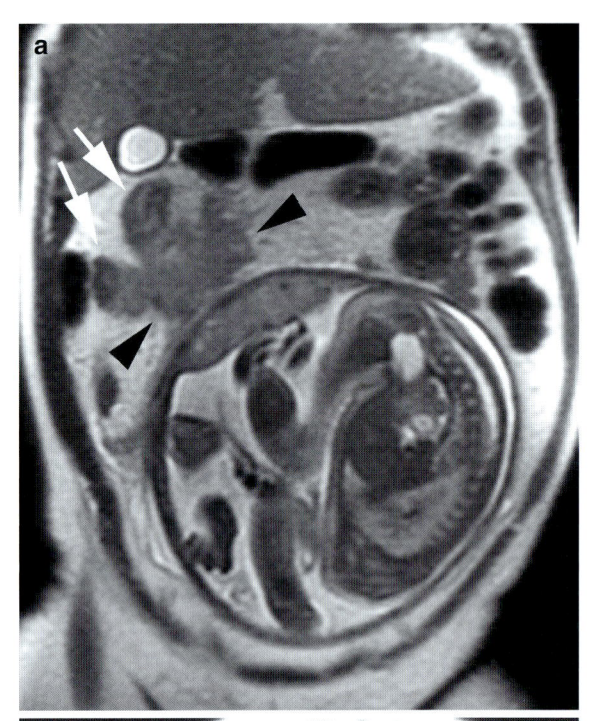

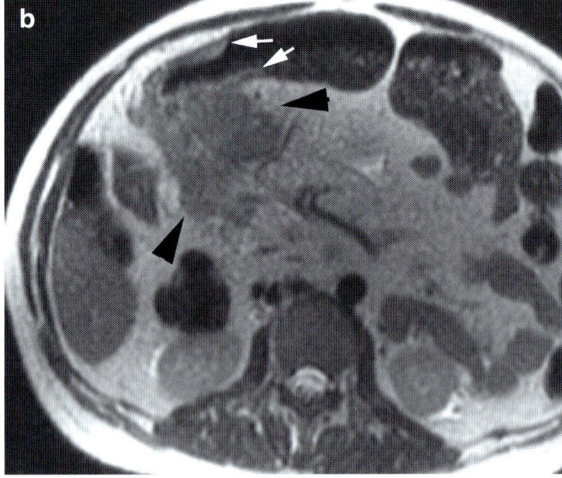

Fig. 17.19. (a) Coronal T2-weighted single-shot FSE image in a 33-year-old pregnant woman at 30-week gestational age with Crohn's disease and new onset of right-sided abdominal pain shows diffuse thickening of the terminal ileum (*white arrows*) and an irregular area of intermediate signal intensity (*black arrowheads*) consistent with phlegmon. (b) Axial T2-weighted single-shot FSE image confirms the presence of a moderate-size phlegmon (*black arrowheads*) and better demonstrates the area of wall thickening (*white arrows*) in the terminal ileum, adjacent to the phlegmon. The presence of extraluminal complications in patients with Crohn's disease is well evaluated with T2-weighted single-shot FSE images without the use of fat saturation because of the excellent soft-tissue contrast achieved between the hyperintense mesenteric fat, the intermediate signal intensity of the bowel wall, and the intraluminal low signal intensity provided by the oral contrast preparation

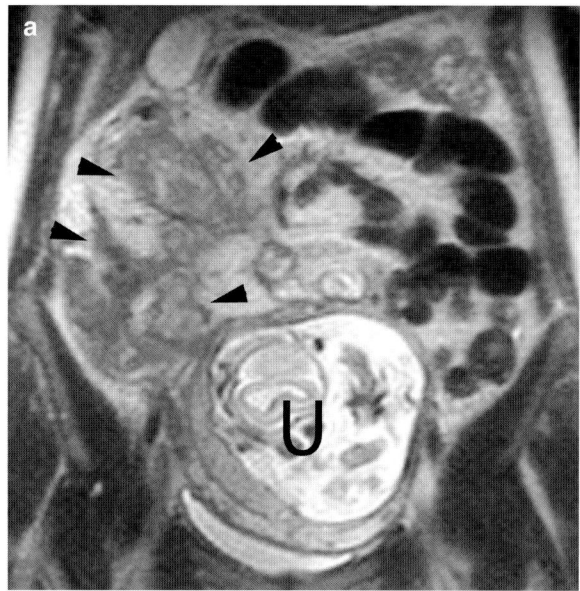

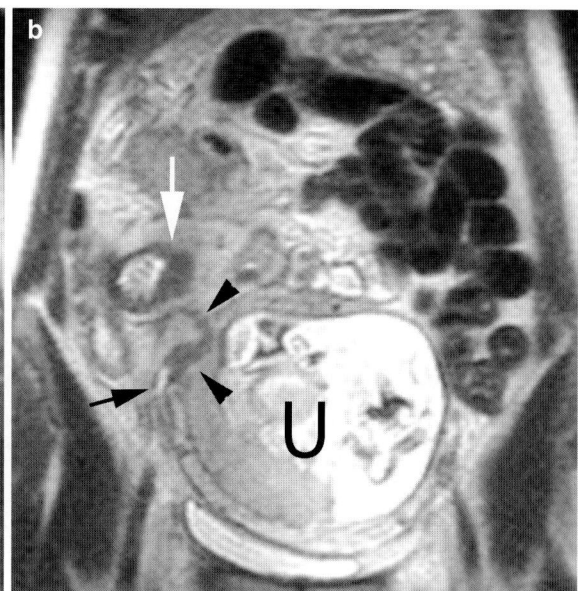

Fig. 17.20. (a) Coronal T2-weighted single-shot FSE image in a 30-year-old pregnant woman with a history of Crohn's disease at 19-week gestational age presenting with right lower quadrant tenderness and fever shows a large area of irregular intermediate signal intensity (*arrowheads*) in the right hemiabdomen consistent with a phlegmon. Note the gravid uterus (*U*). (b) Coronal T2-weighted image from the same acquisition as (a) at a slightly more anterior location, shows diffuse wall thickening of the terminal ileum (*white arrow*) and a thickened appendix (*black arrowheads*) with a fluid-filled, enlarged tip (*black arrow*). MR findings were consistent with an acute flare of Crohn's disease with involvement of the appendix. The patient recovered with conservative management

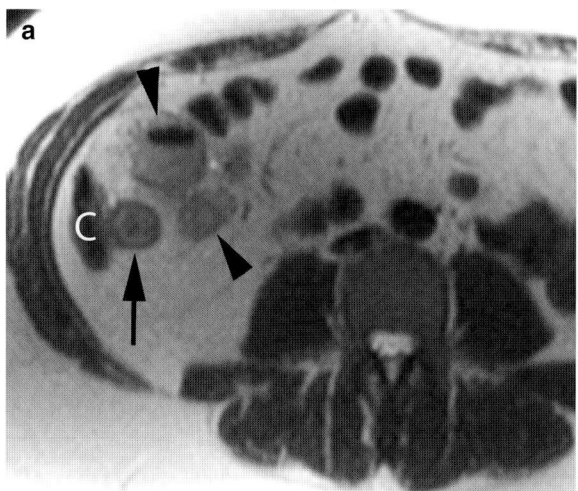

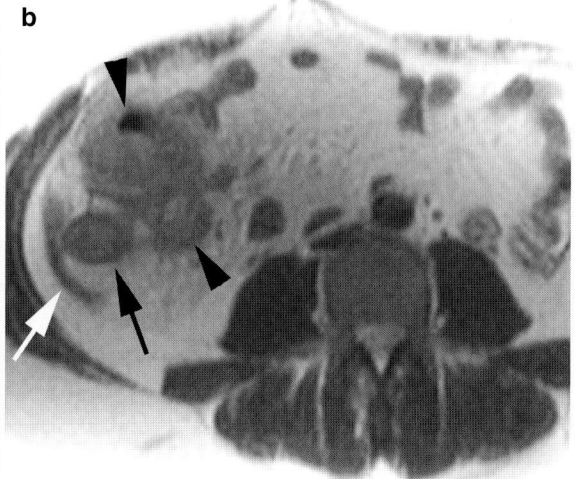

Fig. 17.21. (a) Axial, T2-weighted single-shot FSE image in a 37-year-old pregnant woman at 9-week gestational age with a history of Crohn's disease now presenting with new onset of right lower quadrant pain shows wall thickening of the terminal ileum (*black arrow*) and two adjacent small abscesses (*black arrowheads*) adjacent to the cecum (*C*). The larger, more anteriorly located abscess contains an air-fluid level. The patient was placed initially on antibiotic therapy, but complained of worsening symptoms. On repeat MRI obtained 5 days later, (b) axial, T2-weighted single-shot FSE image confirms enlargement of the abscesses (*black arrowheads*) and persistent thickening of the terminal ileum (*black arrow*). Note the mildly thickened appendix (*white arrow*). The patient underwent percutaneous drainage of the abscesses, and was followed with multiple MR examinations to avoid repeated radiation exposure to her fetus

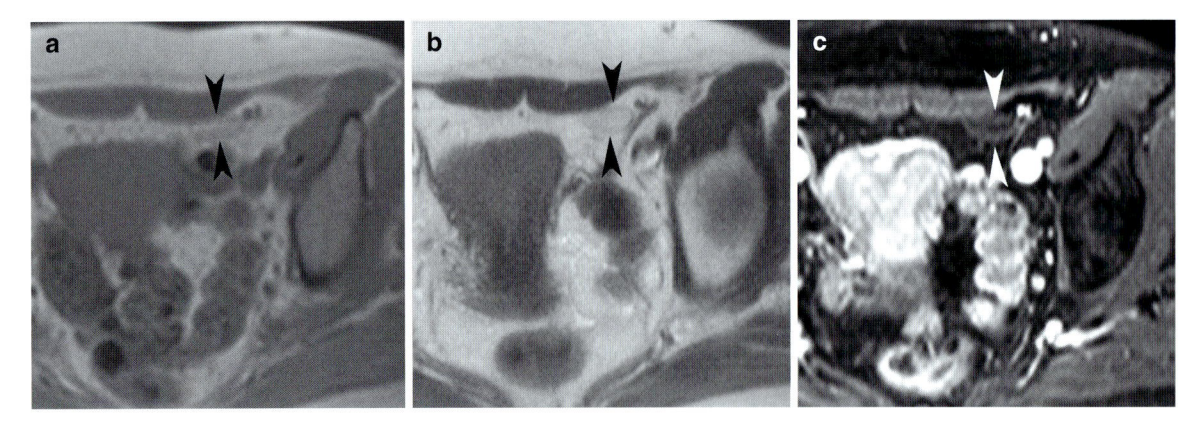

Fig. 17.22. Axial, (**a**) T1-weighted GRE and (**b**) T2-weighted FSE images of the pelvis in a 60-year-old female presenting with left lower quadrant abdominal pain demonstrate an ovoid lesion within the left lower quadrant, adjacent to the sigmoid colon (not pictured), containing central signal intensity corresponding to fat, and a peripheral low signal intensity rim (*arrowheads*). (**c**) Axial, gadolinium-enhanced, 3D fat-saturated, spoiled GRE, T1-weighted image demonstrates enhancement of the rim. Findings were compatible with mild epiploic appendagitis

On T1- and T2-weighted MRI, epiploic appendagitis appears as a pericolonic, oval-shaped lesion containing a low signal intensity rim, and a center that follows the signal intensity of fat (Fig. 17.22) (BARBIER et al. 1998; SIRVANCI et al. 2002). On postgadolinium, T1-weighted fat-suppressed sequences, the rim, which represents the inflamed visceral peritoneum, demonstrates increased enhancement (BARBIER et al. 1998; SIRVANCI et al. 2002). A hypointense central dot on T1- and T2-weighted imaging may be seen within the lesion, likely representing a fibrous septa that has been described in histopathologic specimens (SIRVANCI et al. 2002). Fat-stranding is commonly seen around the inflamed epiploic appendage (BARBIER et al. 1998).

17.3.1.4
Colonic Diverticulitis

Acute diverticulitis is a condition that results from inflammation of colonic diverticula due to decreased perfusion secondary to obstruction or impaction of fecal material (BUCKLEY et al. 2007). Imaging plays an important role in the diagnosis of acute diverticulitis and detecting its complications. While CT has been considered the gold standard for the imaging assessment of diverticulitis, recent studies suggest that MRI can provide high sensitivity and specificity for the diagnosis of this condition. In a prospective study of 55 patients, Heverhagen and colleagues reported MRI to have a sensitivity of 94% and specificity of 88% for diagnosing acute diverticulitis (HEVERHAGEN et al. 2008). These authors used inversion recovery (STIR), balanced steady-state free precession (TrueFISP), and pre- and post-gadolinium T1-weighted fat-suppressed GRE sequences to diagnose the condition. Previously, these authors found that an imaging protocol consisting of only STIR and TrueFISP sequences was sufficient to diagnose colonic diverticulitis. STIR imaging was useful for demonstrating edema, pericolonic exudation, and ascites, while TrueFISP sequences were noted to highlight segmental areas of colonic narrowing. The authors concluded that single-shot FSE imaging provided no additional information (HEVERHAGEN et al. 2001).

On MRI the features of acute diverticulitis include the presence of diverticula, bowel wall thickening, and pericolonic stranding (BUCKLEY et al. 2007). Stranding appears as ill-defined pericolonic areas of high signal intensity on T2-weighted imaging, which appear more conspicuous with fat suppression (Fig. 17.23). The inflamed diverticulum demonstrates mural thickening and marked enhancement on Postcontrast imaging. When the adjacent interfascial planes are inflamed, they appear thickened and hyperenhancing on postgadolinium T1-weighted imaging (Fig 17.24) (HAMMOND et al. 2008).

Clinically, cecal diverticulitis can mimic acute appendicitis, and cross-sectional imaging plays an important role in distinguishing these two entities. While pericecal wall thickening and focal pericolonic inflammation may be seen in both entities, imaging features that favor cecal diverticulitis over acute

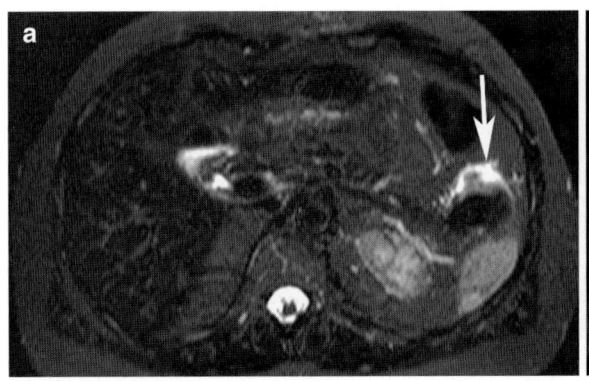

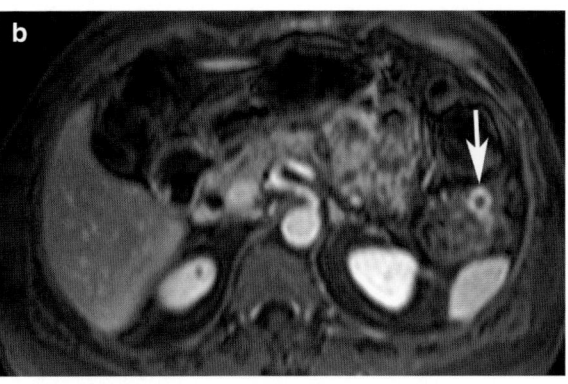

Fig. 17.23. (a) Axial, T2-weighted FSE image with fat suppression in a man with left upper quadrant abdominal pain demonstrates a focal area of high signal adjacent to the splenic flexure compatible with pericolonic inflammation (*arrow*). (b) Axial, gadolinium-enhanced 3D fat-saturated, spoiled GRE T1-weighted image shows avid enhancement within an inflamed diverticulum (*arrow*) in the splenic flexure, compatible with acute diverticulitis

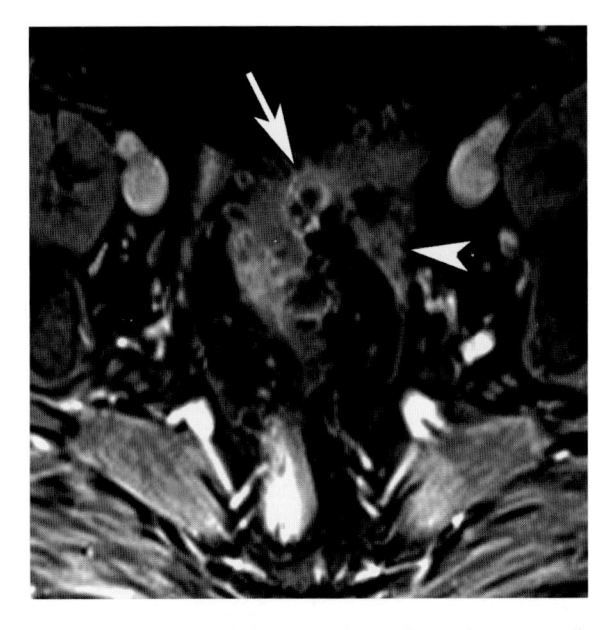

Fig. 17.24 Axial, gadolinium-enhanced 3D fat-saturated, spoiled GRE T1-weighted image obtained in a woman with sigmoid diverticulitis demonstrates numerous diverticula within the sigmoid colon with mural thickening and enhancement of an inflamed diverticulum (*arrow*). Note surrounding fat stranding with thickening and enhancement of the adjacent sigmoid mesocolon (*arrowhead*)

appendicitis include identification of a normal appendix, visualization of diverticula, or the presence of inflammation involving the ascending colon at a level distal to the ileocecal valve (BALTHAZAR et al. 1987; CHINTAPALLI et al. 1999; HOEFFEL et al. 2006).

Complications of acute diverticulitis include phlegmon, abscess, and fistula formation, which can be recognized on MRI. Phlegmons appear as heterogeneous ill-defined areas of mildly increased signal intensity on T2-weighted imaging, and demonstrate prominent enhancement Postcontrast administration (Fig. 17.25). Abscesses appear as pericolonic, rim-enhancing, fluid collections with central low signal on T1-weighted images and high signal on T2-weighted images (PEDROSA and ROFSKY 2003; HAMMOND et al. 2008). Fistulas can appear as enhancing tracts, which may contain fluid. While extraluminal air appears as a signal void on all imaging sequences, the sensitivity of MR for the detection of small collections of extraluminal air is low (PEDROSA and ROFSKY 2003; HAMMOND et al. 2008). While CT has been shown to be an invaluable tool for classifying the severity of acute perforated diverticulitis, thereby helping to guide surgical management, the role of MRI, because of its limited sensitivity for the detection of perforation (i.e. small amounts of extraluminal air), remains unclear for stratifying the degree of perforated diverticular disease (LOHRMANN et al. 2005).

17.3.1.5
Peptic Ulcer Disease

While MRI is not the primary imaging modality used to diagnose peptic ulcer disease, patients present with nonspecific abdominal pain, and may have an MRI performed to evaluate for other suspected disease processes such as pancreatitis. T2-weighted single-shot FSE and gadolinium-enhanced fat-suppressed T1-weighted GRE images have been

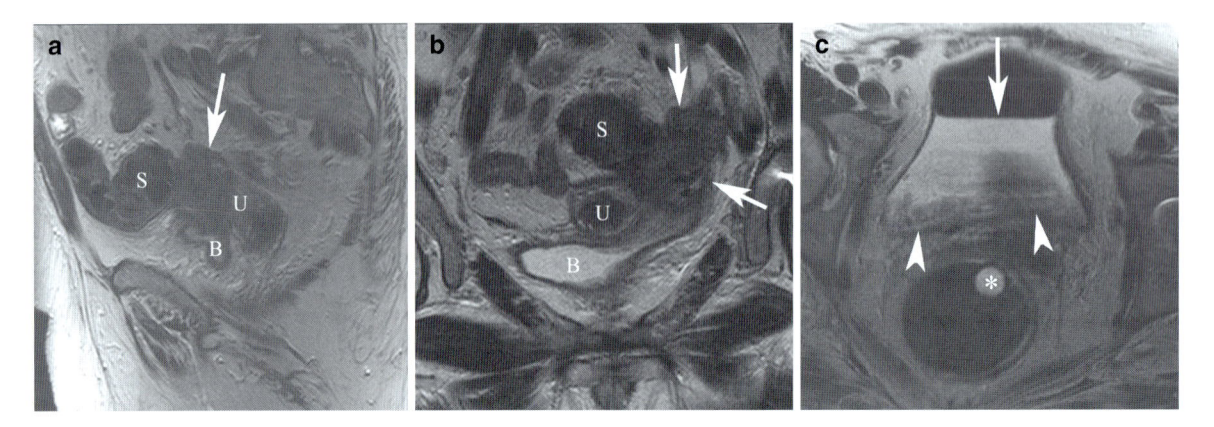

Fig. 17.25. (a) Sagittal and (b) coronal T2-weighted FSE images in a woman with sigmoid diverticulitis complicated by phlegmon and colovesicular fistula formation demonstrate an ill-defined mass-like area of heterogeneous signal within the pelvis (*arrows*) compatible with a phlegmon, involving the sigmoid colon (S), left uterine fundus (U), and bladder (B). (c) Axial T2-weighted FSE image through the bladder shows an air-fluid level within the bladder lumen (*arrow*) with dependent debris (*arrowheads*), findings secondary to the presence of the colovesicular fistula. Incidental note is made of a rectal catheter (*asterisk*)

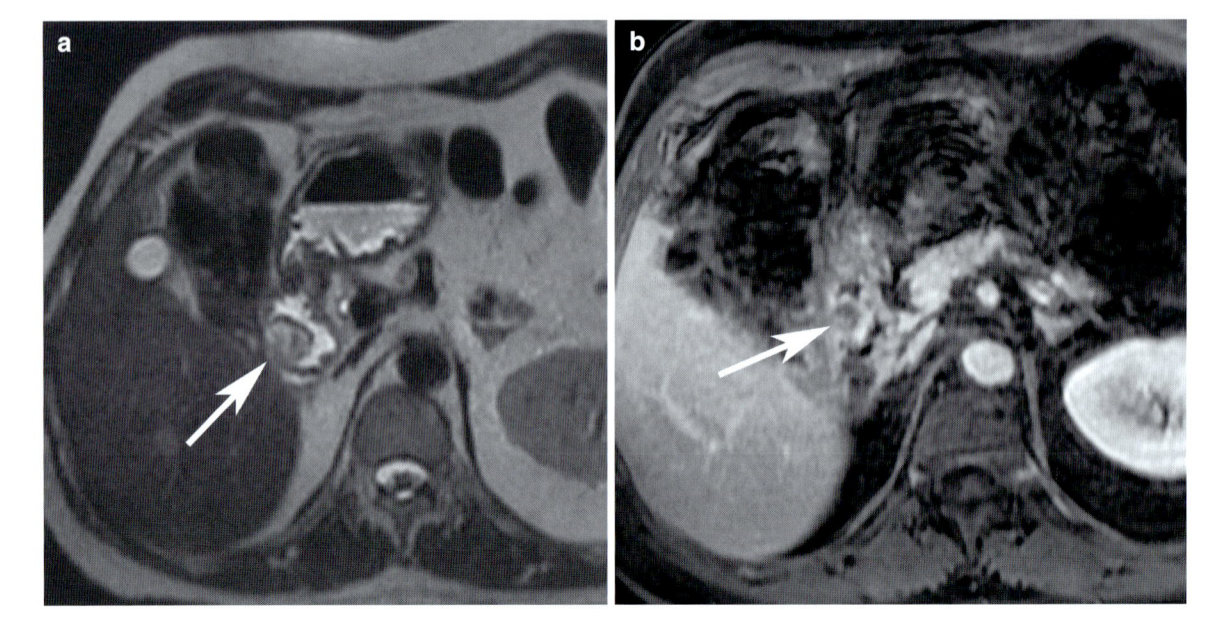

Fig. 17.26. (a) Axial, T2-weighted single-shot FSE image of the first portion of the duodenum in a man with a duodenal bulb ulcer with associated duodenitis confirmed on endoscopy demonstrates a focal area of heaped-up mural thickening within the duodenal bulb, which is heterogeneously hyperintense. (b) On the axial, gadolinium-enhanced 3D fat-saturated, spoiled GRE, T1-weighted image, this region of ulceration and inflammation demonstrates mural enhancement

reported to be helpful for detecting features of peptic ulcer disease, including ulcers, gastritis, and duodenitis (MARCOS and SEMELKA 1999).

Peptic ulcers within the stomach or duodenum may appear as focal areas of wall thickening and edema, appearing as high signal intensity areas on T2-weighted imaging (Fig. 17.26) (HAMMOND et al. 2008). With contrast administration, the ulcerated regions demonstrate enhancement, which is hyperintense relative to normal gastric or bowel wall (MARCOS and SEMELKA 1999). Thickening and edema of the gastric or duodenal wall and folds indicate regions of gastritis or duodenitis, which may be accompanied by surrounding inflammatory stranding (CRONIN et al.

2008). Luminal narrowing may be present in areas of inflamed stomach or duodenum, and gastric outlet obstruction may occur in severe cases (MARCOS and SEMELKA 1999). Perforation may be signaled by the visualization of fluid collections adjacent to regions of ulcerated or inflamed bowel. These fluid collections typically demonstrate hypointense signal on T1-weighted imaging and hyperintense signal on T2-weighted imaging. If hemorrhage is present, however, the collections may appear as areas of high signal intensity on both T1- and T2-weighted imaging (Fig 17.27). Because MRI is limited in its detection of small collections of air, small areas of extraluminal air may be missed.

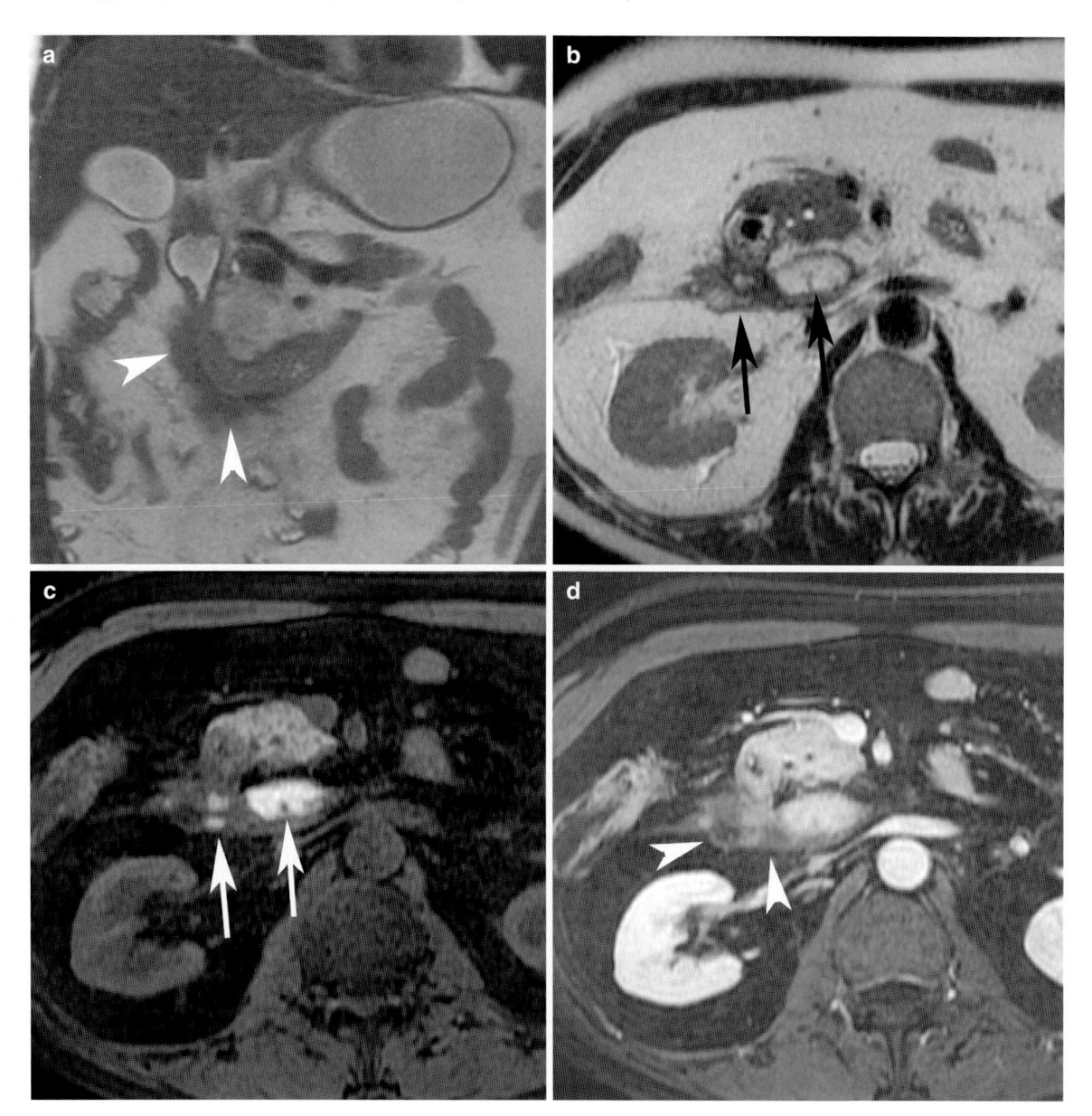

Fig. 17.27. (a) Coronal T2-weighted single-shot FSE in a man with a perforated duodenal ulcer demonstrates mural thickening of the genu of the duodenum with surrounding inflammatory fat stranding (*arrowheads*), compatible with duodenitis. Axial, (b) T2-weighed single-shot FSE and (c) unenhanced, fat-saturated, spoiled GRE, T1-weighted images show several paraduodenal fluid collections (*arrows*) which are high in signal on both T1- and T2-weighted imaging, compatible with hemorrhage within these collections. (d) The axial, gadolinium-enhanced, 3D fat-saturated, spoiled GRE, T1-weighted image depicts enhancement of the wall within the second and third portions of the duodenum and adjacent inflammatory stranding (*arrowheads*)

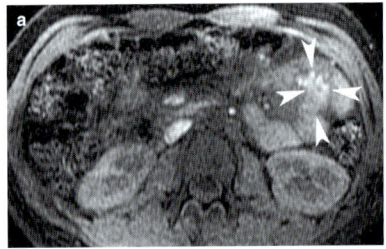

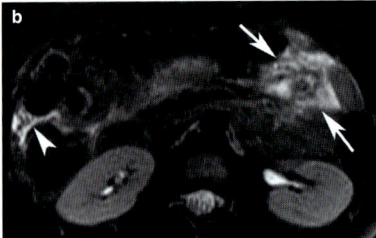

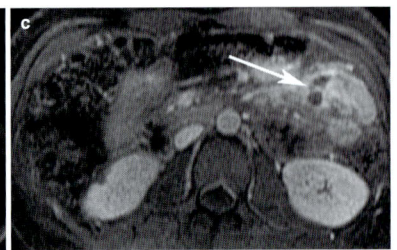

Fig. 17.28. (a) Axial, unenhanced 3D, fat-suppressed, spoiled GRE, T1-weighted image obtained in a 21-year-old female with abdominal pain and elevated amylase and lipase shows a hyperintense mass (*arrowheads*) within the left abdomen, intimately associated with jejunal loops of bowel, with an acinar pattern similar to normal pancreas. (b) Axial, T2-weighted, fat-suppressed, single-shot FSE image demonstrates increased signal within and around the mass, compatible with inflammation and edema (*arrows*). Fluid is also noted within the right hemiabdomen (*arrowhead*). (c) Axial, gadolinium-enhanced, 3D fat-suppressed, spoiled GRE, T1-weighted image depicts increased enhancement of the mass and the surrounding inflammatory changes, with a central nonenhancing bilobed fluid collection (*arrow*). Findings were compatible with ectopic pancreatitis of the jejunum, which was confirmed on surgical and pathologic analysis

17.3.1.6
Ectopic Pancreas

Ectopic or heterotopic pancreas is a rare developmental anomaly where pancreatic tissue is present outside the usual location, anatomically distinct from the main body of the pancreas, with a separate ductal system and blood supply (BARBOSA et al. 1946). The estimated incidence of this condition at autopsy ranges from 0.55 to 13.7% (LAI and TOMPKINS 1986). Ectopic pancreas is most frequently seen within the upper gastrointestinal tract with 70–86.5% involving the stomach, duodenum, or jejunum (BARBOSA et al. 1946; LAI and TOMPKINS 1986). Less commonly, ectopic pancreas can be found within the ileum, bile ducts or gallbladder, umbilicus, splenic hilum, omentum, and mesentery (BARBOSA et al. 1946; LAI and TOMPKINS 1986; SILVA et al. 2006). While this condition is usually asymptomatic, ectopic pancreatic rests within the stomach and duodenum can cause epigastric pain (LAI and TOMPKINS 1986). Additionally, as the aberrant pancreas is susceptible to any pathologic condition that can affect normal pancreas, the ectopic pancreas can produce clinical symptoms when complicated by acute pancreatitis or pancreatic cancer (BARBOSA et al. 1946; RUBESIN et al. 1997; SILVA et al. 2006).

On MRI, the signal intensity and enhancement of the ectopic pancreas parallels that of the normal pancreas on all sequences (LEE et al. 2008a; OKUHATA et al. 2008). Unenhanced, fat-suppressed, T1-weighted images are helpful for highlighting the ectopic pancreatic tissue, as the aberrant pancreas, similar to normal pancreas, will exhibit higher signal intensity when compared to the surrounding mesentery and bowel structures (Fig. 17.28) (OKUHATA et al. 2008). Heavily T2-weighted MR cholangiopancreaticogram sequences have been reported to be useful in identifying the ectopic pancreatic duct, a pathognomonic feature of the aberrant pancreatic rest (SILVA et al. 2006). When acutely inflamed, the ectopic pancreatitis can demonstrate the surrounding fat stranding and edema with adjacent fluid collections. These features are well depicted with T2-weighted imaging with fat suppression, with inflammation and fluid appearing as areas of high signal (Fig. 17.28). With contrast administration, increased enhancement is seen within the ectopic pancreas and surrounding inflamed regions (SILVA et al. 2006). Loops of adjacent bowel may demonstrate wall and fold thickening (RUBESIN et al. 1997).

17.3.2
Acute Neoplastic Conditions of the Gastrointestinal Tract

While MRI has recently become an emerging imaging modality for the detection, diagnosis, and staging of a variety of gastrointestinal tract neoplasms, MRI is also useful for imaging the acute complications of these neoplasms, including hemorrhage, obstruction, ischemia, and bowel inflammation.

Gastrointestinal stromal tumor (GIST) is one subtype of tumor that is prone to ulcerate and hemorrhage, especially when large (MARTIN et al. 2005). High-grade GISTs appear heterogeneous in signal intensity on T1- and T2-weighted imaging, which is reflective of intratumoral hemorrhage and/or liquefactive necrosis, findings characteristic in these neoplasms (MARCOS

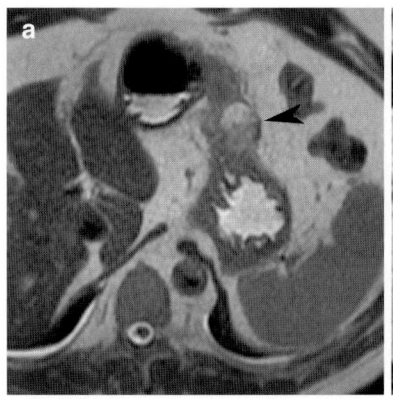

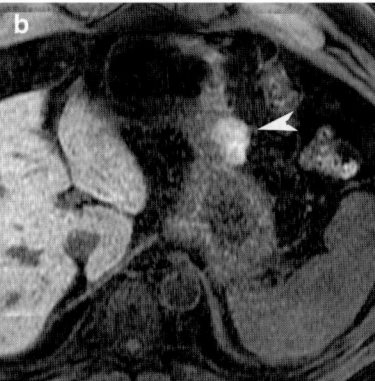

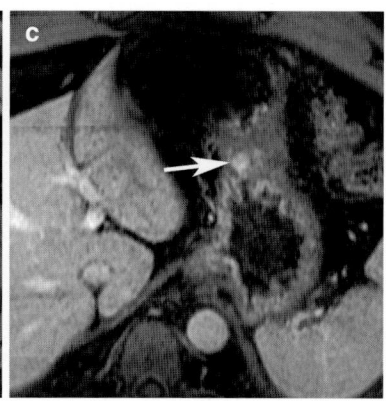

Fig. 17.29. Axial, (**a**) T2-weighted single-shot FSE and (**b**) unenhanced, 3D fat-suppressed, T1-weighted GRE images in a 55-year-old-male presenting with abdominal pain demonstrate a heterogeneously hyperintense region both on T1- and T2-weighted imaging adjacent to the greater curvature of the stomach (*arrowheads*) compatible with a hematoma. (**c**) Axial, gadolinium-enhanced, 3D fat-suppressed, T1-weighted GRE image shows an enhancing subcutaneous nodule (*arrow*) within the greater curvature of the stomach, adjacent to the hematoma, which was revealed to be a gastric GIST complicated by hemorrhage upon surgery and pathologic analysis

and SEMELKA 1999). These tumors tend to be hypervascular, and demonstrate marked arterial enhancement that persists on the equilibrium phase (MARCOS and SEMELKA 1999; MARTIN et al. 2005). Low signal, nonenhancing regions within the tumor indicate necrotic areas. On T1-weighted imaging, particularly with fat-suppression, hemorrhage is highlighted as regions of high signal (Fig. 17.29). By subtracting the precontrast T1-weighted imaging sequence from the Postcontrast imaging sequence, enhancement within regions of hemorrhage can be more easily detected.

Neoplastic involvement of the gastrointestinal tract can also result in an acute clinical presentation due to the surrounding inflammation caused by the malignancy. Ulcerative or large lesions of the gastrointestinal tract can cause wall thickening and enhancement, fat stranding, and adjacent edema (Fig. 17.30). Gastrointestinal tract neoplasms may not only incite bowel inflammation, but also mimic inflammatory bowel disease. Small bowel lymphoma can simulate Crohn's disease and radiologically present on MRI with mural nodularity, symmetric or asymmetric concentric wall thickening, effacement or thickening of the mucosal folds, focal bowel dilation, luminal strictures, ulceration, and mesenteric fat infiltration (Fig. 17.31) (SARTORIS et al. 1984; LOHAN et al. 2008). Finally, acute bowel perforation may occur in patients with primary and secondary neoplastic involvement of the bowel undergoing chemotherapy with targeted therapies. An intact primary tumor, colonoscopy, or sigmoidoscopy carried out within 1 month of starting bevacizumab therapy, prior adjuvant radiotherapy, presence of tumor at the site of perforation, obstruction, intra-abdominal abscess, carcinomatosis, and acute diverticulitis have been identified as potential risk factors for bowel perforation in patients with a variety of tumors undergoing therapy with bevacizumab (Fig. 17.32) (HEDRICK et al. 2006; SUGRUE et al. 2006).

17.3.3
Ischemia and Obstruction of the Gastrointestinal Tract

CT is the imaging modality of choice for evaluating suspected ischemia and bowel obstruction due to its widespread availability, short imaging times, and insensitivity to bowel peristalsis. MRI, however, can be used as an alternative imaging modality for the evaluation of bowel obstruction in patients in whom radiation is not desirable, such as in the pregnant and pediatric populations. Similarly, MRI can provide evaluation of the intra-abdominal vasculature without the need for intravenous contrast, which is particularly advantageous for those patients with contraindications to iodinated contrast administration, such as patients with renal insufficiency and allergies to iodinated contrast media.

Bowel ischemia results from insufficient blood flow to the intestine due to a variety of causes including thromboembolism, nonocclusive etiologies,

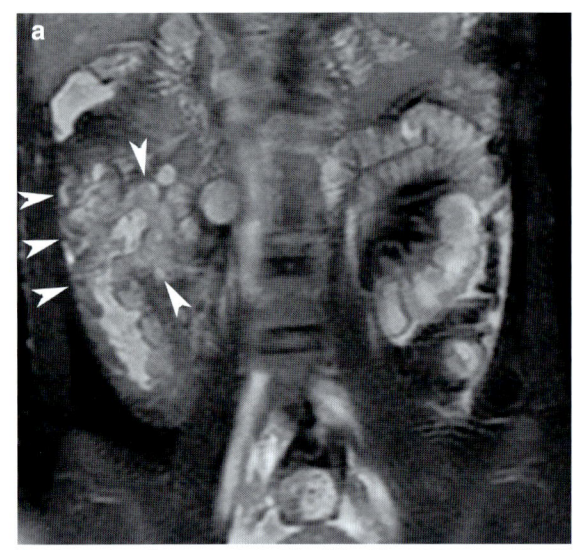

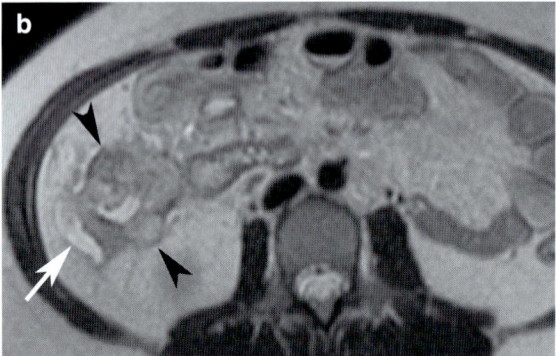

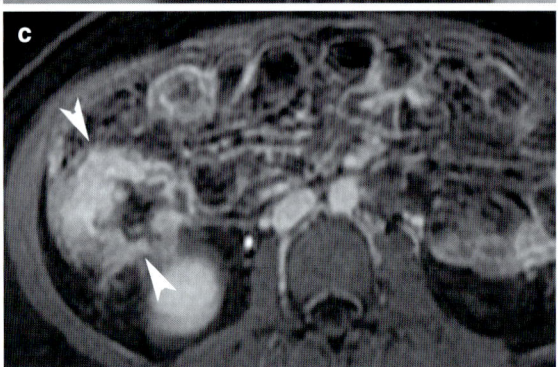

Fig. 17.30. (a) Coronal, fat-saturated T2-weighted single-shot FSE and (b) axial, T2-weighted single-shot FSE images in a 21-year-old female with right lower quadrant pain demonstrate the wall of the ascending colon to be circumferentially thickened. Increased signal intensity within the wall is compatible with mural edema (*arrowheads*), with adjacent hyperintense fluid noted tracking along the right paracolic gutter (*white arrow*). (c) Axial, gadolinium-enhanced, 3D fat-suppressed, T1-weighted GRE image shows increased enhancement within the wall of the right colon (*arrowheads*) with surrounding inflammatory fat stranding and peritoneal enhancement. Adenocarcinoid tumor of the ascending colon was diagnosed at surgery and pathologic analysis

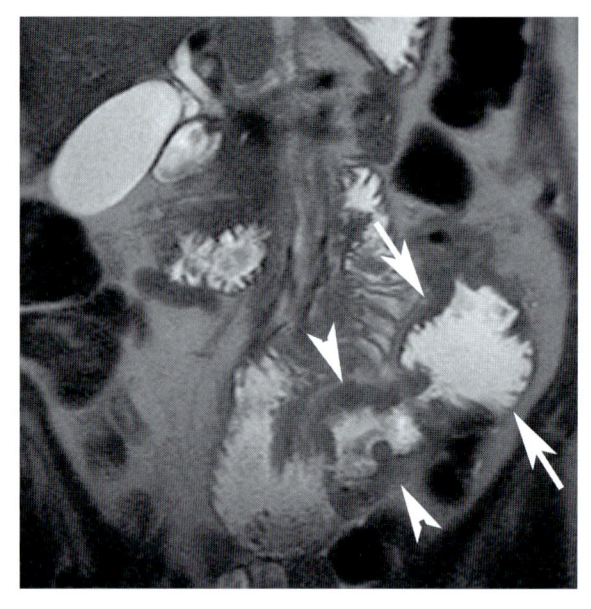

Fig. 17.31. Coronal T2-weighted FSE image in a 58-year-old female presenting with abdominal pain demonstrates an abnormal loop of jejunum in the left lower quadrant with nodularity, wall thickening (*arrowheads*), and focal aneurysmal dilatation (*arrows*). High-grade jejunal B-cell lymphoma was diagnosed at pathology

bowel obstruction, neoplasm, vasculitis, trauma, chemotherapy, inflammatory conditions, radiation, and corrosive injury (Rha et al. 2000). The appearance of bowel ischemia on MRI is often nonspecific, mimicking other inflammatory or infectious processes. Ischemic bowel segments may demonstrate bowel wall thickening and mural stratification ("target" or "halo" sign), with increased signal within the wall on T2-weighted imaging surrounded by a layer of intermediate signal on either side, signifying the presence of mural edema (Fig. 17.33) (Rha et al. 2000; Pedrosa and Rofsky 2003). The involved bowel segment may appear dilated, and adjacent mesenteric edema and fluid can be visualized (Martin et al. 2005). With contrast administration, the ischemic bowel can demonstrate diffuse intense enhancement on the 60–90-s delayed fat-saturated T1-weighted images (Fig. 17.34) (Martin et al. 2005). When infarcted, lack of enhancement may be seen in the affected segments of bowel (Klein et al. 1996). While the detection of pneumatosis on MRI can be extremely difficult, the presence of the blooming effect within the bowel wall on the longer echo time, in-phase images compared to the shorter echo time, opposed-phase images (an echo time scheme commonly used on 1.5 T magnets) can help identify pneumatosis.

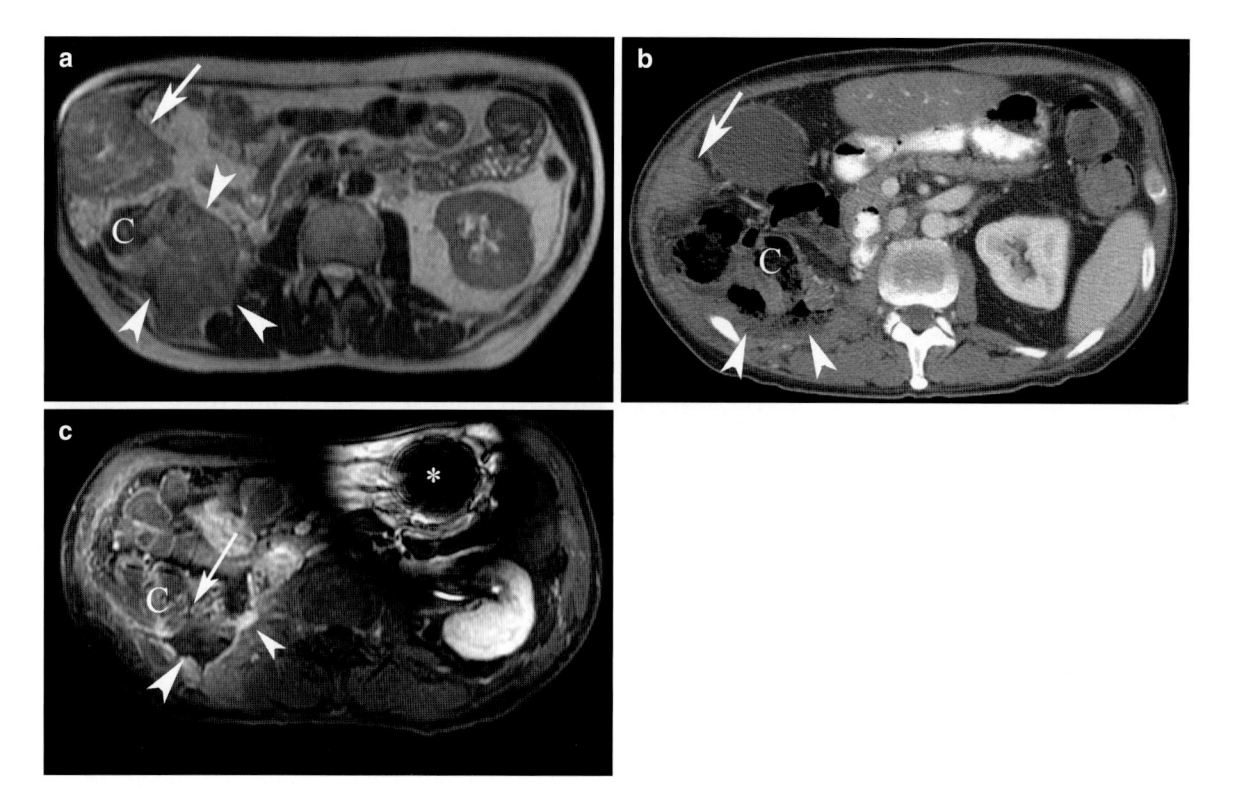

Fig. 17.32. (a) Axial, T2-weighted single-shot FSE image in a 61-year-old man with metastatic renal cell carcinoma status post right nephrectomy demonstrates a large heterogeneous mass (*arrowheads*) within the nephrectomy bed compatible with tumor recurrence, intimately associated with the ascending colon (*C*). A second soft-tissue metastasis is seen within the right anterolateral abdominal wall (*arrow*). Ten days after the initiation of bevacizumab therapy, the patient presented with right-sided abdominal pain and (b) an axial CT image obtained during the portal venous phase of enhancement demonstrates dramatic response to therapy with replacement of the previously seen tumor within the nephrectomy bed with a contained collection of air and fecal material (*arrowheads*) in communication with the ascending colon (*C*). Findings are compatible with ascending colonic perforation and abscess formation. Note the marked reduction in size of the right anterolateral abdominal wall metastasis (*arrow*). (c) Axial, gadolinium-enhanced, 3D fat-suppressed, T1-weighted GRE image from a subsequent MRI obtained a few months later shows communication (*arrow*) of the nonenhancing retroperitoneal fluid collection (*large arrowhead*) with the ascending colon (*C*). Enhancing soft-tissue nodule (*small arrowhead*) at the anteromedial margin of the fluid collection represents residual tumor within the nephrectomy bed. Susceptibility from a gastrostomy tube is present (*asterisk*)

T2-weighted, single-shot FSE imaging can confirm the presence of pneumatosis by demonstrating curvilinear low signal within the bowel wall which is separated from the bowel lumen by the mucosa (Fig. 17.35) (Pedrosa et al. 2007).

Single-shot FSE images are particularly valuable for depicting ischemic bowel in pregnancy. Similar to nonpregnant patients with ischemic bowel, abnormal bowel loops may demonstrate submucosal edema, adjacent mesenteric stranding, and bowel dilation. Like nonpregnant patients, these imaging features, however, are not specific for ischemia (Fig. 17.36).

MRI is also an excellent imaging modality for detecting bowel obstruction (see Chap. 16). The degree and level of small bowel obstruction can be readily demonstrated with T2-weighted single-shot FSE images without the need for oral or intravenous contrast (Regan et al. 1998; Leyendecker et al. 2004). Using only single-shot FSE images, Regan et al. (1998) identified small bowel obstruction in 26 of 29 patients with CT or radiographic evidence of small bowel obstruction, with a sensitivity of 90%. The correct level of obstruction was identified on MRI in 73% of the patients, and the cause of the small bowel obstruction could be visualized in 50% of the patients. A more recent study in 28 patients with bowel obstruction showed MRI, with the use of single-shot FSE imaging only, could diagnose the cause of bowel obstruction in 95% of the cases, and had a sensitivity, specificity, and accuracy of 95, 100, and 96%, respectively, for diagnosing both small and large bowel obstruction (BEALL et al. 2002). The use of multiplanar T2-weighted, single-shot FSE MRI is particularly valuable in evaluating for bowel obstruction in pregnant patients in whom the administration of intravenous contrast is undesirable (Fig. 17.37). Multiplanar TrueFISP imaging without oral or intravenous contrast has also been shown to be helpful in diagnosing small bowel obstruction and identifying the level of obstruction in pregnancy (MCKENNA et al. 2007).

17.3.4
Infection of the Gastrointestinal Tract

In patients with suspected gastrointestinal tract infection, cross-section imaging, namely CT, is usually reserved for the detection of complications related to the infection, including perforation, obstruction, or abscess formation. MRI is rarely used as a primary imaging modality for clinical assessment in these scenarios, and therefore, a paucity of literature exists describing the utility of MRI in the evaluation of gastrointestinal tract infection.

The imaging features of infection involving the gastrointestinal tract on MRI are nonspecific, appearing similar to other inflammatory, neoplastic, and ischemic conditions that affect the bowel (Fig 17.13). Additionally, infection of the gastrointestinal tract from viral, parasitic, or bacterial sources cannot be discerned based on MRI features alone. The imaging appearance of infected segments

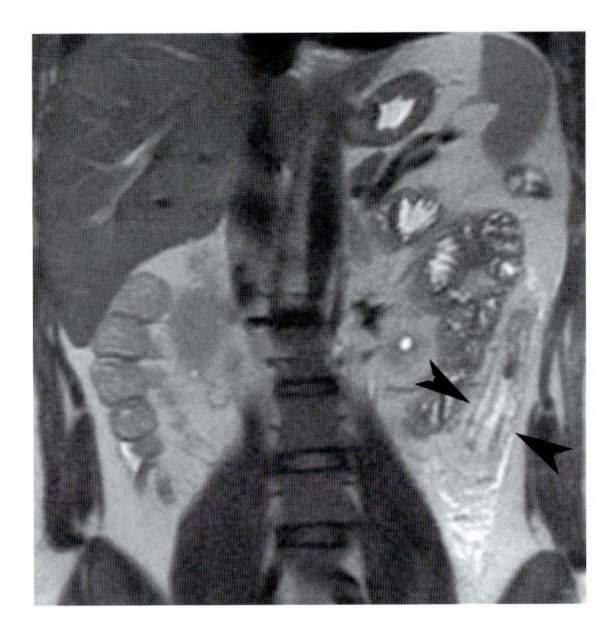

Fig. 17.33. Coronal T2-weighted FSE image in a 29-year-old-man with bloody diarrhea and abdominal pain demonstrates bowel wall thickening and pericolonic stranding and edema of the descending colon. Note colonic mural stratification with central areas of high signal intensity in the wall surrounded by intermediate signal intensity on either side, denoting mural edema (*arrowheads*). The patient underwent colonoscopy and biopsies confirmed ischemic colitis

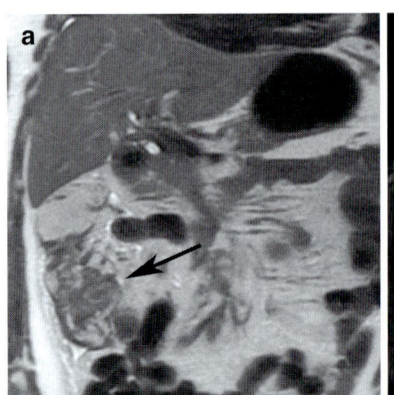

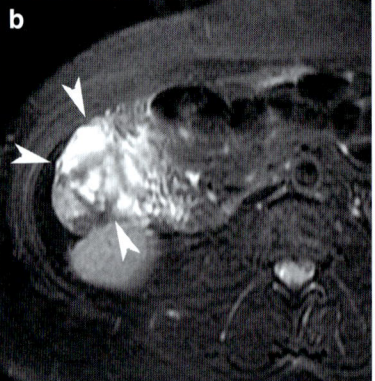

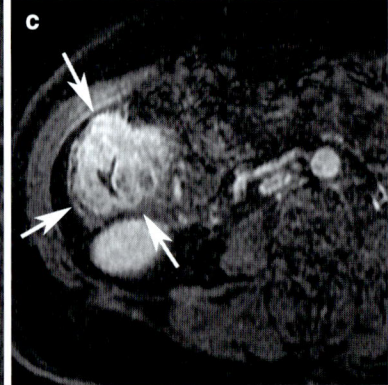

Fig. 17.34. (a) Coronal T2-weighted single-shot FSE image in a 70-year-old-woman presenting with abdominal pain and a history of paroxysmal atrial fibrillation and mitral valve replacement, demonstrates marked circumferential wall thickening of the cecum and ascending colon (*black arrow*). (b) Axial, T2-weighted FSE image with fat suppression demonstrates extensive high signal within the wall of the right colon and surrounding pericolonic fat (*arrowheads*), compatible with edema. (c) Axial, gadolinium-enhanced, 3D fat-suppressed, T1-weighted GRE image obtained during the portal venous phase shows hyperenhancement of the cecal wall (*white arrows*) with luminal narrowing. Right-sided colonic biopsies were obtained, which revealed ischemic colitis

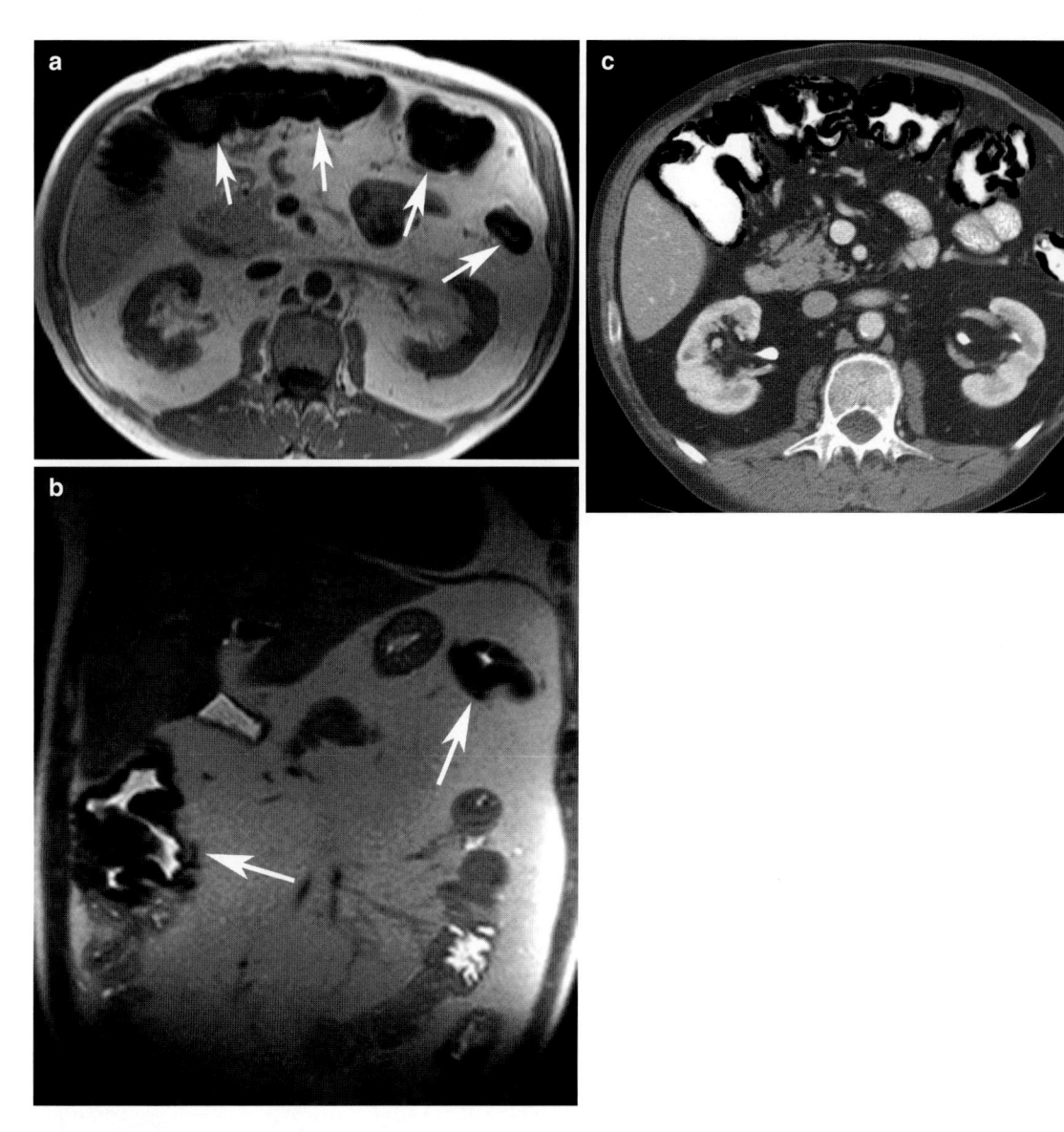

Fig. 17.35. (a) Axial, T1-weighted GRE and (b) coronal, T2-weighted single-shot FSE images in a 58-year-old man with abdominal pain, history of Crohn's disease, and partial colectomy demonstrate extensive, curvilinear areas of low signal within the wall of the colon diffusely (*white arrows*), findings compatible with pneumatosis. (c) Axial CT image obtained during the portal venous phase of enhancement confirms extensive colonic pneumatosis. No free intraperitoneal air, portal venous gas, or dilated loops of bowel were present on either imaging examination to suggest an ischemic etiology, and findings were most suggestive of benign pneumatosis coli. The patient's symptoms quickly improved with conservative management

of bowel or stomach can result in wall thickening, mural edema, and adjacent inflammatory stranding (MARTIN et al. 2005). With contrast administration, infected bowel segments demonstrate increased wall enhancement, which is indistinguishable from other etiologies of mural enhancement (MARTIN et al. 2005).

17.4
Conclusion

The role of MRI in diagnosing acute gastrointestinal conditions continues to expand. The feasibility of evaluating pregnant patients presenting with acute

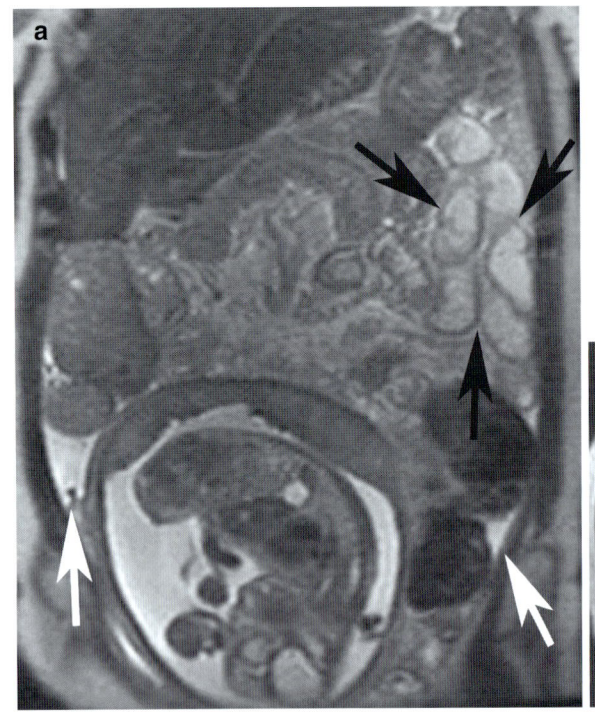

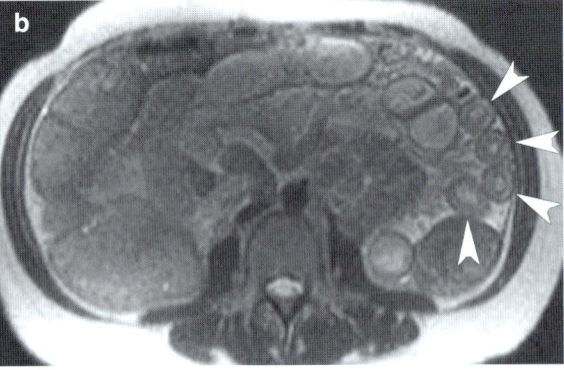

Fig. 17.36. (a) Coronal T2-weighted single-shot FSE image in a 39-year-old pregnant woman at 25-weeks gestation age presenting with severe abdominal pain demonstrates fluid-filled loops of small bowel within the left hemiabdomen (*black arrows*) and free intraperitoneal fluid (*white arrows*). (b) Axial T2-weighted single-shot FSE image shows multiple loops of small bowel within the left hemiabdomen with marked wall thickening and a target appearance (*arrowheads*) indicative of mural edema. At surgery, the patient was found to have a small bowel volvulus secondary to an adhesion, resulting in extensive small bowel ischemia

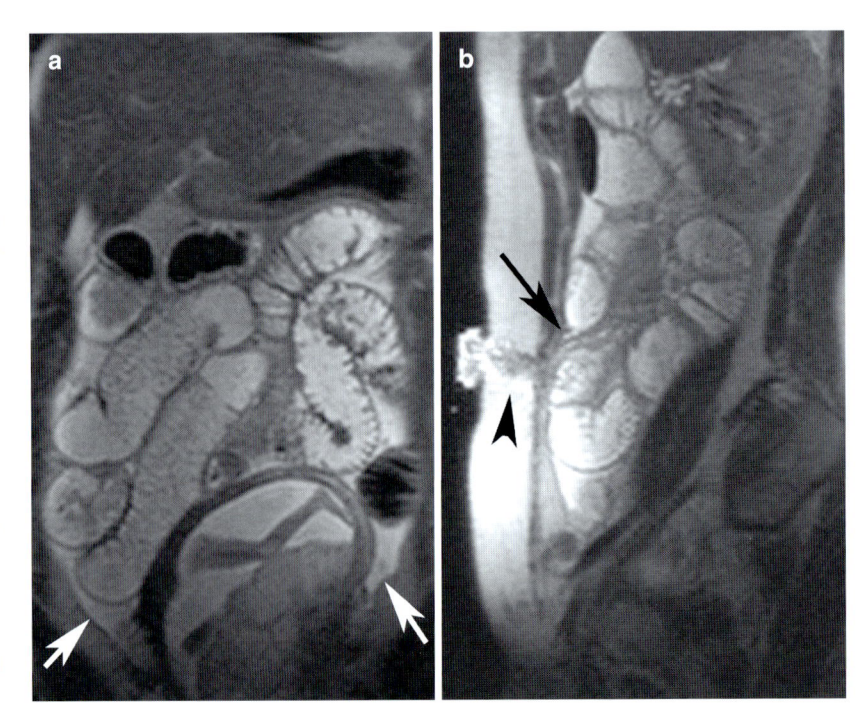

Fig. 17.37. (a) Coronal T2-weighted single-shot FSE image in a 34-year-old pregnant female at 19-week gestational age with a history of ulcerative colitis and total colectomy demonstrates diffusely dilated, fluid-filled loops of small bowel with free fluid noted in the abdominal cavity (*white arrows*), compatible with a high-grade small bowel obstruction. (b) On the sagittal T2-weighted single-shot FSE image, the transition point of the small bowel obstruction is noted at the level of the ostomy (*arrowhead*), as the end ileal loop abruptly tapers due to a stenosis at the ostomy (*black arrow*). This patient underwent balloon dilation of the ostomy with resolution of the bowel obstruction and her symptoms

abdominal pain with MRI has been established; however, its use has not become generalized. Because of the lack of familiarity of MRI among radiologists for these particular applications, combined with the relatively longer examination times of MRI, ultrasound and CT continue to be the preferred imaging modalities for the evaluation of acute abdominal pain in both pregnant and nonpregnant populations in many institutions. Furthermore, the broad applicability of MRI in the evaluation of acute abdominal pain in nonpregnant patients requires further validation. The use of short, tailored MRI protocols, possibly including new MRI techniques such as DWI sequences, may enable its inclusion in the imaging diagnostic algorithms for acute abdominal pain. The lack of sensitivity of MRI for detecting air, however, may represent an important limiting factor in its widespread adoption. Nevertheless, MRI may be advantageous for evaluating specific acute abdominal conditions in both pregnant and nonpregnant patients, including diagnosing acute appendicitis in pregnancy after an inconclusive ultrasound examination, evaluation of inflammatory bowel disease and its complications, diagnosing acute biliary conditions, and offering a non-contrast imaging alternative for the evaluation of vascular pathology.

References

Aho AJ, Heinonen R, Lauren P (1973) Benign and malignant mucocele of the appendix. Histological types and prognosis. Acta Chir Scand 139:392–400
Balthazar EJ, Megibow AJ, Gordon RB, et al (1987) Cecal diverticulitis: evaluation with CT. Radiology 162:79–81
Barbier C, Denny P, Pradoura JM, et al (1998) [Radiologic aspects of infarction of the appendix epiploica]. J Radiol 79:1479–1485
Barbosa JJ, Dockerty MB, Waugh JM (1946) Pancreatic heterotopia: a review of the literature and report of 41 authenticated surgical cases of which 25 were clinically significant. Surg Gynecol Obstet 82:527–542
Beall DP, Fortman BJ, Lawler BC, et al (2002) Imaging bowel obstruction: a comparison between fast magnetic resonance imaging and helical computed tomography. Clin Radiol 57:719–724
Bennett GL, Tanpitukpongse TP, Macari M, et al (2009) CT diagnosis of mucocele of the appendix in patients with acute appendicitis. AJR Am J Roentgenol 192:W103–W110
Bernstein CN, Greenberg H, Boult I, et al (2005) A prospective comparison study of MRI versus small bowel follow-through in recurrent Crohn's disease. Am J Gastroenterol 100:2493–2502
Birchard KR, Brown MA, Hyslop WB, et al (2005) MRI of acute abdominal and pelvic pain in pregnant patients. AJR Am J Roentgenol 184:452–458
Birnbaum BA, Wilson SR (2000) Appendicitis at the millennium. Radiology 215:337–348
Buckley O, Geoghegan T, McAuley G, et al (2007) Pictorial review: magnetic resonance imaging of colonic diverticulitis. Eur Radiol 17:221–227
Carr NJ, McCarthy WF, Sobin LH (1995) Epithelial noncarcinoid tumors and tumor-like lesions of the appendix. A clinicopathologic study of 184 patients with a multivariate analysis of prognostic factors. Cancer 75:757–768
Chan JH, Tsui EY, Luk SH, et al (2001) MR diffusion-weighted imaging of kidney: differentiation between hydronephrosis and pyonephrosis. Clin Imaging 25:110–113
Chintapalli KN, Chopra S, Ghiatas AA, et al (1999) Diverticulitis versus colon cancer: differentiation with helical CT findings. Radiology 210:429–435
Cobben L, Groot I, Kingma L, et al (2009) A simple MRI protocol in patients with clinically suspected appendicitis: results in 138 patients and effect on outcome of appendectomy. Eur Radiol 19:1175–1183
Cobben LP, Groot I, Haans L, et al (2004) MRI for clinically suspected appendicitis during pregnancy. AJR Am J Roentgenol 183:671–675
Cronin CG, Lohan DG, DeLappe E, et al (2008) Duodenal abnormalities at MR small-bowel follow-through. AJR Am J Roentgenol 191:1082–1092
Earls JP, Rofsky NM, DeCorato DR, et al (1997) Hepatic arterial-phase dynamic gadolinium-enhanced MR imaging: optimization with a test examination and a power injector. Radiology 202:268–273
Eyvazzadeh AD, Pedrosa I, Rofsky NM, et al (2004) MRI of right-sided abdominal pain in pregnancy. AJR Am J Roentgenol 183:907–914
Fattahi R, Balci NC, Perman WH, et al (2009) Pancreatic diffusion-weighted imaging (DWI): comparison between mass-forming focal pancreatitis (FP), pancreatic cancer (PC), and normal pancreas. J Magn Reson Imaging 29:350–356
Furukawa A, Saotome T, Yamasaki M, et al (2004) Cross-sectional imaging in Crohn disease. Radiographics 24:689–702
Ganguli S, Raptopoulos V, Komlos F, et al (2006) Right lower quadrant pain: value of the nonvisualized appendix in patients at multidetector CT. Radiology 241:175–180
Garcia K, Hernanz-Schulman M, Bennett DL, et al (2009) Suspected appendicitis in children: diagnostic importance of normal abdominopelvic CT findings with nonvisualized appendix. Radiology 250:531–537
Gourtsoyiannis N, Papanikolaou N, Grammatikakis J, et al (2002) MR enteroclysis: technical considerations and clinical applications. Eur Radiol 12:2651–2658
Greenberg JJ, Esposito TJ (1996) Appendicitis after laparoscopic appendectomy: a warning. J Laparoendosc Surg 6:185–187
Hammond NA, Miller FH, Yaghmai V, et al (2008) MR imaging of acute bowel pathology: a pictorial review. Emerg Radiol 15:99–104
Hedrick E, Kozloff M, Hainsworth J (2006) Safety of bevacizumab plus chemotherapy as first-line treatment of patients with metastatic colorectal cancer: updated results from a large observational registry in the US (BRiTE) [meeting abstracts]. J Clin Oncol 24:3536

Herrmann KA, Michaely HJ, Zech CJ, et al (2006) Internal fistulas in Crohn disease: magnetic resonance enteroclysis. Abdom Imaging 31:675–687

Heverhagen JT, Ishaque N, Zielke A, et al (2001) Feasibility of MRI in the diagnosis of acute diverticulitis: initial results. Magma 12:4–9

Heverhagen JT, Sitter H, Zielke A, et al (2008) Prospective evaluation of the value of magnetic resonance imaging in suspected acute sigmoid diverticulitis. Dis Colon Rectum 51:1810–1815

Higa E, Rosai J, Pizzimbono CA, et al (1973) Mucosal hyperplasia, mucinous cystadenoma, and mucinous cystadenocarcinoma of the appendix. A re-evaluation of appendiceal "mucocele". Cancer 32:1525–1541

Hoeffel C, Crema MD, Belkacem A, et al (2006) Multi-detector row CT: spectrum of diseases involving the ileocecal area. Radiographics 26:1373–1390

Hormann M, Puig S, Prokesch SR, et al (2002) MR imaging of the normal appendix in children. Eur Radiol 12:2313–2316

Incesu L, Coskun A, Selcuk MB, et al (1997) Acute appendicitis: MR imaging and sonographic correlation. AJR Am J Roentgenol 168:669–674

Israel GM, Malguria N, McCarthy S, et al (2008) MRI vs. ultrasound for suspected appendicitis during pregnancy. J Magn Reson Imaging 28:428–433

Kanal E, Barkovich AJ, Bell C, et al (2007) ACR guidance document for safe MR practices: 2007. AJR Am J Roentgenol 188:1447–1474

Kim S, Jain M, Harris AB, et al (2009) T1 hyperintense renal lesions: characterization with diffusion-weighted MR Imaging versus contrast-enhanced MR imaging. Radiology 251:796–807

Klein HM, Klosterhalfen B, Kinzel S, et al (1996) CT and MRI of experimentally induced mesenteric ischemia in a porcine model. J Comput Assist Tomogr 20:254–261

Koh DM, Miao Y, Chinn RJ, et al (2001) MR imaging evaluation of the activity of Crohn's disease. AJR Am J Roentgenol 177:1325–1332

Lai EC, Tompkins RK (1986) Heterotopic pancreas. Review of a 26 year experience. Am J Surg 151:697–700

Landen S, Bertrand C, Maddern GJ, et al (1992) Appendiceal mucoceles and pseudomyxoma peritonei. Surg Gynecol Obstet 175:401–404

Lee JC, Wong KP, Lo SS, et al (2008a) Acute ectopic pancreatitis. Hong Kong Med J 14:501–502

Lee KS, Rofsky NM, Pedrosa I (2008b) Localization of the appendix at MR imaging during pregnancy: utility of the cecal tilt angle. Radiology 249:134–141

Lee SS, Kim AY, Yang SK, et al (2009) Crohn disease of the small bowel: comparison of CT enterography, MR enterography, and small-bowel follow-through as diagnostic techniques. Radiology 251:751

Leyendecker JR, Gorengaut V, Brown JJ (2004) MR imaging of maternal diseases of the abdomen and pelvis during pregnancy and the immediate postpartum period. Radiographics 24:1301–1316

Liebig T, Stoupis C, Ros PR, et al (1993) A potentially artifact-free oral contrast agent for gastrointestinal MRI. Magn Reson Med 30:646–649

Lohan DG, Alhajeri AN, Cronin CG, et al (2008) MR enterography of small-bowel lymphoma: potential for suggestion of histologic subtype and the presence of underlying celiac disease. AJR Am J Roentgenol 190:287–293

Lohrmann C, Ghanem N, Pache G, et al (2005) CT in acute perforated sigmoid diverticulitis. Eur J Radiol 56:78–83

Low RN, Francis IR, Politoske D, et al (2000) Crohn's disease evaluation: comparison of contrast-enhanced MR imaging and single-phase helical CT scanning. J Magn Reson Imaging 11:127–135

Maccioni F, Bruni A, Viscido A, et al (2006) MR imaging in patients with Crohn disease: value of T2- versus T1-weighted gadolinium-enhanced MR sequences with use of an oral superparamagnetic contrast agent. Radiology 238:517–530

Maccioni F, Viscido A, Broglia L, et al (2000) Evaluation of Crohn disease activity with magnetic resonance imaging. Abdom Imaging 25:219–228

Madwed D, Mindelzun R, Jeffrey RB Jr (1992) Mucocele of the appendix: imaging findings. AJR Am J Roentgenol 159:69–72

Mangi AA, Berger DL (2000) Stump appendicitis. Am Surg 66:739–741

Marcos HB, Semelka RC (1999) Stomach diseases: MR evaluation using combined t2-weighted single-shot echo train spin-echo and gadolinium-enhanced spoiled gradient-echo sequences. J Magn Reson Imaging 10:950–960

Martin DR, Danrad R, Herrmann K, et al (2005) Magnetic resonance imaging of the gastrointestinal tract. Top Magn Reson Imaging 16:77–98

McKenna DA, Meehan CP, Alhajeri AN, et al (2007) The use of MRI to demonstrate small bowel obstruction during pregnancy. Br J Radiol 80:e11–e4

Nitta N, Takahashi M, Furukawa A, et al (2005) MR imaging of the normal appendix and acute appendicitis. J Magn Reson Imaging 21:156–165

Okuhata Y, Maebayashi T, Furuhashi S, et al (2008) Characteristics of ectopic pancreas in dynamic gadolinium-enhanced MRI. Abdom Imaging. http://www.springerlink.com/content/kp444564843871v8/. Published December 2, 2008. Accessed May 1, 2009

Oto A, Ernst RD, Ghulmiyyah LM, et al (2009) MR imaging in the triage of pregnant patients with acute abdominal and pelvic pain. Abdom Imaging 34:243–250

Oto A, Ernst RD, Shah R, et al (2005) Right-lower-quadrant pain and suspected appendicitis in pregnant women: evaluation with MR imaging–initial experience. Radiology 234:445–451

Patel SJ, Reede DL, Katz DS, et al (2007) Imaging the pregnant patient for nonobstetric conditions: algorithms and radiation dose considerations. Radiographics 27:1705–1722

Pedrosa I, Lafornara M, Pandharipande PV, et al (2009) Pregnant patients suspected of having acute appendicitis: effect of MR imaging on negative laparotomy rate and appendiceal perforation rate. Radiology 250:749–757

Pedrosa I, Levine D, Eyvazzadeh AD, et al (2006) MR imaging evaluation of acute appendicitis in pregnancy. Radiology 238:891–899

Pedrosa I, Rofsky NM (2003) MR imaging in abdominal emergencies. Radiol Clin North Am 41:1243–1273

Pedrosa I, Zeikus EA, Levine D, et al (2007) MR imaging of acute right lower quadrant pain in pregnant and nonpregnant patients. Radiographics 27:721–743; discussion 743–753

Pickhardt PJ, Levy AD, Rohrmann CA Jr, et al (2002) Primary neoplasms of the appendix manifesting as acute appendicitis: CT findings with pathologic comparison. Radiology 224:775–781

Pickhardt PJ, Levy AD, Rohrmann CA Jr, et al (2003) Primary neoplasms of the appendix: radiologic spectrum of disease with pathologic correlation. Radiographics 23: 645–662

Qizilbash AH (1975) Mucoceles of the appendix. Their relationship to hyperplastic polyps, mucinous cystadenomas, and cystadenocarcinomas. Arch Pathol 99:548–555

Rao PM, Sagarin MJ, McCabe CJ (1998) Stump appendicitis diagnosed preoperatively by computed tomography. Am J Emerg Med 16:309–311

Regan F, Beall DP, Bohlman ME, et al (1998) Fast MR imaging and the detection of small-bowel obstruction. AJR Am J Roentgenol 170:1465–1469

Rha SE, Ha HK, Lee SH, et al (2000) CT and MR imaging findings of bowel ischemia from various primary causes. Radiographics 20:29–42

Rioux M, Langis P (1994) Primary epiploic appendagitis: clinical, US, and CT findings in 14 cases. Radiology 191:523–526

Rofsky NM, Lee VS, Laub G, et al (1999) Abdominal MR imaging with a volumetric interpolated breath-hold examination. Radiology 212:876–884

Rubesin SE, Furth EE, Birnbaum BA, et al (1997) Ectopic pancreas complicated by pancreatitis and pseudocyst formation mimicking jejunal diverticulitis. Br J Radiol 70: 311–313

Sadowski EA, Bennett LK, Chan MR, et al (2007) Nephrogenic systemic fibrosis: risk factors and incidence estimation. Radiology 243:148–157

Sartoris DJ, Harell GS, Anderson MF, et al (1984) Small-bowel lymphoma and regional enteritis: radiographic similarities. Radiology 152:291–296

Shellock FG, Crues JV (2004) MR procedures: biologic effects, safety, and patient care. Radiology 232:635–652

Shin LK, Halpern D, Weston SR, et al (2005) Prospective CT diagnosis of stump appendicitis. AJR Am J Roentgenol 184:S62–S64

Siddiki H, Fidler J (2009) MR imaging of the small bowel in Crohn's disease. Eur J Radiol 69:409–417

Silva AC, Charles JC, Kimery BD, et al (2006) MR Cholangiopancreatography in the detection of symptomatic ectopic pancreatitis in the small-bowel mesentery. AJR Am J Roentgenol 187:W195–W197

Singh AK, Desai H, Novelline RA (2009) Emergency MRI of acute pelvic pain: MR protocol with no oral contrast. Emerg Radiol 16:133–141

Singh AK, Gervais DA, Hahn PF, et al (2005) Acute epiploic appendagitis and its mimics. Radiographics 25:1521–1534

Sirvanci M, Balci NC, Karaman K, et al (2002) Primary epiploic appendagitis: MRI findings. Magn Reson Imaging 20:137–139

Sugrue M, Kozloff M, Hainsworth J (2006) Risk factors for gastrointestinal perforations in patients with metastatic colorectal cancer receiving bevacizumab plus chemotherapy [meeting abstracts]. J Clin Oncol 24:3535

Taouli B, Thakur RK, Mannelli L, et al (2009) Renal lesions: characterization with diffusion-weighted imaging versus contrast-enhanced MR imaging. Radiology 251:398–407

Truty MJ, Stulak JM, Utter PA, et al (2008) Appendicitis after appendectomy. Arch Surg 143:413–415

van Randen A, Bipat S, Zwinderman AH, et al (2008) Acute appendicitis: meta-analysis of diagnostic performance of CT and graded compression US related to prevalence of disease. Radiology 249:97–106

Verswijvel G, Vandecaveye V, Gelin G, et al (2002) Diffusion-weighted MR imaging in the evaluation of renal infection: preliminary results. Jbr-Btr 85:100–103

Walsh DC, Roediger WE (1997) Stump appendicitis–a potential problem after laparoscopic appendicectomy. Surg Laparosc Endosc 7:357–358

Woodfield C, Lazarus E (2008) MR imaging of appendicitis in pregnancy: comparison of appendix visualization without and with oral contrast material administration [abstract]. Radiological Society of North America Scientific Assembly and Annual Meeting Program 518

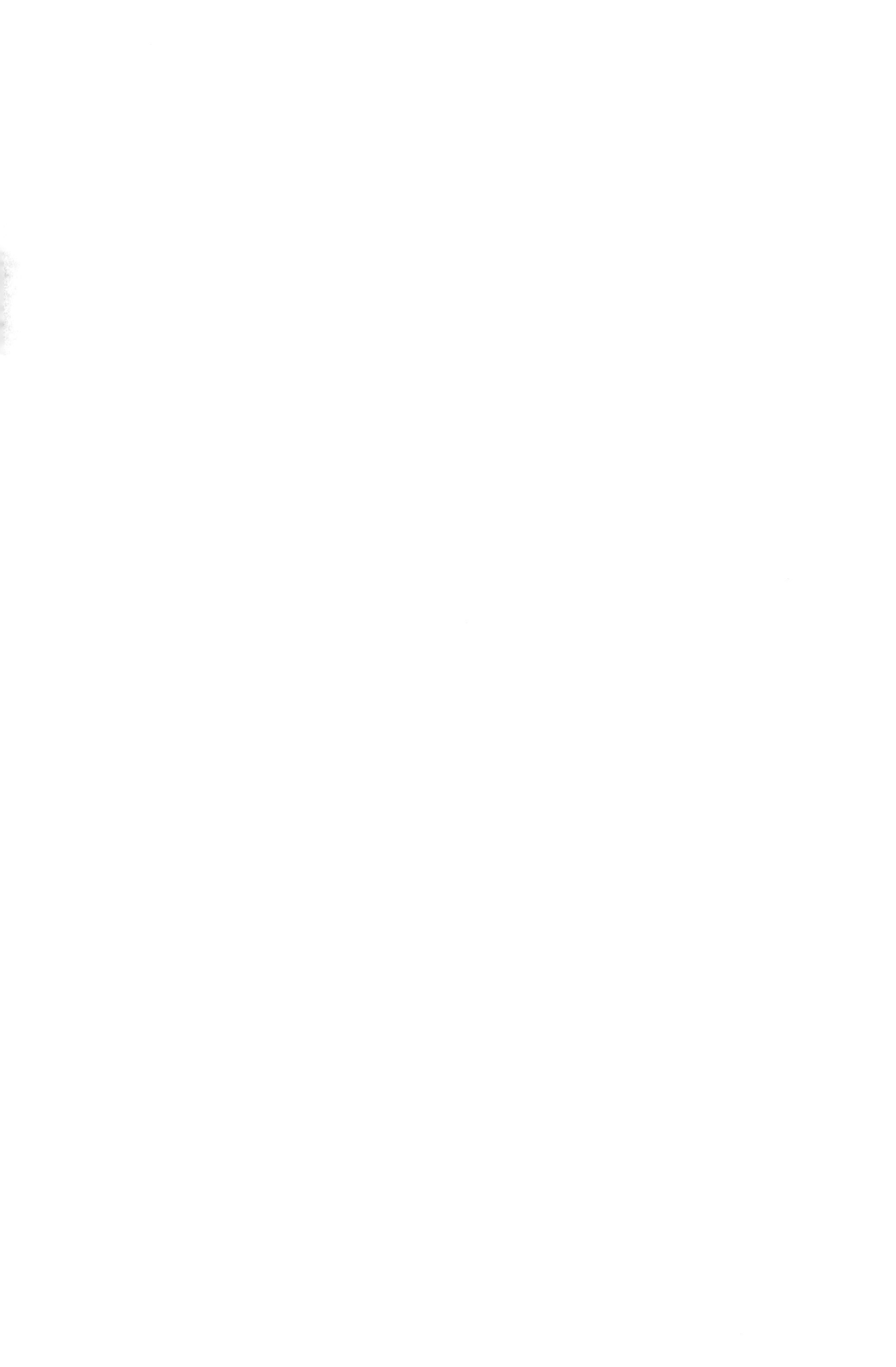

MRI of the Pelvic Floor

CAECILIA S. REINER and DOMINIK WEISHAUPT

CONTENTS

18.1 Introduction 315

18.2 Technical Considerations 316
18.2.1 Patient Positioning 316
18.2.2 Patient Preparation 316
18.2.3 Imaging Technique 317
18.2.4 Image Analysis 318
18.2.5 Normal Findings 318

18.3 Spectrum of Abnormal Findings 319
18.3.1 Rectocele 319
18.3.2 Enterocele 321
18.3.3 Intussusception and Rectal Prolapse 322
18.3.3.1 Intussusception 322
18.3.3.2 External Rectal Prolapse 323
18.3.2 Pelvic Organ Prolapse 323
18.3.2.1 Cystocele 323
18.3.2.2 Utero-Vaginal Prolapse 324
18.3.3 Pelvic Floor Relaxation (Pelvic Floor Descent), Descending Perineal Syndrome 324
18.3.4 Dyssynergic Defecation 324

18.4 Conclusion 326

References 326

CAECILIA S. REINER, MD
Institute of Diagnostic Radiology, University Hospital Zurich, Raemistrasse 100, 8091 Zurich, Switzerland
DOMINIK WEISHAUPT, MD
Division of Radiology, City Hospital Triemli, Birmensdorferstrasse 497, 8063 Zurich, Switzerland

KEY POINTS

The pelvic floor is a complex anatomic and functional unit. Over the past few years MR imaging has gained increasing acceptance as imaging modality for evaluation of the pelvic floor. Using static T2-weighted sequences, the morphology of the pelvic floor can be visualized in great detail. A multicoil array and a rapid half-Fourier T2-weighted, balanced steady-state free precession (bSSFP), or gradient-recalled echo (GRE) sequence are used to obtain sagittal images while the patient is at rest, during pelvic squeeze, during pelvic strain, and to document the evacuation process. On these images the radiologist identifies the pubococcygeal line (which represents the level of the pelvic floor) and the H- and M-Lines (which are helpful for confirming pelvic laxity). Based on these static and dynamic MR imaging sequences, a vast array of morphologic and functional pelvic floor disorders can be depicted.

18.1
Introduction

The pelvic floor is a complex anatomic and functional unit of multiple muscle layers, fascia and ligaments. In clinical routine, a simple anatomic concept of the female pelvic floor has gained acceptance. Especially for treatment planning, the female pelvic floor may be separated into three functional compartments: the anterior compartment (bladder and urethra), the middle compartment (vagina, cervix, uterus, and adnexa), and the posterior compartment (anus and rectum). Intact structure of the pelvic floor is a basic prerequisite for a normal mechanism of defecation and continence. Pelvic floor dysfunction is a complex condition involving some or all of the pelvic organs.

Common clinical symptoms of pelvic floor dysfunction are chronic constipation, pelvic pain, organ prolapse, and fecal incontinence. Underlying causes are often functional disorders including rectocele, rectal prolapse and intussusception, enterocele, abnormal pelvic floor relaxation with pelvic organ prolapse, and dyssynergic defecation.

For evaluation of these pelvic floor disorders, clinicians and surgeons have traditionally relied on physical examination and clinical scoring systems. Although clinical scoring systems are helpful to establish diagnosis, they are less useful for surgical triage and planning, because they do not involve direct assessment of anatomy. To improve surgical outcome and success, preoperative triage and careful planning is necessary.

In recent years, MRI has been introduced to supplement clinical data in selecting surgical candidates and in planning repairs. MRI is not only able to visualize detailed morphology of the pelvic floor in a static imaging mode, but can also be used as a dynamic imaging method for evaluation of the pelvic floor. The latter is also known as dynamic MR imaging of the pelvic floor or MR defecography, if the focus of interest is directed on the posterior pelvic floor compartment.

In this chapter we review the technique and clinical applications of imaging of the pelvic floor with emphasis on the posterior pelvic floor compartment. Static imaging of the anal sphincter is covered in Chap. 19 of this book. This chapter focuses specifically on dynamic MR imaging of the pelvic floor illustrating the MRI features of a vast array of anorectal dysfunctions and pelvic floor prolapse.

18.2
Technical Considerations

18.2.1
Patient Positioning

Dynamic pelvic imaging may be performed in an open-configuration MR system in the sitting position, or in a closed-configuration MR system in the supine position. Although the sitting position is the physiologic position during defecation, MR defecography is usually performed in the supine position, because of the limited availability of open-configuration MR magnets, which would allow examination in the physiologic sitting position. Reports about the influence of body position on defecation are sparse in the literature. A study about patient positioning during MR defecography showed that MR defecography in the supine position and in the seated position is equally effective in identifying most of the clinically relevant abnormalities of the pelvic floor (BERTSCHINGER et al. 2002). The lacking influence of gravity when patients are imaged in supine instead of sitting position may affect the diagnosis of intussusceptions. In the study of BERTSCHINGER et al. (2002) all intussusceptions found in upright positions were missed in supine position. This means, if an intussusception is found in supine position it should be regarded as clinically relevant, and if it is missing in supine position, it cannot be reliably regarded as ruled out. In a study using supine dynamic MR (KRUYT et al. 1991) and sitting conventional defecography, the authors found no differences for the position of the anorectal junction (ARJ) or the measurements of the anorectal angle (ARA) between sitting and prone positions. In contrast, a study using conventional defecography showed significant differences for ARA and perineal descent between left lateral decubitus and seated position during conventional defecography (JORGE et al. 1994). In another study, Rao et al (2006) showed differences in the defecation maneuver for different body positions and different stool characteristics when performing balloon expulsion tests. These possible differences between the two body positions in mind, it is recommendable to employ always the same position for a given diagnostic group.

18.2.2
Patient Preparation

The administration of contrast agent for MRI of the pelvic floor varies in different studies, from use of no contrast agent to filling of the rectum, vagina, urethra, and bladder with contrast agent; placement of markers in the vagina or rectum; or placement of urethral catheters (HEALY et al. 1997; LIENEMANN et al. 1997; YANG et al. 1991). For evaluation of the posterior compartment of the pelvic floor, authorities agree that the rectum should be filled with contrast agent. The rectum is filled with contrast agent not only for better delineation, but also mainly to study the actual act of defecation. This is of importance, as some disorders of the pelvic floor appear in their full size only during defecation, like rectal prolapse or intussusception (LIENEMANN and FISCHER 2003).

Immediately before the examination, the rectum is filled with the rectal enema. The volume of enema used is variable and ranges between 120 and 300 mL (Halligan et al. 2001; Karlbom et al. 1999; Maglinte and Bartram 2007). Some investigators administer contrast agent until the patient feels a sustained desire to defecate. Others use a standardized volume of contrast agent. Although it is not known if the amount of contrast agent administered, influences the extent of structural pelvic floor disorders, in our experience 250–300 mL of enema gives the best results. However, the time needed to evacuate the contrast agent and thus the assessment of the evacuation ability depend on the amount of contrast agent (see Sect. 18.3.4). Therefore, it is necessary to standardize the volume administered. The viscosity of the contrast agent should be similar to that of normal rectum content because the manifestations of pelvic floor pathologies vary with different fecal consistency (Bartram et al. 1988; Karlbom et al. 1999; Solopova et al. 2008). Authors recommend ultrasound gel (Fletcher et al. 2003; Kelvin et al. 2000; Lienemann et al. 1997; Vanbeckevoort et al. 1999) or mashed potatoes (Bertschinger et al. 2002; Dvorkin et al. 2004; Hetzer et al. 2006). Depending on the sequence used for dynamic MR imaging, the rectal enema may be doped with a small amount of standard extracellular gadolinium-based MR contrast agent. In general, neither premedication nor oral or rectal preparation for bowel cleansing is necessary before imaging. In our current imaging protocol, we do not perform retrograde filling of the bladder and we do not perform tagging of the vagina. In order to ensure filling of the bladder we ask the patient not to void the bladder at least 1 h before the examination. With regard to the middle-compartment, the soft-tissue contrast is usually high enough to identify all anatomic landmarks. Therefore, we do not perform any tagging of the vagina. Exceptions may be specific queries before surgery is performed such as reconstruction of the pelvic floor in severe uterus prolapse.

Beside the administration of contrast agent, a clear instruction of the patients about the procedure of the examination is essential. Because most patients might be nervous and intimidated, technicians must be trained in placing patients at ease in the MRI unit and giving clear instructions. Patient cooperation is critical for a useful examination. Therefore, patients need to be instructed about imaging at different pelvic positions, including imaging at rest, at squeezing, at straining, and during defecation, before starting the examination. During the examination, the technicians are coaching the patients using a microphone and headset. In order to protect the scanner from soiling we cover the phased array coil with plastic and ask the patient to wear diapers. As the setting and the retrograde administration of rectal contrast agent is artificial, some have advocated the use of the term evacuation. This is to indicate the difference of this setting to physiologic defecation. In this chapter defecation and MR defecography are used as terms as these are commonly used.

18.2.3
Imaging Technique

MR defecography may be performed in supine position using all commercially available closed- or open-configuration MR systems with horizontal access. When dynamic pelvic MR is performed in these MR systems the patient is placed in supine position and a pelvic phased-array coil is used for signal transmission and/or reception. After filling the rectum the examination starts with a localizer sequence. The examination protocol includes non-fat-suppressed static T2-weighted fast spin-echo (FSE) or fast recovery FSE sequences in the transaxial plane. These sequences are performed to visualize the anatomy of the pelvic floor. Subsequently, dynamic MR imaging is performed. For dynamic MR imaging in the different positions (at squeezing, at straining, and during defecation) various MR sequences can be used with similar results. The basic requirement for the sequence is the necessity for a fast imaging update. Some authors have used T2-weighted single-shot fast spin-echo sequences (SSFSE) in the midsagittal plane obtained at rest, at squeezing, at straining, and during defecation. Alternatively, balanced steady-state free precession (bSSFP) sequences may be used for this purpose. Our current protocol includes (bSSFP) sequences obtained at rest, at squeezing, straining, and after evacuation. For assessment of the defecation bSSFP sequence or alternatively a T1-weighted multiphase GRE sequence may be used. If the T1-weighted multiphase GRE sequence is used, the rectal enema is usually tagged with a small amount of an extracellular gadolinium-based contrast agent. Which sequence is used depends on the scanner. For the evacuation phase, it is important to have a sequence which offers the possibility to acquire images over a long time period without the necessity to reload the sequence. This is in particular important in patients with a long prolongation period.

Filling of bladder, vagina, and rectum may act as a splint preventing prolapse, this is also named crowding. For this reason some have advocated a multi-phasic examination when these organs are filled. In this setting, the cystographic phase is performed before rectal filling, because rectal distention elevates the bladder base and may mask a cystocele (Kelvin and Maglinte 1997).

18.2.4
Image Analysis

Image analysis is performed according to the three-compartment model of the pelvic floor (Roos et al. 2002). The three compartments of the pelvic floor are assessed for morphologic changes at different pelvic floor positions. Beside the qualitative assessment, quantitative evaluation of imaging findings is important, because the extent of the imaging findings may influence further management. The use of reference lines for image evaluation is helpful. The most used reference line is the pubococcygeal line (PCL), which is defined on midsagittal images as the line joining the inferior border of the symphysis pubis to the last or second last coccygeal joint. The distance of the base of the bladder (anterior compartment), the cervix or vaginal vault (middle compartment), and the ARJ (posterior compartment) is measured at a 90° angle to the PCL in the different pelvic floor positions (at rest, squeezing, straining, and evacuation) as shown in Fig. 18.1. The ARJ is defined as the cross point between a line along the posterior wall of the distal part of the rectum and a line along the central axis of the anal canal. To determine pathologic pelvic floor descent the measurements are made on the images, which show maximal organ descent, usually during maximal straining or during evacuation. In addition, the anorectal angle (ARA), which is defined as the angle between the posterior wall of the distal part of the rectum and the central axis of the anal canal, can be measured at rest, squeezing, and straining (Fig. 18.2). It has to be noted that the reproducibility of ARA measurements has been debated and questioned in several studies (Ferrante et al. 1991; Penninckx et al. 1990), whereas other studies found the ARA a consistent and reliable parameter (Choi et al. 2000). Furthermore, the extent of other pathologic conditions such as rectoceles and enteroceles are measured.

Beside the three-compartment-model with the PCL as reference line mainly used by surgeons and gastroenterologists, the second known system for grading pelvic floor abnormalities is the HMO system, which is mainly used by urologists and gynecologists (Comiter et al. 1999). The HMO systems distinguish pelvic organ prolapse and pelvic floor relaxation, which are two separate but often coexistent pathologic entities. In pelvic floor relaxation, the pelvic floor with its active and passive support structures becomes weakened leading to hiatal descent and hiatal widening. The degree of pelvic floor relaxation is measured with two reference lines: the H-line which represents hiatal widening and extends from the inferior aspect of the symphysis pubis to the posterior wall of the rectum at the level of the ARJ and the M-line which represents hiatal descent and extends perpendicularly from the PCL to the posterior end of the H-line (Fig. 18.3). Abnormal pelvic floor relaxation is present, when the H-line exceeds 6 cm, and when the M-line exceeds 2 cm in length (Boyadzhyan et al. 2008).

Pelvic organ prolapse is defined as any organ descent beyond the H-line. The organ descent constitutes the O component of the HMO system and is measured as the shortest distance between the most caudal aspect of a given organ during maximal straining (bladder, vaginal vault, or any part of the remaining cervix in cases with a hysterectomy, small bowel, sigmoid colon) and the H-line (Boyadzhyan et al. 2008; Comiter et al. 1999). Pelvic organ prolapse is graded as small (grade 1, 0–2 cm below the H-line), moderate (grade 2, 2–4 cm), and large (grade 3, >4 cm). Also HMO measurements are performed during maximal straining, when pathologic findings usually show maximal extension.

18.2.5
Normal Findings

At rest, the base of the bladder and the cervix or vaginal vault lies at or above the level of the PCL. The ARJ typically projects at or within 3 cm below the level of the PCL. The rectum is filled with contrast medium and should be smooth in outline, the anal canal is closed and builds an ARA between about 94° and 114° to the rectum (Bartram et al. 1988; Ekberg et al. 1985; Goei et al. 1989; Kruyt et al. 1991). During maximum pelvic floor contraction (squeezing) the pelvic floor is elevated in relationship to the PCL and the ARA is decreased by about 10–23° (Goei et al. 1989; Kruyt et al. 1991). Recording pelvic floor movement when the patient contracts the pelvic floor demonstrates pelvic floor muscle strength. Impaired movement may reflect weakness of the pelvic floor

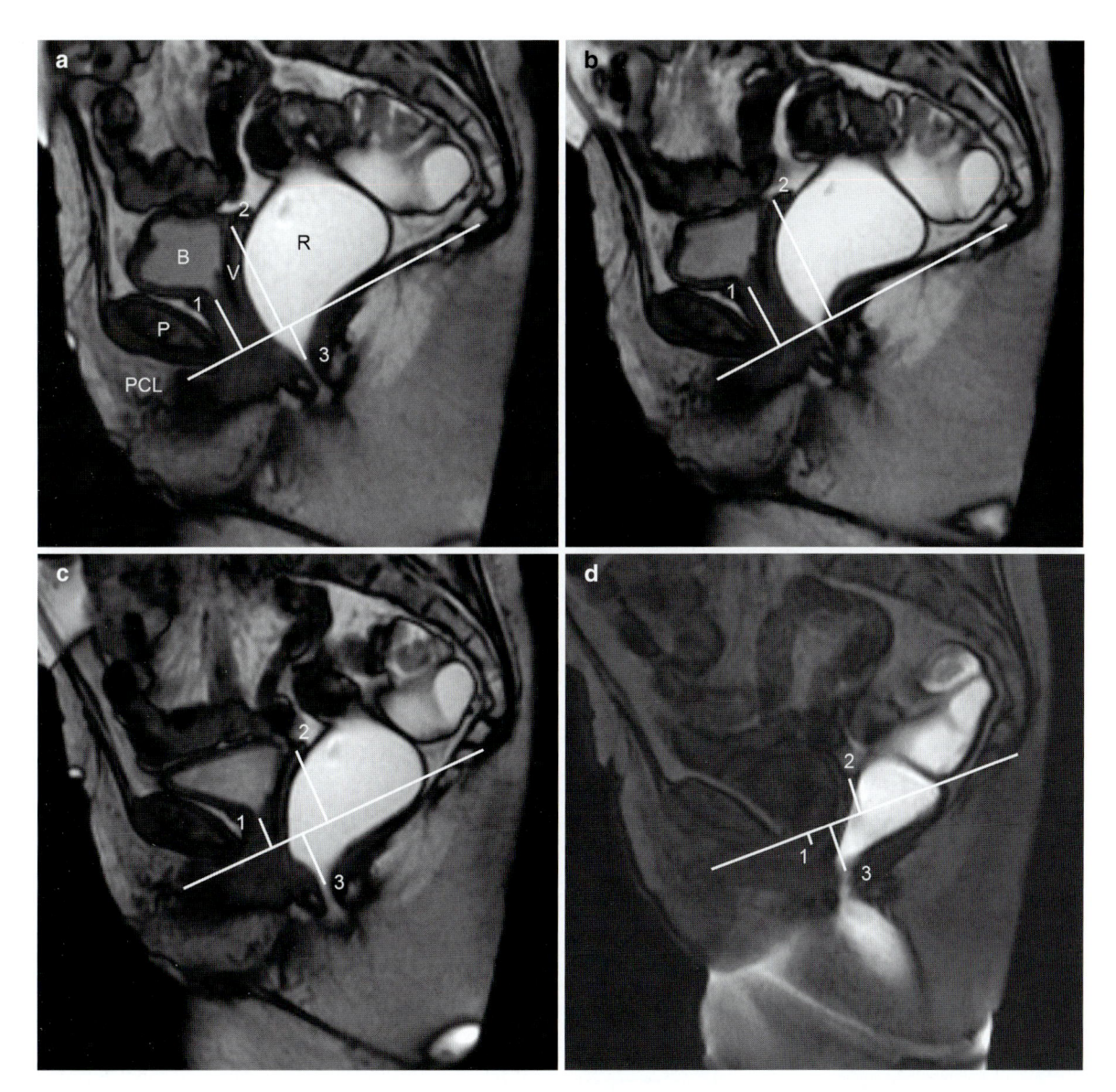

Fig. 18.1. Seventy-nine-year-old female patient with normal findings at MR defecography. On midsagittal balanced steady-state free precession (bSSFP) T2-weighted MR images obtained at rest (**a**), at squeezing (**b**), and at straining (**c**) and on a T1-weighted multiphase gradient recalled echo MR image during evacuation (**d**) the position of the base of the bladder (*1*, anterior compartment), the vaginal vault (*2*, middle compartment), and the anorectal junction (ARJ) (*3*, posterior compartment) is measured at a 90° angle to the PCL. *P* symphysis pubis; *B* bladder; *V* vaginal vault; *R* rectum; *PCL* pubococcygeal line

muscles (BHARUCHA et al. 2005). During straining, the pelvic floor muscles relax and the pelvic floor descends normally <3 cm below the PCL. With the descent of the ARJ, the ARA increases to about 113–135° (BARTRAM et al. 1988; EKBERG et al. 1985; GOEI et al. 1989; KRUYT et al. 1991). Finally, the anal canal opens and the contrast material is evacuated. Normally, two-thirds of the contrast material should be evacuated within 60 s (when about 400 mL of contrast agent are administered) (MINGUEZ et al. 2004).

18.3
Spectrum of Abnormal Findings

18.3.1
Rectocele

Rectoceles are defined as an outpouching of the rectal wall. The anterior wall is most commonly affected, but a rectocele may also be located in the posterior

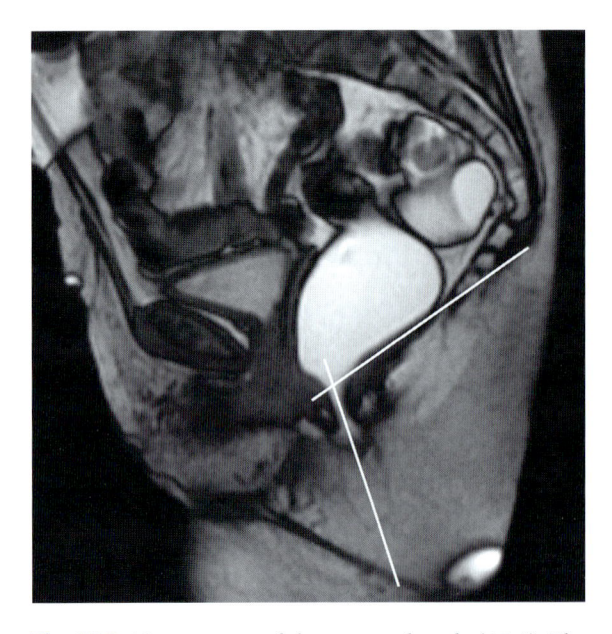

Fig. 18.2. Measurement of the anorectal angle (ARA). The ARA is measured between a line drawn through the posterior border of the distal part of rectum and a line drawn through the central axis of the anal canal

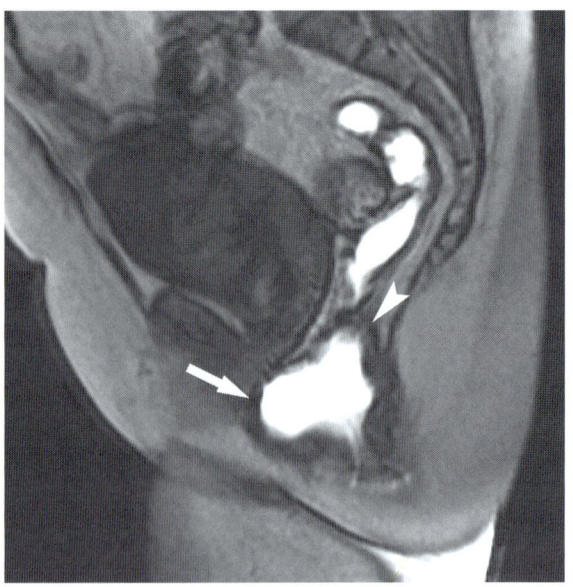

Fig. 18.4. Sixty-one-year-old female patient with chronic constipation. Midsagittal T1-weighted gradient recalled echo MR image during defecation shows bulging of the anterior (*arrow*) and posterior (*arrowhead*) rectal wall, which was graded as moderate anterior and posterior rectocele

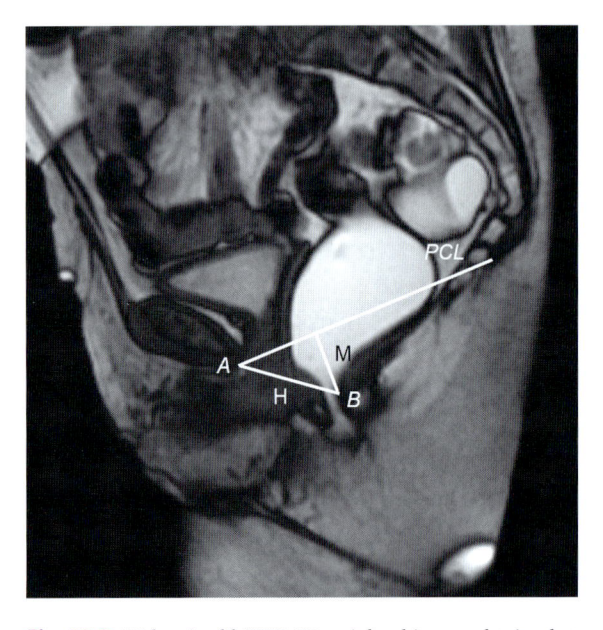

Fig. 18.3. Midsagittal bSSFP T2-weighted image obtained at straining shows landmarks used in the HMO system. The landmarks are the inferior aspect of the symphysis pubis (*A*) and the posterior wall of the rectum at the level of the ARJ (*B*). The H-line (*H*) represents the anteroposterior hiatal width and extends from *A* to *B*. The M-line (*M*) represents hiatal descent and extends perpendicularly from the pubococcygeal line (*PCL*) to the posterior end of the H line

rectal wall (Fig. 18.4), where it is also termed posterior perineal hernia because the defect occurs through the levator plate (Mahieu et al. 1984). Most rectoceles become apparent only during defecation.

Rectoceles are common and some degree of rectocele formation is present in most symptomatic women. Small rectoceles are seen in asymptomatic women and most likely represent normal variation (Shorvon et al. 1989). Rectoceles may develop due to weakness of the rectovaginal fascia, promoted by different factors such as chronic constipation, complicated vaginal delivery, hysterectomy, congenital or constitutional weakness of the pelvic floor, or aging.

A rectocele does not necessarily impede evacuation but retention of stool within a rectocele may lead to a sense of incomplete evacuation (Fig. 18.5). The clinical relevance may be determined by different criteria as the size, retention of contrast medium, the need for evacuation assistance, and the reproducibility of outlet obstruction.

The size, location, and degree of emptying of rectoceles can be assessed with MR defecography. In addition, MR defecography allows for the detection of other pelvic floor pathologies often associated with rectoceles, such as dyssynergic defecation, intussusception, and enterocele. The treatment decision in patients with rectoceles highly depends on these associated imaging findings. According to their maximum sagittal diame-

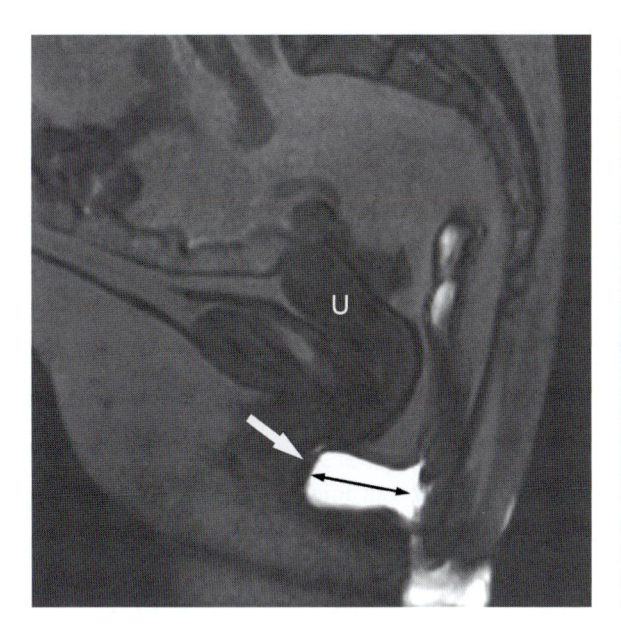

Fig. 18.5. Sixty-three-year-old female patient with feeling of incomplete evacuation. Midsagittal T1-weighted gradient recalled echo MR image obtained during defecation shows and anterior rectocele (*white arrow*). The extension of the anterior rectocele is measured as the maximum wall protrusion beyond the expected margin of the normal anterior rectal wall (*black arrow*). In this case the anterior rectocele was graded as large with a diameter of 4.4 cm and showed retention of contrast medium at the end of defecation. In addition, a peritoneocele is seen with protrusion of peritoneal fat below the pubococcygeal line. *U* uterus

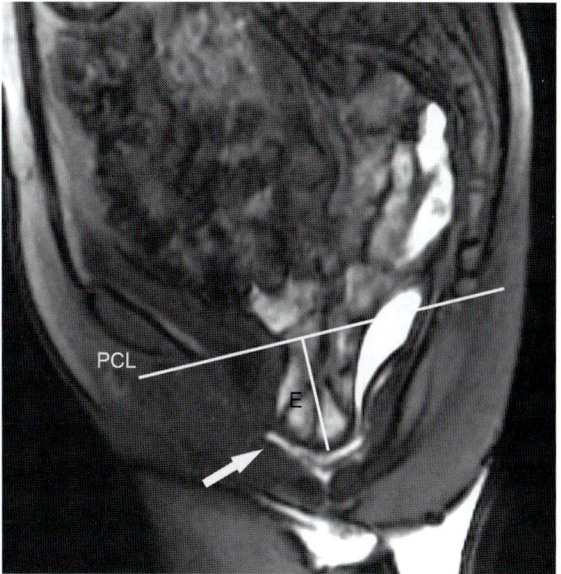

Fig. 18.6. Fifty-five-year-old female patient with clinical symptoms of outlet obstruction after hysterectomy. Midsagittal T1-weighted gradient recalled echo MR image obtained during defecation shows protrusion of a moderate enterocele (4.3 cm) (*E*) into the extended, convex perineum as well as a moderate anterior rectocele (*arrow*). The enterocele leads to a compression of the anorectum resulting in outlet obstruction. *PCL* pubococcygeal line, *E* enterocele

ter, rectoceles are graded as small (<2 cm), moderate (2–4 cm), and large (>4 cm) (Fig. 18.5) (Roos et al. 2002). Anterior rectoceles with a sagittal diameter of up to 2 cm are found in up to 20% of asymptomatic women, thus only anterior rectoceles > 2 cm should be considered abnormal (Shorvon et al. 1989).

18.3.2
Enterocele

An enterocele is defined as a herniation of the peritoneal sac, which contains omental fat (peritoneocele), small bowel (enterocele), or large bowel (sigmoidocele), into the rectovaginal or rectovesical space below the PCL. The prevalence of enteroceles in patients with pelvic floor disorders ranges from 17 to 37% (Hock et al. 1993; Kelvin et al. 1992). Women are more frequently affected and often have a history of vaginal or abdominal hysterectomy (Karasick et al. 1993). Symptoms vary and are largely dependent on size and location of the enterocele. Patients may present with constipation, a feeling of incomplete evacuation, or a sensation of a heavy feeling in the vagina. Large enteroceles may follow the sacral curve and lead to compression of the anorectum resulting in outlet obstruction (Fig. 18.6). Compared to the other forms of pelvic organ prolapse, clinical examination is insufficient for the detection of enteroceles, which are missed in up to 50% at clinical examination compared to conventional defecography. Nevertheless, conventional defecography does not seem to be ideally suited for the detection of enteroceles due to its lacking soft tissue contrast. Even when additional opacification of vagina and bowel is performed, conventional defecography fails to demonstrate up to 20% of enteroceles (Gousse et al. 2000; Lienemann et al. 2000). MR imaging is ideally suited for the evaluation of enteroceles, being superior to conventional cystocolpoproctography (Lienemann et al. 2000). Because of its inherent soft tissue contrast, MR defecography allows for the differentiation between peritoneocele, enterocele, and sigmoidocele without filling the small or large bowel with contrast agent. Furthermore, with the accurate detection of enteroceles, MR defecography identifies patients planned for surgical repair of pelvic prolapse, in whom an additional operative closure of the cul-de-sac is necessary. A more efficient planning prior to surgery becomes possible. Undetected small enteroceles may result in progressive symptoms and in the need for another operation (Kelvin et al. 1992).

Enteroceles are typically seen at the end of defecation as a consequence of increased intraabdominal pressure, and are often concomitant findings of other pathologies of the pelvic floor. The size of an enterocele is usually measured in relation to the PCL. The largest distance between the PCL and the most inferior point of the enterocele is measured with a perpendicular line. Depending on this distance, small (<3 cm), moderate (3–6 cm), and large (>6 cm) enteroceles are distinguished (Roos et al. 2002).

18.3.3
Intussusception and Rectal Prolapse

Rectal prolapse is defined as an infolding of the rectal wall. An inner rectal prolapse (intussusception) is distinguished from an external rectal prolapse (corresponding to the widely used clinical term "rectal prolapse") (Stoker et al. 2001).

18.3.3.1
Intussusception

An intussusception is the infolding of the rectal mucosa occurring during defecation. Depending on the location, an intrarectal intussusception (Fig. 18.7), limited to the rectum, is distinguished from an intraanal intussusception extending into the anal canal. The location of the intussusception may be anteriorly, posteriorly, or circumferentially. The intussusception either involves only the mucosa or the full thickness of the rectal wall. Patients may present with constipation or feeling of incomplete evacuation as their main symptom due to outlet obstruction or with fecal incontinence. Small intussusceptions may be detected in asymptomatic volunteers (Shorvon et al. 1989).

Using MR defecography, the differentiation between a mucosal intussusception and a full-thickness intussusception is possible. This was shown in a study by Dvorkin et al., where two of ten patients diagnosed with full-thickness intussusception at conventional defecography showed only mucosal intussusception at MR defecography (Dvorkin et al. 2004). The differentiation of mucosal and full-thickness intussusception is of clinical relevance, because the two different forms entail different treatment strategies (Mccue and Thomson 1990; Tsiaoussis et al. 1998). In up to 30% of patients with intussusception associated anterior or middle pelvic floor compartment descent has been shown (Dvorkin et al. 2004) (Fig. 18.7). Thus, MR defecography provides useful additional information, especially if surgery is planned. However, as mentioned above MR defecography performed in supine position may miss intussusception most likely due to the lack of gravity. Therefore, with regard to intussusceptions, we recommend to perform conventional defecography in patients with equivocal findings at MR defecography.

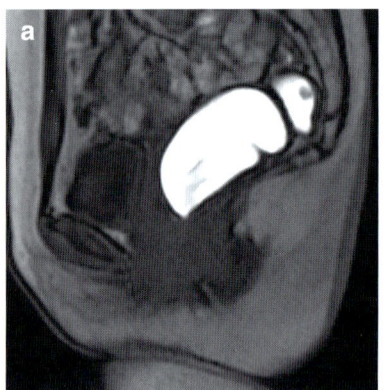

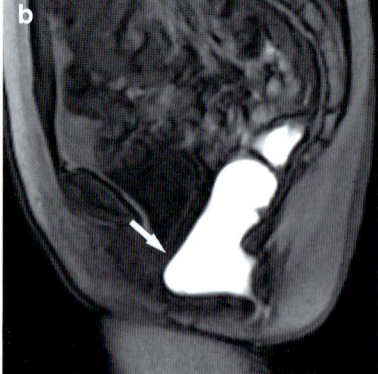

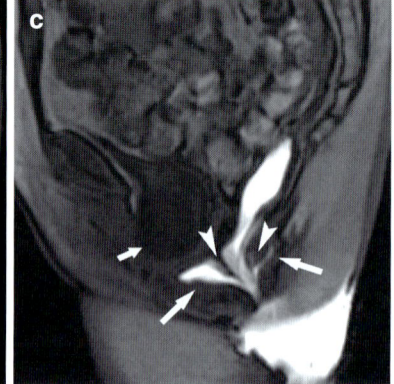

Fig. 18.7. Forty-seven-year-old female patient with pelvic pain, feeling of incomplete evacuation, and need for manually assisted defecation. Midsagittal T1-weighted gradient recalled echo MR images obtained at rest (**a**) show normal configuration of the rectum. MR images at straining (**b**) show a bulging of the anterior rectal wall (*arrow*). During defecation (**c**) a circumferential mural intussusception evolves, which extends into the rectum (full-thickness intrarectal intussusception) (*arrowheads*). Associated moderate anterior and small posterior rectoceles are evident (*large arrows* in **c**). In addition, a cystocele can be seen during defecation (*small arrow* in **c**)

18.3.3.2
External Rectal Prolapse

The external rectal prolapse is defined as an infolding of rectal mucosa, which protrudes through the anal canal outward (Fig. 18.8). The incidence is 4:1,000 and is higher in women than in men (women:men = 6:1) (FENGLER et al. 1997). Common symptoms include constipation, sensation of incomplete evacuation, fecal incontinence, and rectal ulceration with bleeding. External prolapse is a clinical diagnosis, and MR defecography is performed for diagnosing associated pathologies (Fig. 18.8) and surgical planning.

18.3.2
Pelvic Organ Prolapse

18.3.2.1
Cystocele

Cystoceles are the most common pathology of the anterior compartment of the pelvic floor and occur in postmenopausal women. A cystocele is defined as protrusion of the bladder into the anterior vaginal wall and below the PCL. Cystoceles can occur alone or in combination with other pathologies of the pelvic floor (Figs. 18.7–18.9). Patients present with unwanted urinary leakage and incomplete emptying of the bladder. On MR defecography cystoceles are evaluated according to their size, measured from the PCL to the

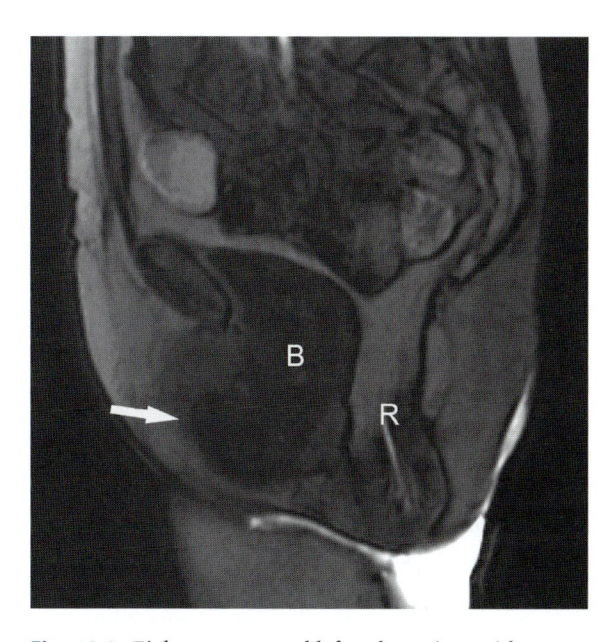

Fig. 18.8. Eighty-two-year-old female patient with recurrence of an external rectal prolapse. Midsagittal T1-weighted gradient recalled echo MR image obtained during defecation shows an external rectal prolapse and an additional large cystocele (*arrow*). *B* bladder, *R* rectum

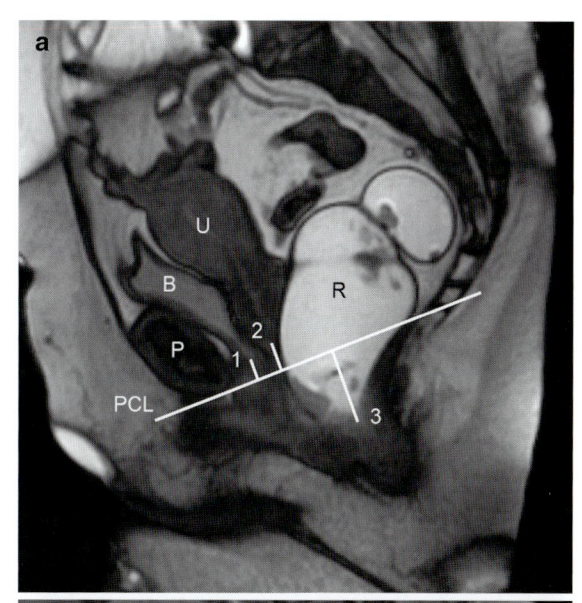

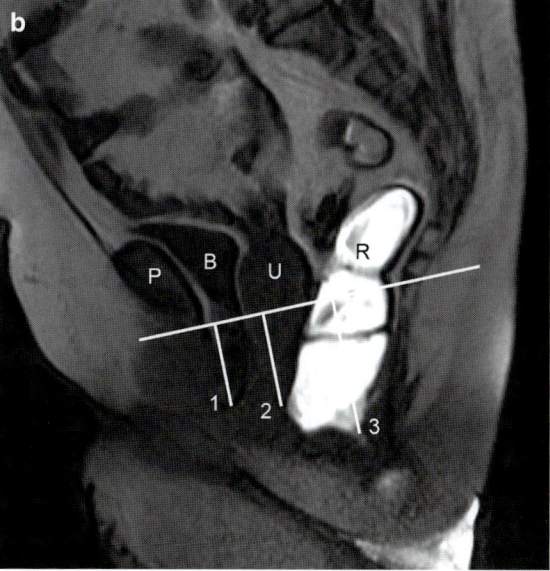

Fig. 18.9. Fifty-seven-year-old female patient with imperative defecation and descending perineum syndrome. (**a**) bSSFP T2-weighted MR image obtained with the patient at rest shows a normal position of the pelvic floor in relation to the PCL with the anterior (*1*) and middle (*2*) compartment above the PCL and the posterior compartment (*3*) 3 cm below the PCL. (**b**) T1-weighted gradient recalled echo MR image obtained during maximal straining shows a bulging of the whole pelvic floor with a moderate descent of the anterior compartment (1: 4.2 cm) and the middle compartment (2: 3.7 cm) and a large descent of the posterior compartment (3: 7 cm). *P* symphysis pubis, *B* bladder, *U* uterus, *R* rectum, *PCL* pubococcygeal line

base of the bladder, and are graded as small (<3 cm), moderate (3–6 cm), or large (>6 cm) (Roos et al. 2002).

18.3.2.2
Utero-Vaginal Prolapse

A descensus of the uterus is commonly due to insufficient uterosacral ligaments, which attach the cranial part of vagina and uterus. The uterus protrudes caudally into the vagina and in severe cases prolapses through the vagina. The utero-vaginal prolapse is usually diagnosed at clinical examination.

18.3.3
Pelvic Floor Relaxation (Pelvic Floor Descent), Descending Perineal Syndrome

The pelvic floor relaxation is defined as pathologic descensus of the pelvic floor at rest or at straining caudal to the PCL. Usually all three compartments of the pelvic floor are involved, but also a descensus only of the anorectum can occur (Roos et al. 2002). Several underlying causes are known, such as multiple vaginal deliveries, gynecological operations, chronic constipation, pudendal nerve neuropathy, or congenital connective tissue disease (Bartolo et al. 1983). Most commonly affected are women, aged 50 years or older (Weber and Richter 2005). Pelvic floor descent is initially characterized by perineal pain and constipation. Incomplete evacuation leads to excessive straining and consecutively to increased denervation and over time to fecal incontinence (Locke et al. 2000).

Although pelvic floor descent sometimes can be already seen at rest, it usually shows the maximal extension at straining and during evacuation (Fig. 18.9). Different quantification and grading systems for pelvic floor descent are described in the literature. A simple method is to measure the descent of the rectum (ARJ), the vaginal vault (or any part of the remaining cervix in case of hysterectomy), and the bladder representing the main structures of the three compartments with respect to the PCL, which is shown in Fig. 18.9. The extent of the pelvic floor descensus is defined as the largest distance between the PCL and the lowest point of the anterior (bladder base), middle (vaginal vault), and posterior pelvic floor compartment (ARJ). A small rectal descent is described when the ARJ is <3 cm below the PCL, a moderate rectal descent when the distance is 3–6 cm, and a large rectal descent when the distance is > 6 cm (Roos et al. 2002). The same grading is used for descent of the anterior and middle pelvic floor compartment.

18.3.4
Dyssynergic Defecation

Dyssynergic defecation produces functional outlet obstruction during defecation and is one of the causes of chronic constipation. Dyssynergic defecation is a functional disorder characterized by either paradoxic contraction or an inability to relax the anal sphincter and/or puborectalis muscle. In the literature, many other terms such as dyskinetic puborectalis muscle (Karasick et al. 1993), nonrelaxing puborectalis syndrome (Jorge et al. 1993), spastic pelvic floor syndrome (Kelvin et al. 1994; Kuijpers and Bleijenberg 1985), pelvic floor dyssynergia (Whitehead et al. 1999) and anismus (Halligan et al. 1995) have been used. In order to take into account that this dysfunction is not confined to a single muscle, an expert group (Rome III) (Bharucha et al. 2006) recently proposed the term "dyssynergic defecation" to appropriately describe the failure of coordination or dyssynergia of the abdominal and pelvic floor muscles involved in defecation.

Patients with dyssynergic defecation present with a variety of symptoms centering on constipation including rectal evacuation difficulties such as excessive straining, sensation of blockage, feeling of incomplete evacuation, need for manually assisted defecation and frequent use of enemas or suppositories (Rao et al. 2004). The exact cause of dyssynergic defecation is still unclear, but there seems to be an association between dyssynergic defecation and pelvic surgery, previous sexual abuse, anxiety, and psychologic stress in some patients (Bolog and Weishaupt 2005).

The diagnosis of dyssynergic defecation is notoriously difficult. Most authorities recommend using a combination of clinical history and diagnostic tests, including electromyography, the balloon expulsion test, manometry, and defecography. The individual weight of each of the tests for the final diagnosis of dyssynergic defecation is not exactly defined.

Functional imaging with conventional or MR defecography is considered to be a useful adjunct in establishing the diagnosis of dyssynergic defecation. Different structural imaging findings in conventional defecography have been described in patients with dyssynergic defecation, which can be also seen on

MR defecography, including prominent impression of the puborectal sling, narrow anal canal, prolonged evacuation, a lack of descent of the pelvic floor, and thus a failure to increase the ARA (Fig. 18.10) (KARLBOM et al. 1995; KUIJPERS and BLEIJENBERG 1985). However, the usefulness of these findings is discussed controversially (HALLIGAN et al. 1995; KARLBOM et al. 1995, 1999). In addition, defecography can be performed to rule out structural rectal abnormalities and provides an estimate of the degree of rectal emptying.

Delayed initiation of evacuation and impaired evacuation, in particular, as seen on conventional defecography are present in patients with dyssynergic (HALLIGAN et al. 1995, 2001). Especially impaired evacuation which was defined by Halligan et al.

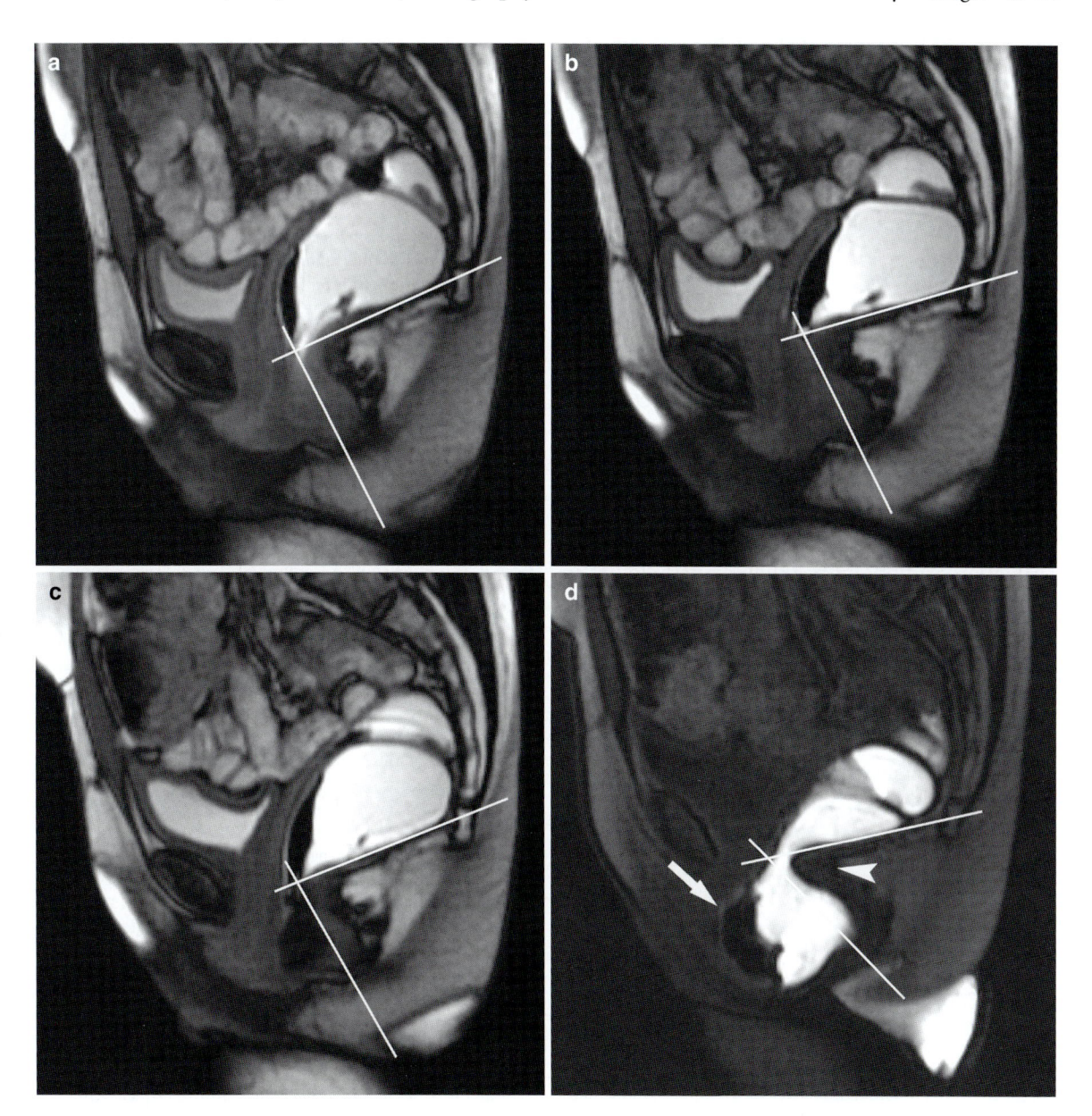

Fig. 18.10. Fifty-four-year-old female patient with clinical suspicion of dyssynergic defecation. On bSSFP T2-weighted MR images obtained at (**a**) rest the ARA measures 93°, whereas the ARA during squeezing is 77° (**b**). (**c, d**) T1-weighted gradient recalled echo MR images show a pathologic decrease of the ARA during straining (79°) (**c**) and during evacuation (55°) (**d**). Paradoxical sphincter contraction is noted with impression of the dorsal anorectal wall during evacuation (*arrowhead* in **d**). After several attempts to defecate a moderate anterior rectocele (*arrow* in **d**) is seen. The patient was able to evacuate only less than two-thirds of the contrast agent

(Halligan et al. 2001) as an inability to evacuate two-thirds of the contrast enema within 30 s is highly suggestive for the presence of dyssynergic defecation. This cut-off value of 30 s for the evacuation of two-thirds of the contrast enema was defined when administering 120 mL of contrast agent. Following the study of Minguez et al., we use a cut-off value of 60 s for the evacuation of two-thirds of the contrast enema, because we administer a larger amount of contrast agent (300 mL). In a study of 31 patients with impaired evacuation at conventional defecography 28 patients (90%) had dyssynergic defecation at subsequent physiologic testing (Halligan et al. 2001).

18.4 Conclusion

MR defecography is a relatively new method, which combines morphologic information of the pelvic floor along with function. Although the primary interest of the examination is the posterior compartment, MR defecography also provides information of the middle and anterior pelvic floor compartment resulting in a global examination of the pelvic floor. MR defecography is recommended as adjunct to clinical examinations and functional tests for the evaluation of different pelvic floor pathologies in patients presenting with symptoms such as constipation or incontinence. Furthermore, MR defecography is a useful diagnostic tool for surgical triage and for planning of specific repairs, especially of the posterior pelvic floor compartment.

For patients with outlet obstruction, MR defecography has been shown to be valuable in the assessment of possible morphologic causes of this disease complex.

References

Bartolo DC, Read NW, Jarratt JA, et al (1983) Differences in anal sphincter function and clinical presentation in patients with pelvic floor descent. Gastroenterology 85:68–75

Bartram CI, Turnbull GK, Lennard-Jones JE (1988) Evacuation proctography: an investigation of rectal expulsion in 20 subjects without defecatory disturbance. Gastrointest Radiol 13:72–80

Bertschinger KM, Hetzer FH, Roos JE, et al (2002) Dynamic MR imaging of the pelvic floor performed with patient sitting in an open-magnet unit versus with patient supine in a closed-magnet unit. Radiology 223:501–508

Bharucha AE, Fletcher JG, Harper CM, et al (2005) Relationship between symptoms and disordered continence mechanisms in women with idiopathic faecal incontinence. Gut 54:546–555

Bharucha AE, Wald A, Enck P, et al (2006) Functional anorectal disorders. Gastroenterology 130:1510–1518

Bolog N, Weishaupt D (2005) Dynamic MR imaging of outlet obstruction. Rom J Gastroenterol 14:293–302

Boyadzhyan L, Raman SS, Raz S (2008) Role of static and dynamic MR imaging in surgical pelvic floor dysfunction. Radiographics 28:949–967

Choi JS, Wexner SD, Nam YS, et al (2000) Intraobserver and interobserver measurements of the anorectal angle and perineal descent in defecography. Dis Colon Rectum 43:1121–1126

Comiter CV, Vasavada SP, Barbaric ZL, et al (1999) Grading pelvic prolapse and pelvic floor relaxation using dynamic magnetic resonance imaging. Urology 54:454–457

Dvorkin LS, Hetzer F, Scott SM, et al (2004) Open-magnet MR defaecography compared with evacuation proctography in the diagnosis and management of patients with rectal intussusception. Colorectal Dis 6:45–53

Ekberg O, Nylander G, Fork FT (1985) Defecography. Radiology 155:45–48

Fengler SA, Pearl RK, Prasad ML, et al (1997) Management of recurrent rectal prolapse. Dis Colon Rectum 40:832–834

Ferrante SL, Perry RE, Schreiman JS, et al (1991) The reproducibility of measuring the anorectal angle in defecography. Dis Colon Rectum 34:51–55

Fletcher JG, Busse RF, Riederer SJ, et al (2003) Magnetic resonance imaging of anatomic and dynamic defects of the pelvic floor in defecatory disorders. Am J Gastroenterol 98:399–411

Goei R, van Engelshoven J, Schouten H, et al (1989) Anorectal function: defecographic measurement in asymptomatic subjects. Radiology 173:137–141

Gousse AE, Barbaric ZL, Safir MH, et al (2000) Dynamic half Fourier acquisition, single shot turbo spin-echo magnetic resonance imaging for evaluating the female pelvis. J Urol 164:1606–1613

Halligan S, Bartram CI, Park HJ, et al (1995) Proctographic features of anismus. Radiology 197:679–682

Halligan S, Malouf A, Bartram CI, et al (2001) Predictive value of impaired evacuation at proctography in diagnosing anismus. AJR Am J Roentgenol 177:633–636

Healy JC, Halligan S, Reznek RH, et al (1997) Magnetic resonance imaging of the pelvic floor in patients with obstructed defaecation. Br J Surg 84:1555–1558

Hetzer FH, Andreisek G, Tsagari C, et al (2006) MR defecography in patients with fecal incontinence: imaging findings and their effect on surgical management. Radiology 240:449–457

Hock D, Lombard R, Jehaes C, et al (1993) Colpocystodefecography. Dis Colon Rectum 36:1015–1021

Jorge JM, Ger GC, Gonzalez L, Wexner SD (1994). Patient position during cinedefecography. Influence on perineal descent and other measurements. Dis Colon Rectum 37(9):927–931

Jorge JM, Wexner SD, Ger GC, et al (1993) Cinedefecography and electromyography in the diagnosis of nonrelaxing puborectalis syndrome. Dis Colon Rectum 36:668–676

Karasick S, Karasick D, Karasick SR (1993) Functional disorders of the anus and rectum: findings on defecography. AJR Am J Roentgenol 160:777–782

Karlbom U, Nilsson S, Pahlman L, et al (1999) Defecographic study of rectal evacuation in constipated patients and control subjects. Radiology 210:103–108

Karlbom U, Pahlman L, Nilsson S, et al (1995) Relationships between defecographic findings, rectal emptying, and colonic transit time in constipated patients. Gut 36:907–912

Kelvin FM, Maglinte DD (1997) Dynamic cystoproctography of female pelvic floor defects and their interrelationships. AJR Am J Roentgenol 169:769–774

Kelvin FM, Maglinte DD, Benson JT (1994) Evacuation proctography (defecography): an aid to the investigation of pelvic floor disorders. Obstet Gynecol 83:307–314

Kelvin FM, Maglinte DD, Hale DS, et al (2000) Female pelvic organ prolapse: a comparison of triphasic dynamic MR imaging and triphasic fluoroscopic cystocolpoproctography. AJR Am J Roentgenol 174:81–88

Kelvin FM, Maglinte DD, Hornback JA, et al (1992) Pelvic prolapse: assessment with evacuation proctography (defecography). Radiology 184:547–551

Kruyt RH, Delemarre JB, Doornbos J, et al (1991) Normal anorectum: dynamic MR imaging anatomy. Radiology 179:159–163

Kuijpers HC, Bleijenberg G (1985) The spastic pelvic floor syndrome. A cause of constipation. Dis Colon Rectum 28:669–672

Lienemann A, Anthuber C, Baron A, et al (1997) Dynamic MR colpocystorectography assessing pelvic-floor descent. Eur Radiol 7:1309–1317

Lienemann A, Anthuber C, Baron A, et al (2000) Diagnosing enteroceles using dynamic magnetic resonance imaging. Dis Colon Rectum 43:205–212; discussion 212–203

Lienemann A, Fischer T (2003) Functional imaging of the pelvic floor. Eur J Radiol 47:117–122

Locke GR III, Pemberton JH, Phillips SF (2000) AGA technical review on constipation. American Gastroenterological Association. Gastroenterology 119:1766–1778

Maglinte DD, Bartram C (2007) Dynamic imaging of posterior compartment pelvic floor dysfunction by evacuation proctography: techniques, indications, results and limitations. Eur J Radiol 61:454–461

Mahieu P, Pringot J, Bodart P (1984) Defecography: II. Contribution to the diagnosis of defecation disorders. Gastrointest Radiol 9:253–261

McCue JL, Thomson JP (1990) Rectopexy for internal rectal intussusception. Br J Surg 77:632–634

Minguez M, Herreros B, Sanchiz V, et al (2004) Predictive value of the balloon expulsion test for excluding the diagnosis of pelvic floor dyssynergia in constipation. Gastroenterology 126:57–62

Penninckx F, Debruyne C, Lestar B, et al (1990) Observer variation in the radiological measurement of the anorectal angle. Int J Colorectal Dis 5:94–97

Rao SS, Kavlock R, Rao S (2006) Influence of body position and stool characteristics on defecation in humans. Am J Gastroenterol 101:2790–2796

Rao SS, Mudipalli RS, Stessman M, et al (2004) Investigation of the utility of colorectal function tests and Rome II criteria in dyssynergic defecation (Anismus). Neurogastroenterol Motil 16:589–596

Roos JE, Weishaupt D, Wildermuth S, et al (2002) Experience of 4 years with open MR defecography: pictorial review of anorectal anatomy and disease. Radiographics 22:817–832

Shorvon PJ, McHugh S, Diamant NE, et al (1989) Defecography in normal volunteers: results and implications. Gut 30:1737–1749

Solopova AE, Hetzer FH, Marincek B, et al (2008) MR defecography: prospective comparison of two rectal enema compositions. AJR Am J Roentgenol 190:W118–W124

Stoker J, Halligan S, Bartram CI (2001) Pelvic floor imaging. Radiology 218:621–641

Tsiaoussis J, Chrysos E, Glynos M, et al (1998) Pathophysiology and treatment of anterior rectal mucosal prolapse syndrome. Br J Surg 85:1699–1702

Vanbeckevoort D, Van Hoe L, Oyen R, et al (1999) Pelvic floor descent in females: comparative study of colpocystodefecography and dynamic fast MR imaging. J Magn Reson Imaging 9:373–377

Weber AM, Richter HE (2005) Pelvic organ prolapse. Obstet Gynecol 106:615–634

Whitehead WE, Wald A, Diamant NE, et al (1999) Functional disorders of the anus and rectum. Gut 45(Suppl 2):II55–59

Yang A, Mostwin JL, Rosenshein NB, et al (1991) Pelvic floor descent in women: dynamic evaluation with fast MR imaging and cinematic display. Radiology 179:25–33

MRI of the Anus

Steve Halligan and Stuart A. Taylor

CONTENTS

19.1 MRI of Fistula-In-Ano 329
19.1.1 Anal Anatomy and the Etiology of Fistula-In-Ano 330
19.1.2 Classification of Fistula-In-Ano 331
19.1.3 Clinical Assessment and Treatment of Fistula-In-Ano 332
19.1.4 MR Imaging of Fistula-In-Ano 333
19.1.5 MRI Technique 334
19.1.6 Image Interpretation 335
19.1.7 Effect of Preoperative MRI on Surgery and Clinical Outcome 339
19.1.8 Differential Diagnosis of Perianal Sepsis 340
19.1.9 Which Patients Should Be Imaged? 341

19.2 MR Imaging to Investigate Anal Incontinence 342
19.2.1 Anal Incontinence 342
19.2.2 MRI Findings in Anal Incontinence 342

19.3 MR Imaging of Anal Malignancy 343

References 345

KEY POINTS

This chapter will detail the clinical utility of MRI of the anus. The main emphasis will be on fistula-in-ano, where MRI is extensively used because it is generally accepted to be the reference standard investigation, surpassing even surgical assessment. The pathogenesis of fistula-in-ano is described, along with the different types of fistula encountered and the principles of surgical treatment. We describe how fistula-in-ano may be imaged with MR and emphasize that precise Preoperative characterization of the anatomical course of the fistula and all associated infection is critical, if surgery is to be most effective. We also detail other clinical scenarios where MRI of the anus has particular clinical utility, namely investigation of anal incontinence and anal malignancy.

19.1
MRI of Fistula-In-Ano

Fistula-in-ano describes an abnormal communication between the anal canal (or occasionally the rectum) and the perianal skin. It is a common condition that has a tendency to recur despite apparently curative surgery. Recurrence after surgery is almost always due to infection that has escaped detection by the surgeon and thus gone untreated. It is now increasingly recognized that Preoperative imaging, notably by MRI, is able to identify fistulas and associated abscesses that would otherwise have been missed. Not only can MRI elegantly display perianal fistulas, Preoperative MRI has been shown to influence subsequent surgery and significantly diminish the chance of recurrent disease as a result. Because of

---

Steve Halligan, MBBS, MD, FRCR, FRCP
Stuart A. Taylor MBBS, BSc, MD, MRCP, FRCR
Department of Specialist Radiology, University College London, University College Hospital, 235 Euston Road, London NW1 2BU, UK

this, Preoperative imaging is becoming increasingly routine, especially in patients with recurrent fistulas. In order to fully understand the role of imaging for fistula-in-ano, an appreciation of their etiology and how the various fistula types are defined by anatomical boundaries is mandatory.

19.1.1 Anal Anatomy and the Aetiology of Fistula-In-Ano

The anal canal is essentially a luminal cylinder surrounded by two muscular sphincters, the internal and external anal sphincters, which are composed of smooth and striated muscle, respectively (Fig. 19.1). The external sphincter merges, proximally with the sling-like puborectalis muscle which itself merges with the levator plate of the pelvic floor. The internal sphincter is the distal termination of the circular muscle of the gut tube. Lying between the external and internal sphincters is the longitudinal muscle, which is the termination of the rectal longitudinal smooth muscle. The longitudinal muscle interdigitates between the internal and external sphincters and terminates in the perianal skin. The longitudinal muscle is thought to bind the structures of the anus together, especially as it has no obvious sphincteric effect. There is a surgical plane of dissection between the internal and external sphincters, known as the intersphincteric space. This space is most frequently found between the longitudinal muscle and external sphincter, and is filled with fat containing loose areolar tissue. The ischioanal fossa lies lateral to the sphincter complex, is filled with fat, and is traversed by a network of fibro-elastic connective tissue. Because this space lies adjacent to the anus (vs. the rectum) and lies immediately below (vs. above) the levator plate of the pelvic floor, the authors prefer the term "ischioanal" fossa rather than "ischiorectal," which is commonly used by surgeons. However, the two terms are interchangeable.

The anal canal is lined with epithelial tissue. The proximal region is lined with rectal columnar epithelium and the distal with squamous epithelium, which merges with the squamous epithelium of the perianal skin. The junction between the two (i.e. the histological ano-rectal junction) is generally in the region of the dentate line, which is an undulating structure formed by the distal aspects of longitudinal anal folds (the columns of Morgagni). The dentate line lies approximately 2 cm cranial to the anal verge and

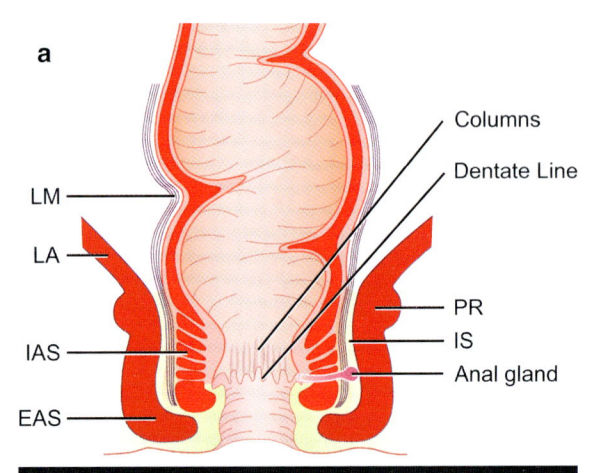

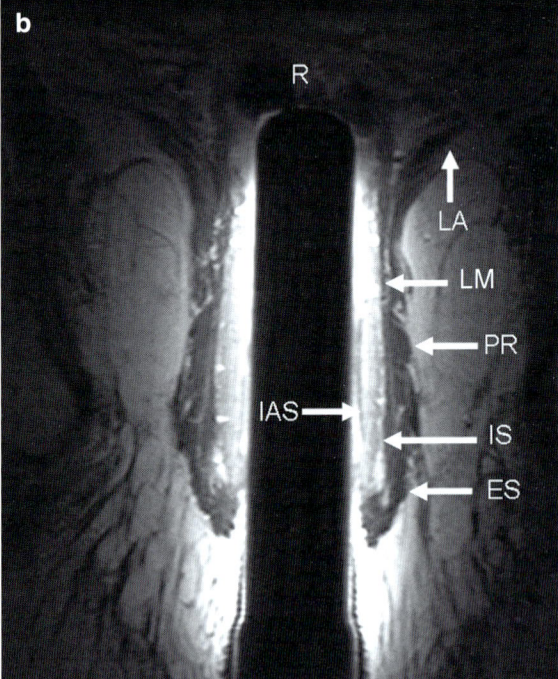

Fig. 19.1. (a) Diagrammatic representation of the anal canal, coronal view. *EAS* external sphincter; *IAS* internal sphincter; *PR* puborectalis muscle, *LA* levator ani, *LM* longitudinal muscle; *IS* intersphincteric plane. (b) Coronal T2-weighted scan showing the same structures (courtesy Jaap Stoker MD)

is a crucial landmark in fistula-in-ano because anal glands communicate with the anal lumen in this region. The anal glands are blind ending sinuses, which are believed to secrete mucus and thus lubricate the anal canal. They are arranged more or less circumferentially around the anus and discharge into the lumen approximately at the level of the dentate line, as described above. They penetrate the surrounding structures to various degrees – some may only reach the subepithelial tissues, others may reach the internal sphincter, and the deepest reach the intersphincteric space (Fig. 19.1). Chiari (1878) was the first to suggest that fistula-in-ano was initiated by infection of the anal glands – the "cryptoglandular hypothesis" (PARKS 1961). It is now believed that the anal glands become infected, perhaps because the draining duct becomes blocked by debris, and that this infection may ultimately result in an acute peri-anal abscess. An acute peri-anal abscess is a common surgical scenario, familiar to all general and colo-proctological surgeons. Treatment is generally by incision and drainage over the most fluctuant part of the abscess, but this procedure does not pay due attention to the source of infection in the intersphincteric space. The result is that as many as 87% patients with an acute peri-anal abscess may subsequently develop a fistula (FUCINI 1991). Acute perianal abscess and fistula-in-ano are therefore likely to be acute and chronic manifestations of the same disease. A fistula develops when intersphincteric infection is allowed to continue unabated. Fistula-in-ano has a prevalence of approximately 0.01%, predominantly affecting young adults (SANIO 1984). It is commoner in men, who dominate in all published series, with a male:female ratio of approximately 2:1. While some fistulas can be entirely asymptomatic, most patients complain of discharge but local pain due to inflammation is also often present.

19.1.2
Classification of Fistula-In-Ano

By definition a fistula describes an abnormal communication between two epithelial surfaces. The anatomical course of the fistula will be dictated by the location of the infected anal gland and the anatomical planes and boundaries that surround it. The internal opening of the fistula will usually be in the anal canal at the level of the dentate line, that is at the original site of the duct draining the infected gland. In the radial plane, the internal opening is usually posterior at 6 o'clock, simply because anal glands are more abundant posteriorly, especially in men. The fistula can reach the perianal skin via a variety of routes, some more tortuous than others and thereby penetrating and involving the muscles of the anal sphincter and surrounding tissues to a variable degree. Fistulas may thus be "classified" according to the route taken by this "primary track," which links the internal and external openings. Furthermore, classification influences treatment very significantly, about which more later. There have been a variety of attempts to classify fistula-in-ano, with various nomenclature, but by far the most widely used is that proposed by Parks and colleagues in 1976 (PARKS et al. 1976). Parks carefully analyzed a consecutive series of 400 patients referred to the surgeon's of St. Mark's Hospital London, a specialist hospital dealing with coloproctological disease, and found that he was able to place all fistulas encountered into one of four broad categories; intersphincteric, transsphincteric, suprasphincteric, and extrasphincteric. Importantly, most of these groupings could be explained by the cryptoglandular hypothesis.

The path of least anatomical resistance for festering intersphincteric infection is straight down the intersphincteric space, creating an intersphincteric fistula, which comprises 45% of Parks' series (Fig.19.2). Importantly, this fistula does not penetrate the adjacent external sphincter, which forms a relative barrier to spread. However, some truculent fistulas do penetrate into the external sphincter, and by doing so reach the ischioanal fossa (Fig. 19.2). This results in a transsphincteric fistula, which comprised 30% of Parks' series. Other fistulas may spread upwards in the intersphincteric space rather than downwards. In order to reach the perianal skin the primary track must then arch over the puborectalis muscle, cross the levator plate, and then traverse the ischioanal fossa. This type, termed a suprasphincteric fistula (Fig. 19.2), comprises 20% of Parks' series.

It is obvious that inter-, trans-, and suprasphincteric fistulas are all predicated by sepsis in the intersphincteric space. However, Parks also noted a fourth type of fistula in 5% of cases, which did not feature intersphincteric infection. Instead, these fistulas penetrated the rectum or anorectal junction directly, bypassing the intersphincteric space completely (Fig. 19.2). Cleary, this type of fistula cannot be

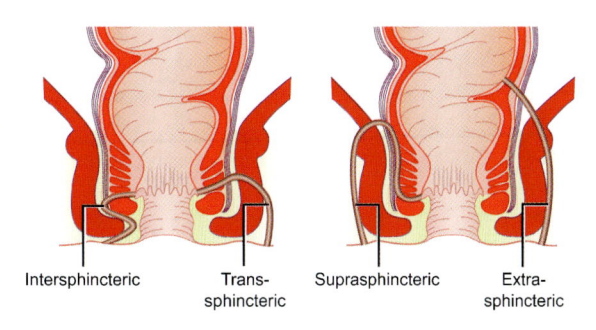

Fig. 19.2. Park's classification of fistula-in-ano showing the four basic types of primary fistula tracks

explained by anal gland infection and Parks hypothesized that these "extrasphincteric" fistulas were instead due to disease originating outside the anal canal. He stressed that primary rectal or pelvic disease should be considered when this type of fistula was encountered, for example diverticular disease, rectal Crohn's disease, carcinoma. It should be noted that Parks' series inevitably suffered spectrum bias owing to the specialized nature of St. Marks Hospital; a bias acknowledged by Parks himself, with the result that complex fistulas were almost certainly overrepresented in his series. For example, Parks did not describe submucus fistulas, which are very superficial and do not involve the sphincter at all.

While most fistulas probably start as a simple, single primary track, unabated infection may result in ramifications (often multiple) that branch away from this. Such secondary tracks are generally termed "extensions" (Fig. 19.3) and are the major factor that underpins recurrent fistulas because they may occur several centimetres away from the primary track and often lie deep in surrounding tissues, thus escaping easy detection. Their distance from the primary track also complicates the surgery needed to treat them adequately (see sections below). Extensions may be intersphincteric, ischioanal, or supralevator (pararectal) and they may take the form of tracks or abscesses. Exactly when a track becomes an abscess has no precise definition but both describe regions of sepsis. The ischioanal fossa is the commonest site for an extension, especially one that arises from the apex of a transsphincteric fistula (Fig 19.3). Extensions also occur in the horizontal plane and are known as "horseshoes" if there is ramification of sepsis on both sides of the internal opening (Fig. 19.3).

Thus the "classification" of a fistula involves description of the path taken by the primary track and the anatomical location of any associated extensions.

19.1.3
Clinical Assessment and Treatment of Fistula-In-Ano

Surgical treatment of fistula-in-ano is usually straightforward and involves laying-open the fistula by incision, usually by cutting down onto a metal probe that has been inserted into the primary track. However this seemingly simple procedure has many unexpected traps waiting for the unwary. Injudicious incision and overenthusiastic exploration can very quickly and convert a simple fistula into a surgical nightmare by creating additional extensions, tracks, and communications, with disastrous consequences for the patient. The prime objectives are to identify the track and any associated extensions, and then eradicate these by draining all associated infection, all without compromising anal continence. It is the right balance between eradication of sepsis and preservation of function that is the art of fistula surgery. In order to achieve this, two surgical questions need to be answered Preoperatively:

- What is the relationship between the fistula and the anal sphincter? That is, can the track be safely laid open without risking postoperative incontinence?
- Are there any extensions from the primary track that need to be treated in order to prevent recurrence? If so, where are they?

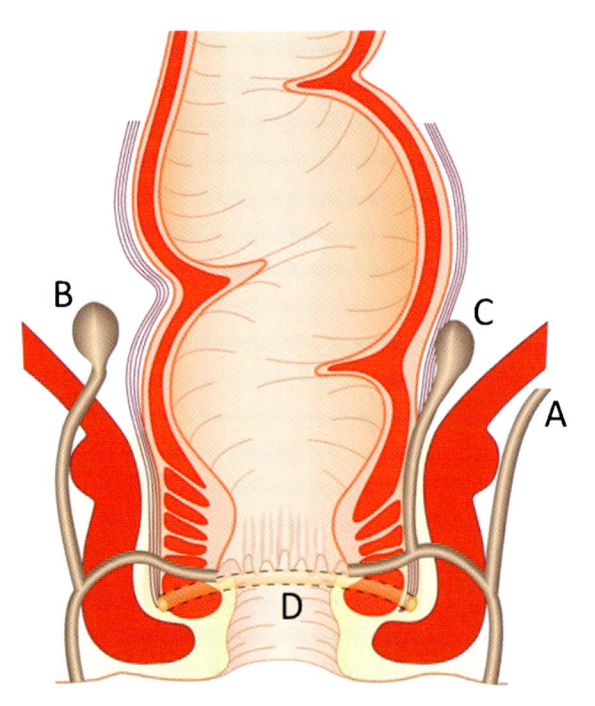

Fig. 19.3. Extensions: there are two transsphincteric primary fistula tracks. (**a**) An extension into the roof of the ischioanal fossa. (**b**) Supralevator extension, piercing the levator plate. (**c**) Supralevator extension via the intersphincteric plane. (**d**) Horseshoe extension in the intersphincteric plane

Surgeons have traditionally relied on examination under (general) anesthesia (EUA) to answer these questions. At EUA, the surgeon attempts to classify the fistula by palpation and probing so as to determine its relationship to the sphincter. However, the surgeon cannot visualize underlying muscles directly and the loss of tone induced by general anesthesia further impairs precise identification. The height of the internal opening relative to the anal canal and sphincters is crucial; the higher the opening is, the more sphincter will be divided when the fistula is laid open. A blunt metal probe is inserted into the external opening and gently directed toward the dentate line in order to find the anal opening. This is not as straightforward as it sounds. For example, the internal opening is frequently very difficult to see but the probe must not be advanced forcefully because doing so is a major cause of unintentional tracks and extensions. For example, forceful probing of a transsphincteric fistula track in the roof of the ischioanal fossa can easily rupture through the levator plate, thereby causing a supralevator extension. In the worst instance, the probe can even rupture into the rectum, converting a transsphincteric fistula into an extrasphincteric fistula, which is very difficult to treat indeed (Parks et al. 1976). Identification of associated extensions at EUA is central to curing the fistula. It is well-recognized that missed extensions are the commonest cause of recurrence, which reaches 25% in some series (Lilius 1968). Extensions require specific treatment and inevitably necessitate more extensive surgery. For example, supralevator extensions are particularly difficult both to diagnose (because they are high above the anal canal) and to treat (because the levator plate forms a barrier to drainage).

The net result is that at EUA it can be very difficult to classify the primary track with confidence, and there is ample opportunity to make matters even worse. Patients with recurrent disease are a particular case in point. They are most likely to harbour foci of missed sepsis but are also the most difficult to assess at EUA. In the context of multiple failed operations previously, digital palpation frequently cannot distinguish between scarring due to repeated surgery and induration due to an underlying extension. Furthermore, this group is also most likely to have extensions that travel several centimetres away from the primary track, which further hampers their detection. The more chronic the fistula, the more complicated associated extensions tend to be. The inevitable result is that these patients become progressively more difficult to treat, with both patient and surgeon becoming ever more exasperated. The key to breaking this loop is accurate Preoperative assessment.

19.1.4
MR Imaging of Fistula-In-Ano

For many years radiologists have attempted to help answer the surgical questions posed in the section above, with varying degrees of success. Contrast fistulography was the first modality employed, and involves catheterizing the external opening with a fine cannula and then gently injecting water-soluble contrast in order to opacify the fistula track. Unfortunately, fistulography suffers from two major drawbacks. First, extensions from the primary track may fail to fill with contrast if they are plugged tract debris, very remote, or if there is excessive contrast reflux from either the internal or external openings. Second, the sphincter muscles themselves are not directly imaged, which means that the relationship between the track and sphincter must be guessed. Furthermore, an inability to visualize the levator plate means that it can be very difficult to decide whether an extension is supra- or infra-levator. The net result is that fistulography is both difficult to interpret and its results are unreliable. While initial reports of computerized tomography (CT) for fistula-in-ano were encouraging, fistula visualization is not enough; they must be classified correctly, and more mature data suggest that CT cannot do this with sufficient accuracy. This is because the attenuation of the anal sphincter and pelvic floor is similar to the fistula itself unless the latter contains air or contrast. This is compounded with an inability to image in the surgically relevant coronal plane.

Anal endosonography (AES) was the first technique to directly visualize the anal sphincter complex in detail and, naturally, AES has been applied to the classification of fistula-in-ano. While AES can be very useful, it is difficult to interpret in the context of fistula disease and highly dependent on the experience of the sonographer. Also, being an ultrasound technique, structures remote from the transducer are difficult to see, with the result that extensions may be easily missed because of variable penetration beyond the sphincter complex. Also, AES cannot reliably distinguish infection from fibrosis since both appear hyporeflective, and this causes particular difficulties in patients with recurrent disease since infected tracks and fibrotic scars frequently occur together. Injection of hydrogen peroxide into the external opening may help differentiate between the two but other limitations persist, especially in patients with extensions and remote tracks. While there is no doubt that AES is a valuable technique in the right hands,

MRI is generally superior: A study comparing AES to digital evaluation and MRI in 108 primary tracks found that digital evaluation correctly classified 61%, AES 81%, and MR imaging 90% (Buchanan et al. 2004). While AES was particularly adept at correctly predicting the site of the internal opening, achieving this in 91% compared to 97% for MRI (Buchanan et al. 2004), there is little doubt that MRI is a superior technique overall.

Over the past decade MRI has emerged as the leading contender for Preoperative classification of fistula-in-ano. This is because, with the right sequences, MRI can vividly separate fistula tracks and extensions from surrounding structures. Furthermore, its ability to image in surgically relevant planes means that the anatomical course of the fistula can be determined easily. Indeed, the ability of MRI to not only accurately classify tracks but also to identify disease that would otherwise have been missed has had a palpable effect on surgical treatment and, ultimately, patient outcome (Halligan and Buchanan 2003; Halligan and Stoker 2006).

19.1.5
MRI Technique

Field strength is not critical for good results. Although higher field strength might provide more elegant images, these do not seem to convey significantly more diagnostic information than lesser machines. Initial reports necessarily used the body coil with good results (Lunniss et al. 1992; Spencer et al. 1996). The introduction of external phased array surface coils increased signal to noise ratio (SNR) and spatial resolution, to good effect (Beets-Tan et al. 2001; Buchanan et al. 2002). The best spatial resolution is achieved using dedicated endoluminal anal coils (Fig 19.1b) (Hussain et al. 1996). It should be stressed that anal endoluminal coils are not the same as rectal coils. Rather, they are smaller in diameter and are intended to cross the anus. While endoanal coils undoubtedly provide the most elegant images of the anal sphincter complex, they suffer the same limitation as AES – the limited field of view means that distant extensions will occasionally be missed (Halligan and Bartram 1998). While the exact choice of coil depends on personal preference, availability, the patient being studied, and the clinical question, it is important that a wide field-of-view is achieved in any patient where a distant extension from the primary track is a possibility. Obvious examples are patients with recurrent fistulas and those with Crohn's disease but potentially any patient with a fistula may have an extension. Because of this, a phased array body or surface coil will usually be the most appropriate choice whereas the high spatial resolution of endoluminal coils makes them ideal for precisely demonstrating the location and height of the internal opening. Endoanal coils may also have a special role for demonstrating ano- or recto-vaginal fistulas, which are notoriously difficult to image.

Various investigators have adopted different strategies regarding the sequences used to image fistula-in-ano. All agree that anatomical precision is needed, so that the course of the fistula with respect to adjacent structures can be judged accurately, and all employ some method by which sepsis (i.e. infection) is highlighted. These aims can be achieved in various ways. Many investigators employ the rapid and convenient fast spin-echo T2-weighted sequence, which provides good contrast between hyperintense fluid (pus) within the track and the hypointense fibrous wall that surrounds it, while simultaneously enabling good discrimination between the muscular layers of the anal sphincter. Fat suppression techniques are very useful. The earliest reports used STIR imaging, with T1-weighted scans for additional anatomical clarification (Lunniss et al. 1992). With subsequent improvements in scanner technology, it is possible to achieve excellent results using STIR sequences alone since anatomical resolution is satisfactory (Buchanan et al. 2002, 2004). Fat suppressed T2-weighted fast spin-echo and/or T1-weighting enhanced by gadolinium contrast are acceptable alternatives or may be used in combination (Spencer et al. 1996). While other approaches have included saline instillation into the external opening, or rectal contrast medium, such measures increase examination complexity in the face of the already excellent results achieved by less invasive procedures, and there is therefore little motivation to adopt them. For the majority of their clinical work the authors use a 1.5-T magnet, a single sagittal T-2 weighted study and two STIR sequences (axial and coronal – see section below), which makes for a very rapid and easy examination (Tables 19.1 and 19.2). Patients do not fast prior to the procedure and the authors do not use a smooth muscle relaxant.

It is central to success that imaging planes are correctly aligned with respect to the anal sphincter. Because the anal canal is tilted forwards from the vertical by approximately 45°, axial and coronal images that are straight with respect to the patient/scanner tabletop will result in oblique images of the

Table 19.1. MR imaging protocols for imaging fistula-in-ano

Imaging planes	Sequence	Fat suppression	TR (ms)	TE (ms)	Echo train length	No. of excitations	Field of view (mm)	Imaging matrix	Slice thickness (mm) [gap]	Bandwidth (kHz)
Sagittal	T2 TSE	no	6,700	97	15	4	200	256	4 [1]	130
Coronal–angled to the anal canal	STIR	No (IR) TI 150	4,520	27	5	1	280	256	4 [1]	132
Axial–angled to the anal canal	STIR	No (IR) TI 150	6,000	28	5	1	200	256	4 [1]	132

The table details the imaging protocols currently used by the authors to image fistula-in-ano. These have been developed using a Siemens 1.5 T magnet and external phased array coils

Table 19.2. MR imaging protocols for imaging anal canal tumors and pelvic floor

Imaging planes	Sequence	Fat suppression	TR (ms)	TE (ms)	Echo train length	No. of excitations	Field of view (mm)	Imaging matrix	Slice thickness (mm) [gap]	Bandwidth (kHz)
Axial-angled to anal canal	T2 TSE	No	5,170	92	15	4	200	256	3 [1]	191
Coronal-angled to anal canal	T2 TSE	No	3,200	92	15	4	180	256	3 [1]	191
Sagittal	T2 TSE	No	7,670	97	15	4	250	256	4 [1]	130

The table details the imaging protocols currently used by the authors to image fistula-in-ano. These have been developed using a Siemens 1.5 T magnet and external phased array coils

anus, and the geography of any fistula will be difficult to ascertain. This is especially so when trying to determine the height of the internal opening. Oblique axial and coronal planes orientated orthogonal and parallel to the anal sphincter are mandatory and are most easily planned from an initial, midline sagittal acquisition through the pelvis (Fig. 19.4). It may be necessary to align supplementary scans to the rectal axis in complex cases with an internal opening high in the rectum, but this is seldom necessary. It is important that the imaged volume extends several centimetres above the levator muscles and also includes the whole pre-sacral space, both of which are common sites for extensions. The entire perineum should also be included. Occasionally, tracks may extend for several centimetres, even leaving the pelvis or reaching the legs, and any track must be followed to its termination if this has not been included on the standard volume. The precise location of the primary track (e.g. ischioanal or intersphincteric) is usually most easily appreciated using axial images and the radial site of the internal opening is also well seen using this plane. Coronal images best visualize the levator plate, which separates supra from infralevator infection. The height of the internal opening may also be best appreciated on coronal images, with the caveat that the anal canal must be imaged along its entire cranio-caudal extent, as explained above.

19.1.6
Image Interpretation

The success of MR imaging for Preoperative classification of fistula-in-ano is a direct result of its sensitivity for tracks and abscesses combined with high anatomical precision. Accurate Preoperative classification is achieved by correctly relating the imaged fistula and any extensions to the anal sphincter. All reports should include the following information: The radial location and classification of the primary track, the radial location and level of the internal opening, and a description of any extensions including abscesses.

Active tracks are filled with pus and/or granulation tissue, and thus appear as hyperintense longitu-

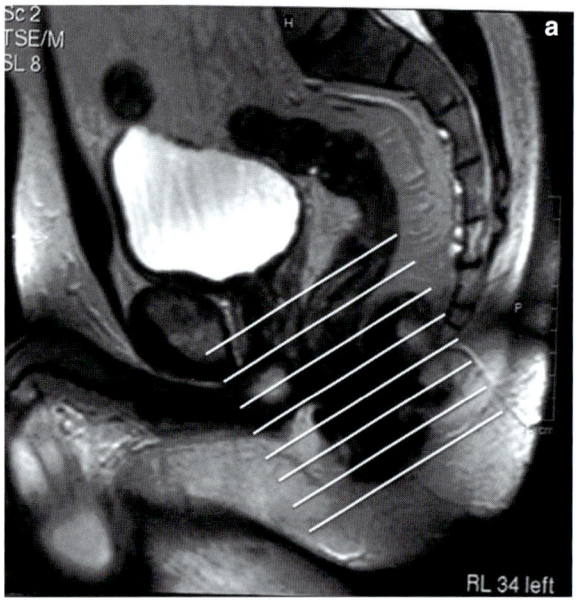

Fig. 19.4. Sagittal T2-weighted planning scan showing the orientation of the anal canal and the oblique axis to which the axial (a) and coronal (b) scans must be aligned. Images should extend well into the supralevator compartment and also cover the entire presacral space

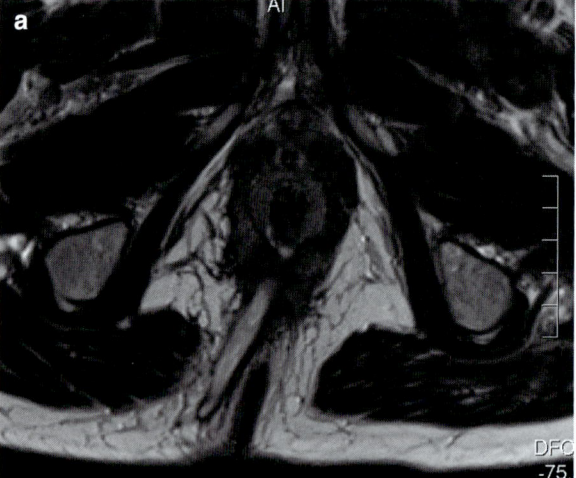

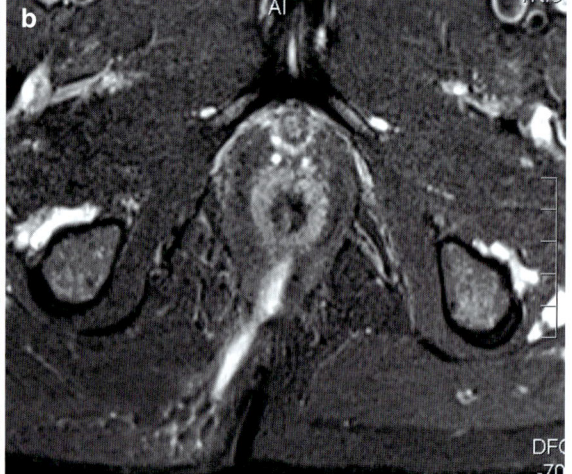

Fig. 19.5. Male patient with a transsphincteric fistula-in-ano. (a) T2-weighted axial image at mid anal canal level. (b) Corresponding STIR image. There is a transsphincteric fistula in the right posterior quadrant, which is clearly penetrating the external sphincter to reach an internal opening at 6 o'clock posterior

dinal structures on T2-weighted (Fig. 19.5a) or STIR sequences (Fig. 19.5b). If thought clinically relevant, gadolinium contrast can be used to distinguish between pus and granulation tissue *per se*. Active tracks are often surrounded by hypointense fibrous walls (Fig. 19.5a), which can be relatively thick, especially in patients with recurrent disease and previous surgery. Occasionally some hyperintensity within this fibrous area may be seen, probably reflecting edema. Hyperintensity may also extend beyond the track and its fibrous sleeve, representing adjacent inflammation and edema.

The external anal sphincter is clearly visualized on MRI. It is relatively hypointense and its lateral border contrasts sharply against the fat within the ischioanal fossa, on both STIR (Fig. 19.5b) and especially on

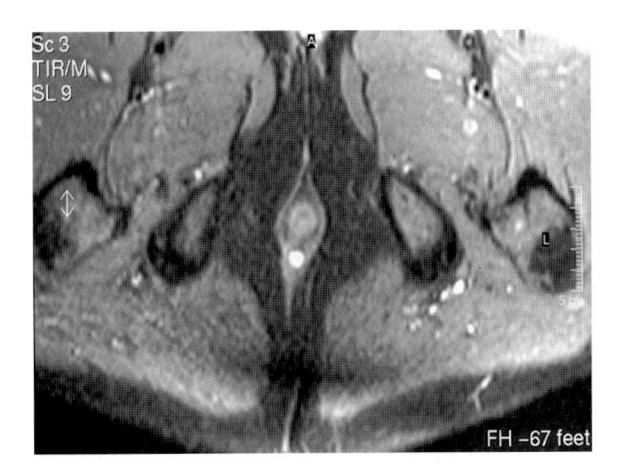

Fig. 19.6. Axial STIR MR images in a man with a posterior intersphincteric fistula. Note that the fistula is contained by the external sphincter; there is no sepsis in the ischioanal fossa

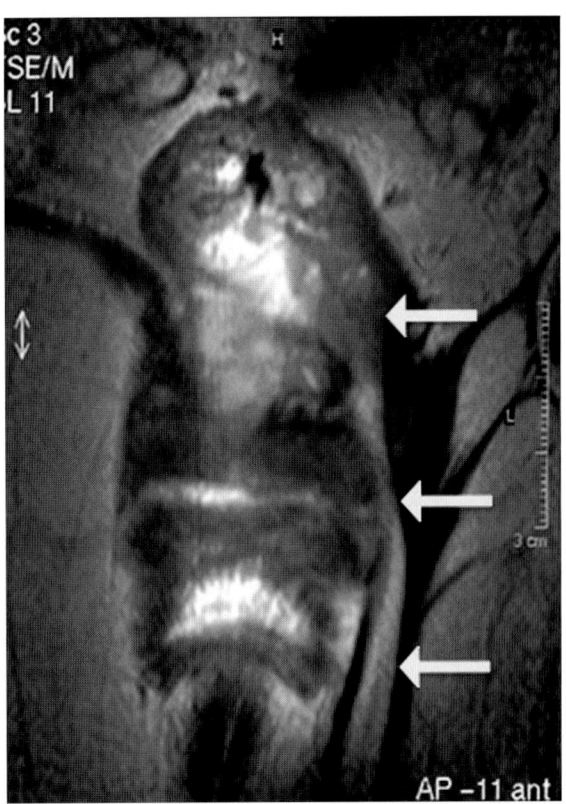

Fig. 19.7. Coronal T2-weighted MR image in a man with an extrasphincteric fistula. Note that the primary fistula track (*arrows*) enters the rectum at the level of the levator plates. There is no opening in the anal canal

T2-weighted studies (Fig. 19.5a). This result is that it is relatively easy to determine whether a fistula is constrained by the external sphincter or has extended beyond it. If a fistula remains constrained by the external sphincter throughout its course, then it is highly likely to be intersphincteric (Fig. 19.6). While any evidence of a track in the ischioanal fossa effectively excludes an intersphincteric fistula, transsphincteric, suprasphincteric, and extrasphincteric fistulas all share this feature – it is the level of the internal opening and the level at which the fistula crosses the sphincter complex that differentiates between these latter types. A transsphincteric fistula will be the commonest cause of a track in the ischioanal fossa (Fig. 19.5) simply because it is much more frequent than either supra- or extrasphincteric types.

The exact anatomical location of the internal opening can be difficult to define. Two questions need to be answered: what is the radial site of the internal opening and what is its level? The vast majority of anal fistulas open into the anal canal at the level of the dentate line, commensurate with the cryptoglandular hypothesis of fistula pathogenesis. Furthermore, most fistulas also enter posteriorly, at 6 o'clock. Unfortunately, the dentate line cannot be identified as a discrete anatomical entity, even when using endoanal receiver coils, but its general position can be estimated with reasonable precision: The dentate line lies at approximately mid-anal canal level. This is generally midway between the superior border of the puborectalis muscle and the most caudal extent of the subcutaneous external sphincter. These landmarks define the "surgical" anal canal (as distinct from the "anatomical" anal canal, which is shorter, and defined as the canal caudal to the anal valves). Dentate level is undoubtedly best estimated using coronal views, which allow the entire cranio-caudal extent of the puborectalis muscle and external sphincter to be appreciated, but its location can be estimated from axial views with reasonable precision given sufficient prior experience. It should be noted that in many patients the puborectalis muscle is rather gracile, unlike the bulky muscle suggested in many anatomical illustrations. Notably, the puborectalis frequently blends imperceptibly into the external sphincter, which hampers precise identification of the mid-anal canal level. Nevertheless, this can be overcome with experience. It may be helpful to trace the course of the puborectalis from its anterior anchorage on the pubis, back toward the sphincter complex, which helps differentiate it from the external sphincter. Any track that penetrates the pelvic floor above the level of the puborectalis muscle is potentially a suprasphincteric or extrasphincteric fistula. The level of the internal opening distinguishes between these, being anal in the former and rectal in the latter (Fig. 19.7).

Transsphincteric fistulas penetrate the external sphincter directly, a feature that can be easily appreciated on axial (Fig. 19.5) or coronal views. However, recent MR studies have revealed that a transsphincteric track may cross the sphincter at a variety of angles (BUCHANAN et al. 2003a, b). For example, it may arch upwards as it passes through the external sphincter and thus cross the muscle at a higher level than would be deduced merely from inspecting the level of the internal opening. This is important because such tracks will require a greater degree of sphincter incision during fistulotomy, with a correspondingly increased risk of postoperative incontinence. Coronal MRI is best placed to estimate the precise angulation of the tract with respect to the surrounding musculature (BUCHANAN et al. 2003b).

The radial site of the internal opening is simple to identify if the fistula track can be traced right to the anal mucosa but this appearance is very unusual since the internal opening is rarely widely patent – rather it is more often compressed and can be very difficult to see, even during direct inspection at EUA. Consequently, it is typically impossible to trace a fistula right up to the anal mucosa, unless an endoanal coil has been used. It follows that an intelligent deduction must be made as to where the internal opening is likely to be. This is best achieved by looking to where there is maximal intersphincteric sepsis, since the internal opening is likely to lie adjacent or very close to this (Fig. 19.8). The intersphincteric space and longitudinal layer is often seen as a low-intensity ring lying between the internal and external sphincter. The internal sphincter is hyperintense on both T2-weighted fast spin echo and STIR sequences. The radial position of the internal opening is reported with respect to a clock face, with 12 o'clock being directly anterior with the patient in the supine position. It should be noted that the patient's position on the operating table may differ from this depending on the surgical approach taken (e.g., prone jacknife). The surgeon needs to understand that the radiological report refers to the patient in the supine standard anatomical position.

The major advantage of MR imaging is the facility with which it can image any extensions associated with the primary track. Morphologically, extensions frequently take the form of complex track systems, regions of which are often dilated to create an abscess (although a precise radiological definition of when a track becomes an abscess and vice versa remains elusive). Extensions are revealed as hyperintense regions on T2-weighted and STIR sequences and also enhance further if intravenous contrast is given. Again, collateral inflammation can be present to variable extent. The commonest type of extension is one that arises from the apex of a transsphincteric track and extends into the roof of the ischioanal fossa (Fig. 19.9).

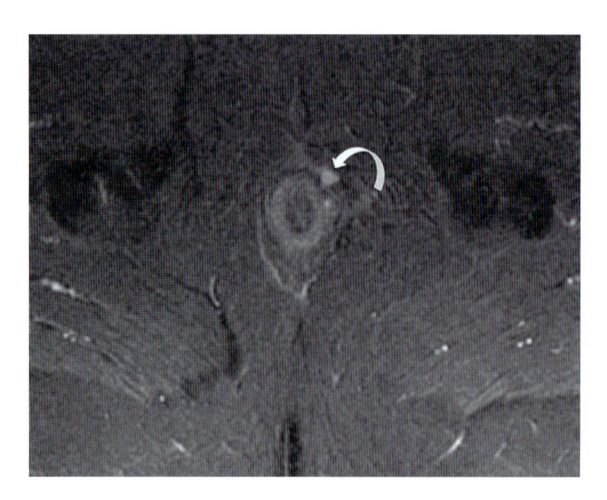

Fig. 19.8. Axial STIR image in a man with a transsphincteric fistula. The epicentre of sepsis is in the intersphincteric plane at 1–2 o'clock (*curved arrow*). This indicates the radial position of the internal communication with the anal lumen

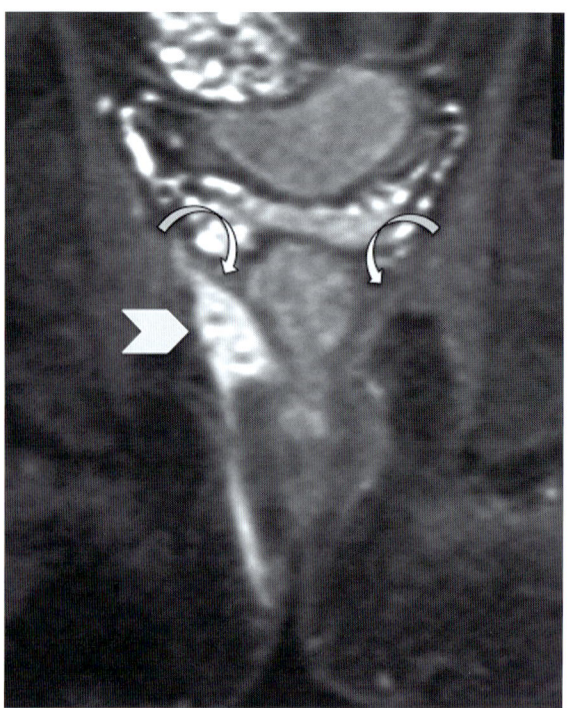

Fig. 19.9. Coronal STIR MR image in a patient with a transsphincteric fistula and extension (*arrowhead*) into the roof of the right ischio-anal fossa. The extension is below the levator plates (*curved arrows*)

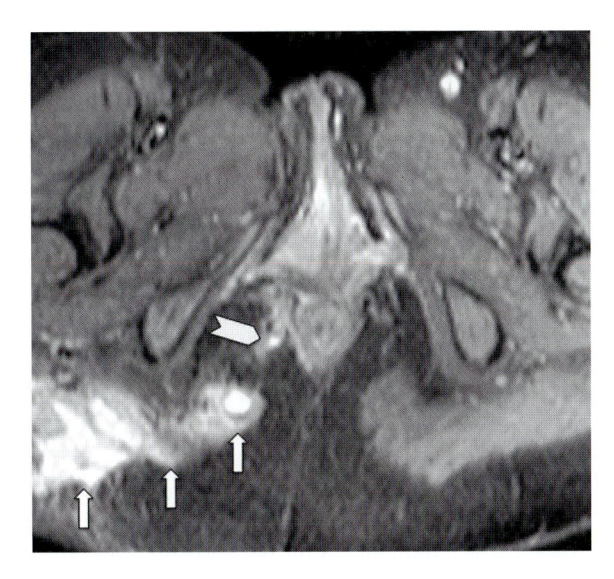

Fig. 19.10. Axial STIR image in a woman with a primary transsphincteric fistula-in-ano (*arrowhead*). Preoperative MR imaging reveals a very substantial extension into the right buttock (*arrows*), which was unsuspected

The major benefit of preoperative MRI is that it can alert the surgeon to extensions that would otherwise be missed during EUA. This is especially the case when extensions are either contralateral to the primary track or when they are several centimetres away from it (Fig. 19.10). It is especially important to image supralevator extensions (Fig. 19.11) since these are not only particularly difficult for the surgeon to detect but they also pose specific difficulties with treatment. Horseshoe extensions spread either side of the internal opening and are recognized on MRI by their unique configuration (Fig. 19.12). Horseshoes may be intersphincteric, ischioanal, or supralevator. Complex extensions are especially common in patients with recurrent fistula-in-ano or those who have Crohn's disease.

19.1.7
Effect of Preoperative MRI on Surgery and Clinical Outcome

Over the past decade MRI has revolutionized the treatment of patients with fistula-in-ano. As stated in the sections above, this is because MRI can Preoperatively classify fistulas with high accuracy, alerting the surgeon to disease that would otherwise have been missed. While there are reports of the technique dating from 1989 (Koelbel et al. 1989) it was

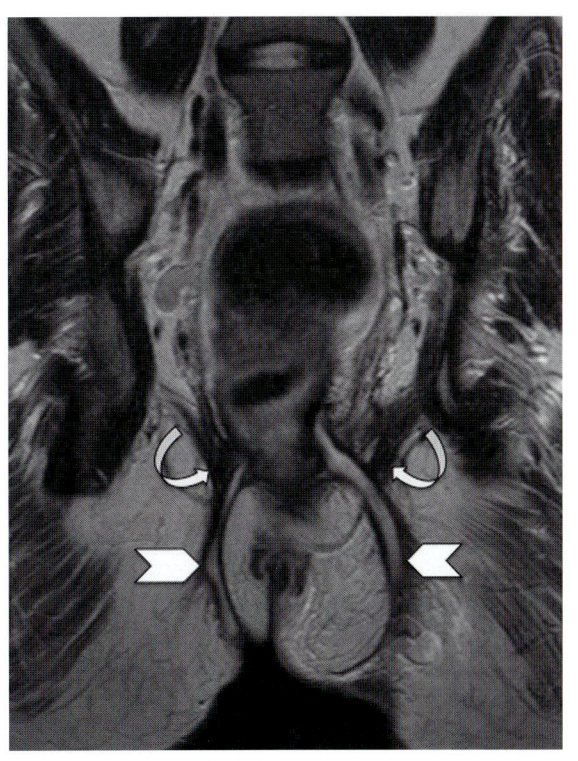

Fig. 19.11. Coronal T2-weighted MR image in a patient with bilateral fistulas (*arrowheads*). There are bilateral supralevator extensions – the tracks penetrate the levator plates (*curved arrows*) to reach the supralevator space

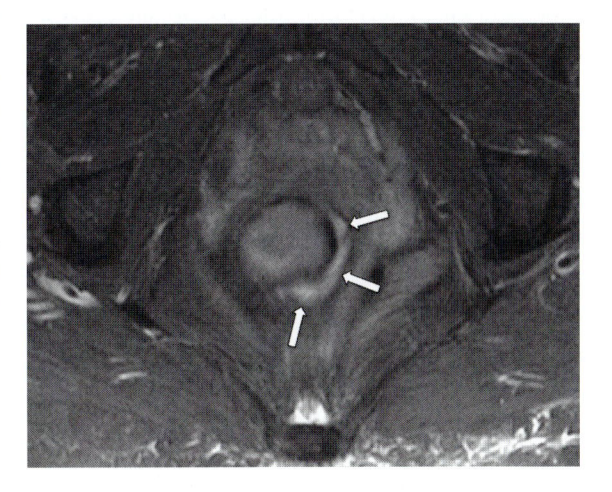

Fig. 19.12. Axial STIR MR image showing a horseshoe extension (*arrows*)

not until the description by Lunniss et al. (1992) that the true potential of MRI was appreciated fully. Lunniss imaged 16 patients with cryptoglandular fistula-in-ano and compared the classification achieved by MRI with that obtained at subsequent EUA. MR imaging proved correct in 14 of the 16 cases (88%), immediately suggesting that it was by far the most accurate Preoperative assessment available at the time. However, the remaining two patients, in whom MRI had suggested disease but where EUA had been normal, represented subsequently with disease at the site initially indicated by MRI. The clear implication was that EUA had missed disease that had been detected by MR. This led the authors to conclude, "MRI is the most accurate method for determining the presence and course of anal fistulae" (Lunniss et al. 1992).

Lunnis' work was rapidly confirmed by other workers and subsequently elaborated on. For example, Spencer and colleagues independently classified 37 patients into those with simple or complex fistulas on the basis of MRI and EUA, and found that MRI was the better predictor of clinical outcome, with positive and negative predictive values of 73% vs. 57% and 87% vs. 64% for MRI and surgery, respectively (Spencer et al. 1998). This study implied clearly that MRI and clinical outcome were closely related, and again raised the possibility that Preoperative MRI could help identify features that caused post-operative recurrence. Beets-Tan and colleagues extended this hypothesis by investigating the therapeutic impact of Preoperative MRI; the MRI findings in 56 patients were revealed to the operating surgeon after they had completed an initial EUA (Beets-Tan et al. 2001). MRI provided important additional information that precipitated further surgery in 12 of the 56 patients (21%), predominantly in those with recurrent fistulas or Crohn's disease (Beets-Tan et al. 2001). Buchanan and co-workers hypothesized that the therapeutic impact and thus beneficial effect of Preoperative MRI would be greatest in patients with recurrent fistulas, since these had the most chance of harboring occult infection while simultaneously being the most difficult to evaluate clinically (Buchanan et al. 2002). After an initial EUA they revealed the findings of Preoperative MRI in 71 patients with recurrent fistulas, and left any further surgery in the light of the MRI findings to the discretion of the operating surgeon. The clinical course of each patient was then followed subsequently. They found that postoperative recurrence was only 16% for surgeons who always acted when MRI suggested they had missed areas of sepsis, whereas recurrence was 57% for those surgeons who always chose to ignore imaging, believing their own assessment to be superior (Buchanan et al. 2002). Furthermore, of the 16 patients who needed further surgery, MRI predicted the site of this disease correctly in all cases (Buchanan et al. 2002).

Ever since Lunnis's work suggested that EUA might be an imperfect reference standard with which to judge MRI (Lunniss et al. 1992), comparative studies have been plagued by the lack of a genuine reference standard. It is now well-recognized that surgical findings at EUA are often incorrect, especially if the fistula is complex. In particular, false-negative diagnoses are relatively frequent. In a recent comparative study of endosonography, MRI and EUA in 34 patients with fistulas due to Crohn's disease, Schwartz and co-workers found that a combination of the results of at least two modalities was necessary in order to arrive at a correct classification (Schwartz et al. 2001). Lunnis' was the earliest work to suggest that many surgical false-negatives will only reveal themselves over the course of long-term clinical follow-up and others have confirmed this observation (Spencer et al. 1998; Buchanan et al. 2002; Schwartz et al. 2001). At this point in time, comparative studies that ignore clinical outcome are likely to be seriously flawed. Recognizing this, Buchanan and co-workers examined 108 primary tracks by digital examination, anal endosonography and MRI, and then followed patients' clinical progress to establish an enhanced reference standard for each patient who was based on ultimate clinical outcome rather than EUA (Buchanan et al. 2004). The authors found that digital evaluation correctly classified 61% of primary tracks, AES 81%, and MR imaging 90% (Buchanan et al. 2004). While endosonography was particularly adept at predicting the site of the internal opening correctly, achieving this in 91%, MRI achieved this in 97% and was superior to endosonography in all assessments investigated by the authors (Buchanan et al. 2004). While endosonography is undoubtedly a useful tool for investigating fistula-in-ano, it cannot compete with MRI for detection of extensions, which is undoubtedly the most important role for Preoperative imaging. MRI is also more generally available and less operator dependent.

19.1.8
Differential Diagnosis of Perianal Sepsis

Not all perianal sepsis is caused by fistula-in-ano. For example, acne conglobata, hidradenitis suppurativa, pilonidal sinus, actinomycosis, tuberculosis, proctitis, human immunodeficiency virus, lymphoma, and anal and rectal tumors may all cause peri-anal infection. While clinical examination is often conclusive, this is not always the case and imaging may help clarify the differential diagnosis. As noted in the sections above, the cardinal feature of fistula-in-ano is intersphincteric infection, which is not generally found in other conditions. Whenever imaging suggests that infection is superficial rather than deep-seated, and there is no sphincteric involvement, then other conditions such as hidradenitis suppurativa should be considered. For example, a study comparing patients with pilonidal sinus and fistula-in-ano found that MRI could reliably distinguish between the two on the basis of intersphincteric infection and an enteric opening, both of which were always absent in pilonidal sinus (Fig. 19.13) (Taylor et al. 2003).

The possibility of underlying Crohn's disease should always be considered in patients who have particularly complex fistulas, especially if the history is relatively short. Indeed, a perianal fistula is the presenting symptom in approximately 5% of patients with Crohn's disease and 30–40% will experience anal disease at some time (Schwartz et al. 2002). MRI can be extended cranially to encompass the small bowel when Crohn's disease is suspected and the possibility of underlying pelvic disease should be considered in any patient with an extraphincteric fistula, whether thought to be due to Crohn's disease or otherwise.

19.1.9
Which Patients Should Be Imaged?

While most patients with fistula-in-ano are simple to both diagnose and treat, a proportion will benefit from detailed and accurate Preoperative investigation. Where there is easy access to MRI, it could be argued that all patients should be imaged Preoperatively. For example, while the therapeutic impact of Preoperative MRI is undoubted in patients with complex disease (Beets-Tan et al. 2001; Buchanan et al. 2002), it has been estimated that the therapeutic impact of MR imaging is 10% in patients presenting for the first time with seemingly simple fistulas (Buchanan et al. 2003a, b). However, where access to imaging is more restricted, the clinician and radiologist will need to select those patients who are most likely to benefit. Since there is now overwhelming evidence that MRI alters surgical therapy and improves clinical outcome in patients with recurrent disease, MRI should be performed routinely in such cases. Patients presenting for the first time with a fistula that appears complex on clinical examination should also be referred, as should patients with known Crohn's disease since the preponderance of complex fistulas is increased in this subgroup.

The benefit of MRI is not restricted to surgical assessment. The advent of monoclonal antibody to human tumor necrosis factor alpha has impacted dramatically upon the medical management of patients whose fistulas are due to Crohn's disease, especially those with chronic disease. However, therapy is contraindicated if an abscess is present and MRI may be used to search for this. Indeed, MRI may be used to monitor therapy since it seems that fistulas may persist in the face of clinical findings that suggest remission. For example, MRI studies in patients whose external opening has closed have revealed that underlying sepsis is often still present, indicating a need for continuing therapy (Bell et al. 2003). A recent study of fistula enhancement following gadolinium enhancement in patients with Crohn's disease found that pixel-by-pixel analysis was able to differentiate between differing levels of systemic disease activity, raising the possibility that this approach could be used to titrate medical therapy (Horsthuis et al. 2009)

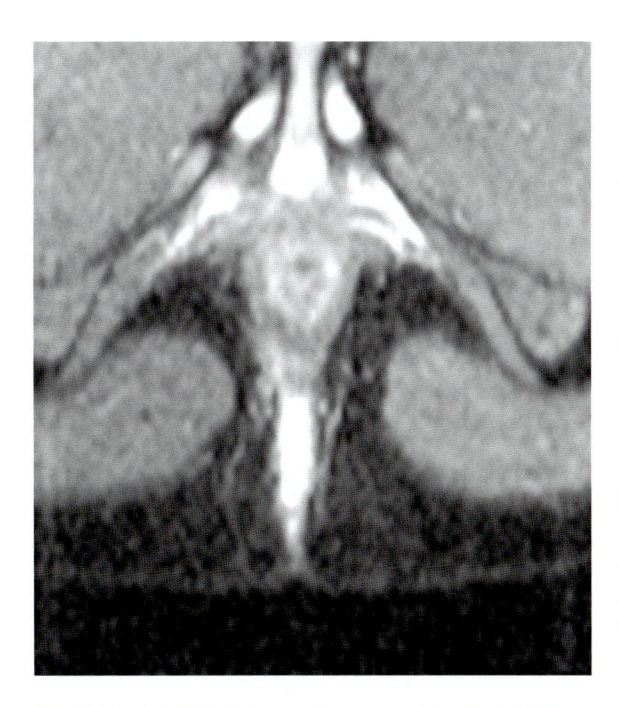

Fig. 19.13. Axial STIR image in a man with pilonidal sinus disease in whom a fistula was suspected clinically. There is a track posteriorly at 6 o'clock, which penetrates deep enough to contact the posterior aspect of the external sphincter but there is no penetration into the sphincter and no intersphincteric sepsis. No internal opening was found at EUA

19.2
MR Imaging to Investigate Anal Incontinence

19.2.1
Anal Incontinence

Anal incontinence is common, especially in women. It is particularly debilitating from a social perspective and its prevalence increases with age. Etiology can be broadly divided into two groups: Incontinence due to sphincter degeneration or atrophy (due to age for example) and incontinence due to loss of integrity of the anal sphincter ring. The latter occurs most commonly in women following childbirth by vaginal delivery. While anal sphincter laceration during childbirth was previously thought to be a relatively rare event because it could only be identified clinically in one per 200 vaginal deliveries, studies using anal endosonography (AES) immediately postpartum have suggested an incidence closer to one-third of all vaginal deliveries: A prospective, endosonographic study of 202 unselected consecutive women pre- and postvaginal delivery revealed anal sphincter tears in 28 of 79 of primiparous subjects (35%) and 21 of 48 of multiparous subjects (44%) (Sultan et al. 1993). Symptoms of anal incontinence may occur immediately after delivery if trauma is sufficient but many women present later in life, presumably because cumulative effects of multiple deliveries, progressive neuropathy, aging, and the menopause overcome their compensation mechanisms (Reay Jones et al. 2003). Many are also too embarrassed to complain or they, or their doctors, believe that the condition is incurable.

Minor degrees of anal incontinence can often be satisfactorily managed with dietary manipulation, pharmacological treatment, or physiotherapy and biofeedback. However, if this proves unsatisfactory, then more aggressive treatment is warranted. While there are many modalities available to investigate anal sphincter function, for example measurement of anal squeeze pressures and pudendal nerve latency, it is imaging that has assumed the central role in the investigation of anal incontinence. This is simply because imaging most accurately identifies whether the anal sphincter ring is intact or not. Patients whose external sphincter has been disrupted by childbirth can be treated surgically by a sphincter repair, the aim of which is to restore mechanical integrity to the sphincter ring. If the sphincters are found to be intact on imaging, then the etiology of the patient's incontinence is likely to be degenerative or neurogenic in origin and surgical sphincter repair has nothing to offer – in such cases, sacral nerve stimulation (Jarrett et al. 2008) or surgical implantation of an artificial anal sphincter may be necessary (Vaizey et al. 1998).

19.2.2
MRI Findings in Anal Incontinence

Anal endosonography was the first imaging modality able to visualize the separate components of the anal sphincter complex with sufficient clarity for clinical utility (Law and Bartram 1989). Obstetric sphincter lacerations are diagnosed simply by an anterior discontinuity in the muscles of the external sphincter complex. As described in the sections above, AES is generally inferior to MRI for assessment of fistula-in-ano, principally because the depth of penetration is limited by the probe frequency. However, assessment of anal sphincter integrity only requires that the sphincter be imaged with precision – depth of penetration is a secondary concern. For this reason, AES is used extensively in the diagnostic work-up of patients with anal incontinence, especially since it is cheap and relatively simple to perform, and has been proven to be extremely accurate (Malouf et al. 2000).

An alternative to AES is MRI using a dedicated endoanal receiver coil, which allows the sphincter complex to be resolved with a spatial resolution sufficient to diagnose sphincter defects. Clinical studies using such coils were first described over a decade ago and comparisons were made with AES. Stoker and colleagues found MRI to be superior (Rociu et al. 1999) whereas Halligan and co-workers found the opposite (Malouf et al. 2000). These data probably reflect differing preferences and familiarity with the modalities being tested – there is no doubt that both have clinical utility for the detection of sphincter tears. Subsequent larger comparative studies have found no significant difference between the two techniques for the detection of sphincter tears (Dobben et al. 2007). There is one area where MRI is almost certainly superior however, and that is for the assessment of external sphincter atrophy. This describes replacement of the striated muscle of the external sphincter by fat, and is believed to arise as a consequence of neuropathy, possibly initiated by childbirth. It is well recognized that external sphincter laceration and neuropathy can coexist several years following vaginal delivery – in this context the presence of atrophy prejudices the

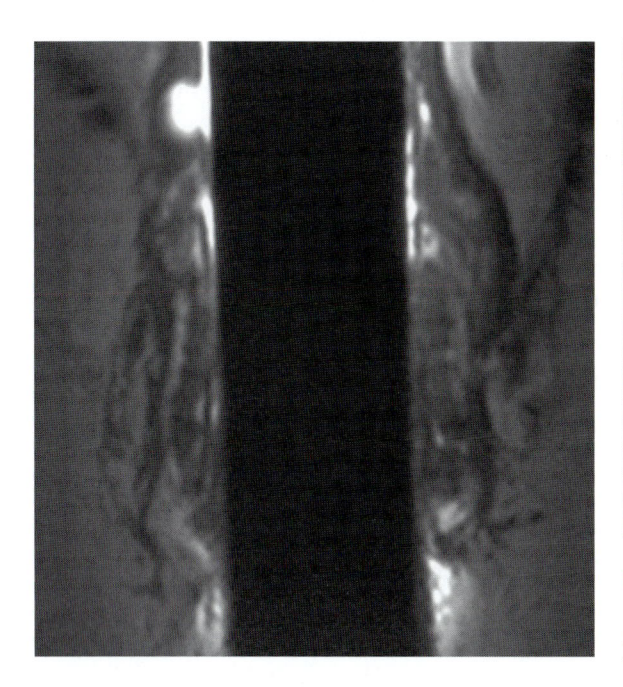

Fig. 19.14. Coronal T2-weighted images from an endoanal receiver coil showing extensive sphincter atrophy

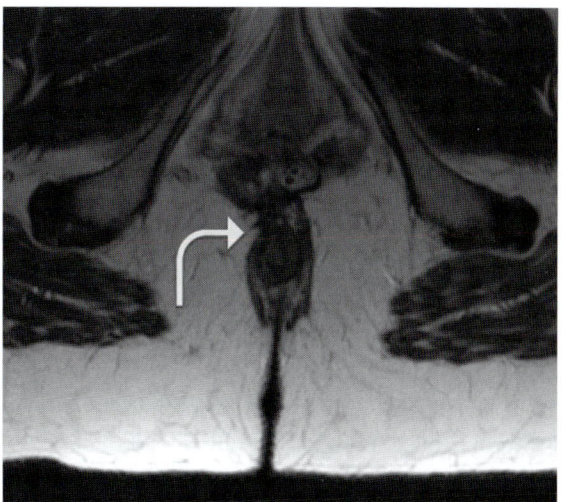

Fig. 19.15. Axial T2-weighted image showing a right anterior quadrant external anal sphincter tear (*arrow*) and perineal scarring (compare to normal left side) following vaginal delivery

results of external sphincter repair because the muscle is of poor quality (Briel et al. 1999).

Endoanal coils are housed within a rigid plastic cylinder (as opposed to inflatable rectal coils) that is designed to cross the anal sphincter, and the diameter varies between 7 and 19 mm, with smaller diameters being used to image paediatric sphincters (deSouza et al. 1997). While this design affords the highest spatial resolution, advances in pelvic phased-array coil technology mean that the anal sphincter complex can be visualized in detail using these, and the need for an endo-anal coil has diminished (Terra et al. 2005). Irrespective of the coil used, most workers use a T2-weighted sequence (e.g. turbo spin-echo) since this affords good contrast between the various components of the sphincter complex while also providing excellent anatomical visualization. It is particularly suited for distinguishing between fat and striated muscle and thus is effective in external sphincter atrophy (Fig. 19.14). A combination of axial and coronal T2-weighted sequence is sufficient (Tables 19.1 and 19.2). The internal sphincter is relatively hyperintense whereas the external sphincter, puborectal muscle, and levator muscles are relatively hypointense. In patient with sphincter tears following obstetric injury, these are revealed by discontinuity of the external sphincter ring anteriorly (Fig. 19.15). Depending on the severity of the tear, the internal sphincter may also be involved. In clinical practice, it is usual for both sphincters to be lacerated. Tears usually involve the full length of the anal canal. Partial tears are less common but convey less functional disturbance (Williams et al. 2001).

A study of 30 patients who both underwent external phased array and endoanal MRI found that they did not differ significantly in their ability to depict external sphincter atrophy (Williams et al. 2001). However, as ever, accuracy was contingent on observer experience and authors have concluded that both techniques could only be recommended if sufficient expertise for interpretation was available (Terra et al. 2006). A study of 200 incontinent patients found that MR features of external sphincter atrophy on phased-array imaging correlated with impaired anal squeeze pressures as assessed by anal manometry, implying that MR could be used to identify patients whose muscle quality was poor (Terra et al. 2006).

19.3
MR Imaging of Anal Malignancy

Anal tumors are very rare and account for <1% of large bowel tumors. In contrast to colorectal tumors, which are nearly always adenocarcinomas, anal tumors tend to be epidermal in origin, for example squamous cell carcinoma. The anus is however one of the most pluripotential sites for tumors (because it is a junctional zone anatomically) and many cell types can be encountered, including melanomas, Paget's and anal gland carcinoma. Like cervical carcinoma, there is a strong association with human papillomavirus infection. HIV infection and smoking are also associated with increased relative risk.

Anal tumors typically spread upwards, into the rectum, with the result that they may be difficult to distinguish from rectal cancers on clinical grounds. It should also be borne in mind that a tumor in the anal canal is more likely to be due to caudal spread of a rectal cancer than a primary anal carcinoma, simply because rectal cancer is vastly more common. Some cases of primary anal tumors may also be misclassified as squamous carcinoma of the skin. Cranial extension of anal carcinoma may result in direct invasion of local structures deeper to the anal sphincter, notably the musculature of the pelvic floor and the prostate or vagina. Local nodal spread is to the mesorectal nodes and, importantly, the inguinal nodes, which should be encompassed in the imaging field. Metastatic spread tends to be to the liver, lungs, and bone.

Treatment of anal tumors is radically different from that of rectal carcinoma. Specifically, combined modality therapy using chemoradiation is the mainstay of treatment. In complete contrast to rectal cancer therapy, surgery has relatively little to offer, and is reserved for treatment of very early superficial tumors (so that prolonged chemo-radiotherapy can be avoided) and to excise relapsed local disease where this is possible – normally by abdominoperineal excision of the anus and rectum or more extensive pelvic exenteration.

The role of MRI is thus to stage the primary tumor and to define its margins for the radiotherapist, so that all malignant tissue is encompassed in the treatment field, and to assess the effects of treatment. These aims are best achieved using pelvic phased-array imaging since insertion of an endoanal coil may

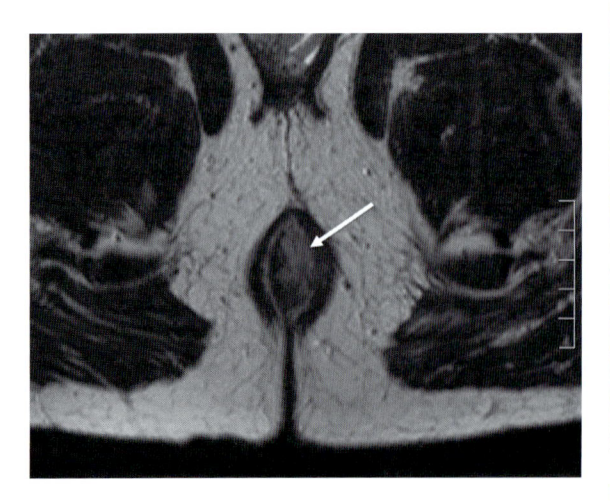

Fig. 19.16. Axial T2-weighted image at mid anal canal level in a man with anal carcinoma. The tumor (*arrow*) has penetrated through the internal sphincter and intersphincteric plane but is still confined by the external anal sphincter

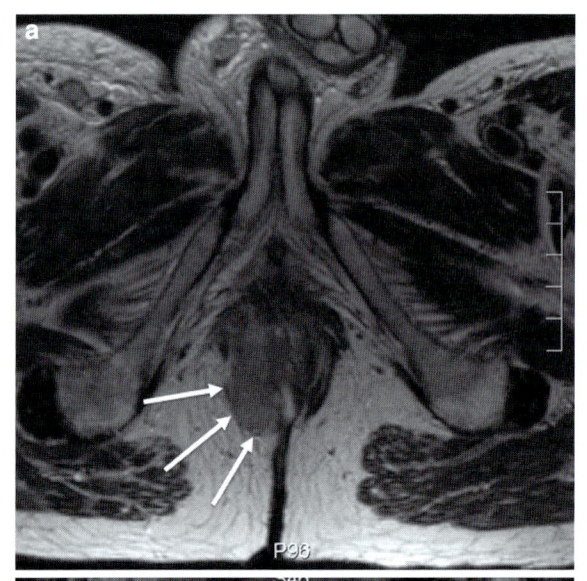

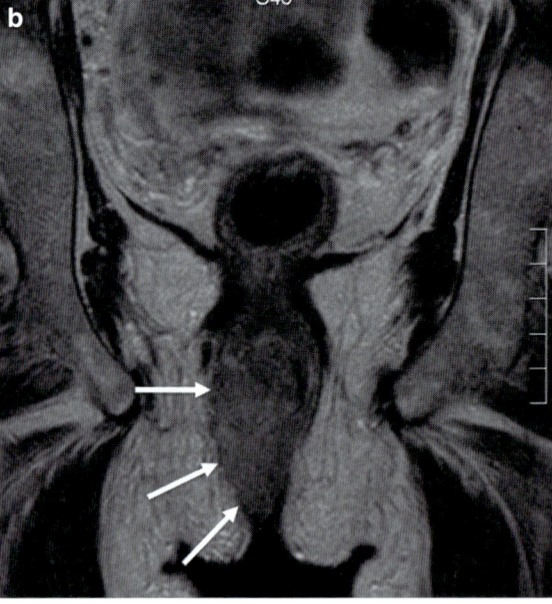

Fig. 19.17. (a) Axial T2-weighted image and (b) coronal T2-weighted image in a man with anal carcinoma (*arrows*). In contrast to the patient in Fig. 19.16, this tumor has penetrated through all layers of the anal sphincter complex to reach the right ischio-anal fossa

be difficult, painful, and field of view limitations may prevent detection of disease remote from the anal lumen (Koh et al. 2008). T2-weighted axial and coronal images, aligned with anal canal, should be sufficient to delineate the primary tumor and local extent (Figs. 19.16 and 19.17) (Tables 19.1 and 19.2).

References

Beets-Tan RG, Beets GL, van der Hoop AG, et al (2001) Imaging of anal fistulas: does it really help the surgeon? Radiology 218:75–84

Bell SJ, Halligan S, Windsor ACJ, et al (2003) Response of fistulating Crohn's disease to infliximab treatment assessed by magnetic resonance imaging. Aliment Pharmacol Ther 17:387–393

Briel JW, Stoker J, Rociu E, et al (1999) External anal sphincter atrophy on endoanal magnetic resonance imaging adversely affects continence after sphincteroplasty. Br J Surg 86:1322–1327

Buchanan G, Halligan S, Bartram CI, et al (2004) Clinical examination, endosonography, and magnetic resonance imaging for preoperative assessment of fistula-in-ano: comparison to an outcome derived reference standard. Radiology 233:674–681

Buchanan G, Halligan S, Williams A, et al (2002) Effect of MRI on clinical outcome of recurrent fistula-in-ano. Lancet 360:1661–1662

Buchanan GN, Halligan S, Williams AB, et al (2003a) Magnetic resonance imaging for primary fistula in ano. Br J Surg 90:877–881

Buchanan GN, Williams AB, Bartram CI, et al (2003b) Potential clinical implications of direction of a trans-sphincteric anal fistula track. Br J Surg 90:1250–1255

Chiari H (1878) Uber die analen divertikel der rectumschleimhaut und ihre beziehung zu den anal fisteln. Wien Med Press 19:1482–1483

deSouza NM, Gilderdale DJ, MacIver DK, et al (1997) High resolution MR imaging of the anal sphincter in children: a pilot study using endoanal receiver coils. AJR Am J Roentgenol 169:201–206

Dobben AC, Terra MP, Slors JF, et al (2007) External anal sphincter defects in patients with fecal incontinence: comparison of endoanal MR imaging and endoanal US. Radiology 242:463–471

Fucini C (1991) One stage treatment of anal abscesses and fistulae. Int J Colorect Dis 6:12–16

Halligan S, Bartram CI. (1998) MR imaging of fistula in ano: are endoanal coils the gold standard? AJR Am J Roentgenol 171:407–412

Halligan S, Buchanan G (2003) Imaging fistula-in-ano. Eur J Radiol 42:98–107

Halligan S, Stoker J (2006) Imaging fistula-in-ano: state-of-the-art. Radiology 239:18–33

Horsthuis K, Lavini C, Bipat S, et al (2009) Perianal Crohn disease: evaluation of dynamic contrast-enhanced MR imaging as an indicator of disease activity. Radiology 251: 380–387

Hussain SM, Stoker J, Schouten WR, et al (1996) Fistula in ano: endoanal sonography versus endoanal MR imaging in classification. Radiology 200:475–481

Jarrett ME, Dudding TC, Nicholls RJ, et al (2008) Sacral nerve stimulation for fecal incontinence related to obstetric anal sphincter damage. Dis Colon Rectum 51:531–537

Koelbel G, Schmiedl U Majer MC, et al (1989) Diagnosis of fistulae and sinus tracts in patients with Crohn disease: value of MR imaging. Am J Roentgenol 152:999–1003

Koh DM, Dzik-Jurasz A, O'Neill B, et al (2008) Pelvic phased-array MR imaging of anal carcinoma before and after chemoradiation. Br J Radiol 81:91–98

Law PJ, Bartram CI. (1989) Anal endosonography. Technique and normal anatomy. Gastrointest Radiol 14:349–353

Lilius HG (1968) Investigation of human foetal anal ducts and intramuscular glands and a clinical study of 150 patients. Acta Chir Scand Supp 383:88

Lunniss PJ, Armstrong P, Barker PG, et al (1992) Magnetic resonance imaging of anal fistulae. Lancet 340:394–396

Malouf AJ, Williams AB, Halligan S, et al (2000) Prospective assessment of accuracy of endoanal MR imaging and endosonography in patients with fecal incontinence. AJR Am J Roentgenol 175:741–745

Parks AG (1961) The pathogenesis and treatment of fistula-in-ano. Br Med J 5224:463–469

Parks AG, Gordon PH, Hardcastle JD (1976) A classification of fistula –in-ano. Br J Surg 63:1–12

Reay Jones NH, Healy JC, King LJ, et al (2003) Pelvic connective tissue resilience decreases with vaginal delivery, menopause and uterine prolapse. Br J Surg 90:466–467

Rociu E, Stoker J, Eijkemans MJ, et al (1999) Fecal incontinence: endoanal US versus endoanal MR imaging. Radiology 212:453–458

Sanio P (1984) Fistula-in-ano in a defined population: incidence and epidemiological aspects. Acta Chir Gynaecol 73:219–224

Schwartz DA, Loftus EV Jr, Tremaine WJ, et al (2002) The natural history of fistulizing Crohn's disease in Olmsted County, Minnesota. Gastroenterology 122:875–880

Schwartz DA, Wiersema MJ, Dudiak KM et al (2001) A comparison of endoscopic ultrasound, magnetic resonance imaging, and exam under anesthesia for evaluation of Crohn's perianal fistulas. Gastroenterology 121:1064–1072

Spencer JA, Chapple K, Wilson D, et al (1998) Outcome after surgery for perianal fistula: predictive value of MR imaging. AJR Am J Roentgenol 171:403–406

Spencer JA, Ward J, Beckingham IJ, Adams C, Ambrose NS (1996) Dynamic contrast-enhanced MR imaging of perianal fistulas. Am J Roentgenol 167:735–741

Sultan AH, Kamm MA, Hudson CN, et al (1993) Anal sphincter disruption during vaginal delivery. New Engl J Med 329:1905–1911

Taylor SA, Halligan S, Bartram CI (2003) Pilonidal sinus disease: MR imaging distinction from fistula in ano. Radiology 226:662–667

Terra MP, Beets-Tan RG, van Der Hulst VP, et al (2005) Anal sphincter defects in patients with fecal incontinence: endoanal versus external phased-array MR imaging. Radiology 236:886–895

Terra MP, Beets-Tan RG, van der Hulst VP, et al (2006) MRI in evaluating atrophy of the external sphincter in patients with fecal incontinence. AJR Am J Roentgenol 187: 991–999

Terra MP, Deutekom M, Beets-Tan RG, et al (2006) Relationship between external anal sphincter atrophy at endoanal magnetic resonance imaging and clinical, functional, and anatomic characteristics in patients with fecal incontinence. Dis Colon Rectum 49: 668–678

Vaizey CJ, Kamm MA, Gold DM, et al (1998) Clinical, physiological, and radiological study of a new purpose-designed artificial bowel sphincter. Lancet 352:105–109

Williams AB, Bartram CI, Halligan S, et al (2001) Anal sphincter damage after vaginal delivery using three-dimensional endosonography. Obstet Gynecol 97(5 Pt 1):770

Subject Index

A

Acute appendicitis, 287–293
Acute conditions, 283–311. *See also* Acute appendicitis; Diverticulitis; Peptic ulcer disease; Small bowel obstruction
- inflammatory bowel disease, 293–299
- protocols, 284–287
Adhesions, 165, 271–281
- cine MRI, 272–275
- imaging criteria, 273–275
Ampullary tumors, 103–105
Anal incontinence, 5, 18, 232, 316, 322–324
- anal endosonography, 342
- external sphincter atrophy, 342, 343
- MRI findings, 342–343
- sphincter defect, 342
Anal tumors, 343–344
Annular pancreas, 105
Anorectal fistulas. *See* Perianal fistula (Fistula-in-Ano)
Anus, 329–345. *See also* Anal incontinence; Anal tumors; Perianal fistula (fistula-in-ano)
- anatomy, 330–331

B

Balanced fast field echo (FFE), 9–10
Balanced steady state free precession (b-SSFP), 9–10, 30
- balanced FFE, 9–10
- banding artifact at 3T, 26, 27
- FIESTA, 9–10
- true-FISP, 9–10
Barium sulfate preparations, 43
Bezoars, 280
B1-inhomogeneity artefacts, 24
Blueberry juice, 43
Bowel distension, 41–42. *See also* Contrast media
- bright lumen, 38–39
- dark lumen, 39–40
- gadolinium-based agents for intravenous use, 44–46
- general requirements, 36–37
- osmolarity, 41–42
- paramagnetic agents, 36
- relaxivity, 37–38
- superparamagnetic particles, 36 (3.4)
- T1 and T2 agents, 36

Bowel motility, 229–246
- data analysis, 237–240
- dynamic MRI, 240–245
- impact of drugs, 241–242
- impedance measurement, 232–233
- inflammatory bowel diseases, 242–244
- manometry, 232, 245
- MR motility imaging, 245–246
- normal motility, 241
- postoperative ileus, 241
- preparation, 233–235
- scintigraphy, 231–232, 245
- sequences, 235
- ultrasound, 245
Breath-hold interpolated 3D T1W (VIBE, LAVA, FAME, THRIVE), 11–12

C

Carcinoid, 146
Celiac disease, 129, 159–160
Chemical shift artifacts, 23–24
Choledococele, 103, 109
Cine MRI, 272–275
- adhesions, 272–275
Clinical assessment, 332–333
Coils, 4–5, 69–71
- endoanal coils, 343
- endoluminal coils, 5, 70–71, 75–78
Colonography. *See* MR colonography
Contrast agents, 33–47, 118–120, 136, 234, 247, 250. *See also* Bowel distension
- barium sulfate preparations, 43
- biphasic agents, 42–43
- general concepts, 34–38
- intraluminal contrast media, 118, 136–137
- isphagula/psyllium Husk Fiber, 43
- locust bean gum, 43
- mannitol, 42
- methyl cellulose, 43
- oral contrast agent, 84
- pineapple and blueberry juice, 43
- polyethylene glycol (PEG), 42
- sorbitol, 42
Contrast media, 118–120. *See* Contrast agents

Crohn's disease, 123–129, 141–145, 155–159
- abscess, 125–126, 143
- active *vs.* elective evaluation, 151–152
- bowel preparation and tubes, 150–151
- bowel wall stratification, 124
- bowel wall thickening, 123–124, 142
- capacity and hardware, 152
- CD disease activity assessment, 126
- clinical role of imaging, 155–159
- cobblestoning, 142
- comb sign, 125
- creeping fat, 126
- disease activity assessment, 143–145, 157
- disease stage, 152
- early lesions, 141
- enhancement after intravenous contrast administration, 124
- extra enteric assessment, 152
- fistula, 125–126, 143
- ileocolonoscopy, 157, 158
- inflammatory bowel disease, 155–159
- lymph nodes, 125, 143–145
- MR enterography/enteroclysis, 152–153, 155
- preparation, 150–151
- radiation, 150
- radiology/endoscopy, 155
- role enterography, 123–129
- signal intensity of the bowel wall, 124
- small bowel barium examinations, 157
- small bowel obstruction, 279
- stenosis, 126, 138
- ulcerations, 124–125
- ulcers, 142
- wireless capsule endoscopy, 150
Cystocele, 323–324

D

Descending perineal syndrome, 324
Desmoid tumors, 161
Diffusion-weighted MRI (DWI), 15–16, 56–58, 221
- clinical studies, 60–61
- diffusion tensor imaging, 58–59
- enterography, 121
- histological validation, 59
- image analysis, 58
- perfusion MRI, 221
- reproducibility, 59
- technical parameters, 57–58
Diverticular disease, 198–199
Diverticulitis, 198–199, 290, 300–301
Duodenal, 96–103
- adenocarcinoma, 99–101
- carcinoids, 102
- diverticula, 96
- duplication, 96–97
- hematoma, 98
- lipoma, 97–98
- lymphoma, 101–102
- metastases, 102
- stromal tumors, 98
Duodenum, 93–114
- findings, 96–114
- MRI compared to CT, 107–108
- technique, 94–96
Dynamic acquisition, 14–15
Dynamic contrast-enhanced MRI (DCE-MRI), 52–56
- clinical studies, 56
- histopathological validation, 55–56
- kinetic modelling, 53–55
- measurement reproducibility, 56
- technical parameters, 52–53
Dyssynergic defecation, 324–326

E

Echoplanar imaging (EPI), 6
Ectopic pancreas, 304
Endometriosis, 131, 167
- rectum, 224–225
- small bowel, 167
Enteroclysis, 117, 135–147. See also Crohn's disease; Small bowel
- anti-spasmolytic agents, 120
- benign small bowel neoplasms, 129–130
- CD disease activity assessment, 126
- celiac disease, 129
- cine imaging, 122
- Crohn's disease, 123–129, 141–145
- diffusion-weighted imaging (DWI), 121
- duodenal intubation, 136
- intraluminal contrast agents, 136–137
- intravenous contrast agents, 118, 120
- malignant small bowel neoplasms, 130–131
- normal appearances, 140–141
- patient acceptance, 120
- patient position, 120
- patient's position, 137
- pulse sequences, 121–122, 137–140
- sequences, 121–122
- small bowel lymphomas, 130
- small bowel neoplasms, 145–146
Enterocoele, 321–322
Enterography, 117–132
Esophagus, 67–78
- conventional MRI, 69, 72–73
- external surface coil, 69–70
- high-resolution MRI, 69–71, 73–76
- normal anatomy, 71–72
- patient preparation, 69
- staging, 72–78
External rectal prolapse, 323

F

Familial adenomatous polyposis (FAP), 160–162
Familial mediterranean fever, 131–132
Fast acquisition with multiphase EFGRE3D (FAME), 11–12
Fast imaging employing steady state acquisition (FIESTA), 9–10
Fast imaging with steady precession (True-FISP), 9–10
Fast spin-echo (FSE), 6
Fat suppression, 13–14
– short tau inversion recovery (STIR), 13
– spectral fat suppression, 13
Fecal incontinence. See Anal incontinence
Fistula-in-Ano. See Perianal fistula

G

Gastrointestinal cancers, 259
Gastrointestinal stromal tumor (GIST), 304

H

High-field strength, 21–30
– colonography, 182
– contrast agents, 23
– parallel imaging, 28
– SAR limitations, 24–25
– SSFP banding artifacts, 25–28
Hydrographic projection imaging, 12–13

I

Inflammatory bowel disease (IBD), 155–159, 194–198, 242–244, 293–298. See also Crohn's disease
– MR colonography, 195–198
Intramural intestinal hemorrhage, 280
Intussusception, 280, 322
Ischemia, 305–308
Isphagula/psyllium husk fibre, 43

K

Kinetic modelling, 53–55
– T1-weighted sequences, 53–55
– T2*-weighted sequences, 55

L

Liver acquisition with volume acceleration (LAVA), 11–12
Locust bean gum, 43
Lymphoma, 129–131, 278

M

Malabsorption disorders, 146–147
Malrotation, 280–281
Mannitol, 42
Mesenteric adenitis, 257
Mesenteric paniculitis, 256
Mesothelioma, 265–266
Methylcellulose, 43
MR colonography, 173–183
– analysis, 174, 181–182
– bowel cleansing, 175–176
– bowel distention, 177–179
– bowel preparation, 175–177
– Crohn's disease, 196
– detection of precursors of colorectal cancer, 186–194
– diverticular disease, 198–199
– diverticulitis, 198–199
– fecal tagging, 176–177
– hardware, 174–175
– high field, 182
– image contrast, 179–180
– image interpretation, 188
– incomplete colonoscopy, 199, 200
– inflammatory bowel disease, 195–198
– intermediate and large polyps, 193, 194
– patient acceptance, 200–201
– performance, 180–181
– post processing, 181–182
– results, 185–202
– results in high-prevalence colorectal cancer populations, 188–190
– results in low prevalence colorectal cancer populations, 194
– screening, 194
– spasmolytic agents, 178–179
– technique, 173–183
MR-fluoroscopy/cine imaging, 83–86, 122
MR hydrography, 40–43

N

Nuclear medicine examinations, 157–158

O

Occult GI bleeding, 163–165
Oral contrast agent, 84
Ovarian cancer, 261–263

P

Paraduodenal pancreatitis, 105–107
Parallel imaging, 5

– sensitivity encoding (SENSE), 5
– spatial harmonics (SMASH), 5
Pelvic floor, 315–326
– cystocele, 323–324
– descending perineal syndrome, 324
– dyssynergic defecation, 324–326
– external rectal prolapse, 323
– image analysis, 318
– image technique, 317, 318
– intussusception, 322–323
– normal findings, 318–319
– patient positioning, 316
– patient preparation, 316, 317
– pelvic floor relaxation, 324
– pelvic organ prolapse, 323–324
– protocol, 317
– rectocele, 319–321
– relaxation, 324
– utero-vaginal prolapse, 324
Pelvic organ prolapse, 323–324
Peptic ulcer disease, 301–303
Perfusion imaging, 16
Perianal fistula (fistula-in-ano), 222, 329–341
– aetiology, 330–331
– anal endosonography (AES), 333–334
– anorectal fistulas, 222–224
– benefit of MRI, 339–341
– classification, 331–332
– clinical assessment, 332–333
– computed tomography (CT), 333
– differential diagnosis, 340–341
– effect on clinical outcome, 339–340
– examination under (general) anaesthesia, 332–333
– fistulography, 333
– image interpretation, 335–339
– technique, 334–335
Peritoneal carcinomatosis, 278
Peritoneal tumor spread, 259–261
Peritoneum, 249–267
– anatomy, 253–256
– benign diseases, 256–259
– image interpretation, 252–253
– intraluminal contrast material, 250–251
– malignant diseases, 259–267
– protocol, 251–252
Peritonitis, 257
Peutz–Jeghers syndrome (PJS), 129, 130, 161–162
Pilonidal sinus, 340, 341
Pineapple and blueberry juice, 43
Polyethylene glycol (PEG), 42–43
Primary epiploic appendagitis, 298–300
Primary peritoneal cancer, 266–267
Pseudomyxoma peritonei, 263–265

R

Radiation enteritis, 165–166
Radiation enteropathy, 279–280
Rapid acquisition with relaxation enhancement (RARE; TSE, FSE), 6–8
Rectal cancer
– circumferential resection margin (CRM), 212–214
– clinical background, 205–208
– computed tomography, 220–221
– diffusion-weighted MRI, 221
– endorectal ultrasound (EUS), 220
– extramesorectal lymph nodes, 215–216
– lymph nodes, 214–216
– MR protocol, 208–209
– perfusion MRI, 221
– PET-CT, 221
– recommendations for rectal cancer management, 222
– restaging, 216–220
– risk assessment with MR imaging, 211–216
– T-stage, 212
Rectocoele, 319–321
Rectum, 205–225. See also Anorectal fistulas; Endometriosis; Rectal cancer
– anatomy, 209–211
– enterocoele, 321–322

S

Scleroderma/progressive systemic sclerosis, 131, 159–160
Sclerosing encapsulating peritonitis, 258–259
Sequences, 5–16
Small bowel, 117–128. See also Clinical role, Enteroclysis, Enterography
– benign neoplasms, 129–130
– familial polyposis, 130
– malignant neoplasms, 279
– Peutz–Jeghers syndrome (PJS), 129, 130
– physiology, 229–231
Small bowel lymphomas, 130
Small bowel malignancy, 162–163
Small bowel obstruction, 146, 275–281, 291, 305
– appendicitis, 279
– bezoars, 280
– Crohn's disease, 279
– diverticulitis, 279
– extrinsic masses, 278, 279
– hernia, 276–278
– intraabdominal adhesions, 276
– intramural intestinal hemorrhage, 280
– intussusception, 280
– lymphoma, 278
– malrotation, 280–281

– peritoneal carcinomatosis, 278
– radiation enterpathy, 279–280
Sorbitol, 42
Specific absorption rate (SAR), 24–25, 29
Spoiled gradient echo (FLASH, SPGR, T1FFE), 10–11
Stomach, 67–78
– conventional MRI, 69, 72–73
– external surface coil, 69–70
– high-resolution MRI, 69–71, 73
– normal anatomy on MRI, 71–72
– patient preparation, 69
– staging, 72–78
Susceptibility, 22–23

T

Tissue relaxation rates, 22
Treatment, 332–333
True-FISP, 9–10
Tuberculous peritonitis, 257–258
Turbo spin-echo (TSE), 6–8
T2*-weighted sequences, 55
T1W high resolution isotropic volume examination (THRIVE), 11–12

U

Upper GI tract motility, 81–90
– abnormal findings, 87–88
– esophageal motility, 85–86
– gastric motility, 88–89
– MR-fluoroscopy, 83–86
– normal findings, 87
– oral contrast agent, 84
– oro-pharyngeal motility, 87
– physiology of deglutition, 82–83
Utero-vaginal prolapse, 324

V

Volume interpolated breath hold examination (VIBE), 11–12

W

Wireless capsule endoscopy (WCE), 158
– Crohn's disease, 158
– occult GI bleeding, 163
– small bowel tumors, 163

List of Contributors

REGINA G.H. BEETS-TAN, MD
Department of Radiology
Maastricht University Medical Center
The Netherlands
P. Debyelaan 25
6229 HX Maastricht
The Netherlands

Email: r.beets.tan@mumc.nl

ARNE S. BORTHNE, MD, PhD
Diagnostic Imaging Center
Akershus University Hospital
1478 Lørenskog
Norway

Email: aborth@broadpark.no

JOHANNES M. FROELICH, PhD
Institute of Diagnostic
Interventional and Pediatric Radiology
University Hospitel
Inselspital Bern
Freiburgstrasse 10
3010 Bern
Switzerland

VICKY GOH, MD
Paul Strickland Scanner Centre
Mount Vernon Hospital
Northwood
Middlesex HA6 2RN
UK

Email: vicky.goh@stricklandscanner.org.uk

SONIA I. GONÇALVES, PhD
Department of Radiology
Academic Medical Center
University of Amsterdam
Meibergdreef 9
1105 AZ Amsterdam
The Netherlands

SOFIA GOURTSOYIANNI, MD
Department of Radiology
University Hospital of Heraklion
University of Crete
Medical School
Stavrakia
71111, Heraklion, Crete
Greece

Email: sgty76@gmail.com

STEVE HALLIGAN, MD, MRCP, FRCR
Department of Imaging
University College London Hospital
2F Podium
235 Euston Road
London NW1 2BU
UK

Email: s.halligan@ucl.ac.uk

SONJA KINNER, MD
Department of Diagnostic and Interventional
Radiology and Neuroradiology
University Hospital Essen
Hufelandstrasse 55
45122 Essen
Germany

Email: Sonja.Kinner@uni-due.de

SONJA KIRCHHOFF, MD
Klinikum der Universität München
Campus Großhadern
Institut für Radiologie
Marchioninistrasse 15
81377 München
Germany

Email: sonja.kirchhoff@med.uni-muenchen.de

Andrea Laghi, MD
Department of Radiological Sciences
University of Rome "La Sapienza"
ICOT Hospital
Polo Pontino, Latina
Via Franco Faggiana 34
04100 Latina
Italy

Email: andlaghi@gmail.com

Doenja M.J. Lambregts, MD
Department of Radiology
Maastricht University Medical Center
P. Debyelaan 25
6229 HX Maastricht
The Netherlands

Thomas C. Lauenstein, MD
PD, Department of Radiology
University Hospital Essen
Hufelandstrasse 55
45122 Essen
Germany

Email: Thomas.lauenstein@uni-due.de

Karen S. Lee, MD
Department of Radiology
Beth Israel Deaconess Medical Center
330 Brookline Avenue
Boston, MA 02215
USA

Email: kslee@bidmc.harvard.edu

Andreas Lieneman, MD
Radiologie Mühleninsel
Mühlenstrasse 4
84028 Landshut
Germany

Email: 4u2c1@gmx.de

David J. Lomas, MD
Department of Radiology
University of Cambridge and Addenbrooke's Hospital
Hills Road
Cambridge
CB2 0QQ
UK

Email: djl15@radiol.cam.ac.uk

Russel N. Low, MD, PhD
Sharp and Children's MRI Center
7901 Frost Street
San Diego
CA 92123
USA

Email: rlow53@yahoo.com

Monique Maas, MD
Department of Radiology
Maastricht University Medical Center
The Netherlands
P. Debyelaan 25
6229 HX Maastricht
The Netherlands

Celso Matos, MD
Department of Radiology
Hopital Erasme
Université Libre de Bruxelles
Route de Lennik 808
1070 Brussels
Belgium

Email: cmatos@ulb.ac.be

Aart J. Nederveen, PhD
Department of Radiology
Academic Medical Center
University of Amsterdam
Meibergdreef 9
1105 AZ Amsterdam
The Netherlands

Email: a.j.nederveen@amc.uva.nl

Valeria Panebianco, MD
Department of Radiological Sciences
"Sapienza" University of Rome
ICOT Hospital
Polo Pontino, Latina
V.le Regina Elena 324
00161 Rome
Italy

Email: valeria.panebianco@uniroma1.it

Nickolas Papanikolaou, PhD
Department of Radiology
University Hospital of Heraklion
University of Crete
Medical School, Stavrakia
71111 Heraklion, Crete
Greece

Email: npapan@med.uoc.gr

MICHAEL A. PATAK, MD
Institute of Diagnostic
Interventional and Pediatric Radiology
University Hospital
Inselspital Bern
Freiburgstrasse 10
3010 Bern
Switzerland

Email: michael.patak@insel.ch

GIUSEPPE PELLE, MD
Department of Radiological Sciences
"Sapienza" University of Rome
ICOT Hospital
Polo Pontino, Latina
V.le Regina Elena
324, 00161 Rome
Italy

IVAN PEDROSA, MD
Department of Radiology
Beth Israel Deaconess Medical Center
330 Brookline Avenue, Boston
MA 02215
USA

Email: ipedrosa@bidmc.harvard.edu

MARTINA PEZZULLO, MD
Department of Radiology
MR Imaging Division
Cliniques Universitaires de Bruxelles
Hôpital Erasme
Université Libre de Bruxelles
Route de Lennik 808
1070 Brussels
Belgium

CLAUDE PIERRE-JEROME, MD, PhD
Emory University
Atlanta, GA
USA

Email: cpierrejerome@msn.com

CAECILIA S. REINER, MD
Institute of Diagnostic Radiology
University Hospital Zurich
Raemistrasse 100
8091 Zurich
Switzerland

ANGELA M. RIDDELL, MD, FRCS, FRCR
Department of Radiology
The Royal Marsden Hospital
NHS Foundation Trust
Fulham Road
London SW3 6JJ
UK

Email: Angela.Riddell@rmh.nhs.uk

JAAP STOKER, MD, PhD
Department of Radiology
Academic Medical Center
University of Amsterdam
Meibergdreef 9
1105 AZ Amsterdam
The Netherlands

Email: j.stoker@amc.uva.nl

N. JANE TAYLOR, PhD
Paul Strickland Scanner Centre
Mount Vernon Hospital
Northwood, London
UK

STUART A. TAYLOR, MD, MRCP, FRCR
Department of Imaging
University College Hospital
2F Podium, 235 Euston Road
London NW1 2BU
UK

Email: csytaylor@yahoo.co.uk

DAMIAN J.M. TOLAN, MD, MBChB, FRCR
Department of Clinical Radiology
Jubilee Wing
Leeds General Infirmary
Leeds Teaching Hospitals NHS Trust
Great George Street, Leeds
West Yorkshire LS1 3EX
UK

Email: djmtolan@doctors.org.uk

RADU TUTUJA, MD
Institute of Nuclear Medicine
University Hospital
Geneva
Switzerland

Dominik Weishaupt, MD
Division of Radiology
City Hospital Triemli
Birmensdorferstrasse 497
8063 Zurich
Switzerland

Email: dominik.weishaupt@triemli.stzh.ch

Klaus-Ulrich Wentz, MD
Institute of Radiology
Kantonspital
Münsterlingen
Switzerland

Constantin von Weymarn, PhD
Institute of Diagnostic
Interventional and Pediatric Radiology
University Hospital
Inselspital Bern
Freiburgstrasse, Bern
Switzerland

Michael Wissmeyer, MD
Clinic for Visceral Surgery and Medicine
University Hospitel
Inselspital Bern
Freiburgstrasse 10
3010 Bern
Switzerland

Manon L.W. Ziech, MD
Department of Radiology
Academic Medical Center
University of Amsterdam
Meibergdreef 9
1105 AZ Amsterdam
The Netherlands

Email: m.l.ziech@amc.uva.nl

Frank M. Zijta, MD
Department of Radiology
Academic Medical Center
University of Amsterdam
Meibergdreef 9
1105 AZ Amsterdam
The Netherlands

Email: F.M.Zijta@olvg.nl

MEDICAL RADIOLOGY Diagnostic Imaging and Radiation Oncology

Titles in the series already published

DIAGNOSTIC IMAGING

Radiological Imaging of Sports Injuries
Edited by C. Masciocchi

Modern Imaging of the Alimentary Tube
Edited by A. R. Margulis

Diagnosis and Therapy of Spinal Tumors
Edited by P. R. Algra, J. Valk and
J. J. Heimans

Interventional Magnetic Resonance Imaging
Edited by J. F. Debatin and G. Adam

Abdominal and Pelvic MRI
Edited by A. Heuck and M. Reiser

Orthopedic Imaging
Techniques and Applications
Edited by A. M. Davies and H. Pettersson

Radiology of the Female Pelvic Organs
Edited by E. K. Lang

**Magnetic Resonance of the Heart
and Great Vessels**
Clinical Applications
Edited by J. Bogaert, A. J. Duerinckx,
and F. E. Rademakers

Modern Head and Neck Imaging
Edited by S. K. Mukherji and J. A. Castelijns

Radiological Imaging of Endocrine Diseases
Edited by J. N. Bruneton
in collaboration with B. Padovani and
M.-Y. Mourou

Radiology of the Pancreas
2nd Revised Edition
Edited by A. L. Baert. Co-edited by
G. Delorme and L. Van Hoe

Trends in Contrast Media
Edited by H. S. Thomsen, R. N. Muller,
and R. F. Mattrey

Functional MRI
Edited by C. T. W. Moonen and
P. A. Bandettini

Emergency Pediatric Radiology
Edited by H. Carty

Liver Malignancies
Diagnostic and Interventional Radiology
Edited by C. Bartolozzi and R. Lencioni

Spiral CT of the Abdomen
Edited by F. Terrier, M. Grossholz, and
C. D. Becker

Medical Imaging of the Spleen
Edited by A. M. De Schepper and
F. Vanhoenacker

Radiology of Peripheral Vascular Diseases
Edited by E. Zeitler

Radiology of Blunt Trauma of the Chest
P. Schnyder and M. Wintermark

Portal Hypertension
Diagnostic Imaging and Imaging-Guided Therapy
Edited by P. Rossi.
Co-edited by P. Ricci and L. Broglia

**Virtual Endoscopy and
Related 3D Techniques**
Edited by P. Rogalla, J. Terwissscha
van Scheltinga and B. Hamm

Recent Advances in Diagnostic Neuroradiology
Edited by Ph. Demaerel

**Transfontanellar Doppler Imaging
in Neonates**
A. Couture, C. Veyrac

Radiology of AIDS
A Practical Approach
Edited by J. W. A. J. Reeders and
P. C. Goodman

CT of the Peritoneum
A. Rossi, G. Rossi

Magnetic Resonance Angiography
2nd Revised Edition
Edited by I. P. Arlart, G. M. Bongartz,
and G. Marchal

**Applications of Sonography
in Head and Neck Pathology**
Edited by J. N. Bruneton
in collaboration with C. Raffaelli,
O. Dassonville

3D Image Processing
Techniques and Clinical Applications
Edited by D. Caramella and
C. Bartolozzi

Imaging of the Larynx
Edited by R. Hermans

Pediatric ENT Radiology
Edited by S. J. King and A. E. Boothroyd

**Imaging of Orbital and
Visual Pathway Pathology**
Edited by W. S. Müller-Forell

Radiological Imaging of the Small Intestine
Edited by N. C. Gourtsoyiannis

Imaging of the Knee
Techniques and Applications
Edited by A. M. Davies and
V. N. Cassar-Pullicino

Perinatal Imaging
From Ultrasound to MR Imaging
Edited by F. E. Avni

**Diagnostic and Interventional
Radiology in Liver Transplantation**
Edited by E. Bücheler, V. Nicolas,
C. E. Broelsch, X. Rogiers
and G. Krupski

Imaging of the Pancreas
Cystic and Rare Tumors
Edited by C. Procacci and
A. J. Megibow

Imaging of the Foot & Ankle
Techniques and Applications
Edited by A. M. Davies,
R. W. Whitehouse and J. P. R. Jenkins

Radiological Imaging of the Ureter
Edited by F. Joffre, Ph. Otal and
M. Soulie

Radiology of the Petrous Bone
Edited by M. Lemmerling and
S. S. Kollias

Imaging of the Shoulder
Techniques and Applications
Edited by A. M. Davies and J. Hodler

Interventional Radiology in Cancer
Edited by A. Adam, R. F. Dondelinger,
and P. R. Mueller

**Imaging and Intervention in
Abdominal Trauma**
Edited by R. F. Dondelinger

**Radiology of the Pharynx
and the Esophagus**
Edited by O. Ekberg

**Radiological Imaging
in Hematological Malignancies**
Edited by A. Guermazi

Functional Imaging of the Chest
Edited by H.-U. Kauczor

**Duplex and Color Doppler Imaging
of the Venous System**
Edited by G. H. Mostbeck

Multidetector-Row CT of the Thorax
Edited by U. J. Schoepf

Radiology and Imaging of the Colon
Edited by A. H. Chapman

Multidetector-Row CT Angiography
Edited by C. Catalano and R. Passariello

Focal Liver Lesions
Detection, Characterization, Ablation
Edited by R. Lencioni, D. Cioni,
and C. Bartolozzi

**Imaging in Treatment Planning
for Sinonasal Diseases**
Edited by R. Maroldi and P. Nicolai

Clinical Cardiac MRI
With Interactive CD-ROM
Edited by J. Bogaert, S. Dymarkowski,
and A. M. Taylor

**Dynamic Contrast-Enhanced Magnetic
Resonance Imaging in Oncology**
Edited by A. Jackson, D. L. Buckley, and
G. J. M. Parker

Contrast Media in Ultrasonography
Basic Principles and Clinical Applications
Edited by E. Quaia

Paediatric Musculoskeletal Disease
With an Emphasis on Ultrasound
Edited by D. Wilson

MR Imaging in White Matter Diseases of the Brain and Spinal Cord
Edited by M. Filippi, N. De Stefano, V. Dousset, and J. C. McGowan

Imaging of the Hip & Bony Pelvis
Techniques and Applications
Edited by A. M. Davies, K. Johnson, and R. W. Whitehouse

Imaging of Kidney Cancer
Edited by A. Guermazi

Magnetic Resonance Imaging in Ischemic Stroke
Edited by R. von Kummer and T. Back

Diagnostic Nuclear Medicine
2nd Revised Edition
Edited by C. Schiepers

Imaging of Occupational and Environmental Disorders of the Chest
Edited by P. A. Gevenois and P. De Vuyst

Virtual Colonoscopy
A Practical Guide
Edited by P. Lefere and S. Gryspeerdt

Contrast Media
Safety Issues and ESUR Guidelines
Edited by H. S. Thomsen

Head and Neck Cancer Imaging
Edited by R. Hermans

Vascular Embolotherapy
A Comprehensive Approach
Volume 1: *General Principles, Chest, Abdomen, and Great Vessels*
Edited by J. Golzarian. Co-edited by S. Sun and M. J. Sharafuddin

Vascular Embolotherapy
A Comprehensive Approach
Volume 2: *Oncology, Trauma, Gene Therapy, Vascular Malformations, and Neck*
Edited by J. Golzarian.
Co-edited by S. Sun and M. J. Sharafuddin

Vascular Interventional Radiology
Current Evidence in Endovascular Surgery
Edited by M. G. Cowling

Ultrasound of the Gastrointestinal Tract
Edited by G. Maconi and G. Bianchi Porro

Parallel Imaging in Clinical MR Applications
Edited by S. O. Schoenberg, O. Dietrich, and M. F. Reiser

MRI and CT of the Female Pelvis
Edited by B. Hamm and R. Forstner

Imaging of Orthopedic Sports Injuries
Edited by F. M. Vanhoenacker, M. Maas and J. L. Gielen

Ultrasound of the Musculoskeletal System
S. Bianchi and C. Martinoli

Clinical Functional MRI
Presurgical Functional Neuroimaging
Edited by C. Stippich

Radiation Dose from Adult and Pediatric

Multidetector Computed Tomography
Edited by D. Tack and P. A. Gevenois

Spinal Imaging
Diagnostic Imaging of the Spine and Spinal Cord
Edited by J. Van Goethem, L. van den Hauwe and P. M. Parizel

Computed Tomography of the Lung
A Pattern Approach
J. A. Verschakelen and W. De Wever

Imaging in Transplantation
Edited by A. Bankier

Radiological Imaging of the Neonatal Chest
2nd Revised Edition
Edited by V. Donoghue

Radiological Imaging of the Digestive Tract in Infants and Children
Edited by A. S. Devos and J. G. Blickman

Pediatric Chest Imaging
Chest Imaging in Infants and Children
2nd Revised Edition
Edited by J. Lucaya and J. L. Strife

Color Doppler US of the Penis
Edited by M. Bertolotto

Radiology of the Stomach and Duodenum
Edited by A. H. Freeman and E. Sala

Imaging in Pediatric Skeletal Trauma
Techniques and Applications
Edited by K. J. Johnson and E. Bache

Image Processing in Radiology
Current Applications
Edited by E. Neri, D. Caramella, C. Bartolozzi

Screening and Preventive Diagnosis with Radiological Imaging
Edited by M. F. Reiser, G. van Kaick, C. Fink, S. O. Schoenberg

Percutaneous Tumor Ablation in Medical Radiology
Edited by T. J. Vogl, T. K. Helmberger, M. G. Mack, M. F. Reiser

Liver Radioembolization with ^{90}Y Microspheres
Edited by J. I. Bilbao, M. F. Reiser

Pediatric Uroradiology
2nd Revised Edition
Edited by R. Fotter

Radiology of Osteoporosis
2nd Revised Edition
Edited by S. Grampp

Gastrointestinal Tract Sonography in Fetuses and Children
A. Couture, C. Baud, J. L. Ferran, M. Saguintaah and C. Veyrac

Intracranial Vascular Malformations and Aneurysms
2nd Revised Edition
Edited by M. Forsting and I. Wanke

High-Resolution Sonography of the Peripheral Nervous System
2nd Revised Edition
Edited by S. Peer and G. Bodner

Imaging Pelvic Floor Disorders
2nd Revised Edition
Edited by J. Stoker, S. A. Taylor, and J. O. L. DeLancey

Coronary Radiology
2nd Revised Edition
Edited by M. Oudkerk and M. F. Reiser

Integrated Cardiothoracic Imaging with MDCT
Edited by M. Rémy-Jardin and J. Rémy

Multislice CT
3rd Revised Edition
Edited by M. F. Reiser, C. R. Becker, K. Nikolaou, G. Glazer

MRI of the Lung
Edited by H.-U. Kauczor

Imaging in Percutaneous Musculoskeletal Interventions
Edited by A. Gangi, S. Guth, and A. Guermazi

Contrast Media. Safety Issues and ESUR Guidelines
2nd Revised Edition
Edited by H. Thomsen, J.A.W. Webb

Inflammatory Diseases of the Brain
Edited by S. Hähnel

Imaging of Bone Tumors and Tumor-Like Lesions - Techniques and Applications
Edited by A.M. Davies, M. Sundaram, and S.J. James

MR Angiography of the body
Technique and Clinical Applications
Edited by E. Neri, M. Cosottini and D. Caramella

Virtual Colonoscopy
A Practical Guide
Edited by P. Lefere and S. Gryspeerdt

Diffusion-Weighted MR Imaging
Applications in the Body
Edited by D.-M. Koh and H.C. Thoeny

MRI of the Gastrointestinal Tract
Edited by J. Stoker

Digital Mammography
Edited by U. Bick and F. Diekmann

Springer

MEDICAL RADIOLOGY Diagnostic Imaging and Radiation Oncology
Titles in the series already published

RADIATION ONCOLOGY

Lung Cancer
Edited by C. W. Scarantino

Innovations in Radiation Oncology
Edited by H. R. Withers and L. J. Peters

Radiation Therapy of Head and Neck Cancer
Edited by G. E. Laramore

Gastrointestinal Cancer – Radiation Therapy
Edited by R. R. Dobelbower, Jr.

Radiation Exposure and Occupational Risks
Edited by E. Scherer, C. Streffer, and K.-R. Trott

Interventional Radiation
Therapy Techniques – Brachytherapy
Edited by R. Sauer

Radiopathology of Organs and Tissues
Edited by E. Scherer, C. Streffer, and K.-R. Trott

Concomitant Continuous Infusion
Chemotherapy and Radiation
Edited by M. Rotman and C. J. Rosenthal

Intraoperative Radiotherapy – Clinical Experiences and Results
Edited by F. A. Calvo, M. Santos, and L. W. Brady

Interstitial and Intracavitary Thermoradiotherapy
Edited by M. H. Seegenschmiedt and R. Sauer

Non-Disseminated Breast Cancer
Controversial Issues in Management
Edited by G. H. Fletcher and S. H. Levitt

Current Topics in Clinical Radiobiology of Tumors
Edited by H.-P. Beck-Bornholdt

Practical Approaches to Cancer Invasion and Metastases
A Compendium of Radiation Oncologists' Responses to 40 Histories
Edited by A. R. Kagan with the Assistance of R. J. Steckel

Radiation Therapy in Pediatric Oncology
Edited by J. R. Cassady

Radiation Therapy Physics
Edited by A. R. Smith

Late Sequelae in Oncology
Edited by J. Dunst, R. Sauer

Mediastinal Tumors. Update 1995
Edited by D. E. Wood, C. R. Thomas, Jr.

Thermoradiotherapy and Thermochemotherapy
Volume 1: *Biology, Physiology, and Physics*

Volume 2: *Clinical Applications*
Edited by M. H. Seegenschmiedt, P. Fessenden and C. C. Vernon

Carcinoma of the Prostate
Innovations in Management
Edited by Z. Petrovich, L. Baert, and L. W. Brady

Radiation Oncology of Gynecological Cancers
Edited by H. W. Vahrson

Carcinoma of the Bladder
Innovations in Management
Edited by Z. Petrovich, L. Baert, and L. W. Brady

Blood Perfusion and Microenvironment of Human Tumors
Implications for Clinical Radiooncology
Edited by M. Molls and P. Vaupel

Radiation Therapy of Benign Diseases
A Clinical Guide
2nd Revised Edition
S. E. Order and S. S. Donaldson

Carcinoma of the Kidney and Testis, and Rare Urologic Malignancies
Innovations in Management
Edited by Z. Petrovich, L. Baert, and L. W. Brady

Progress and Perspectives in the Treatment of Lung Cancer
Edited by P. Van Houtte, J. Klastersky, and P. Rocmans

Combined Modality Therapy of Central Nervous System Tumors
Edited by Z. Petrovich, L. W. Brady, M. L. Apuzzo, and M. Bamberg

Age-Related Macular Degeneration
Current Treatment Concepts
Edited by W. E. Alberti, G. Richard, and R. H. Sagerman

Radiotherapy of Intraocular and Orbital Tumors
2nd Revised Edition
Edited by R. H. Sagerman and W. E. Alberti

Modification of Radiation Response
Cytokines, Growth Factors, and Other Biolgical Targets
Edited by C. Nieder, L. Milas and K. K. Ang

Radiation Oncology for Cure and Palliation
R. G. Parker, N. A. Janjan and M. T. Selch

Clinical Target Volumes in Conformal and Intensity Modulated Radiation Therapy
A Clinical Guide to Cancer Treatment
Edited by V. Grégoire, P. Scalliet, and K. K. Ang

Advances in Radiation Oncology in Lung Cancer
Edited by B. Jeremi´c

New Technologies in Radiation Oncology
Edited by W. Schlegel, T. Bortfeld, and A.-L. Grosu

Multimodal Concepts for Integration of Cytotoxic Drugs and Radiation Therapy
Edited by J. M. Brown, M. P. Mehta, and C. Nieder

Technical Basis of Radiation Therapy
Practical Clinical Applications
4th Revised Edition
Edited by S. H. Levitt, J. A. Purdy, C. A. Perez, and S. Vijayakumar

CURED I · LENT
Late Effects of Cancer Treatment on Normal Tissues
Edited by P. Rubin, L. S. Constine, L. B. Marks, and P. Okunieff

Radiotherapy for Non-Malignant Disorders
Contemporary Concepts and Clinical Results
Edited by M. H. Seegenschmiedt, H.-B. Makoski, K.-R. Trott, and L. W. Brady

CURED II · LENT
Cancer Survivorship Research and Education
Late Effects on Normal Tissues
Edited by P. Rubin, L. S. Constine, L. B. Marks, and P. Okunieff

Radiation Oncology
An Evidence-Based Approach
Edited by J. J. Lu and L. W. Brady

Primary Optic Nerve Sheath Meningioma
Edited by B. Jeremi´c, and S. Pitz

Function Preservation and Quality Life in Head and Neck Radiotherapy
Edited by P.M. Harari, N.P. Connor, and C. Grau

Nasopharyngeal Cancer
Edited by J.J. Lu, J.S. Cooper and A.W.M. Lee

Springer

Printing and Binding: Stürtz GmbH, Würzburg